CONVENTIONAL WARFARE
BALLISTIC, BLAST, AND BURN INJURIES

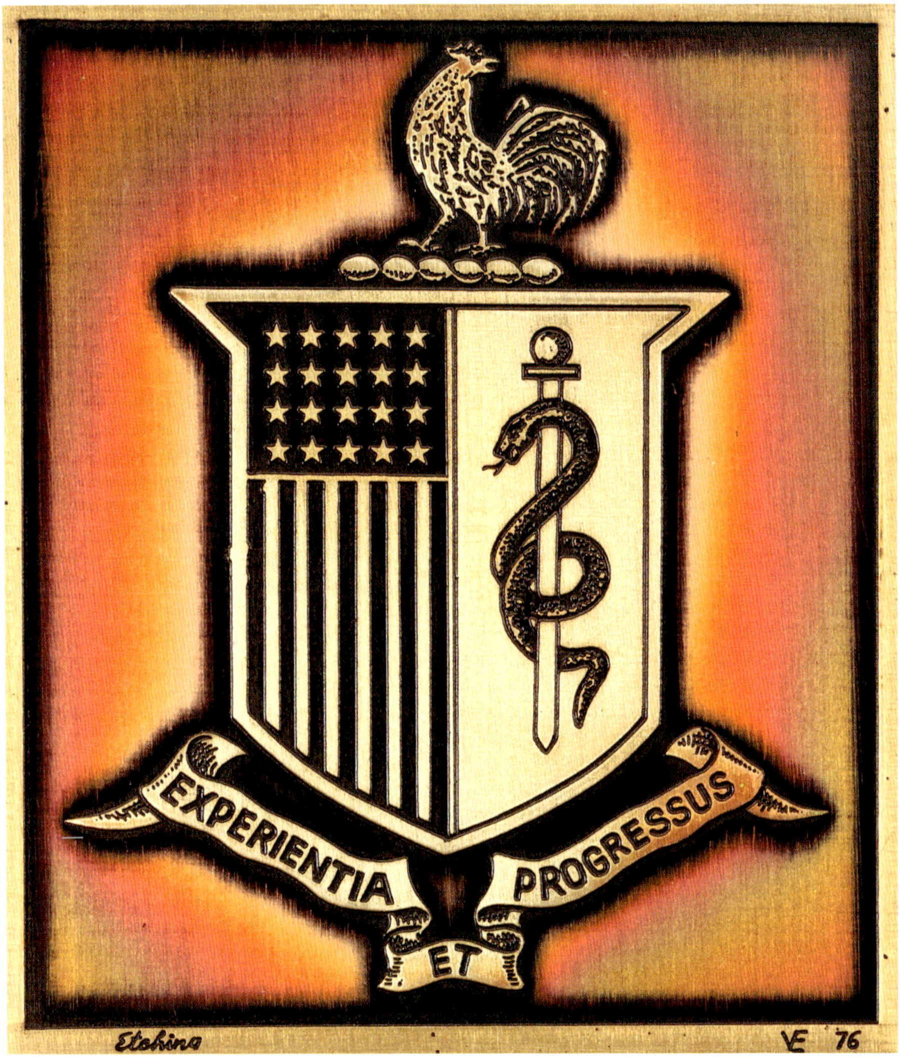

The Coat of Arms
1818
Medical Department of the Army

A 1976 etching by Vassil Ekimov of an
original color print that appeared in
The Military Surgeon, Vol. XLI, No. 2, 1917

The first line of medical defense in wartime is the combat medic. Although in ancient times medics carried the *caduceus* into battle to signify the neutral, humanitarian nature of their tasks, they have never been immune to the perils of war. They have made the highest sacrifices to save the lives of others, and their dedication to the wounded soldier is the foundation of military medical care.

Textbook of Military Medicine

SERIES ON COMBAT CASUALTY CARE

Published by the

Office of the Surgeon General
Department of the Army, United States of America

Editor in Chief

Colonel Russ Zajtchuk, MC, U.S. Army
Deputy Commander
Walter Reed Army Medical Center
Professor of Surgery, Uniformed Services University of the Health Sciences

Managing Editor

Donald P. Jenkins, Ph.D.
Director, Center of Excellence
Walter Reed Army Medical Center
Associate Professor of Surgery, Georgetown University
Visiting Associate Professor of Anatomy,
Uniformed Services University of the Health Sciences

Associate Editor

Colonel Ronald F. Bellamy, MC, U.S. Army
Acting Chief, Department of Surgery, Walter Reed Army Medical Center
Associate Professor of Military Medicine ,
Associate Professor of Surgery,
Uniformed Services University of the Health Sciences

Editor

Colleen Mathews Quick
TMM Publications, Center of Excellence
and the American Registry of Pathology

The TMM Series

Part I. *Warfare, Weaponry, and the Casualty*

Volume

1 BATTLEFIELD ENVIRONMENT

2 MEDICAL CONSEQUENCES OF NUCLEAR WARFARE

3 MEDICAL CONSEQUENCES OF BIOLOGICAL WARFARE

4 MEDICAL CONSEQUENCES OF CHEMICAL WARFARE

5 CONVENTIONAL WARFARE: BALLISTIC, BLAST, AND BURN INJURIES

6 COMBAT STRESS

Part II. *Principles of Medical Command and Support*

Volume

1 MEDICAL COMMAND AND SUPPORT IN AIRLAND BATTLE

2 MEDICINE IN LOW-INTENSITY CONFLICT

Part III. *Military Preventive Medicine and the Environment*

Volume

1 MOBILIZATION AND DEPLOYMENT

2 OCCUPATIONAL HEALTH: THE SOLDIER IN THE INDUSTRIAL BASE

3 THE NATURAL ENVIRONMENT: ALTITUDE, COLD, AND HEAT

Part IV. *Surgical Combat Casualty Care*

Volume

1 THE CASUALTY

2 ANESTHESIA AND CRITICAL CARE

3 MEDICAL IMAGING

4 HEAD AND NECK SURGERY

5 OPHTHALMIC SURGERY AND NEUROSURGERY

6 CARDIOTHORACIC SURGERY

7 ABDOMINAL AND UROGENITAL SURGERY

8 ORTHOPEDIC SURGERY

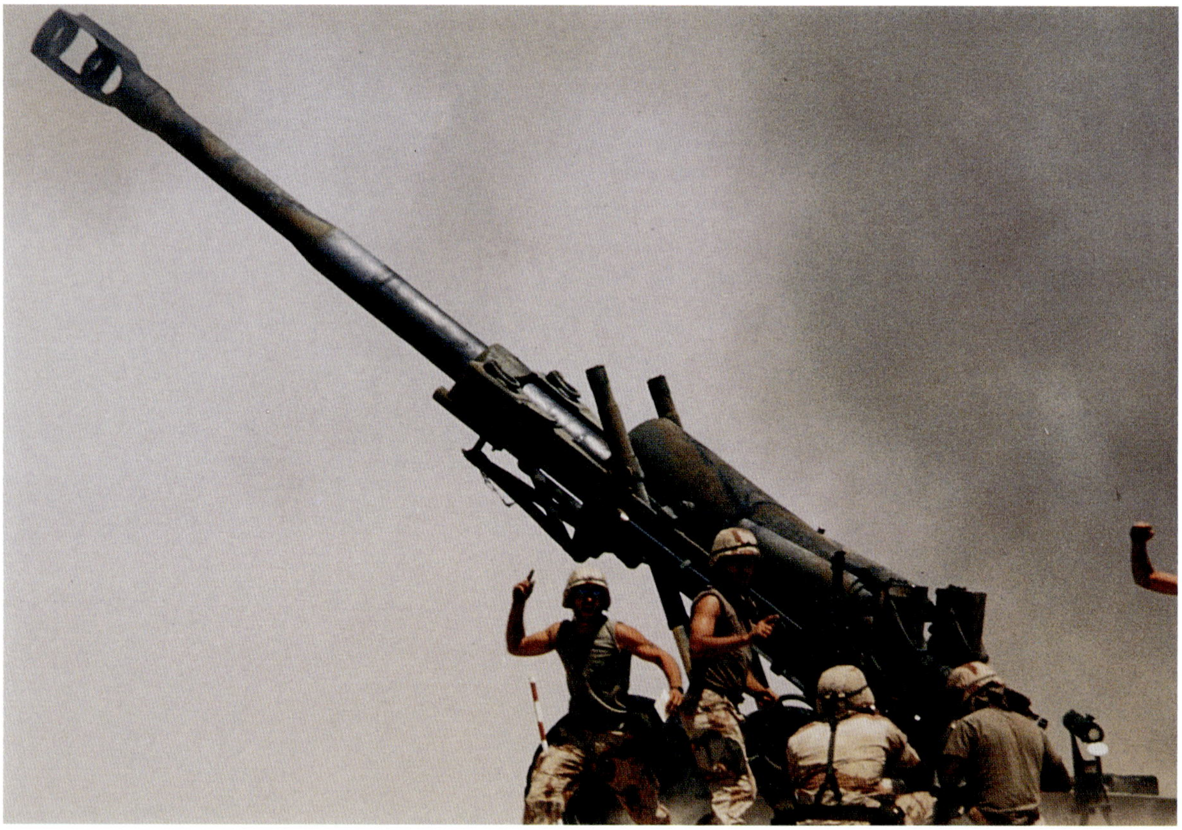

Be slowly lifted up, thou long black arm,
Great gun towering t'ward Heaven, about to curse

—Lieutenant Wilfred Owen
Royal Army
Killed in action in France, 1918

American soldiers, members of the Third Field Artillery, stand by as an M-198 155-mm howitzer is fired during the multinational joint service exercise "Bright Star" in Gabel Mamza, Egypt, in 1985.

CONVENTIONAL WARFARE
BALLISTIC, BLAST, AND BURN INJURIES

Specialty Editors

RONALD F. BELLAMY
RUSS ZAJTCHUK

Contributing Authors

TERESA M. BUESCHER
WILLIAM G. CIOFFI, Jr.
ANTHONY J. JOHNSON
YANCY Y PHILLIPS III
BASIL A. PRUITT, Jr.
DONALD R. RICHMOND
LORING W. RUE III
DOUGLAS D. SHARPNACK
JAMES H. STUHMILLER
JOAN T. ZAJTCHUK

Walter Reed Army Medical Center
Walter Reed Army Institute of Research
Washington, D.C.

Uniformed Services University of the Health Sciences
Bethesda, Maryland

United States Army Institute for Surgical Research
San Antonio, Texas

Assistant Editor for Medicine and Surgery
Captain Cheryl Crowley Moore, MC, U.S. Army
Department of Surgery, Walter Reed Army Medical Center
Fellow, Center of Excellence

Published by the Office of the Surgeon General at TMM Publications,
Center of Excellence in Military Medical Research and Education
Walter Reed Army Medical Center
Washington, D.C. 20307-5000

Library of Congress Cataloging in Publication Data

For sale by the Superintendent of Documents, U.S. Government Printing Office,
Washington, D.C. 20402

Conventional Warfare: Ballistic, Blast, and Burn Injury

Includes index.
1. Weaponry of conventional warfare. 2. Ballistic injury and treatment. 3. Blast injury and treatment. 4. Burn injury and treatment. (eds.) Zajtchuk, R., Jenkins, D. P., Bellamy, R. F., Quick, C. M.
I. Bellamy, Ronald F. II. Zajtchuk, R.

PRINTED IN THE UNITED STATES OF AMERICA

98 97 96 95 94 93 92 91 5 4 3 2 1

Contents

Foreword

Far too often the lessons learned from past wars have been forgotten at great cost to human life. A complacency in our society that armed conflicts will not occur may prevail. Operation Desert Shield, however, has accentuated the importance of military medical operations in times of presumed peace throughout the world. Regardless of our natural tendency to concentrate on peacetime health care, the conflict in the Persian Gulf indelibly imprints the fact that we must be ready to care for those who fight for peace. Armed conflict to resolve political differences among nations will occur despite the dramatic technological, social, and economic progress of the twentieth century.

As those of us in military medicine prepare to support our forces in the Persian Gulf, we must be ready for the challenges presented by modern warfare in this current situation, and later as we proceed into the next century. Because modern warfare will continue to rely on soldier-to-soldier fighting, conventional munitions will be a significant source of casualties regardless of the sophisticated weaponry. Ballistic, blast, and burn injuries in austere settings will continue to demand the attention of the medical corps in order to provide the best possible care and to save lives.

To meet these challenges, the Army Medical Department has embarked on an ambitious readiness initiative. This new doctrine focuses on far-foward surgical care, increased intensive-care capabilities, a policy of returning soldiers to duty as far foward as possible, improved ground and air evacuation capabilities, new medical logistics systems that incorporate blood-distribution networks, and improved management of combat stress. Our goals are to maintain our momentum as we conserve fighting strength and to support our soldiers and their families both in peacetime and in time of war. We cannot afford to forget them.

The military health-care system is the largest comprehensive health-care organization in the United States. Because the vast majority of our patients are not active-duty military personnel, it may seem that our day-to-day activities are far removed from those we would be required to perform during a time of war. Our highest priority is to be able to deploy a highly trained medical corps to any area of the world, however. To be effective, we must maintain the highest standards of technical competence and also be prepared to use our skills creatively and courageously in situations that may be primitive, dangerous, or unknown.

It is my hope that you will find this volume of the *Textbook of Military Medicine* series a useful addition to your readiness training programs, and that it will stimulate you to think about and plan for what will be required of each of us should the need arise again to make a transition from peace to war.

Lieutenant General Frank F. Ledford, Jr.
The Surgeon General
U.S. Army

December 1990
Washington, D.C.

Preface

I would say that two contrary laws seem to be wrestling with each other nowadays: the one, a law of blood and death, ever imagining new means of destruction and forcing nations to be constantly ready for the battlefield—the other a law of peace, work, and health ever evolving new means of delivering man from the scourges which beset him. Which of these two laws will ultimately prevail God alone knows.

—*Louis Pasteur*

Of the thousands of years of human history, few have been free of some type of war. The destructive lessons that warriors learn on the battlefield manage to be easily incorporated into the next confrontation. Civilizations have fallen, empires have rotted from within, and primitivism has cyclically triumphed over artifice, yet weapons technology has never regressed. For better or worse, the characterization of man as a maker of weapons seems to have been consistently borne out.

Unfortunately, the concurrent lessons of war—those that are lifesaving rather than life-destroying—are often forgotten from one conflict to the next. Time after time, medical innovations that affect the management of injuries, the logistics of evacuation, and the operation of far-forward medical facilities are allowed to become irrelevant as soon as a conflict is over.

The recent buildup of forces in the Middle East has reaffirmed the need for a highly trained medical corps that is able to deploy rapidly to any area of the world. Under such conditions, medical personnel will not have the time to learn combat-unique management techniques at their leisure, and civilian surgical manuals will not be adequate reference tools. This volume of the *Textbook of Military Medicine* deals with conventional warfare and addresses in detail conventional weapons, their effects, and the treatment of the casualties that they generate. It reviews the historical significance of these injuries and explains the basic scientific principles underlying the injuring mechanisms so that the medical officer will have a fundamental understanding of the injuries they are called upon to treat.

Colonel Russ Zajtchuk
U.S. Army

December 1990
Washington, D.C.

The current medical system to support the U.S. Army at war is a continuum from the forward line of troops through the continental United States; it serves as a primary source of trained replacements during the early stages of a major conflict. The system is designed to optimize the return to duty of the maximum number of trained combat soldiers at the lowest possible level. Far-forward stabilization helps to maintain the physiology of injured soldiers who are unlikely to return to duty and allows for their rapid evacuation from the battlefield without needless sacrifice of life or function.

Medical Force 2000 (MF2K)
PATIENT FLOW IN A THEATER OF OPERATIONS

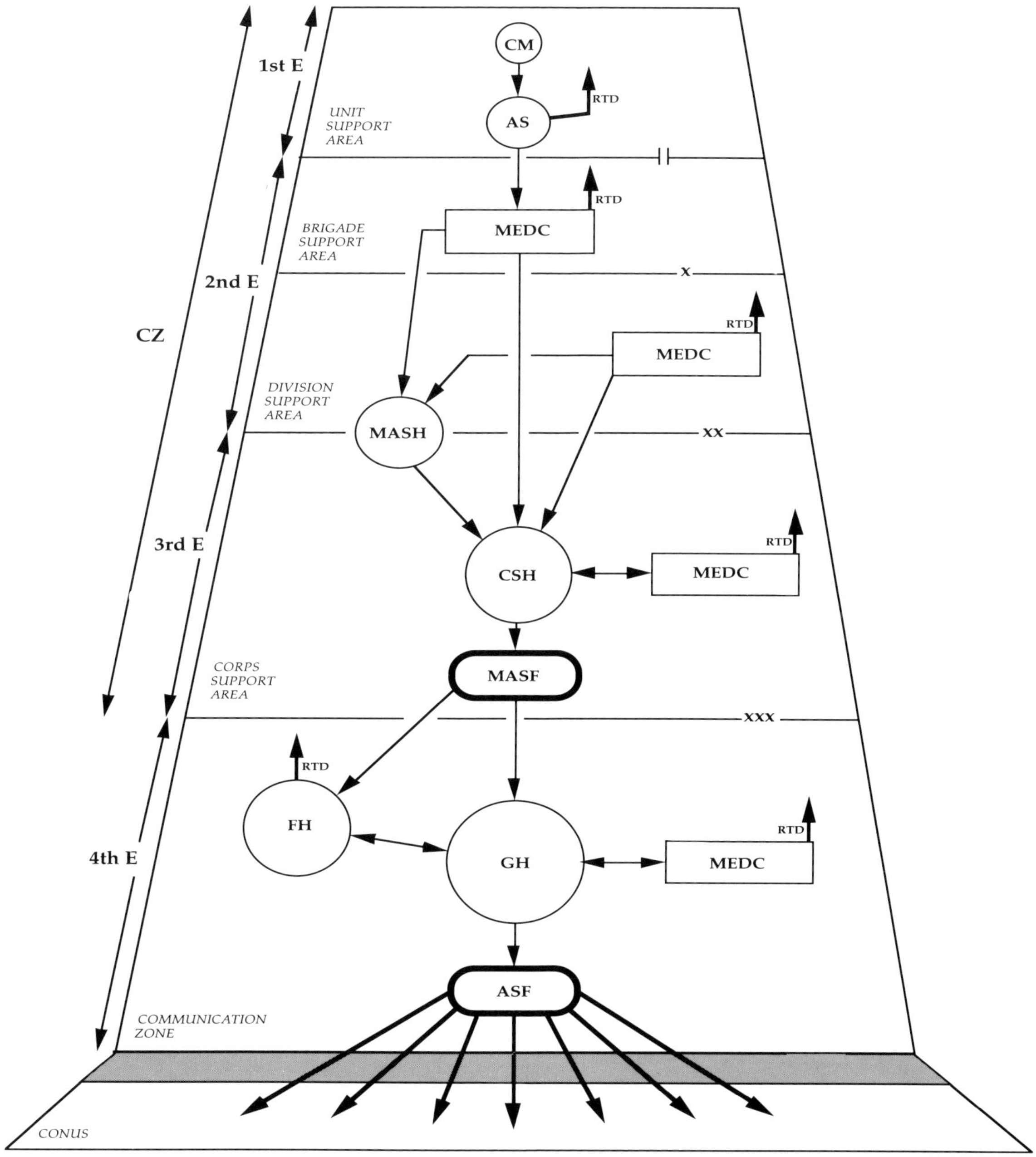

AS: Aid Station
ASF: Aeromedical Staging Facility, *USAF*
CM: Combat Medic
CSH: Combat Support Hospital
CZ: Combat Zone
E: Echelon
FH: Field Hospital
GH: General Hospital
MASF: Mobile Aeromedical Staging Facility, *USAF*
MASH: Mobile Army Surgical Hospital
MEDC: Medical Company
RTD: Return to Duty

Chapter 1

THE WEAPONS OF CONVENTIONAL LAND WARFARE

RONALD F. BELLAMY, M.D., FACS* AND RUSS ZAJTCHUK, M.D., FACS**

*Colonel, United States Army; Acting Chief, Department of Surgery, Walter Reed Army Medical Center, Washington, D.C. 20307-5001
**Colonel, United States Army; Deputy Commander, Walter Reed Army Medical Center, Washington, D.C. 20307-5001

INTRODUCTION

If, as Karl von Clausewitz said, "war is only a continuation of state policy by other means,"[1] then the nature of the "other means"—the weapons of war and their use—becomes the essential subject matter for the military officer. Medical officers have traditionally ignored weaponry, perhaps believing either that such knowledge has no therapeutic benefit for the casualty or that it is in some way incompatible with their ethical obligations. Nevertheless, there are cogent reasons why medical officers should understand weapons and their effects:

- Knowledgeable medical officers will be better able to treat the casualties who are their patients. For example, surgeons who know that wounds made by bullets from high-velocity rifles frequently do not contain massive soft-tissue destruction may be less likely to debride excessively. Similarly, surgeons who know that bullets of a certain design tend to fragment in tissue will be alert to the probable need for extensive surgical exploration. An elementary knowledge of the design and construction of weapons may be useful in unexpected ways as well. For example, an American soldier was thought to have been deliberately shot by one of his own men during a firefight in Vietnam, but the presence of the radiopaque cylinder (typical of the steel core of a Russian-made M43 bullet fired from the Kalashnikova assault rifle) on his roentgenogram indicated that the wound resulted from enemy action (Figure 1-1).
- Medical officers are responsible for protecting the casualties in forward medical units in the combat zone. They will be better able to discharge this responsibility if they can effectively and safely use weapons.
- A surgeon may need to remove an unexploded munition lodged within a casualty's body, and an ordnance expert may not always be available to advise the physician how to proceed safely. What should be done, for example, to treat a casualty who has been struck by a projectile fired at close range and whose gaping soft-tissue wound contains a grenadelike foreign body?
- Medical officers need a knowledge of weapons and their effects in order to predict accurately the number and types of casualties that are likely to result from a combat action.
- The medical officer who is familiar with weapons effects will be more likely to recognize wounds caused by novel enemy weapons. Early in World War II, for example, Soviet military medical authorities recognized that a weapon of unusual design—later identified as the German-made Nebelwerfer, the earliest rocket artillery weapon—caused the distinctive pulmonary injury that is now recognized as *blast lung* (described in the blast section of this textbook.)
- An understanding of weapons effects can lead to the development of protective equipment. For example, Israeli medical officers helped to develop fireproof clothing and the Merkava tank to reduce the incidence of burns to tank crews.

The terminology used in weapons development reflects the relatively rapid development of this field. Words that had a particular meaning in the nineteenth century may now be used to refer to a modern munition that evolved from the original concept but may look nothing like its ancestors. The word *gun* is an example. In the broadest sense, a gun is any weapon that is closed at one end and ejects a projectile from the other. (Thus, by strict definition, what is now called a *recoilless gun* is not really a gun at all, because it is open at both ends.) Over the years, two families of weapons have come to be known by the civilian community as guns: *(a)* small arms and *(b)* heavy weapons used by artillery forces. These weapons operate by the same principles but differ vastly in size, objective, and specialized design refinements. The military community, however, uses the word very specifically to refer only to the heavy weapon, and this textbook will do the same.

Ammunition is defined as the various projectiles (together with their fuses, propellants, and primers) that are fired from firearms; *munition* means a material used in war for defense or attack. This chapter will discuss the three types of wounding agents that are most common in conventional warfare: *(a)* ammuni-

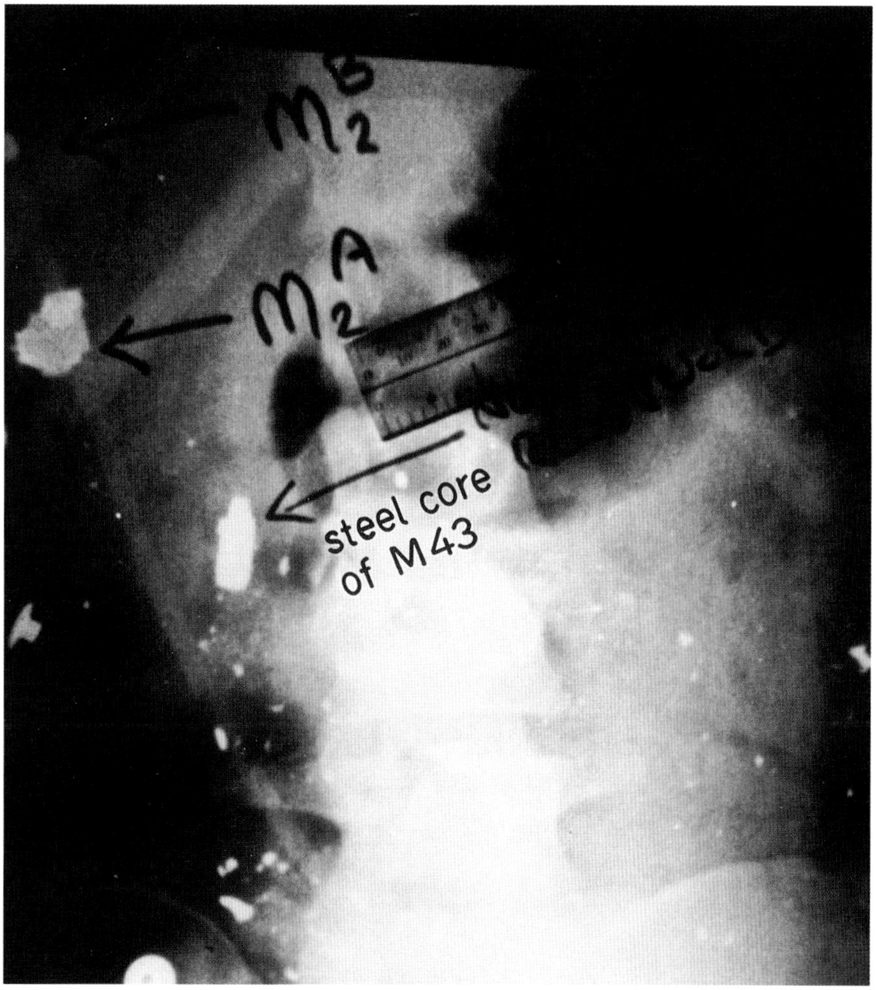

Fig. 1-1. The large metal cylinder shown in this abdominal roentgenogram is the soft steel core of a 7.62 x 39-mm round from a Kalashnikova assault rifle.
Source: Wound Data and Munitions Effectiveness Team

tion that is fired from small arms, *(b)* explosive munitions, and *(c)* flame and incendiary munitions. Because the first two categories of munitions not only cause most battlefield casualties but also present treatment problems that are not likely to be common in nonmilitary medical contexts, they will be discussed at some length in this chapter. The biophysics and the clinical implications of the effects of all three categories of munitions will be discussed in greater detail in this textbook's sections on ballistic, blast, and burn injuries.

Another term that is applied to both small-arms ammunition and heavy explosive munitions is *round.* A round is simply a unit of ammunition that is fired by a weapon. It comprises all of the parts that are necessary either to fire that one shot, or, if the ammunition is designed to do more than act as an inert projectile, to allow it also to travel through air and function successfully when it arrives at the target. Technically, a round can be as simple as one stone hurled from a slingshot. Given modern technology, however, rounds may be even more complex than the weapons that fire them. Depending on their designs, rounds might include any number of refinements, such as sophisticated fuses, fragmenting submunitions, flight stabilizers, tracking devices, or specialized propellants.

The terms *effective range* and *effective radius* are not interchangeable. In this text, the effective range of a weapon will refer specifically to the distance between the point at which the projectile is fired, thrown, or launched and the furthest point at which it can do damage to a certain percentage of combatants. (Depending on the munition, this may mean either a target or a detonation site.) The effective radius refers to the area around an explosive munition's detonation site within which a certain percentage of casualties can be expected.

CHARACTERISTICS OF SMALL ARMS

Small arms are weapons that are used by individual soldiers or small crews primarily to injure or kill enemy personnel.

Small-Arms Ammunition

Small arms fire solid projectiles that have diameters smaller than 20 mm. The typical round of small-arms ammunition consists of *(a)* the bullet and *(b)* the cartridge, which contains the propellant powder and primer and into which the bullet is inserted. Several factors are relevant to the description and assessment of small-arms ammunition.

Measurement. A complete round is characterized by *(a)* the diameter of the bullet, known as the *caliber* and measured in millimeters or, occasionally, in *caliber units* (one caliber equals 1/100 inch) and *(b)* the length of the cartridge (also in millimeters). Thus, the complete rifle round shown in Figure 1-2 would be designated as 5.56 (the caliber) x 45 mm (the length), and the pistol round would be 9 x 19 mm.

It is not sufficient to refer to small-arms ammunition by bullet caliber alone. A given weapon is designed to fire a cartridge of unique size and shape as well as a bullet of defined caliber. Both NATO and Warsaw Pact forces field 7.62-mm bullets, but because the cartridges are quite different, the rounds are not interchangeable.

Velocity. All other factors being equal, the larger the cartridge is (that is, the more propellant powder it contains), the higher the bullet velocity will tend to be at any given point on its path, and the greater its effective tactical range and penetration will be as well. Not surprisingly, the bullet from the rifle round shown in Figure 1-2 has an appreciably higher muzzle velocity (3,200 feet/second [fps]) than does the bullet from the pistol round (1,100 fps).

Significant differences in velocities may exist even among rounds that have the same caliber bullets but different cartridges (Figure 1-3). When fired by the appropriate weapons, the bullet from the Soviet-made 7.62 x 39-mm round has a muzzle velocity of 2,350 fps, whereas the one-third larger cartridge of the Soviet-made 7.62 x 54R-mm round gives its bullet a muzzle velocity of about 2,850 fps. (The "R" signifies that the cartridge has a rim.)

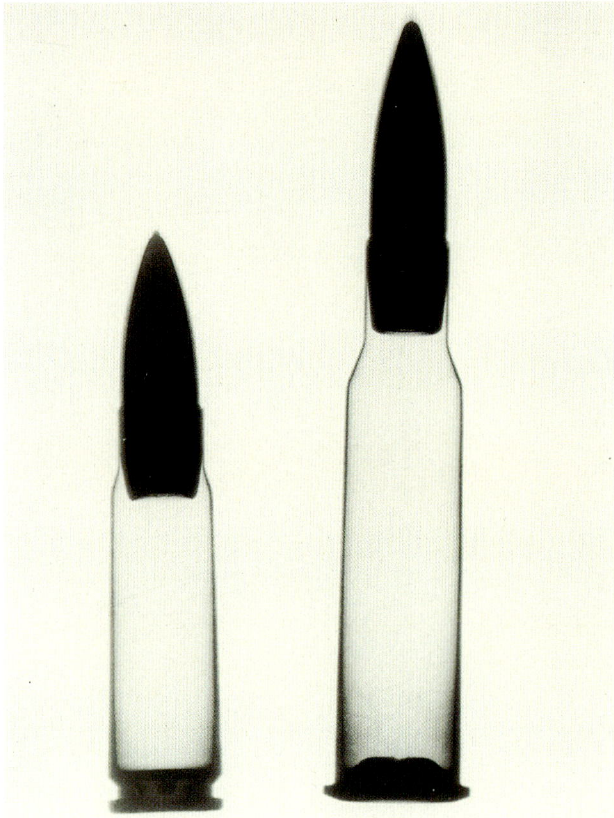

Fig. 1-3. The smaller 7.62 x 39-mm round on the left was one of the first intermediate-power rounds to be developed during World War II, after the old full-power rounds (such as the 7.62 x 54R-mm round on the right) proved to be unsuited to the fully automatic rifles then being developed. Source: P. M. Dougherty

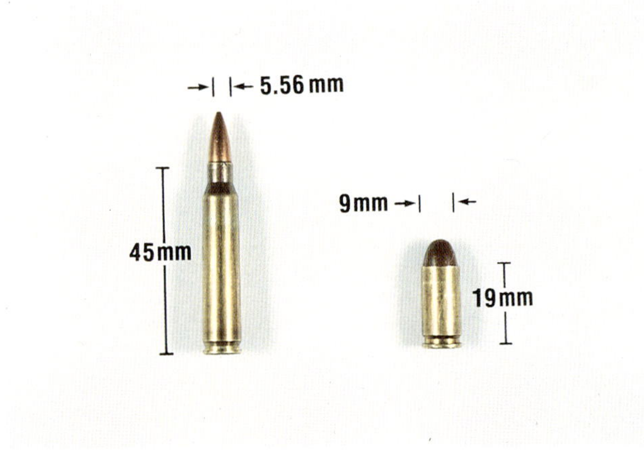

Fig. 1-2. The M193 round fired by an M16 assault rifle is on the left; the Parabellum round fired by the Beretta model M9 pistol is on the right.

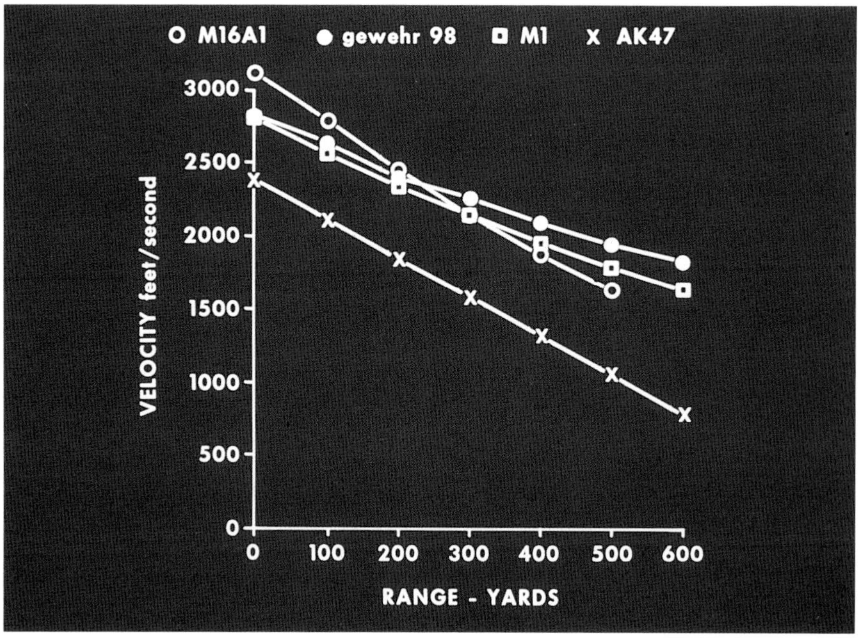

Fig. 1-4. Velocity as a function of muzzle distance for four military rifles: the German-made Gewehr 98 used in World War I (• • •), the American-made M1 used in World War II (■■■), the Soviet-made AK47 (x x x), and the American-made M16 (ooo).
Source: Data estimated by M. L. Fackler from reference 2

Tactical Conditions. How useful a particular round will be in combat depends on more than its velocity, however. For example, when it is used in an automatic weapon, the smaller, slower round shown in Figure 1-3 is more useful to the soldier. Not only can it be fired more accurately than the larger cartridge that it replaced, but the lighter weight of the new round also allows the soldier to carry as much as 50% more ammunition without increasing his load.

Because the velocity of the bullet in flight is related to its distance from the muzzle, tactical conditions determine the distances at which small arms are likely to be most effective (Figure 1-4).[2] An M16A1, for example, is designed to fire high-velocity bullets and to hit targets at a tactical distance of 500 m. On the other hand, an AK47 (the Russian-made Kalashnikova assault rifle) is usually used tactically to spray lower-velocity bullets over a wider area within a much closer range, about 50–100 m. Yet by the time the high-velocity M16 bullet reaches its designed tactical distance, it may actually be traveling more slowly than the lower-velocity AK47 bullet will be when the latter reaches the perimeter of its spray-gun range.

Military Objective. Depending on the objectives they are intended to achieve, even bullets that look alike may be quite different (Figure 1-5). The most common military bullet, known as *ball ammunition,* consists of a metal jacket filled with lead; it is designed to injure or kill personnel.

Specialty rounds have been designed to perform specific functions. The *tracer round* contains pyrotechnic chemicals that trace the flight of the bullet, a valuable aid to accuracy in combat. The *armor-piercing round* contains a dense metal rod within the bullet's jacket that is designed to penetrate soft-skin vehicles, such as trucks. When the bullet comes in contact with the vehicle, its jacket is peeled back and the exposed penetrating rod continues on through the target wall.

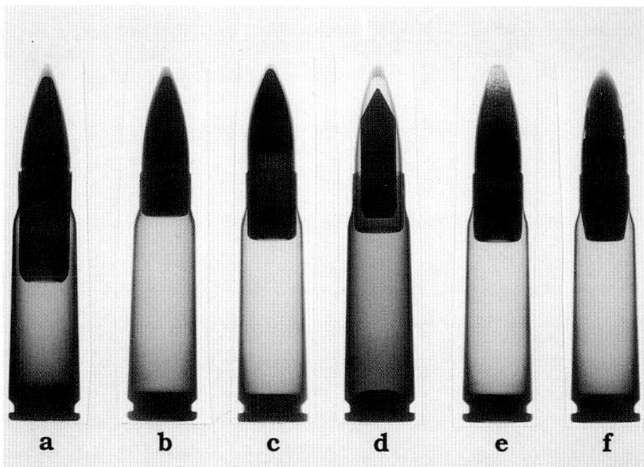

Fig. 1-5. All of the rounds shown in this roentgenogram have dimensions of 7.62 x 39 mm and are similar in appearance (except for their color coding, which cannot be seen on the roentgenogram): *(a)* a Soviet-made tracer-incendiary round; *(b)* a Yugoslavian-made ball-proof round; *(c)* a Soviet-made tracer round (note the metal cylinder, which contains the tracer material, at the bottom of the bullet); *(d)* a Finnish-made armor-piercing round; *(e)* a Soviet-made two-piece tracer-incendiary round; and *(f)* a Soviet-made armor-piercing incendiary round.
Source: P. M. Dougherty

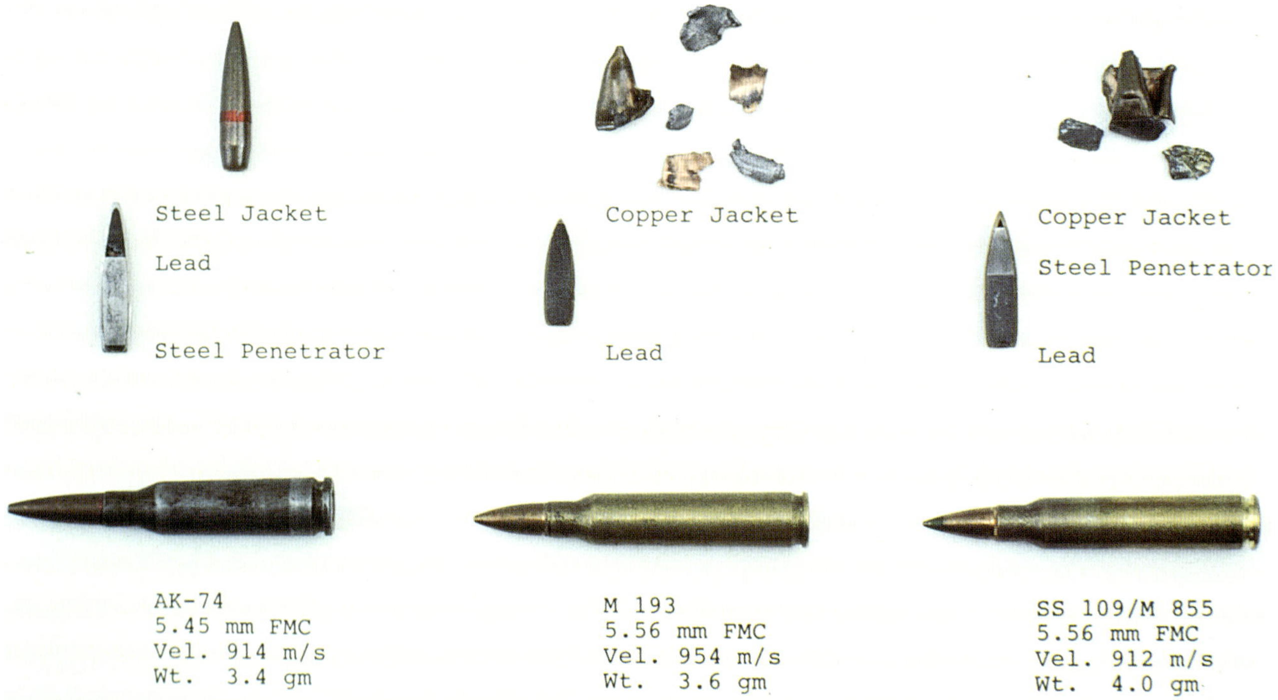
Steel Jacket
Lead
Steel Penetrator
Copper Jacket
Lead
Copper Jacket
Steel Penetrator
Lead
AK-74
5.45 mm FMC
Vel. 914 m/s
Wt. 3.4 gm
M 193
5.56 mm FMC
Vel. 954 m/s
Wt. 3.6 gm
SS 109/M 855
5.56 mm FMC
Vel. 912 m/s
Wt. 4.0 gm

Fig. 1-6. From bottom to top, the intact round, a cutaway showing the internal construction, and the bullet as it appeared after striking a soft-tissue simulant are shown for a bullet fired from a Soviet AK74 (left), an M193 bullet fired from an M16A1 (center), and an M855 bullet fired from an M16A2 or an M249 Squad Automatic Weapon (SAW) (right).
Source: Letterman Army Institute of Research

The *incendiary round* is designed to ignite combustibles, such as gasoline.

Whether specialty rounds create unique casualty-care problems is doubtful. For example, tracers do not contain white phosphorus (contrary to common belief), and ordinary bullet-wound management is appropriate for casualties who have been hit by them. Human tissues hit by an armor-piercing round are usually not resistant enough to strip the jacket from the bullet and therefore the penetrating rod is not exposed. There is no evidence that incendiary rounds cause unusual treatment problems.

Design and Construction. The bullet's design and construction determine the kind of wound that it will cause. The wounding effects of deforming hollow-point and soft-nose hunting ammunition are quite different from those of nondeforming bullets. The Hague Declaration of 1899 prohibited the use of any "bullet which expands or flattens easily in the human body."[3] To meet this requirement, bullets that are designed for military use must be completely covered by a metal jacket. Designers of military small arms have therefore used alternatives, such as fragmenting bullets, that cause equivalent tissue effects. In Figure 1-6, the two copper-jacketed bullets on the right have broken up into many small fragments, whereas the bullet on the left (which has a much stronger steel jacket) has neither broken up nor become deformed. The copper-jacketed bullets may cause more severe tissue damage.

Historical Development of Small Arms

Until the middle of the nineteenth century, soldiers relied on muzzle-loading smooth-bore muskets as their individual small arms. These weapons fired a solid spherical lead shot that traveled at low velocity and was not very accurate. The muskets were also difficult and dangerous to load: The soldier had to stand up to ram the shot down a 3- or 4-foot-long barrel. The time that elapsed between the loading and the firing of the shot was several seconds, very slow by today's standards.

Single-shot Rifle. The introduction of the rifled musket and its spin-stabilized conoidal bullet (such as the Minié) in the 1850s may have had the greatest immediate and measurable impact on war of any new weapon before or since.[4] Modification of the rifle continued throughout the nineteenth century and led to such weapons as the Mauser Infanteriegewehr Model 1898—the Gewehr 98 (Figure 1-7)—a variant of which was Germany's standard rifle in World War I.

The Gewehr 98 was a heavy, cumbersome, single-shot, bolt-action rifle that fired a powerful 7.92 x 59-mm round. It was accurate well beyond 1,000 m in the hands of a well-trained soldier in the benign environment of the rifle range, although such an extensive range was rarely possible in battle. In the trenches of the western front of World War I, the performance of the Gewehr 98 and similar weapons proved to be less than optimal. There, the tactical mission was to saturate an enemy position at close range with overwhelming firepower. One weapon that performed this mission well was the *machine gun.*

Machine Gun. Like the single-shot rifle that it replaced in World War I, the machine gun fires full-power cartridges, but it is *fully automatic* (that is, while its trigger is depressed, it continues to fire until its ammunition supply is depleted). The largest and heaviest of all small arms, this weapon is *crew-served* (that is, it is operated by a team of two or three soldiers).

Machine guns are usually categorized as *(a)* light, *(b)* general purpose, or *(c)* heavy. Examples of Soviet-made machine guns and their ammunition in each category include the light RPK 74 (5.45 x 39 mm); the general purpose RPK (7.62 x 39 mm) and PKS (7.62 x 54R mm) (Figure 1-8); and the heavy machine guns, like the 50-caliber NSV-12.7 (12.7 x 108 mm) and the KPV (14.5 x 114 mm). The heavy machine guns are more often used against matériel; in fact, one of the

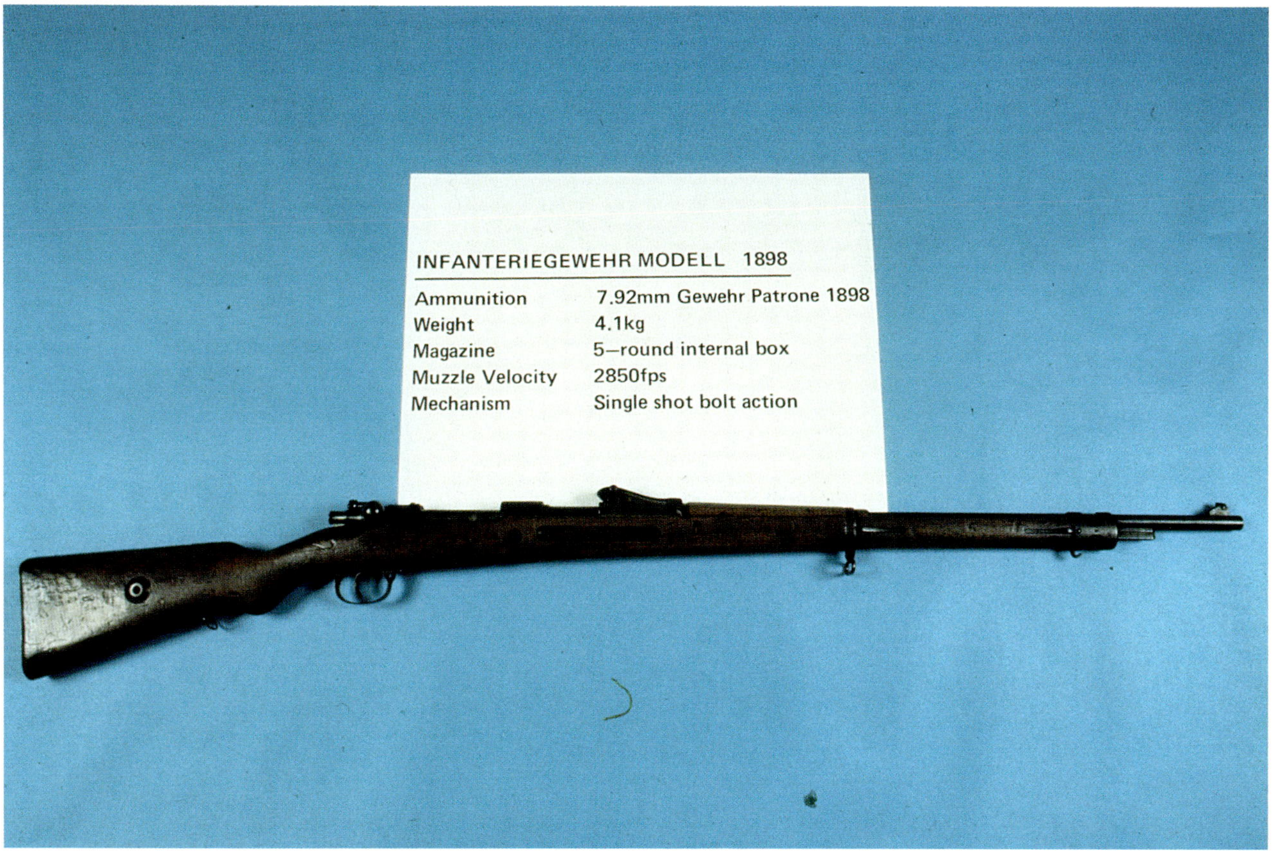

Fig. 1-7. The Gewehr 98
Source: Presidio of San Francisco Army Museum

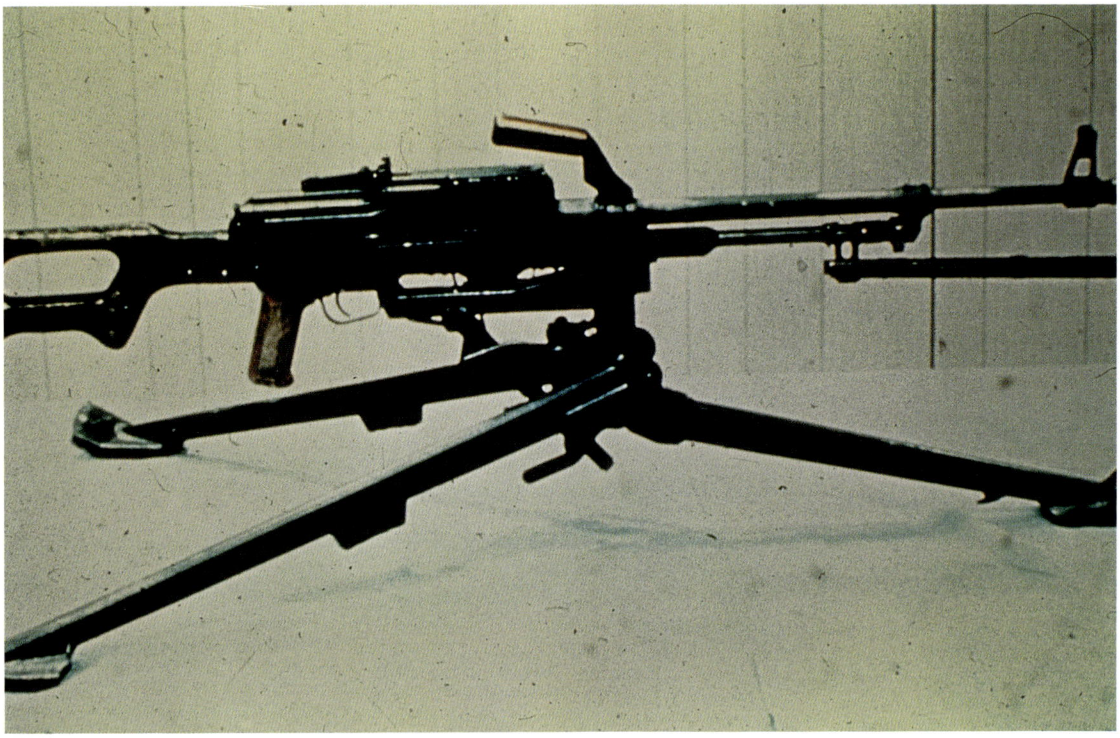

Fig. 1-8. The PKS is a general-purpose machine gun that weighs about 9 kg and has a cyclic rate of fire of 650 rounds/minute.
Source: Letterman Army Institute of Research

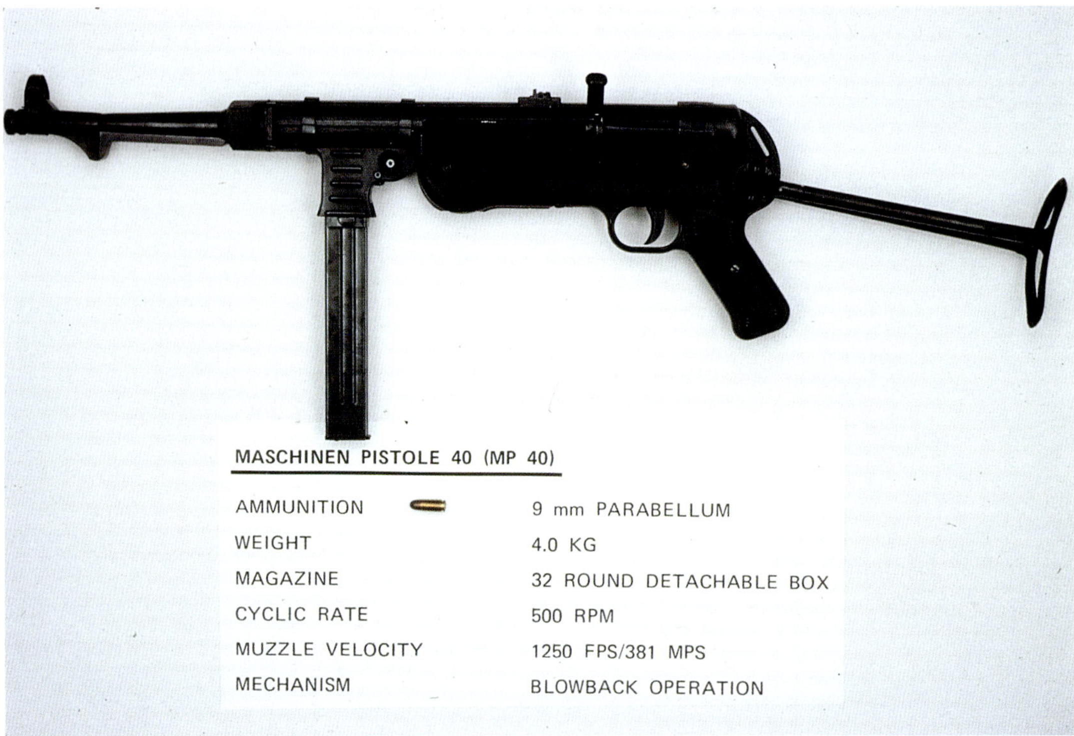

Fig. 1-9. The Maschinenpistole 40 (Schmeisser)

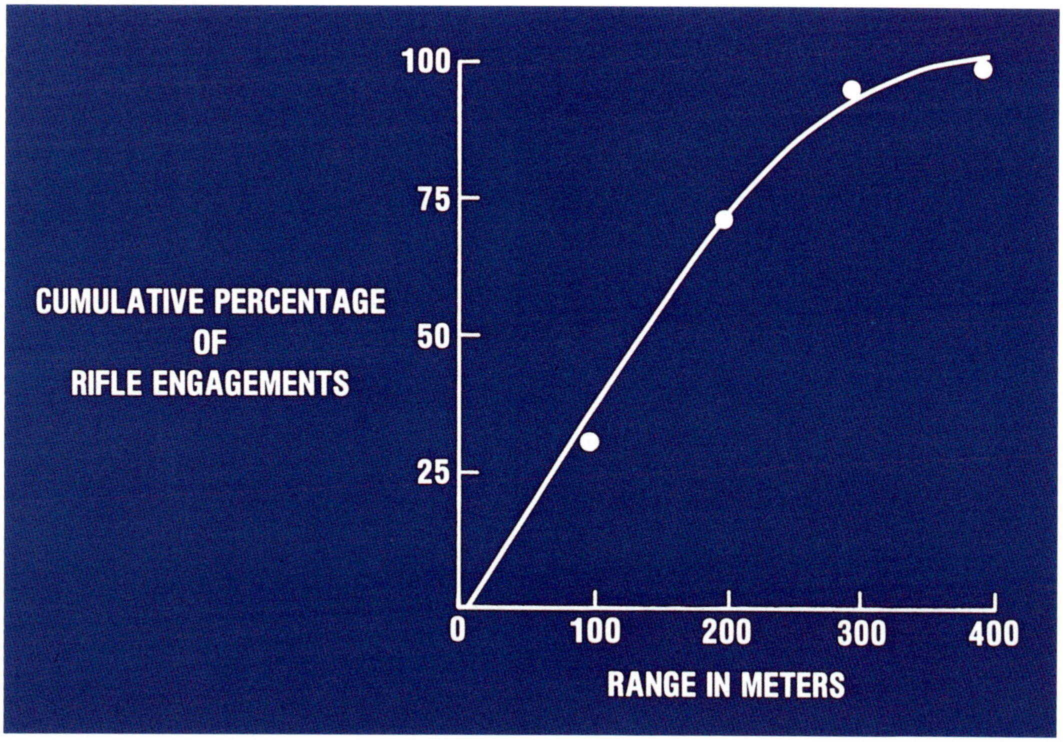

Fig. 1-10. The tactical distances for representative small-arms actions fought by American troops during and since World War II
Sources: Redrawn from data in references 5 and 6

design requirements for the American-made M2- and M3-series Bradley Fighting Vehicles was armor that could withstand the 60-g bullets fired by the KPV.

The relationship between the modern machine gun and the *assault rifle* (described below) is complementary. Like the assault rifle, the machine gun is used to suppress enemy fire rather than to hit specific targets. It is specifically used as a fixed base to provide fire cover for the maneuver elements who are armed with assault rifles. By virtue of its more robust construction and the better heat-dissipating properties of its barrel, the machine gun can sustain more prolonged fire with more powerful cartridges than the assault rifle can, but its heaviness and large size, which make it so useful as a fixed weapon, also create a burden for the soldiers who carry it.

Submachine Gun (Machine Pistol). The need for a lightweight equivalent of a machine gun was not met on a large scale until the appearance in World War II of the *machine pistol*, better known in English-speaking countries as the *submachine gun*. The classic example of this type of weapon is the Maschinenpistole 38/40, or, as it is better known, the Schmeisser (Figure 1-9). Unlike the single-shot rifle or the machine gun, both of which fired full-power cartridges, the submachine gun fired pistol ammunition, which has much less power, a short effective range, and lower lethality. Like the machine gun, however, its action was controllable and fully automatic.

Fully Automatic Rifle (Assault Rifle). The next step in the development of the soldier's individual weapon was the fully automatic rifle, but its design required ammunition that was intermediate in power between the old full-power round of the Gewehr 98 and the pistol ammunition used by the submachine gun. Gewehr 98 ammunition could not be used because—when even a single round was fired—its recoil was so violent that the weapon was difficult to control; when used as a fully automatic weapon, only the first shot was likely to be accurate. Nor was such power really necessary. As was the case in World War I, most ground actions involving small arms still tend to occur at distances of 200 m or less under most combat conditions (Figure 1-10).[5,6]

In 1943, the Germans developed an intermediate-power round measuring 7.92 x 29 mm by cutting the cartridge of the 7.92 x 59-mm round in two. This made possible the design of the first truly useful automatic rifle, the Sturmgewehr 44 (literally, *assault rifle*). At the same time, the Soviets developed an intermediate-power round with dimensions of 7.62 x 39 mm, and began to design a weapon similar to the Sturmgewehr. The result was the famous Avtomat Kalashnikova 1947g, better known as the AK47 (Figure 1-11), which was perfected after World War II.

The first American-made assault rifle, now known as the M16, appeared almost 15 years later. This weapon was not designed by the military; a civilian weapons designer based it on hunting ammunition that was commercially available at the time (the Remington 0.222-inch round modified to 5.56 x 45 mm). The army adopted the M16 after making certain modifications, some of which were later seen to be deleterious.[5] The most important of these was to use more powerful powder, which, by increasing the cyclic rate of fire, also left more powder residue and increased the likelihood that the weapon would jam.

The assault rifle is now the infantry soldier's principal weapon. With its increasing use, military medical personnel have seen more casualties with multiple gunshot wounds sustained at a range of less than 100 m (Figures 1-12 and 1-13). In addition, the close range of the combatants means that first aid will have to be provided in the midst of the firefight, exposing the caregiver to mortal danger.

By combining the large-volume firepower of the submachine gun with the lethality and some of the range of the single-shot rifle, the assault rifle has made both of these weapons obsolete except for specialty missions. For example, the submachine gun is used by antiterrorist units (as well as by terrorists) because its small size makes it useful in confined spaces. Most armies continue to use the single-shot rifle as a sniper's weapon (Figure 1-14).

In addition to its more lethal ammunition, the assault rifle has a relatively long effective range of about 400 m (Figure 1-15).[7] However, it is more frequently used to suppress close-range enemy fire than to hit specific distant targets.

Pistol. The role of the *pistol* on the modern battlefield remains one of conjecture. Although pistols are issued to officers and specialists for personal defense, they have a very short effective range, fire a bullet of modest lethality, and thus are infrequently used. Military personnel who want a truly effective personal weapon are more likely to opt for an assault rifle, a submachine gun, or even a shotgun.

The planned replacement of the venerable Colt .45 (which has a 250-grain, 800-fps bullet) with the Beretta M9 (which has a 115-grain, 1,100-fps bullet) is sure to

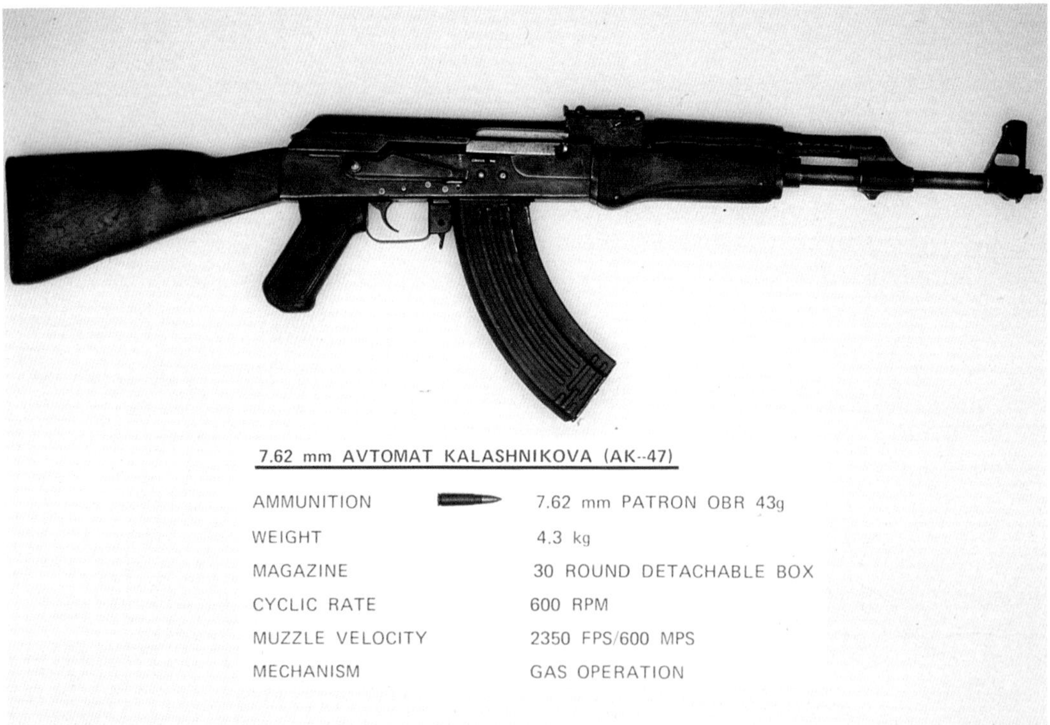

Fig. 1-11. The AK47
Source: Letterman Army Institute of Research

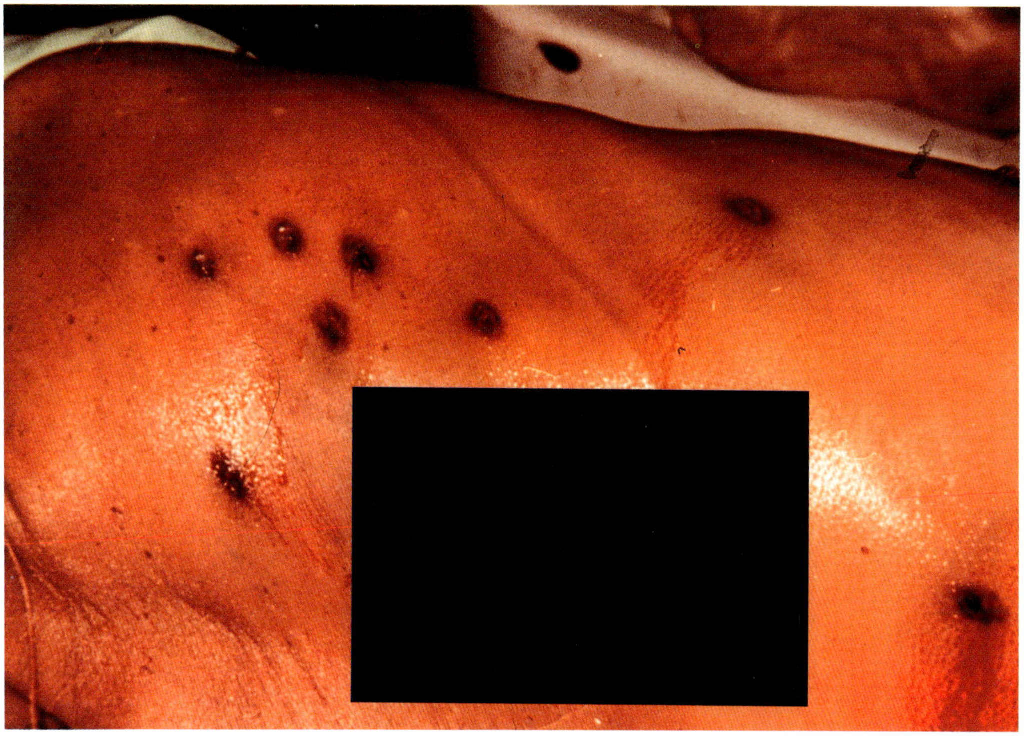

Fig. 1-12. This soldier was killed during a firefight in which the enemy was armed with AK47 assault rifles. There are eight wounds of entry in the right posterior trunk.
Source: Wound Data and Munitions Effectiveness Team

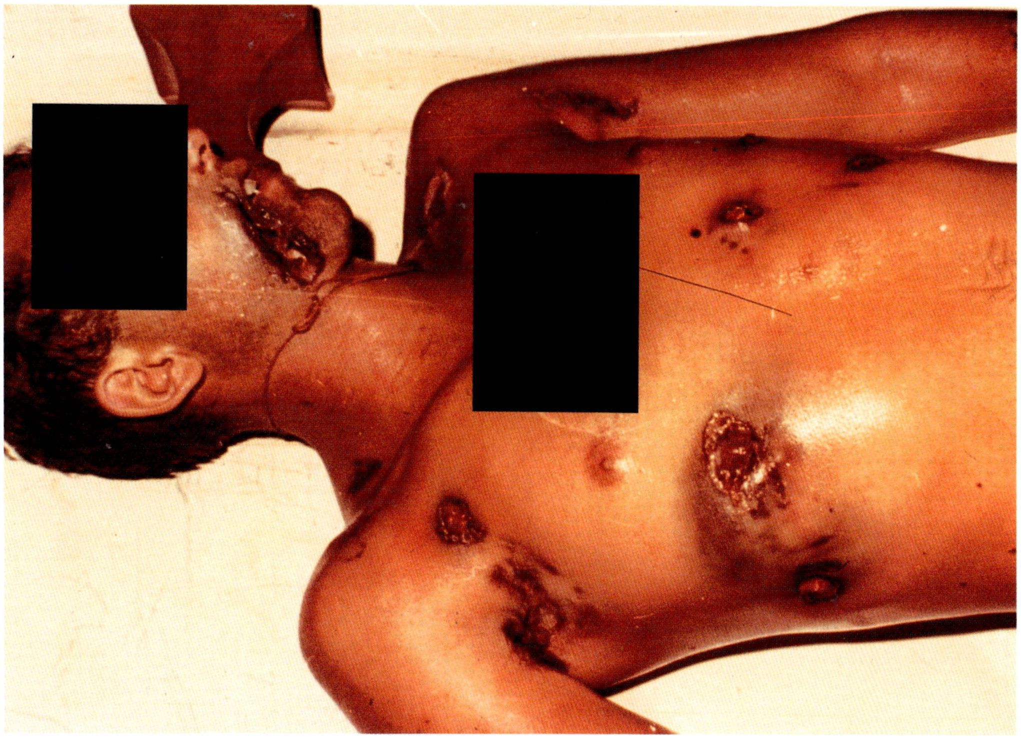

Fig. 1-13. The soldier's anterior wounds of exit are considerably larger than his wounds of entry.
Source: Wound Data and Munitions Effectiveness Team

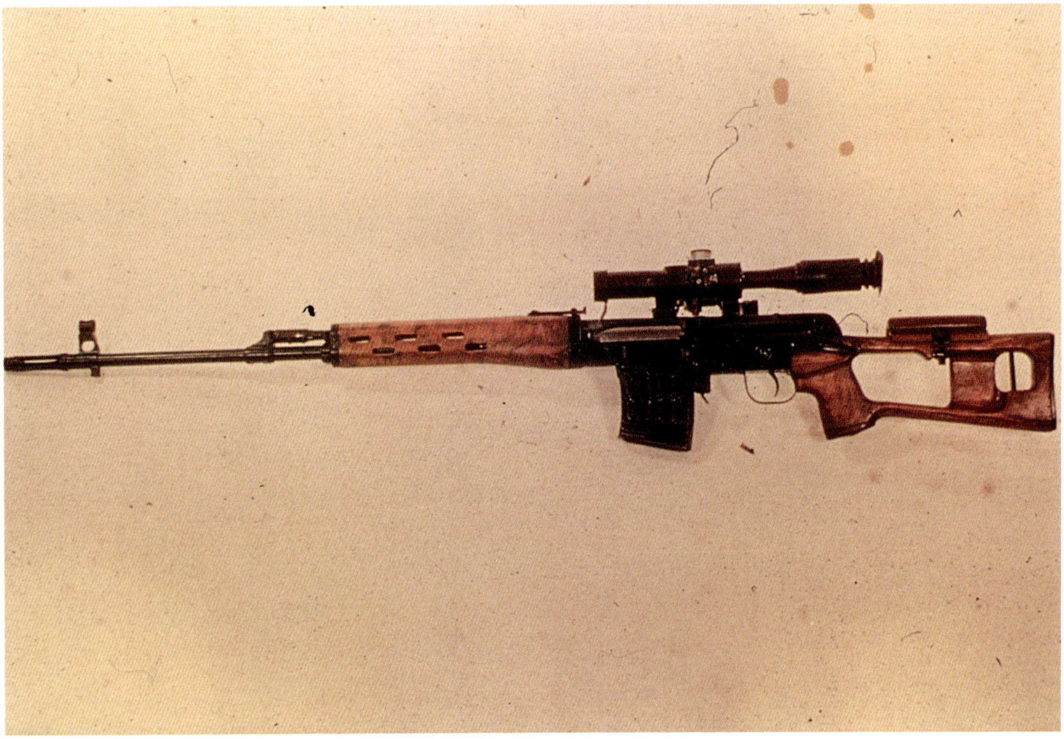

Fig. 1-14. The 7.62-mm Snayperskaya Vintovka Dragunova (SVD) is a semiautomatic gas-operated rifle that fires the 7.62 x 54R round shown in Figure 1-3. Its telescopic sights make it an excellent sniper's weapon.
Source: Letterman Army Institute of Research

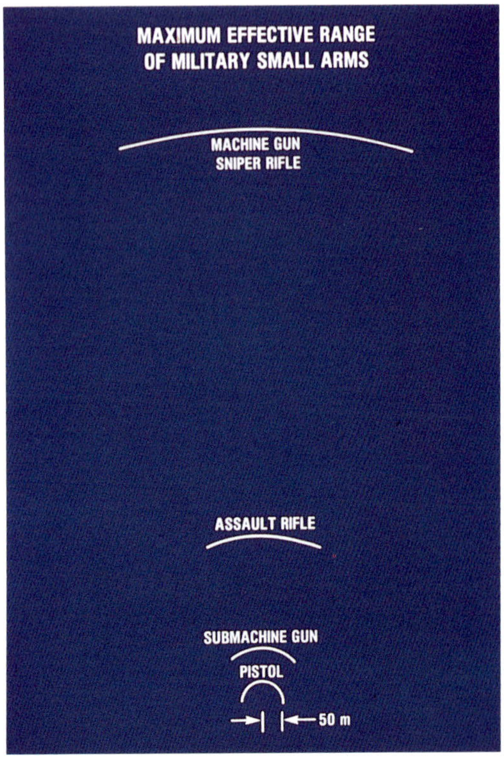

Fig. 1-15. The maximum effective ranges of various classes of military small arms
Source: Reference 7

stir up arguments about the comparative effectiveness of slow, heavy bullets versus fast, light bullets. Proponents of the Colt .45 might say that its larger bullet has more knock-down power. Proponents of the Beretta might say that its faster bullet causes more tissue damage. In any event, this controversy is probably more relevant to civilian law-enforcement authorities than to the military.

Mechanisms and Operations of Small Arms

Small arms are complicated pieces of machinery. They have many small parts that need to work in precise sequences and interactions in order to fire a round safely and effectively.

The Parts of a Small Arm. In very simplified terms, a modern small arm consists of the following parts:

- The *barrel* is a metal tube, open at one end, through which the bullet travels after it is fired. On the inside surface of the barrel are spiral grooves (or *rifling*) that make the bullet spin on its longitudinal axis as it passes through the barrel, giving it a point-forward stability in air. The diameter of the inside of the barrel (called the *bore*) and the diameter of the bullet that passes through it are equivalent; thus, the diameter of a small arm's barrel is usually expressed as its *bore caliber*. The *muzzle* is the open end at the front of the barrel, and the *breech* is the opening at the rear of the barrel into which the round is inserted (or *chambered*).

- The *bolt* is a piece of metal that mechanically closes the breech. This complex movement is brought about in different ways, depending on the design of the weapon. After the round is fired, the bolt is moved away from the breech. This movement not only opens the breech, but also mechanically extracts the spent cartridge.
- The *trigger* is a mechanical device that, in a complicated sequence of events, strikes a *firing pin*, which in turn hits the primer on the base of the chambered cartridge, which then ignites the propellant charge.
- In some weapons, the small arm's operating mechanisms (that is, the bolt and the breech) are covered by a protective metal covering known as the *housing*. In some—but by no means all—weapons, the barrel, too, is fixed to the housing.

The Firing Sequence of a Small Arm. In all small arms—whether they are single-shot, semiautomatic, or fully automatic—several steps occur in sequence each time the weapon is fired: *(a)* the round is chambered in the breech; *(b)* the breech is closed by the bolt; *(c)* the trigger is pulled, which fires the round; *(d)* the bolt is moved away from the breech, which extracts the cartridge in the same movement; and *(e)* a new round is chambered.

With a manually operated single-shot rifle, such as the Gewehr 98, the energy for each step is provided by the soldier, who manually both closes the bolt after the round is chambered and opens the bolt to extract the spent cartridge.

In a semiautomatic weapon, such as the Colt .45 pistol, the energy for extracting one round and chambering the next is supplied by the combustion of the powder in the cartridge. This method of operation is called semiautomatic, but because each firing requires the soldier to pull the trigger to chamber the next round, the term *self-loading* is more accurate.

In a fully automatic weapon, the firing cycle is repeated automatically until the trigger is released or until the *magazine* is empty.

The *cyclic rate of fire* is the maximum rate at which the firing sequence can be carried out. In manually operated weapons, the cyclic rate of fire is usually much too slow to be relevant. In automatic weapons, however, the cyclic rate of fire is an important measure of the weapon's performance. Although the M16 is said to be capable of a cyclic rate of fire of 700–800 rounds/minute, a much slower but more sustained rate of fire (about 12–15 rounds/minute) is more correct; at higher sustained rates, the barrel gets too hot to operate properly, and a soldier cannot load ammunition fast enough to keep up with the rate of fire.

There are three different ways in which fully and semiautomatic weapons use the energy released by the combustion of the powder in the cartridges to replace manual energy in performing some or all of the steps in the firing sequence. These mechanisms are *recoil, blow-back,* and *gas operation* (Figure 1-16).

Recoil Operation. All small arms recoil. Many small-arm weapons designs (including the Colt .45 and some machine guns) use this property as the basis of their firing mechanism. In recoil operation, the small arm's barrel and bolt are locked together as the round is chambered. When the round is fired, the bullet is propelled out of the barrel while an equal but opposite force moves the barrel and bolt backwards in a recoil motion. This motion simultaneously compresses two powerful springs: *(a)* the *barrel spring*, which encircles the barrel and is attached in front of the fixed housing, and *(b)* the *return spring*, which is located

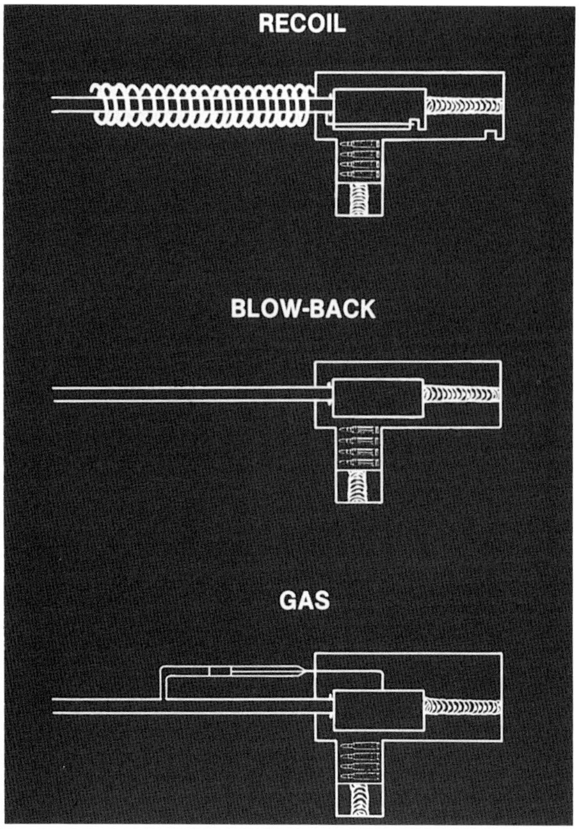

Fig. 1-16. The three basic mechanisms that are used to operate semiautomatic and fully automatic small arms

between the bolt and the back of the housing.

After recoiling several inches backward, the bolt unlocks from the barrel. The barrel rapidly reverses direction and is propelled forward by the energy stored in the barrel spring. At the same time, the bolt and the spent cartridge continue moving backward, and the spent cartridge is ejected. A new round is inserted automatically into the gap between the breech end of the barrel and the bolt. The bolt is then forced forward by the energy stored in the return spring, and this motion both chambers the new round and closes the breech. The new round is now ready to be fired.

Although this mechanism reliably fires without jamming, it is complicated and heavy. Like all weapons, it is also inherently less accurate when fired rapidly.

Blow-back Operation. This is the simplest firing mechanism, and is used in many submachine guns, including the Schmeisser and the Israeli-made Uzi.

With the blow-back mechanism, the barrel is fixed to the housing. The bolt closes the breech, but is not locked to the barrel as it would be in a recoil operation. As the round is fired, the energy from the exploding cartridge propels the bullet out the barrel and simultaneously starts to move the bolt backward. However, in this design, the bolt must be heavy enough to stay in position for a split second longer than it takes for the bullet to be ejected from the barrel. The bolt's backward movement compresses a powerful return spring that connects the rear of the bolt to the housing. (Unlike recoil-operated weapons, the barrel does not move relative to the weapon during this sequence; instead, the bolt and return spring absorb the energy of the recoil.) A new cartridge is inserted into the breech and is chambered when the bolt is driven forward by the energy stored in the return spring.

The blow-back mechanism needs few moving parts, but, because the barrel and bolt are not locked together, this firing mechanism is not commonly used with high-power cartridges. If such cartridges were used, the pressure of the gas that was created when the powder detonated would force open the breech and escape before it exerted its maximum force to propel the bullet out of the barrel. The French, however, have solved this problem and have fielded their FA MAS 5.56-mm high-power automatic assault rifle, which uses the blow-back mechanism.

Gas Operation. Designers of military small arms are focusing on a third mechanism, known as gas operation, which is used by the greatest number of automatic weapons fielded today.

As the round is fired, some of the gas from the exploding powder passes out of the barrel through a small port proximal to the muzzle. The port leads to a tube that extends along the length of the barrel, and, depending on the design, affects the bolt in one of two ways. In some gas-operated weapons, such as the AK47, the pressure of the gas compresses a small piston located at the front end of the tube. A backward-moving piston rod then mechanically moves the bolt away from the breech. In other gas-operated weapons, such as the M16, the pressure of the gas traveling through the unobstructed tube moves the bolt away from the breech.

The latter mechanism has the virtue of simplicity, but—as was shown in Vietnam—may be subject to fouling and consequent jamming unless the weapon is kept clean. The advantages of a gas-operated weapon are its *(a)* low weight, *(b)* ability to function with a high-power cartridge, and *(c)* high cyclic rate of fire.

Trends in Small-Arms Development

The trend in military small-arms development is to design and field weapons that are capable of generating more casualties. If a victim receives multiple random wounds from a weapon, the likelihood that a critical organ will be injured is greater than if the victim were hit with only one projectile. In addition, weapons that make multiple wounds require the opponent to use more resources and personnel to evacuate and treat their casualties.

Weapons designers are experimenting with ways to increase the number of wounds that a small arm can produce. This research is taking three directions:

One approach is to update the shotgun. Firing many projectiles from a single cartridge increases the likelihood that a person within a given range will receive multiple wounds. However, shotgun pellets and similar projectiles have relatively poor aerodynamic properties and do not travel very far. Combat shotguns that use tiny, aerodynamically superior *fléchettes* (literally, tiny arrows) within such rounds are a possible solution.

A second approach is to dispense entirely with inert bulletlike projectiles and instead to fire explosive munitions from small arms. For example, weapons designers are working on lighter and more easily deployed grenade launchers.

A third approach is to develop small arms that have much higher cyclic rates of fire than currently fielded weapons have. But there is a trade-off inherent in automatic weapons: The higher the rate of fire, the less accurate the weapon will be because of its recoil. For example, modern assault rifles have cyclic rates of fire of 600–700 rounds/minute, but the soldier cannot hold even a well-designed weapon steadily enough to completely overcome its recoil. As a result, beyond a range of 200–300 m, the bullets may be so widely dispersed that the probability of the shooter's scoring a hit will be even less than it would have been had a well-aimed single-shot rifle been used. Firing a salvo of lightweight projectiles (like fléchettes) would be one way to overcome the recoil problem, but fléchettes tend not to cause as much physical damage as other projectiles can. Another solution might be to fire a burst of conventional bullets so rapidly that they will have left the barrel before the recoil action becomes apparent to the shooter. There are two ways to do this: *(a)* a tandem round can be used, in which two or three bullets fit one behind the other within the cartridge in such a way that, when the round is fired, the equivalent of three rounds are propelled out of the barrel; or *(b)* caseless ammunition can be used, in which the propellant is molded around the bullet and the cartridge is completely eliminated. This shortens the operating cycle of the weapon by making the cartridge-extraction step of the firing process unnecessary. The German-made Heckler & Koch G11 automatic rifle is an example of a weapon that uses caseless ammunition; it fires a three-round burst of 4.8-mm bullets in 60 msec, too short a time for the weapon's recoil to spoil the shooter's aim.

EXPLOSIVE MUNITIONS

The generic prototype of the exploding munition is the *shell*, which originally was a hollow casing made of metal. Explosive powder was packed into the shell, along with a *fuse* to ignite the powder, and—depending on the design—various kinds of fragments, projectiles, chemicals, or other agents that were designed to spew out when the shell exploded (Figure 1-17).[8] In the older designs, the fragments of the shell casing did most of the damage.

From this basic concept came the more specialized modern exploding munitions, such as grenades, rockets, bombs, and mines.

Like small-arms munitions, explosive munitions that are fired from weapons are often called rounds. An exploding-munition round is larger and more complicated than a small-arm round, although the design principles are similar. The *warhead* corresponds to the bullet, but—unlike that inert projectile—is usually designed to explode. In smaller exploding munitions, the propellant-filled cartridge case will be attached to the warhead, just as the cartridge case is attached to the bullet in small-arms munitions. In very large exploding munitions, however, the warhead and the bags of propellant are loaded into the weapon separately.

The fuses in these weapons have also become much more reliable and sophisticated over time, and now commonly allow detonation to be preset for *(a)* impact, *(b)* a designated time delay, or *(c)* an altitude of several feet to several yards above the ground. Impact fuses rely on a metal rod that is driven into a primer of high-explosive material, which in turn detonates the main charge. Some impact fuses are designed to have a delay of 0.15–0.35 seconds, which allows the exploding munition to penetrate the target before the firing pin is activated. A designated time-delay fuse uses an electronic timer that has been preset to detonate the primer at a designated moment. The altitude (or proximity) fuse relies on a small radar that measures the distance either from the ground or from the target; when a preset distance is reached, the primer is detonated. Other modern munitions use fuses that are

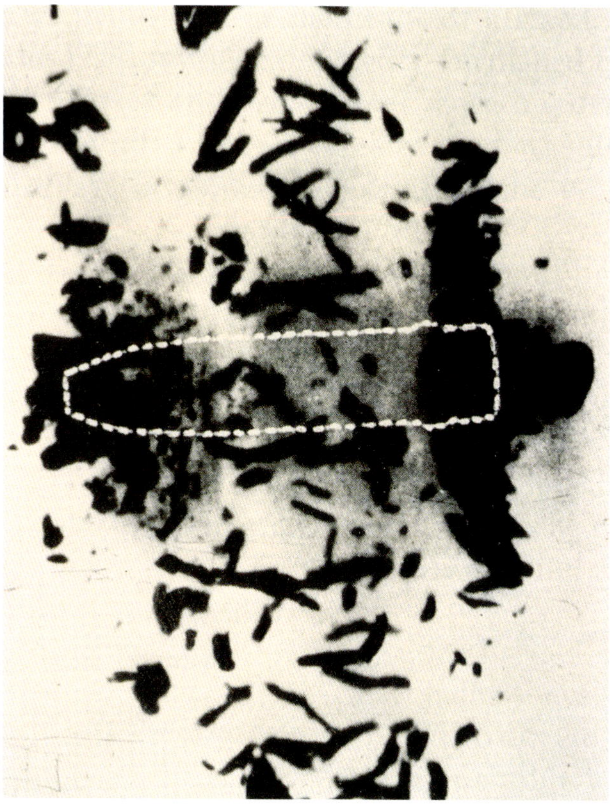

Fig. 1-17. A 20-mm cannon shell at the moment of its detonation
Source: Reference 8

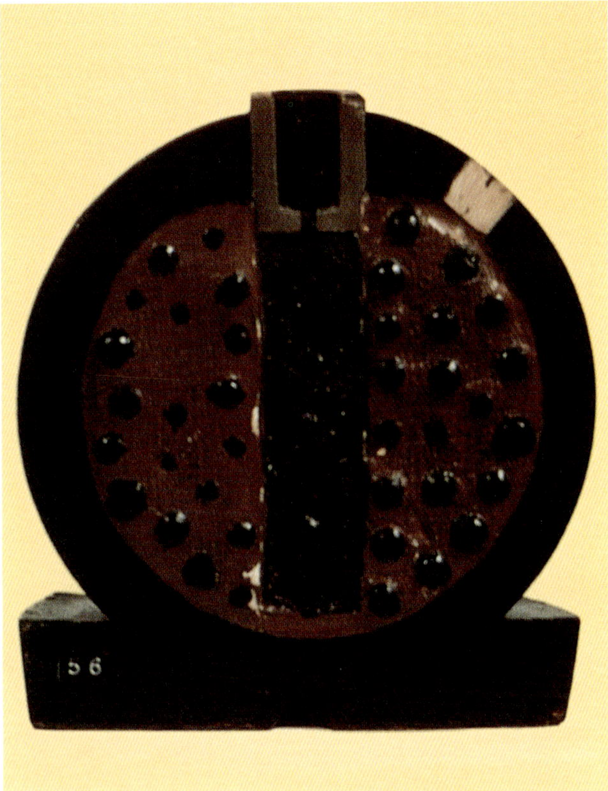

Fig. 1-18. Spherical shrapnel ball (circa 1830). With the addition of sophisticated fuses, today's fragmenting munitions are almost identical in concept.
Source: Reference 9

even more specialized than these relatively common ones.

Depending on its design, an exploding munition can be used against personnel or matériel or both.

Antipersonnel Exploding Munitions

In the nineteenth century, when facing increasingly powerful infantries armed with rifled muskets, artillery forces began to use *shrapnel* to increase the effectiveness of their explosive munitions (Figure 1-18).[9] In addition to its explosive, a shrapnel ball contained many small lead spheres (the actual shrapnel) packed in resin. The lead spheres were blasted out of the shell at detonation, greatly increasing the number of projectiles that an explosive munition could be counted on to produce.

The usual objective of explosive munitions used against personnel is to make multiple hits (Figure 1-19), taking advantage of the penetrating injuries caused by the *ballistic effects* of the fragments flying out from the exploding shell. The two other components of such a detonation are the *blast effects* from the force of the explosion and the *thermal effects* from the explosion's heat.

These three effects generate wounds according to the victim's distance from the epicenter of the explosion (Figure 1-20). Casualties who are close to the detonation are likely to show evidence of all three effects, while casualties who are farther away will sustain only penetrating injury. Even casualties who are some distance from the epicenter are likely to be blown over by the blast; the closer they are to an exploding munition, however, the less likely they are to survive or even to enter the medical-treatment system. Casualties who have received combined ballistic, blast, and thermal injuries usually suffer mutilating blast injury (Figure 1-21) and are unlikely to survive.

Because the radius for ballistic injury retracts more slowly than do the corresponding radii for blast and thermal effects, munitions designers capitalize on the ballistic effects by ensuring that weapons have a ready supply of potential fragments. The simplest way to do this is to build the munition with a thicker wall. This

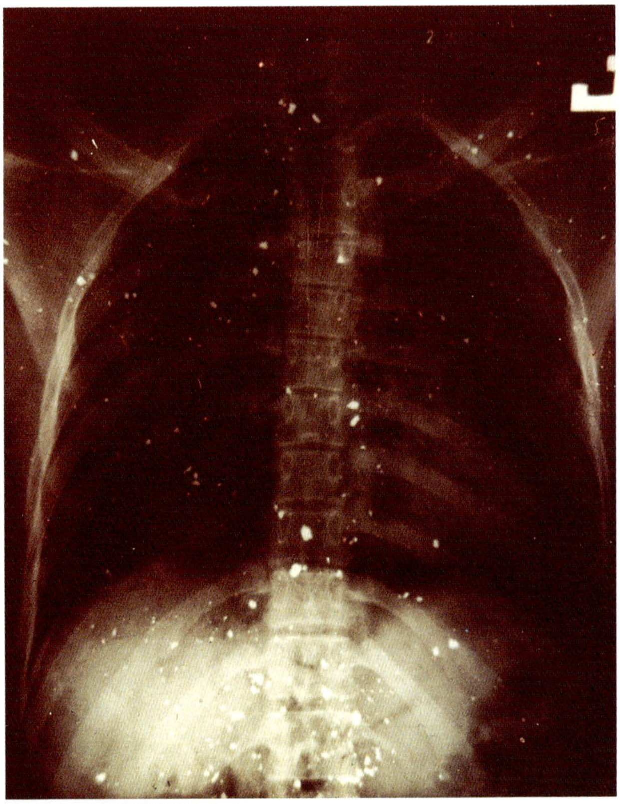

Fig. 1-19. This roentgenogram shows the chest of a casualty who was killed by an 82-mm mortar bomb. Unlike small arms, which usually make few hits, modern explosive munitions usually cause multiple fragmentation wounds.
Source: Wound Data and Munitions Effectiveness Team

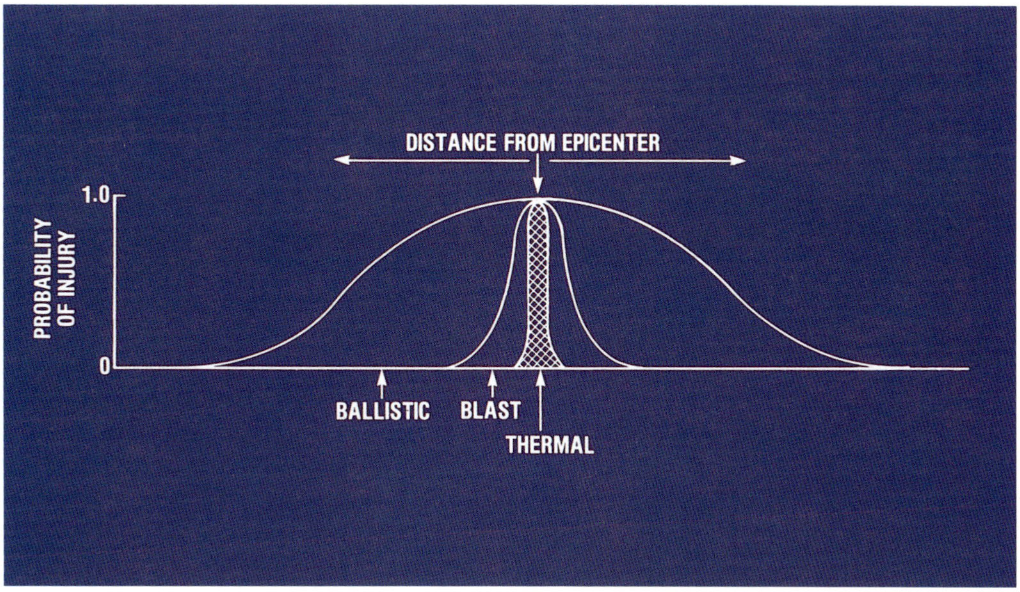

Fig. 1-20. The probability of sustaining a given trauma is related to the casualty's distance from the epicenter of the detonation.

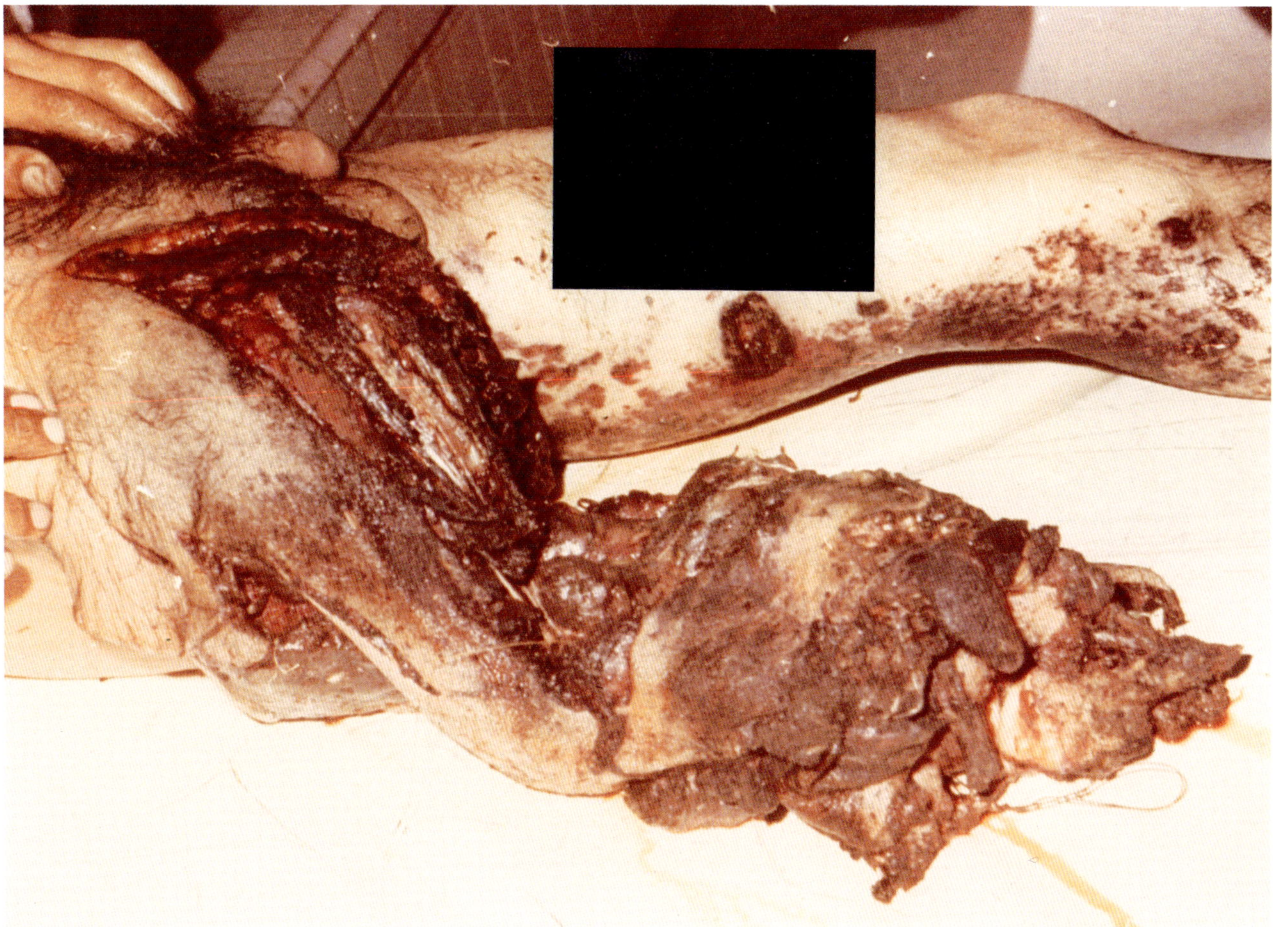

Fig. 1-21. This soldier was killed by a 105-mm shell that detonated several feet from his body. Penetrating ballistic injuries have obviously occurred, and there is evidence of burns. The blast wave also caused some of the tissue mutilation.
Source: Wound Data and Munitions Effectiveness Team

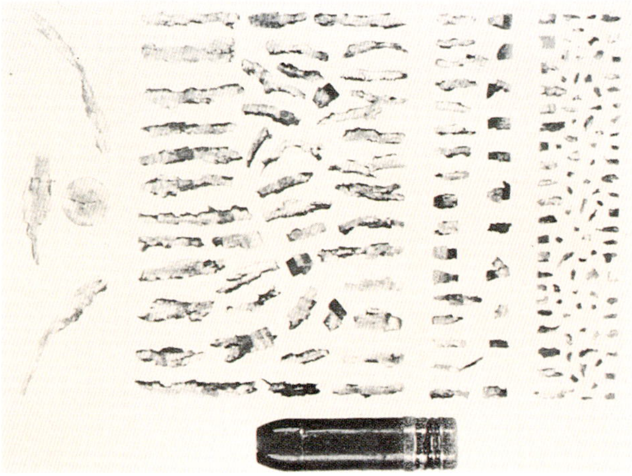

Fig. 1-22. The explosion of a conventional random-fragmentation high-explosive shell yields fragments of various sizes and shapes.
Source: Reference 8

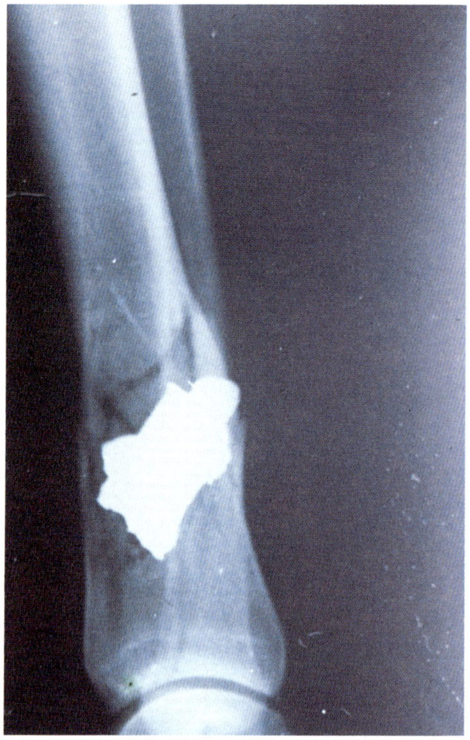

Fig. 1-24. The roentgenogram shows a large fragment from an 82-mm mortar round that has fractured the casualty's tibia.
Source: Wound Data and Munitions Effectiveness Team

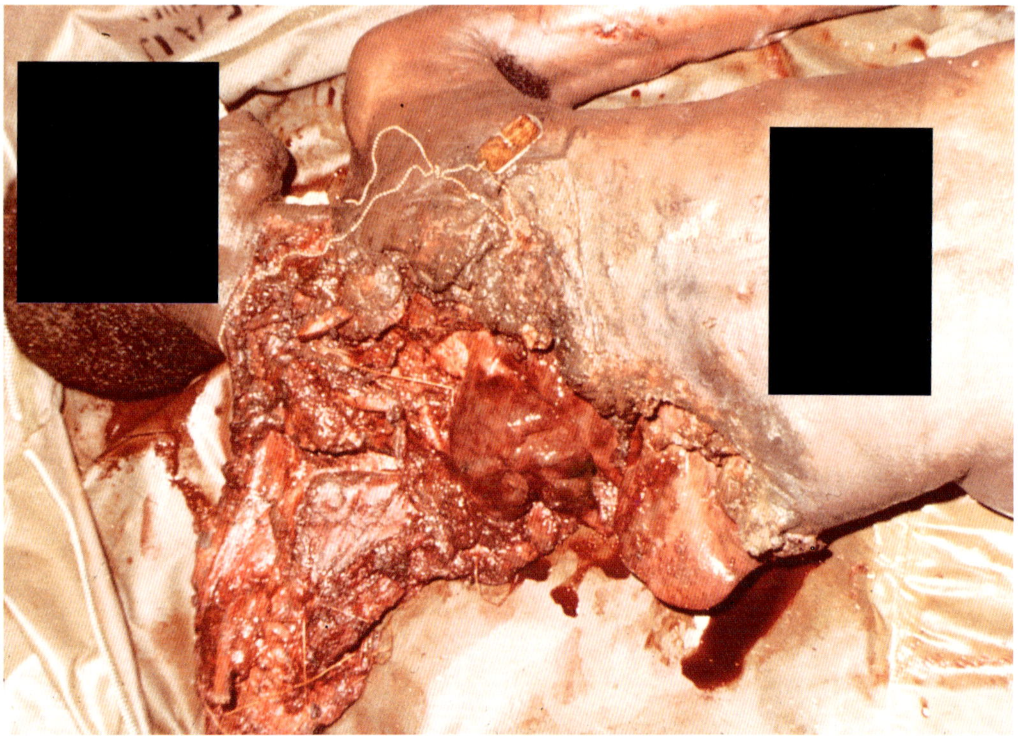

Fig. 1-23. This soldier was hit by an unusually large fragment from a random-fragmentation munition.
Source: Wound Data and Munitions Effectiveness Team

will reduce its blast effects somewhat, but will also increase the likelihood that the exploding wall's fragments will have enough mass to injure the nearby personnel who are hit by them.

Random-Fragmentation Munitions. The shell of a random-fragmentation munition splinters unpredictably, and the resulting fragments vary in size, shape, and velocity (Figure 1-22). A large fragment is usually lethal (Figure 1-23), although the casualty may survive if its velocity is low and the body part struck is not a vital one (Figure 1-24).

Even small fragments can seriously wound a soldier. An explosive spray of a greater number of fast-moving, smaller fragments would be more likely to hit more personnel, and thus would be more efficient than a spray of fewer, larger, and slower chunks (Figure 1-25), which would not only hit fewer personnel, but would do so with more destructive force than would be necessary to incapacitate them. Because a random-fragmentation munition breaks apart unevenly, much of its power is wasted.

Improved-Fragmentation Munitions. Two modern designs have improved the effectiveness of fragmentation munitions (Figure 1-26). The first is the *improved-fragmentation munition,* which can *(a)* be made of a fragmentable material that breaks up in a con-

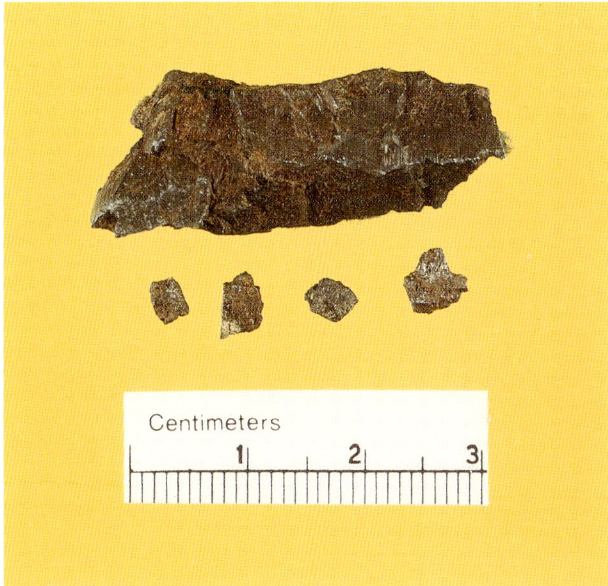

Fig. 1-25. These are random fragments. The larger chunk weighs 15.5 g and is typical of the fragmentation munitions used in World War I; the smaller pieces weigh 100–200 mg and are typical of those used in Vietnam.
Sources: Author and Wound Data and Munitions Effectiveness Team

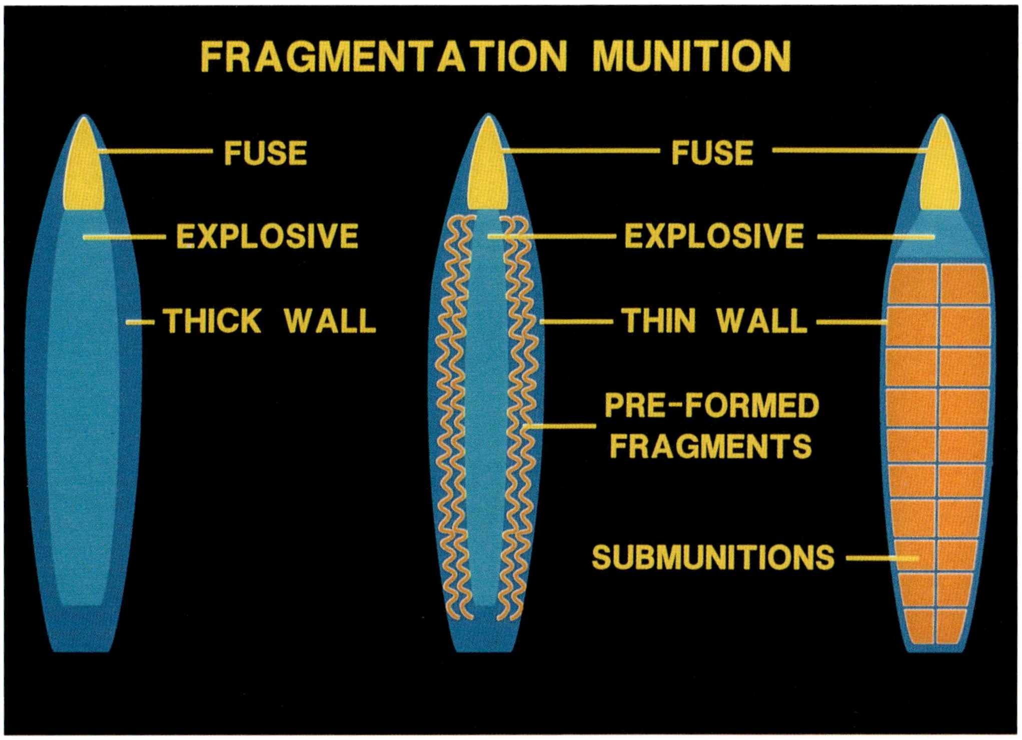

Fig. 1-26. Three varieties of fragmentation weapons are *(a)* the conventional thick-walled, random-fragmentation shell on the left, *(b)* the improved-fragmentation shell in the center, in which preformed fragments are stored between the explosive charge and the outer casing, and *(c)* the cluster munition on the right, in which each submunition is a small explosive bomb.

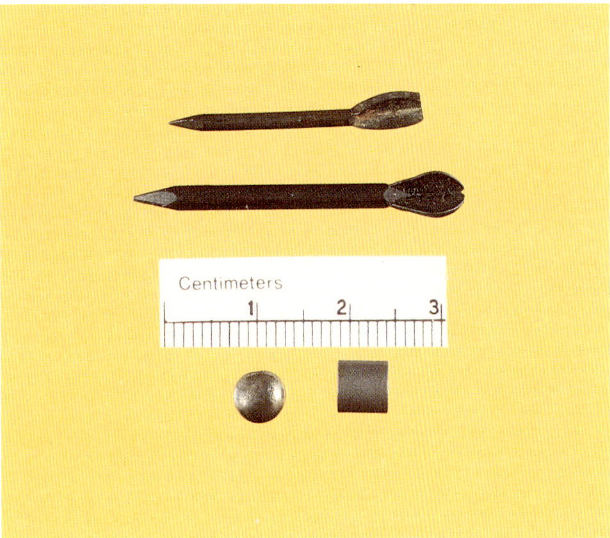

Fig. 1-27. These are typical preformed fragments. The smaller American-made fléchette, which was extracted from a casualty, is bent and is missing a fin. Fléchettes occasionally deform in tissue; such a deformation vastly increases their wounding potential. The smaller fléchette weighs 550 mg; the larger Soviet-made fléchette weighs 1.3 g. The ball and rod weigh 0.7 and 1.0 g, respectively.
Sources: Authors and Wound Data and Munitions Effectiveness Team

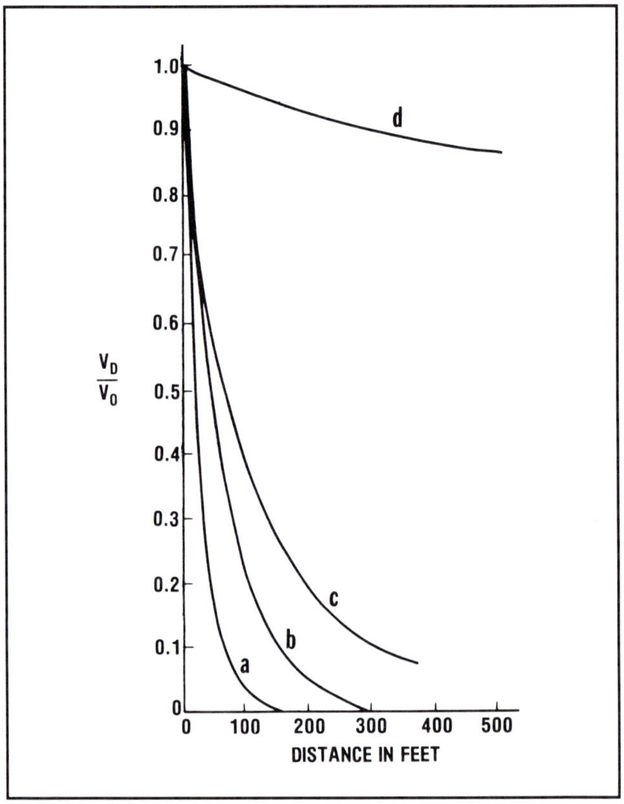

Fig. 1-28. Relative velocity as a function of range for three types of forged-steel missiles and a fléchette found in explosive munitions: (1) a 65-mg forged-steel irregular fragment, (2) a 600-mg forged-steel irregular fragment, (3) a 6.5-g forged-steel irregular fragment, and (4) a nontumbling fléchette. The abscissa represents the distance from the detonation site. The ordinate represents the ratio of the velocity at this given distance (VD) divided by the initial velocity at the detonation's origin (VO). Initial absolute velocities measured close to the munition can be as high as 6,000 fps for the sphere and irregular fragment, but are much lower for the fléchette.
Source: Reference 10

trolled fashion along preformed notches or *(b)* be filled with preformed fragments.

In the first improved-fragmentation model, the shell wall breaks up along preformed notches when the munition is detonated, just as a sheet of postage stamps will tear along its perforations. A typical fragment from a 105-mm improved-fragmentation shell will weigh only about 600 mg, compared to an average fragment from a conventional random-fragmentation shell of the same caliber, which will weigh about 2 g. Because the two whole munitions weigh about the same, three times as many fragments may be created when the improved-fragmentation shell explodes, with a consequent increase in the probability of either hitting many targets or making multiple hits on a given target.

In the second improved-fragmentation model, fragments of optimal size are inserted into the munition when it is manufactured (Figure 1-27). These fragments will be widely disseminated upon detonation. Common types of preformed fragments are *(a)* fléchettes, which have a streamlined shape and stabilizing fins and, thus, superior ballistic properties, *(b)* preformed rods, and *(c)* preformed spheres. The velocity degradations of fléchettes and random fragments are compared in Figure 1-28.[10]

One example of an improved-fragmentation munition that is filled with fléchettes is the 105-mm antipersonnel round, commonly known as a *beehive round* (Figure 1-29). The small cans contain a total of 8,800 fléchettes that are released from the shell at a time determined by the fuse setting. The beehive round is especially effective when fired defensively at opposing forces within 100 m.

Because the fléchette is fin-stabilized, it flies straight in air without needing to spin on its long axis (unlike a rifle bullet, which acquires gyroscopic stability from the rifling spin it receives in the spiral grooves of the barrel). This aerodynamic property also allows the fléchette to pass through helmets and armored vests more easily than bullets can. Paradoxically, the streamlined shape may actually work to the casualty's

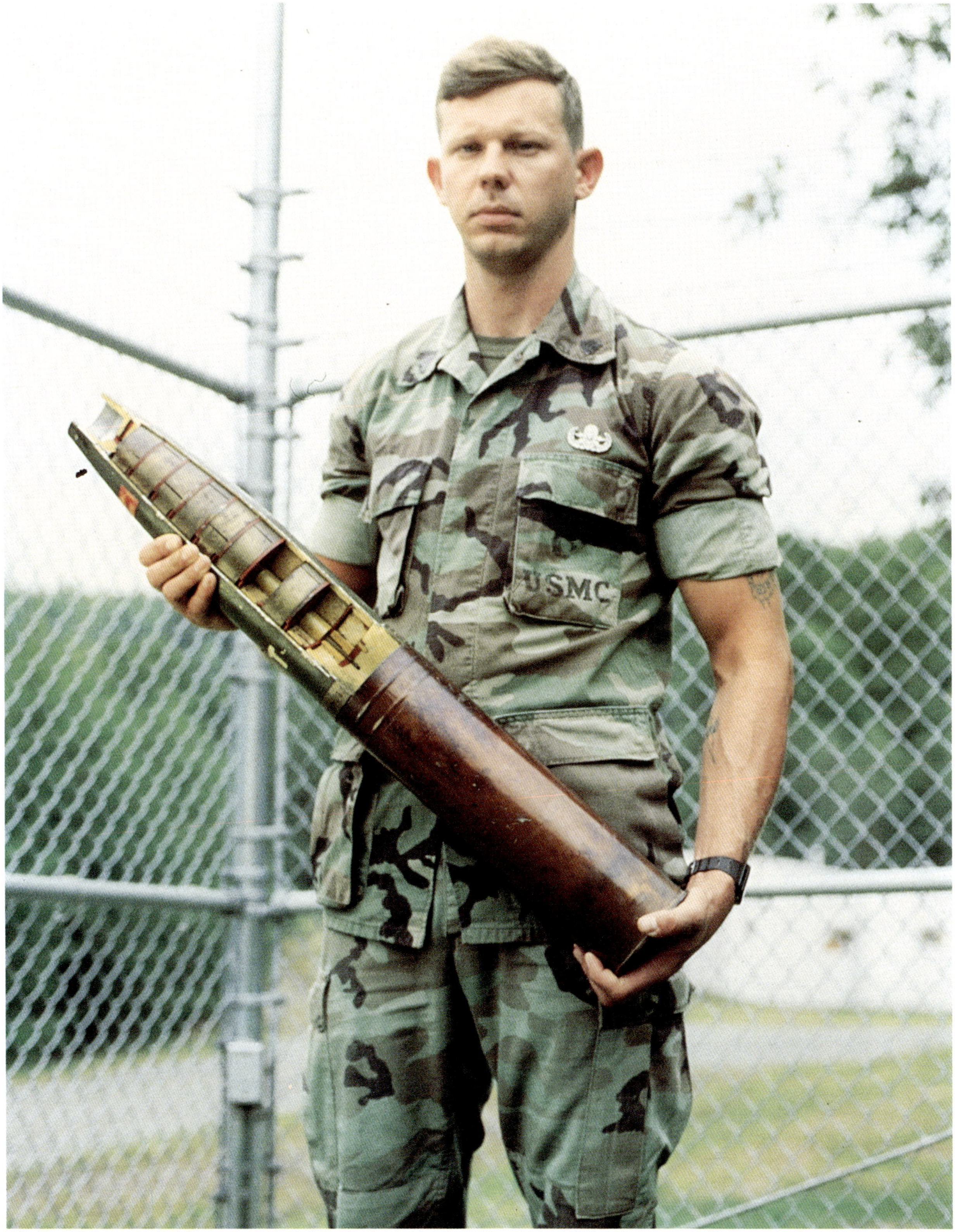

Fig. 1-29. The marine holds a cutaway demonstration model of a 105-mm improved-fragmentation munition (called a beehive round) that is loaded with fléchette-filled containers.
Source: Explosive Ordnance Disposal Group, Quantico Marine Corps Base, VA

advantage. Unlike a chunky shell fragment or even a rifle bullet, which lose their point-forward stability and tend to become unstable when they enter a denser-than-air medium, the fléchette penetrates deep and straight into tissue, creating an extremely narrow pathway, and thus may cause a less severe injury. The easily overlooked wounds of entrance and exit that the point-forward fléchettes create are tiny cruciate slits only a few millimeters long.

In Soviet-made weapons, the fléchettes are packed so that they will all be expelled in a point-forward position. However, some American designs maximize the number of fléchettes that can be packed into a carrier by loading half of them point forward and half of them fin forward. Those that are fin-forward when they are expelled will not have good aerodynamic stability in flight. They will straighten out to a point-forward position by the time they have traveled a few hundred feet, but if they hit a target before then, the force of impact—which may be strong enough to break off the fléchettes' stabilizing fins—will cause a much more severe injury and be more likely to embed the fléchettes in tissue.

Whereas irregular fragments from random-fragmentation munitions fly out at high velocities but have casualty-generating ranges measured only in hundreds of feet, the casualty-generating range of fléchettes is measured in thousands of feet. The superior range of fléchettes is of limited value, however, because most wounding by explosive munitions occurs at very short range. In the Vietnam War, for example, the median distance between a casualty and the site of detonation was only 10 m.[11]

Some improved-fragmentation munitions are filled with preformed rods—hardened steel bits that are packed inside the munition and are expelled when the casing explodes. Preformed rods are less aerodynamic but easier to manufacture than the farther-ranging fléchettes are. Their range and effectiveness are better than those of random fragments. A *cannister shot* is a shotgun-like container that can hold thousands of preformed rods (called *slugs*).

Mortar bombs and grenades commonly have a spiral coil of thick wire notched at 1-cm intervals inserted between the explosive charge and the thin outer case of the munition. Technically, these bits of wire are not preformed fragments because the wire does not break apart until the moment of detonation. But the effect is the same: Small, lightweight, equally sized fragments will be spewed out, causing similar kinds of injuries (Figure 1-30).

Like their nineteenth-century counterparts, some

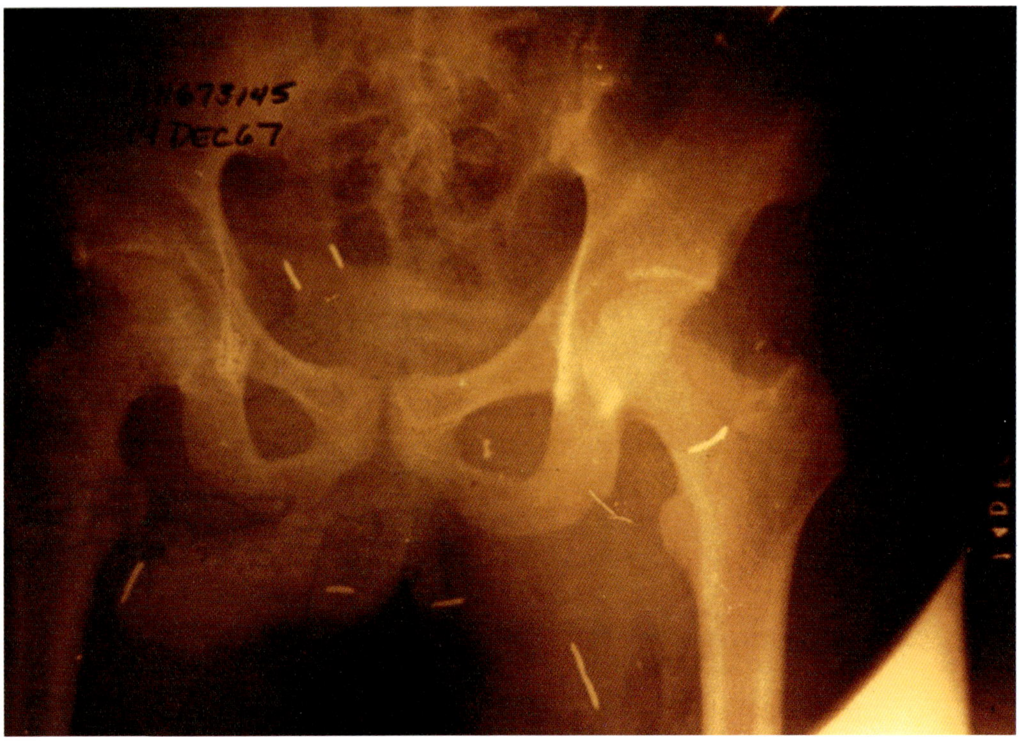

Fig. 1-30. Prenotched wire fragments from an M26 grenade perforated the small bowel and rectum of the casualty shown in this roentgenogram. The average weight of the fragments was 200 mg.
Source: Wound Data and Munitions Effectiveness Team

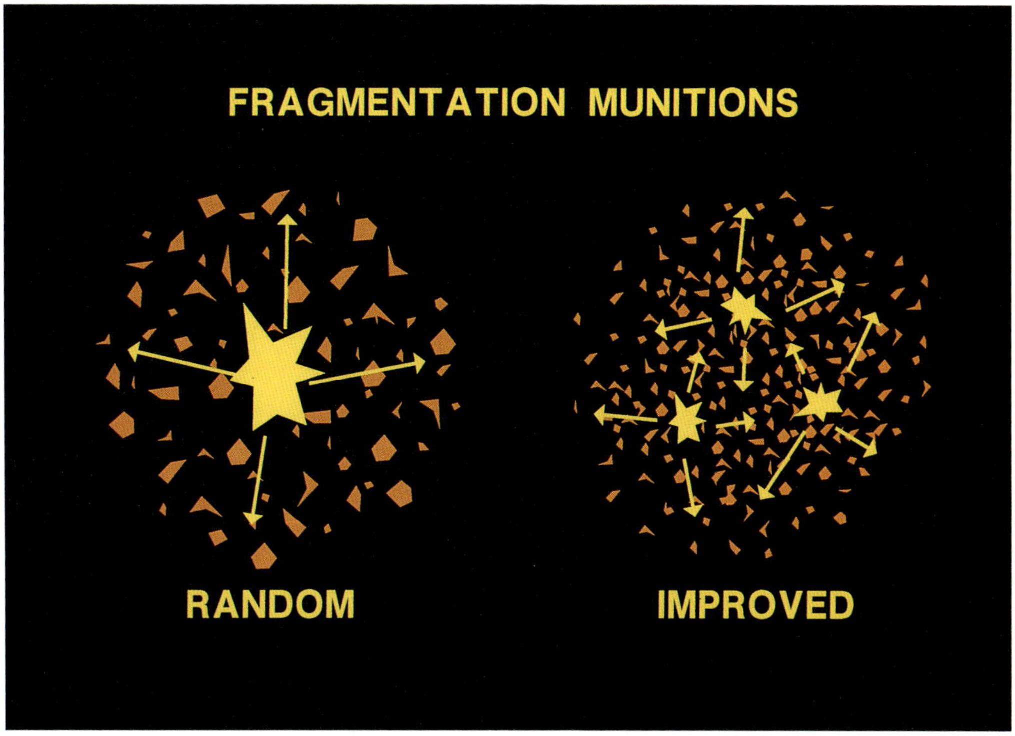

Fig. 1-31. The random-fragmentation munition on the left produces a powerful blast effect and a limited number of relatively large fragments. The cluster munition on the right produces many small fragments, which—although less lethal individually—may generate more casualties because they hit more individual targets many times.

modern improved-fragmentation munitions rely on preformed spheres (still called shrapnel) to do their damage. With the exception of their fuses—the old shrapnel ball used a primitive, often unreliable fuse to ignite its explosive powder—the principle of these weapons has remained unchanged.

Cluster (or Cargo-Carrying) Munitions. Another way to increase the effectiveness of a fragmenting munition is to load a number of smaller explosive munitions into a larger cargo-carrying munition. When a cluster munition is detonated (either before or upon the carrier's impact), its submunitions or bomblets are disseminated over the surrounding terrain. When they explode in turn, fragments are dispersed over a much wider area than would have been affected if the same mass of potential fragments had been derived from a single thick-walled shell casing (Figure 1-31).

These two modern developments—improved-fragmentation munitions and cluster munitions—are not incompatible; indeed, cluster munitions depend upon the improved-fragmentation submunitions for their source of wounding agents (Figures 1-32 and 1-33).

The concept of the cluster munition is not new. In two among many examples, cluster bombs were used extensively by the Germans in the battle of the Kursk Salient on the eastern front in 1943[12] and were implicated in a 1944 accident at an English air station.[13]

Almost every weapon system in modern conventional warfare uses improved-fragmentation or cluster munitions. The absolute radii of these munitions from their detonation point may not be as great as that of random-fragmentation munitions, simply because their fragments may not travel as far as the fewer but heavier random fragments might. But the nature of combat is such that most casualties are generated at relatively close distances. Thus, the effectiveness of improved-fragmentation and cluster munitions will be greater, because their smaller, more uniform fragments—albeit perhaps lacking the mass and velocity to kill distant personnel outright—will be much more numerous in the vicinity of most of the combatants (Figure 1-34). Consequently, many more soldiers are likely to be hit and at least incapacitated (Figure 1-35). The surgical resources required to treat so many injured personnel would be severely strained.

Secondary Missiles. A primary projectile may strike or blast apart rocks, trees, buildings, sand, or other materials with a force sufficient to create *secondary missiles* out of them, and they, in turn, may have the velocity necessary to wound personnel in their paths. Such wounds (like a face peppered with sand, for

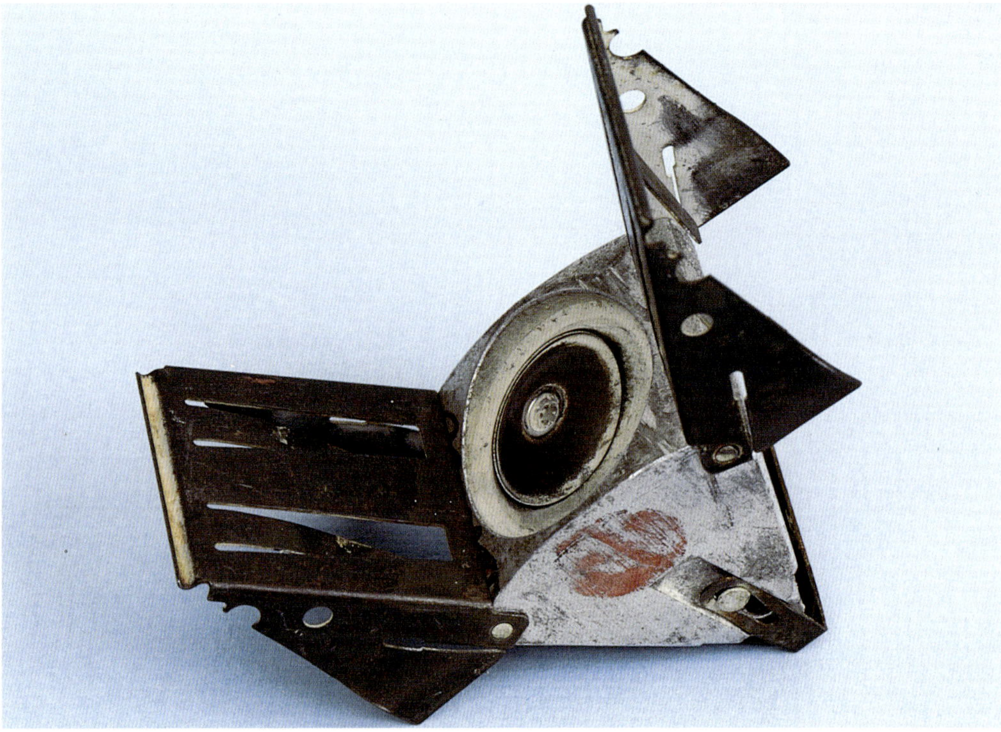

Fig. 1-32. Cluster munitions carry smaller submunitions, such as this aptly named *Dragon Tooth,* an early design that was used during World War II. It was designed to explode on impact.
Source: Explosive Ordnance Disposal Group, Quantico Marine Corps Base

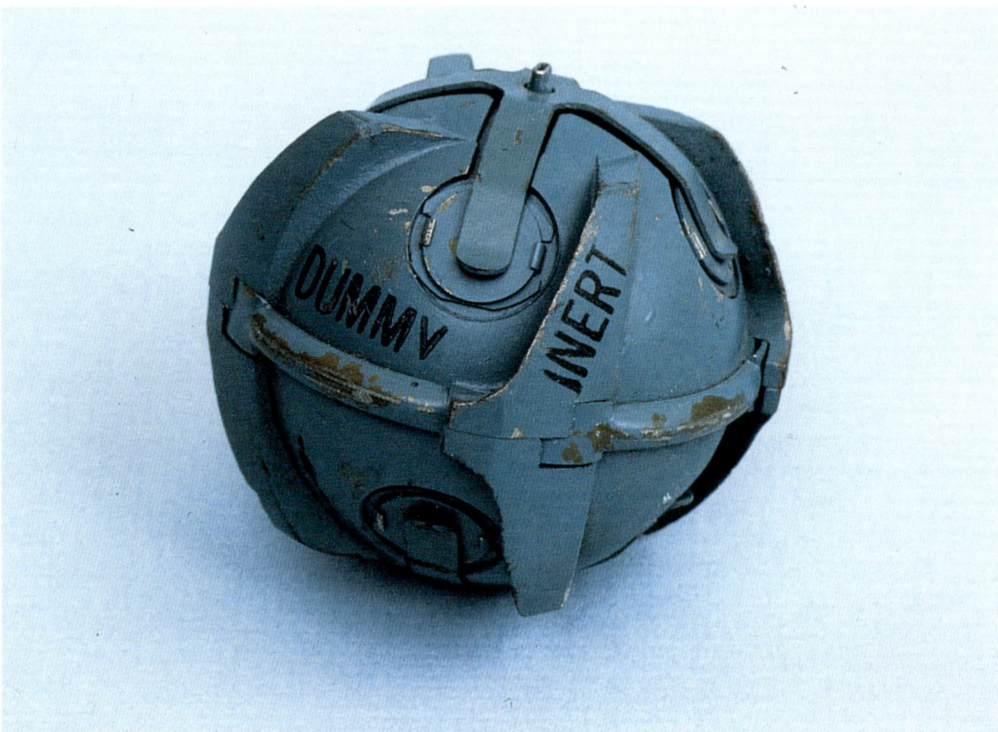

Fig. 1-33. A cluster bomb may contain dozens of these grenadelike *bomb-launched units* (BLUs). A preset BLU may explode after delays of up to several days and, once set, cannot be deactivated.
Source: Explosive Ordnance Disposal Group, Quantico Marine Corps Base

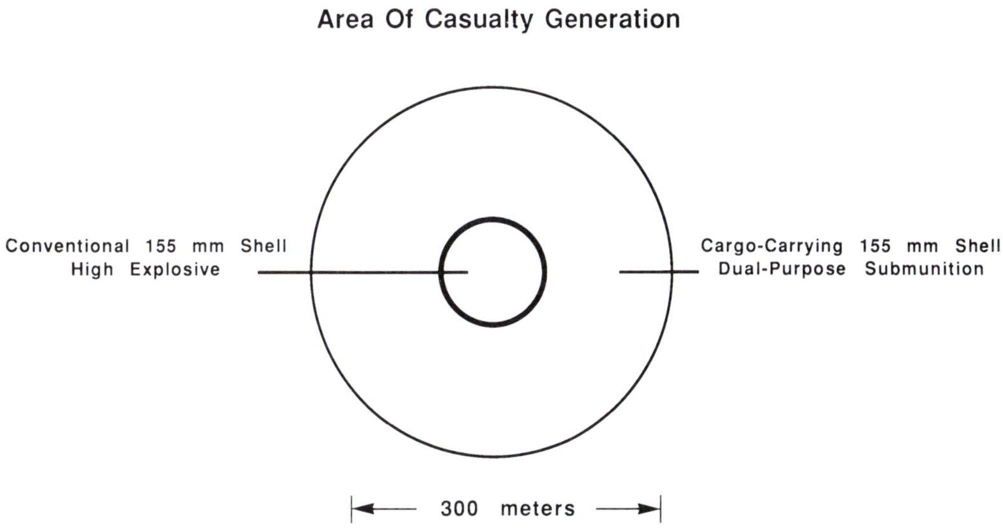

Fig. 1-34. The effective radii for conventional and cluster munitions

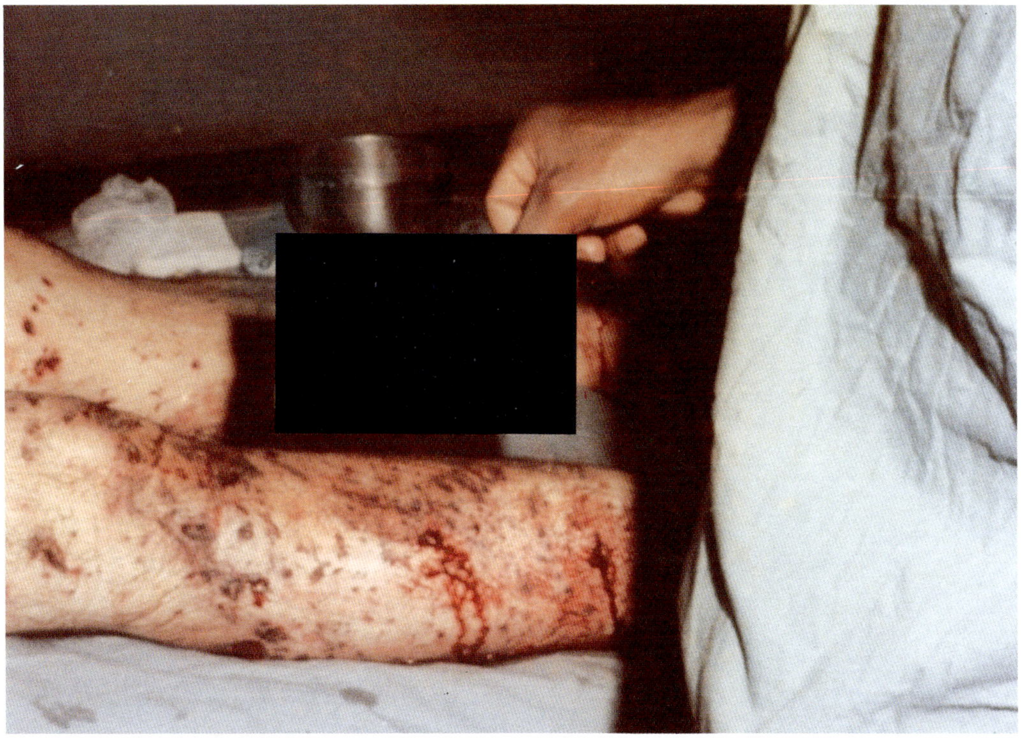

Fig. 1-35. Modern exploding munitions have changed the nature of injuries in warfare. This casualty has received many small penetrating wounds from one cluster munition, unlike most casualties in World Wars I and II who would have presented with one (or a few) relatively large penetrating wounds, such as those in Figures 1-23 and 1-24.
Source: Wound Data and Munitions Effectiveness Team

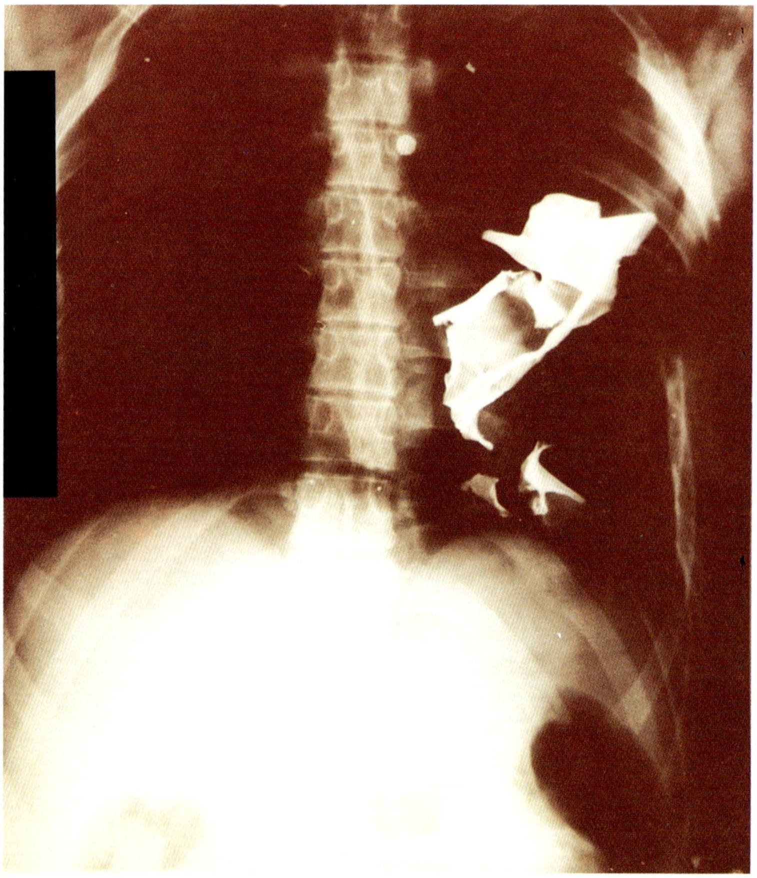

Fig. 1-36. The soldier shown in this roentgenogram was killed by a secondary missile (a piece of metal roofing that was blown off by a rocket).
Source: Wound Data and Munitions Effectiveness Team

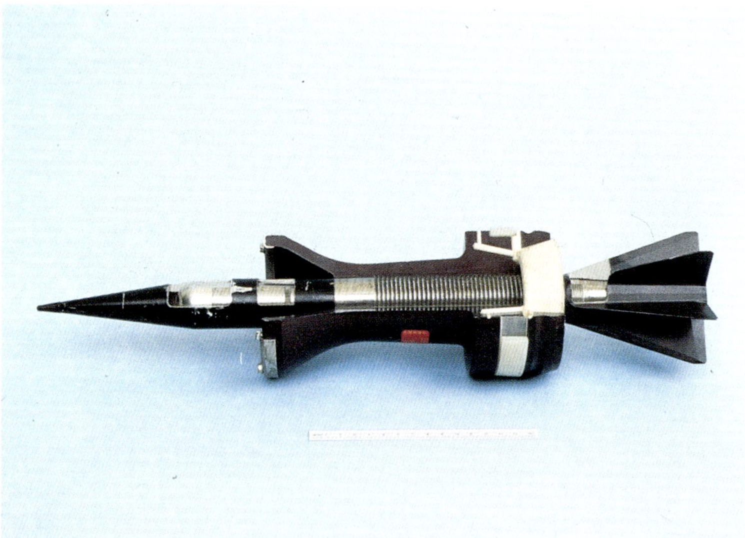

Fig. 1-37. This 105-mm APDSFS antitank projectile has a sabot (the cylinder around the middle of the arrow-like penetrator).
Source: Explosive Ordnance Disposal Group, Quantico Marine Corps Base

example) may be relatively trivial but debilitating enough to keep a soldier out of combat for some time; others that involve heavier secondary missiles, such as bricks, may be much more serious (Figure 1-36).

In the aerial bombing of cities, secondary missiles probably produce more casualties than all other causes of injury combined. Flying glass is particularly dangerous, even at a considerable distance from the source of the blast; its thin, sharp shards can easily penetrate flesh, and the more glass breaks into small pieces, the more wounds it can cause.

Wounds may also be badly contaminated by secondary missiles. A landmine, for example, creates high-velocity secondary missiles from the ground in which it is buried, making it likely that the severe wounds it causes will be filled with dirt, pebbles, and even chunks of plants.

Antimatériel Munitions That Have Antipersonnel Effects

Antimatériel munitions are designed to penetrate targets, such as buildings or fortifications, and to destroy (or render inoperative) armored fighting vehicles. Their warheads work on either of two principles: *(a)* they punch a hole through armor, because they travel at very high speeds and therefore have great kinetic energy, or *(b)* they depend upon explosive effects, such as fragmentation or blast. To be effective, fragmentation warheads must produce fragments that are much larger than those resulting from antipersonnel exploding munitions. Personnel who are caught in the path of an antimatériel exploding munition's effects will almost always be injured or killed.

When these penetrating warheads hit armored vehicles and similar enclosures, the crews are exposed to reflected (and thus greatly enhanced) blast waves known as *complex blast waves.* Antitank munitions that can produce significant blast effects behind armor include *(a)* kinetic-energy warheads, and *(b)* explosive antimatériel warheads.

Kinetic-Energy Antimatériel Warheads. Usually these munitions are fired from heavy guns, which have barrels that are long enough to give these warheads the velocities they need to be effective. The names of these munitions—such as *long-rod penetrators, APFSDS (armor-piercing, fin-stabilized, discarding-sabot) rounds,* and *composite rigid shots*—reflect essential aspects of their design. The mechanisms of armor penetration in these kinetic-energy weapons, however, are the same.

The long-rod penetrator operates on the same principle as the armor-piercing round used by small arms, but on a much larger scale. Its muzzle velocity may exceed 5,000 fps (much faster than the velocity of a bullet from an M16, for example, which is 3,200 fps).

The APFSDS round has several unusual characteristics (Figure 1-37). First, its arrow like penetrating warhead is *subcaliber* (that is, it is much smaller than the bore caliber of the weapon that fires it). Second, the warhead is encircled by a cylindrical *sabot* (literally, shoe) that has the same diameter as the bore of the barrel. The sabot not only positions the penetrating warhead steadily in the barrel, but also is exactly wide enough to receive the full thrust of the separately loaded propellant when the weapon is fired. This ensures that the projectile will be traveling at a maximum velocity when it leaves the barrel. Third, when the projectile and its sabot are propelled free of the barrel, the sabot falls away from the projectile, greatly reducing the aerodynamic drag on the penetrator. Fourth, the penetrator has fins so that it does not lose any of its kinetic energy by becoming unstable during its flight. Finally, the density of the tungsten or depleted-uranium rod inside its streamlined nose cone facilitates the penetration of the target.

The composite rigid shot resembles the APFSDS round, but its outer layer is not discarded. Instead, the area between the penetrator and the barrel is filled with a lightweight metal (such as aluminum) and the whole munition stays together in flight.

When the rod from one of these munitions reaches armor, its enormous kinetic energy is applied to a small target area. It penetrates the armor, blowing out a cloud of fragmentation debris (called *spall*) from the inside wall of the hull or turret, along with a plug of armor, followed by the residual portion of the rod. Because these objects are traveling at supersonic speeds, the shock waves produce a blast overpressure that is enhanced when the waves are reflected from the vehicle's inner walls.

The principal injuring mechanisms of the kinetic-energy warhead are fragments and secondary fires. This warhead will kill any people in its path, whether they are inside or outside an armored vehicle.

Explosive Antimatériel Warheads. The best-known explosive antitank warhead is the *shaped-* or *hollow-charge warhead.* Unlike the kinetic-energy warhead, a shaped-charge warhead can cause several distinctive kinds of injuries. An explanation of its operating principles may clarify the etiology of these unusual wounds.

Shaped-charge warheads contain a high explosive that has been cast or pressed into a cylinder. Late in the nineteenth century, munitions designers found that the energy released by a warhead's detonation could be focused by hollowing out the front of the explosive into a cone-shaped cavity with an apex that faced the middle of the cylinder. During World War I, they learned that lining the face of the cavity with a nonferrous, low-melting-point metal (called a *melt sheet*) focused the energy even more.

The charge is detonated at the base of the explosive cylinder. As the detonation wave travels through the explosive, it causes the cavity's metal liner to collapse on its axis of symmetry, beginning with the cone's apex. About 20% of the liner—together with the gas from the explosive's combustion—is forced into a high-velocity jet, which takes the shape of a long, thin rod. The front of the jet may reach a velocity of 20,000 fps, while the rear of the jet travels at about 6,000 fps. The jet's velocity allows the warhead to perforate monolithic steel plate that is about 5.5 times the diameter of the explosive cylinder. Thus, a weapon like the American-made TOW2 that has a 6-inch warhead can penetrate steel armor that is more than 33 inches thick (Figure 1-38).[14]

Among the first shaped-charge weapons to appear in World War II—which are now known as *light antitank weapons* (LAWs)—included the American-made bazooka (which fired a shaped-charge warhead propelled by a rocket) and the German-made Panzerfaust (a shaped-charge warhead fired from a recoilless gun). Since then, a variety of *high-explosive antitank (HEAT) weapons* utilizing shaped-charge warheads have appeared, many of which are used directly against personnel (Figure 1-39).

Because armor penetration by a shaped-charge warhead does not depend upon the warhead's impact velocity, the munition need not be fired from a large, heavy gun to be effective. In fact, these warheads are fielded in a great variety of sizes, and can be fired from small arms or even thrown by hand. Because of their versatility, shaped-charge warheads can be used very effectively as antipersonnel weapons.

Unlike the effects of any other weapon used in conventional war, the effects of a shaped-charge warhead on body tissues are a complicated mix of ballistic, blast, and thermal traumas.

As the metallic jet passes into an armored vehicle, it produces fragments, a bright flash, heat, smoke, and blast overpressure. The blast levels and expanding gases are usually sufficient to blow the vehicle hatches open, and personnel who are sitting in openings may be propelled out of the vehicle. Anyone in the path of the high-temperature jet will suffer catastrophic burns. As American medical officers in the Vietnam War and their Israeli counterparts in the Yom Kippur War noted, these injuries often looked as though they had been

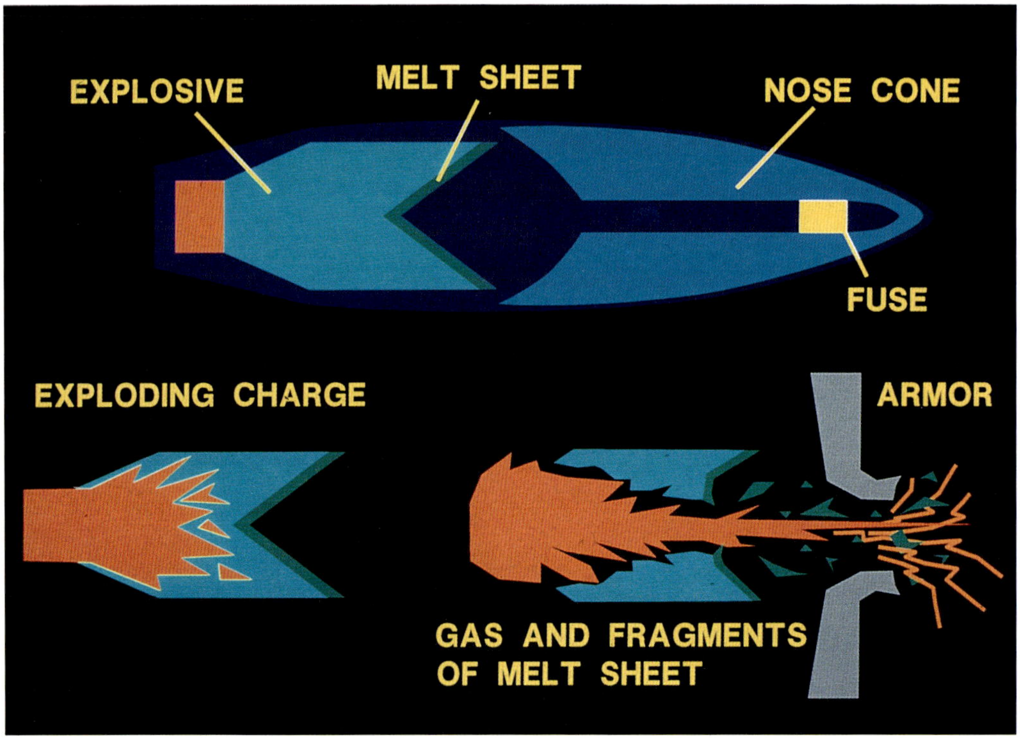

Fig. 1-38. In a shaped-charge warhead, the thermal and kinetic energies of the explosive detonation are focused by both the shape of the charge and the melt sheet that lines it. Although the resulting jet of gas and molten metal has a temperature that may exceed 5,000° C, it is the jet's tremendous kinetic energy, rather than its temperature, that allows it to penetrate armor that is more than 1 foot thick.

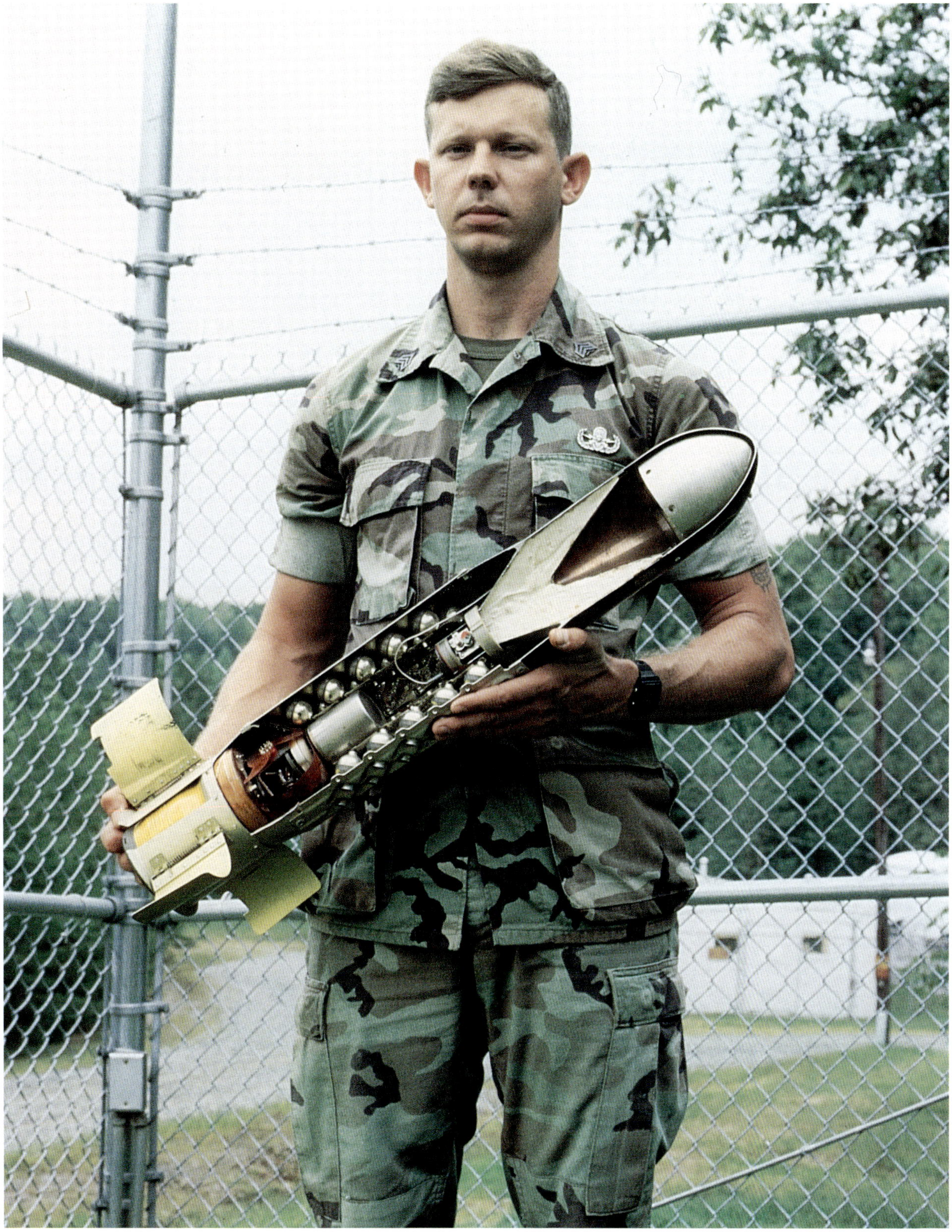

Fig. 1-39. The marine holds a cutaway version of a Dragon medium antitank missile, in which the characteristic hollow shape can be clearly seen.
Source: Explosive Ordnance Disposal Group, Quantico Marine Corps Base

created by a blowtorch (Figures 1-40 and 1-41).

While perhaps not as predominant as the catastrophic injuries caused by the jet, fragmentation wounds are common with shaped-charge warheads. The fragments come from three different sources: *(a)* the nonferrous metal melt sheet of the warhead, *(b)* the nose cone and casing of the warhead, and *(c)* the target itself.

Fragments from the melt sheet exist transiently as globules of hot metal, which may cause deep burns (Figure 1-42).

Fragments from the nose cone and casing are usually small; like the melt sheet, they are made of nonferrous metal and are difficult to detect in a casualty by standard imaging techniques (Figure 1-43). They are most likely to hit those personnel who are off to the sides of the projectile's path. These casualties will tend to be injured by the fragments rather than by burns from the hot metal.

Most of the fragments come from the target itself. When an antitank warhead perforates an armored wall, the wall produces a shower of spall fragments that range in size from small, dustlike particles to large chunks. These fragments scab off in a cone-shaped pattern on the interior side of the armored wall, resulting in multiple fragmentation injuries to anyone within that cone-shaped area (Figure 1-44). In addition, the dustlike particles may burn rapidly in air, a phenomenon known as the *vaporific effect*. Anyone who is exposed to these particles may incur small but deep localized burns (Figure 1-45).

In World War II, injuries were caused primarily by fragmentation. The kinetic-energy penetrator of the shaped-charge warhead tended to break up into many fragments. American forces in Vietnam were more likely to be injured by spall.

Some warheads can do great damage even without penetrating the armor. Unlike the shaped-charge warhead (in which spalling was just one of the damaging effects), a *high-explosive squash-head antiarmor warhead* relies completely on spall as its damaging mechanism. This warhead forms a large blob of plastic explosive when it is squashed against the target at the moment of impact. The ensuing detonation creates a

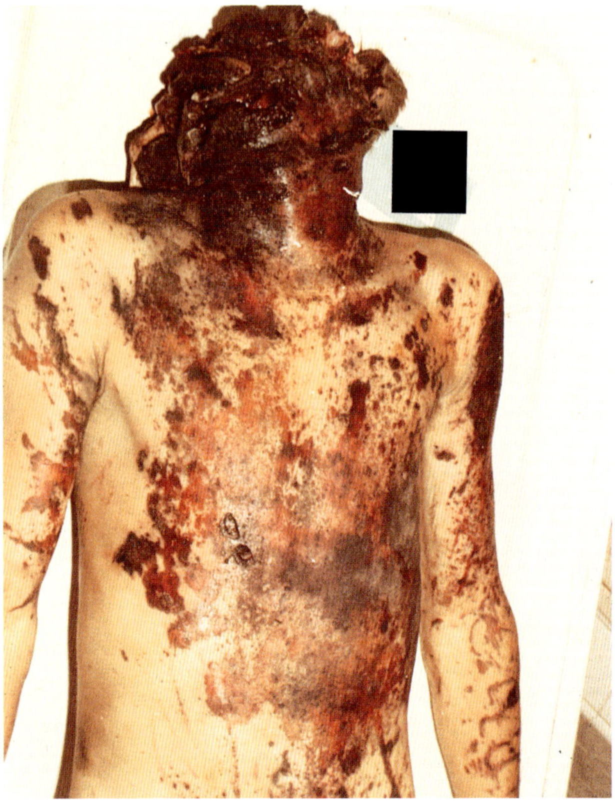

Fig. 1-40. This casualty, who was killed inside an armored personnel carrier, suffered the characteristic mutilation that a shaped-charge antitank warhead (in this case, a Soviet-designed RPG-2) may inflict.
Source: Wound Data and Munitions Effectiveness Team

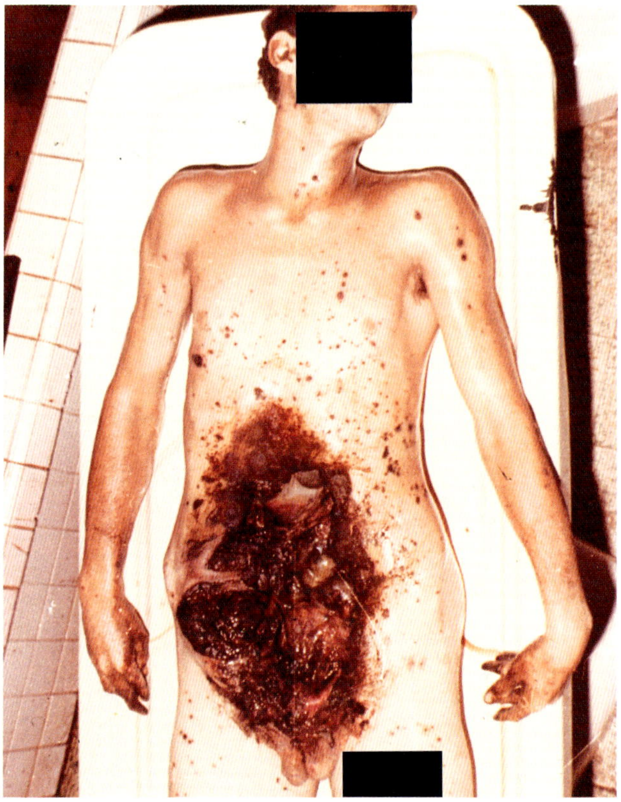

Fig. 1-41. This casualty was killed by a small shaped-charge warhead that was fired from a grenade launcher.
Source: Wound Data and Munitions Effectiveness Team

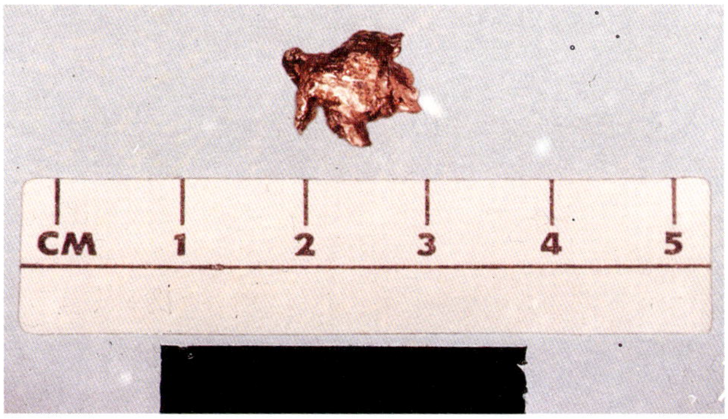

Fig. 1-42. This copper globule came from the melt sheet of an RPG-2 and was found embedded in the casualty's brain.
Source: Wound Data and Munitions Effectiveness Team

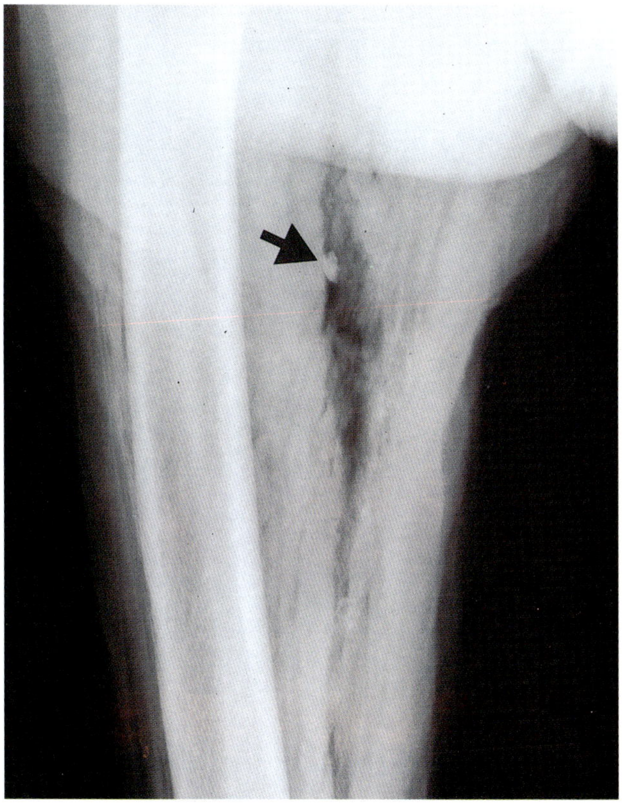

Fig. 1-43. Only the largest of six aluminum casing fragments from a shaped-charge warhead, ranging in size from 2 mm to 6 mm, can be seen in this roentgenogram of soft tissue.
Source: Explosive Ordnance Disposal Group, Quantico Marine Corps Base

shock wave that passes through the armored wall and throws off large scabs of metal spall when the shock wave reaches the wall's far side. Even though the armor is not penetrated, the effects of the shock wave not only damage or destroy the matériel, but also cause secondary explosions and fires involving any munitions that are contained within.

Ordnance Utilizing Explosive Munitions

The three categories of weapons that fire explosive or larger-projectile munitions are cannons, mortars, and guns.

Other munitions (such as bombs, rockets, grenades, and mines) use explosive devices as well, but these are dropped, launched, thrown, or planted rather than fired by artillery ordnance.

Cannons. A cannon is like a large machine gun that uses a recoil automatic-firing mechanism. Its firing trajectory is relatively flat, and its range may reach 1–2 km. Unlike a machine gun, a cannon fires 20–40-mm explosive rounds instead of inert bullets (Figure 1-46). Because it is also much larger than a machine gun, the cannon is mounted on an armored fighting vehicle, which takes the brunt of the weapon's punishing recoil.

Cannons are not big enough to be used against tanks but are usually too big to be used against personnel, and so they have a relatively small role on the battlefield. They are intended to be used primarily against aircraft and lightly protected armored vehicles. In Vietnam, however, the opposing forces had few of these matériel targets, and therefore the American forces found that twin-mounted 40-mm cannons were effective as ad hoc antipersonnel weapons.

Some cannons use the *Gatling gun* principle. Unlike most cannons, which have one barrel, the Gatling gun has six barrels arranged in a circle, and operates like six small arms put together in one weapon. Each barrel is at a different stage of the firing sequence at any given instant, and thus the loading, firing, and extracting processes can be continuous and extremely rapid—6,000 rounds/minute is not an unusual rate of fire. The original model of the Gatling gun used a gas-operated firing mechanism, but modern versions use electric motors. They fire cannon shells or antiarmor projectiles containing tungsten rods.

Mortars. Unlike cannons, mortars are ubiquitous on the battlefield. This muzzle-loading weapon has a relatively short, stubby barrel (called a *tube*), the bore of which varies from 60–240 mm (bore calibers of 81 or 82 mm and 120 mm are the most common). Its light weight and small size allow it to be carried by a small crew of two or three soldiers, yet the World War II

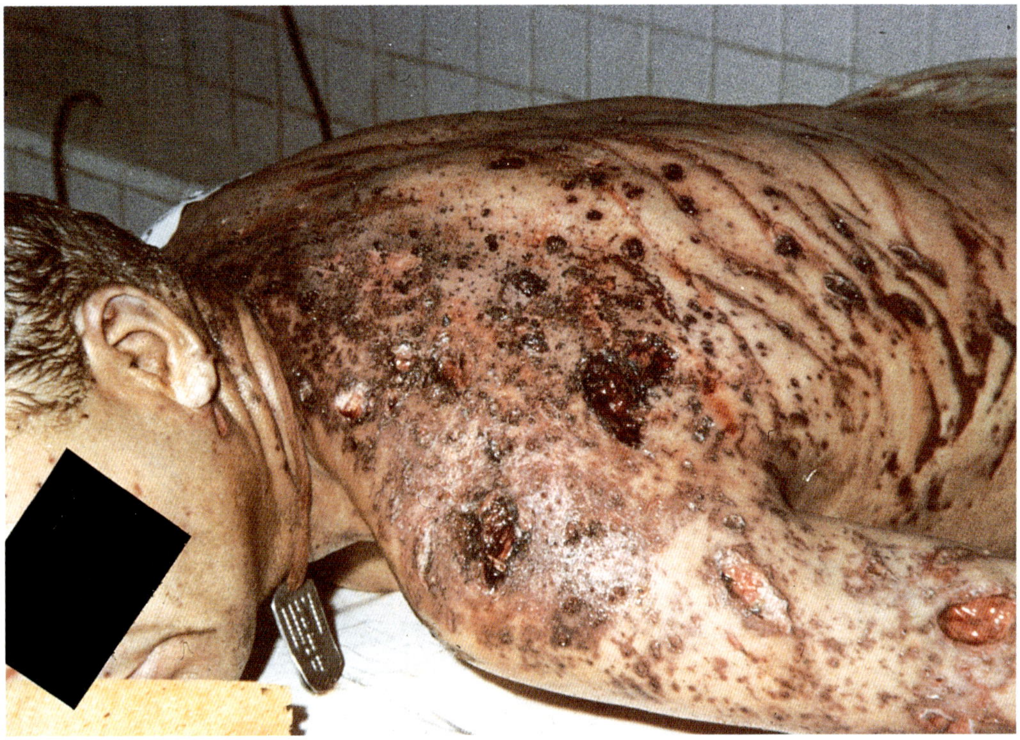

Fig. 1-44. This casualty was killed by spall from the hull of an armored personnel carrier when it was struck by a shaped-charge warhead. Other munitions, including the squash-head warhead and the kinetic-energy penetrator, also create spall.
Source: Wound Data and Munitions Effectiveness Team

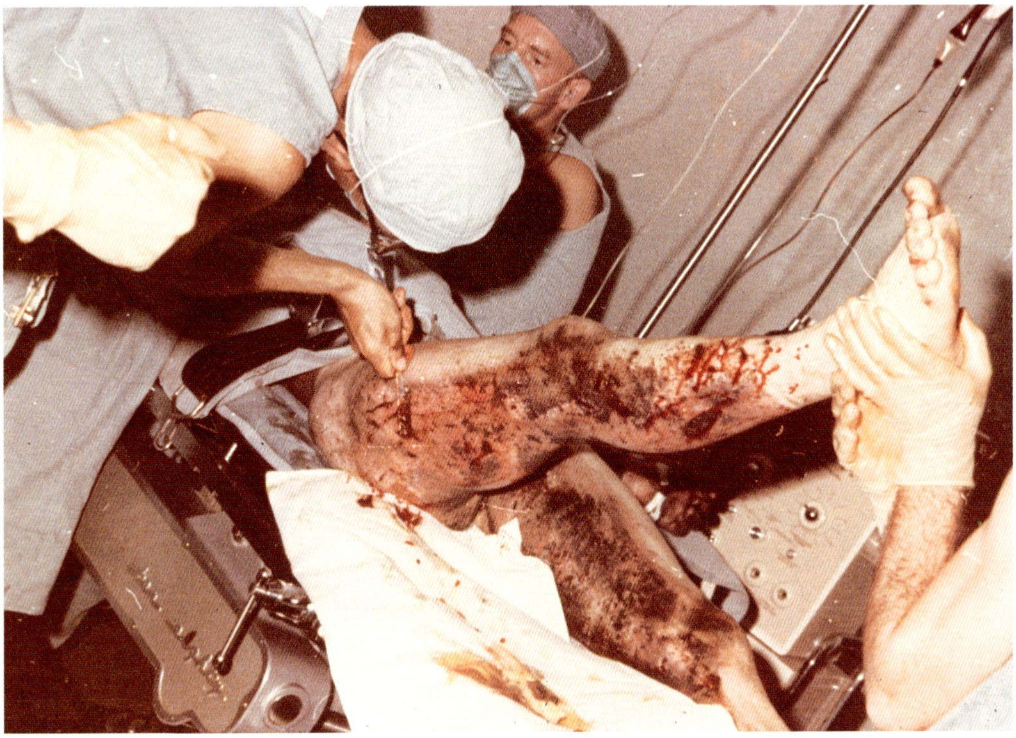

Fig. 1-45. This casualty's many tiny, deep burns were caused by small particles of burning aluminum that were created when a shaped-charge warhead struck the hull of an armored vehicle.
Source: Wound Data and Munitions Effectiveness Team

experience showed that one 81-mm mortar had the casualty-generating potential of three general-purpose machine guns, which would be served by a total of six to eight soldiers. Because its recoil is directed into the ground rather than controlled by a mechanism in the weapon itself, the mortar is one of the simplest of weapons to operate.

The primary mission of a mortar is to cover those units that are not covered by artillery fire. Mortars are designed to fire an explosive projectile at an angle between 45° and 80°. Once the crew has identified the target, they consult a table to determine at what angle the mortar should be set and the size of the explosive charge that should be loaded with the projectile. By varying the height of the parabolic trajectory, the mortar crew can select ranges between several hundred meters and several kilometers.

A mortar characteristically has a high rate of fire; in fact, short-time rates of 20–25 rounds/minute are not unusual. It fires explosive munitions that are conventionally called *bombs* (Figure 1-47). Although these are not true bombs because they are not dropped from aircraft, their tailfins resemble those of true bombs.

Guns. In the context of the artillery forces, a gun is a weapon that *(a)* is crew-served, *(b)* has a mechanism to control recoil, *(c)* has a bore caliber greater than 40 mm, and *(d)* has a barrel length greater than twenty times the bore caliber. The structure of a heavy gun resembles that of its small-arm counterpart, except that in a heavy gun the bolt is called a *breech block.* Depending on the gun's design, the sequence of loading the round and extracting the spent cartridge may be done either manually or mechanically, but—because the energy from the firing of one round is not used to chamber the next—not automatically. These heavy guns come in a variety of sizes and shapes, and can be either towed by tractors or trucks or propelled under their own power using their own tracks.

Most heavy guns are used primarily as indirect-fire weapons (that is, the crew cannot see the targets). When this is their mission, they may fire either antimatériel or antipersonnel munitions. However, guns may sometimes be used directly against specific, visible targets, such as armored fighting vehicles. In this situation, they usually fire antimatériel warheads, such as kinetic-energy penetrators.

Unlike small arms, in which the barrel length is relatively unimportant, the barrel length of heavy guns affects the muzzle velocity of the projectile. The longer the barrel, the greater the gun's range, but also

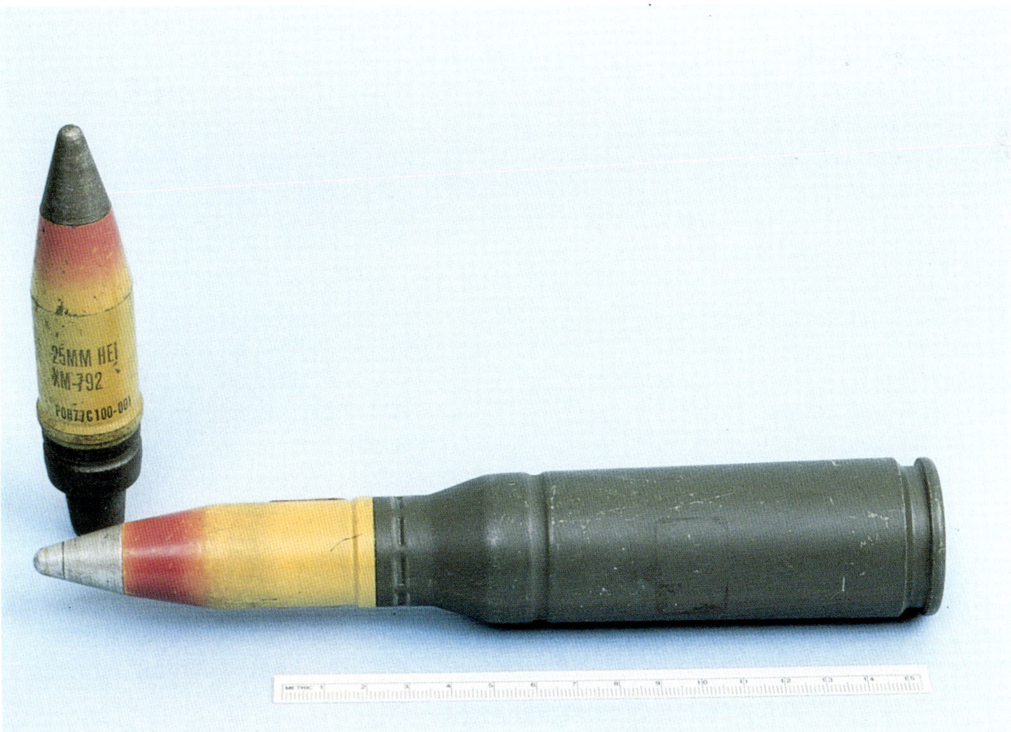

Fig. 1-46. This 25-mm round fired by the M242 cannon of the Bradley Fighting Vehicle is a high-explosive incendiary round. An armor-piercing round is also available.
Source: Explosive Ordnance Disposal Group, Quantico Marine Corps Base

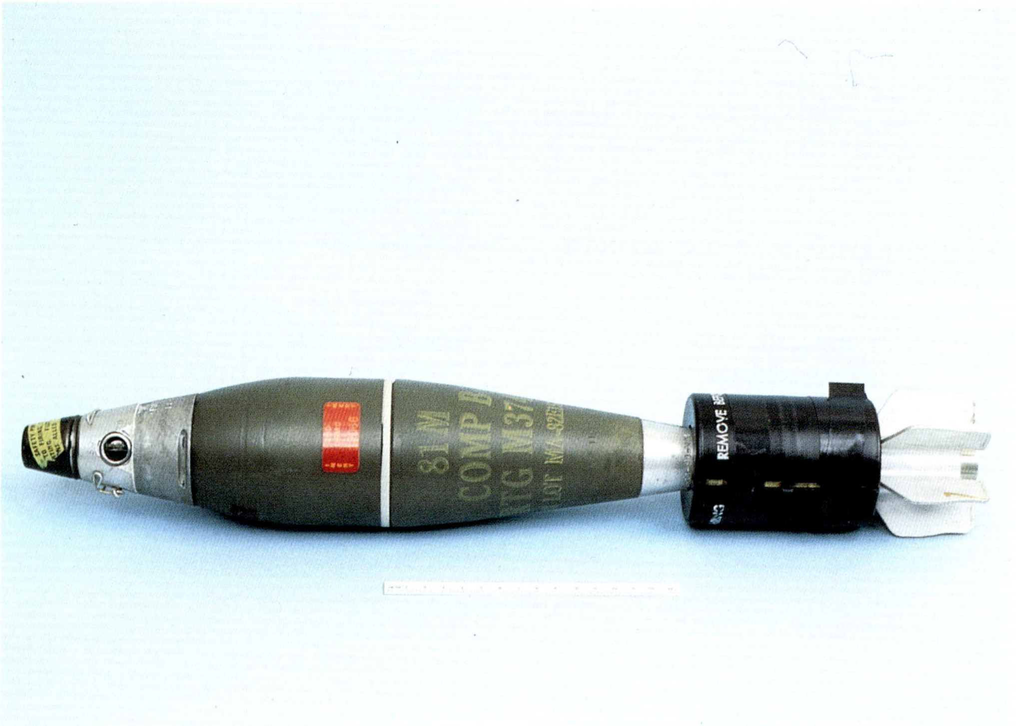

Fig. 1-47. The propellant of this 81-mm mortar bomb consists of *(a)* a shotgunlike cartridge within the tail and *(b)* an auxiliary charge, which is the black incremental-propellant container wrapped around the tail. The weight of the mortar bomb totals about 3.5 kg, one-third of which is the weight of the explosive charge. The controlled breakup of a prenotched metal coil under the thin external case creates fragments.
Source: Explosive Ordnance Disposal Group, Quantico Marine Corps Base

the greater its weight and size. Until recently, barrel length was a convenient distinguishing factor between two classes of guns: *(a)* those with barrel lengths of 40 or more calibers, and *(b)* those with barrel lengths of less than 40 calibers (called *howitzers*). This distinction has gradually faded, however; howitzers have been given longer barrels, and guns with longer barrels (such as the 175-mm M109, which has a barrel length of 58 calibers) have been replaced by rockets.

Heavy guns can fire a variety of rounds, including all types of specialty rounds. Regardless of its type, the warhead of an artillery round is usually called a shell. Shells fired by the 105-mm and 155-mm howitzers weigh 15 kg and 43 kg, respectively. Although both are usually used to attack bunkers and other field fortifications, a shell from the larger weapon will clearly have greater casualty-producing potential.

The casualty-generating potentials of guns and mortars differ, based on several factors:

- The most commonly fielded heavy guns have bore calibers of 105 mm and 152 or 155 mm, although the Soviets have supplied many clients with guns having calibers of 122 mm and 130 mm. These bore calibers resemble those of mortars, but because guns have much longer barrel lengths than mortars do, they are able to fire their projectiles much farther.
- Although mortars and heavy guns may have bore calibers that are similar, most guns fire projectiles that are wider, longer, and heavier than those fired by most mortars.
- The rate of fire in guns—particularly in large guns—will tend to be slower than the rate of fire in mortars. Unlike the round fired by the 105-mm gun (such as the beehive round that was shown in Figure 1-29), in which the cartridge and shell are joined together and loaded into the weapon as a single piece, the propellant charge and warhead of the 155-mm gun are separate and must be individually loaded into the breech. Gun rounds also tend to weigh much more than mortar bombs do, and are correspondingly more difficult to load manually.
- Because mortar bombs have a much higher trajectory than do shells from guns, they tend to strike the ground nearly vertically, whereas shells from guns usually strike more ob-

liquely. Consequently, the area of fragmentation around the detonation point of a mortar bomb will be relatively circular, whereas the fragments from a gun-fired munition that lands obliquely will be expelled outwards in a projection that resembles a butterfly's wings around the detonation site (Figure 1-48). There will be few casualty-producing fragments disseminated either to the front or to the rear of the gun-fired shell; the fragments in front tend to go high into the air, and the fragments to the rear tend to go into the ground (Figure 1-49).

Bombs and Rockets. Although rockets and bombs differ in their modes of delivery, they both contain an explosive within a thin-walled case. The greater the ratio of the explosive mass of the munition to the mass of its wall, the greater will be the blast effects and the more numerous will be the small fragments.

Modern bombs are munitions that are dropped from aircraft. General-purpose aerial bombs may have cases that are so thin that more than 50% of the bomb's weight can be devoted to the explosive. In comparison, conventional explosive projectile shells must have thick walls to withstand the enormous stress of being shot through a barrel. For example, an older random-fragmentation munition that had a thick, heavy case (and therefore a proportionately smaller explosive charge) would have produced relatively few, albeit large, fragments, and may have been able to devote only 5%–10% of its weight to the explosive.

The design of a bomb depends on its objective. An antimatériel bomb may weigh 500–4,000 pounds, and if most of that weight is devoted to the explosive, then the detonating blast's effects on both matériel and personnel may be significant. Secondary missiles created by the blast, as well as large fragments of thin casing from the munition itself, may result in the additional danger of ballistic injury to personnel. Modern bombs that are used primarily against personnel, however, do not depend upon blast effects, but rather have warheads that are designed to injure by fragmentation. Because of their considerable size, these bombs are effective cluster munitions.

Rockets are munitions that are propelled to their targets by self-contained reaction motors. Examples of modern artillery rockets are the Soviet-made BM 21 launcher and the new American-made *Multiple-Launch Rocket System* (MLRS). The MLRS can fire a salvo of as many as twelve 230-mm rockets as far as 30 km. Its rocket is an especially sophisticated example of modern ordnance designed to be used against both personnel and light matériel. Each munition carries 644 warheads, any one of which could kill dozens of people. These dual-purpose warheads are actually shaped-charge warheads that have thick casings, thus combining an antimatériel penetrating function with the antipersonnel fragmentation function. Dual-purpose submunitions are becoming increasingly common in combat (Figure 1-50).

Blast effects were especially prominent with the German-made Nebelwerfer and the Soviet-made Katyusha, the first free-flight artillery rockets designed to be fired in salvo that were extensively used in war. The Nebelwerfer was originally designed to fire large, thin-walled, rocket-propelled projectiles that were supposed to be filled with toxic chemicals or obscurants but were actually fielded with high-explosive charges. The effects of the 15-cm Nebelwerfer 41 were noted in 1942:

> The shell fragments were large and thin and it was clear that the purpose of the projectiles was not to produce shrapnel but to create a blast effect. The presence of so many dead showing no external signs of injury seemed to support this theory. The rapid and successive detonations produced during a Nebelwerfer barrage produced such rapid variations in air pressure within the bombarded zone that many victims suffered extensive damage to their lungs which killed them.[15]

This description of a lung-contusion trauma that is now identified as *blast lung* may mark the first premeditated use of an enhanced-blast munition—in this instance, a *fuel-air explosive* (FAE).

To achieve the FAE effect, all rockets but one in a seven-rocket Nebelwerfer salvo were filled with propane; the remaining rocket was filled with a high explosive. The propane-filled rockets would break apart, releasing the fuel into the air above the target area; ideally, the detonation of the high-explosive rocket would cause the explosive combustion of the fuel-air mixture. Frequently, however, the fuel-air mixture was inexact, resulting in the propane's slow combustion rather than an explosion.

FAE munitions have become sophisticated and prevalent in recent years. A typical FAE device now consists of *(a)* a cylindrical container of a liquid fuel, such as ethylene oxide or propylene oxide, the walls of which are scored so that the container can break apart in a controlled manner, and *(b)* a burster charge, located at the center, which extends along the long axis of the fuel container.

First, the burster charge detonates, and the contents of the fuel container are dispersed as a mistlike, disk-shaped fuel-air cloud over the ground. The diameter of this cloud may range from 50 feet (from an 80-

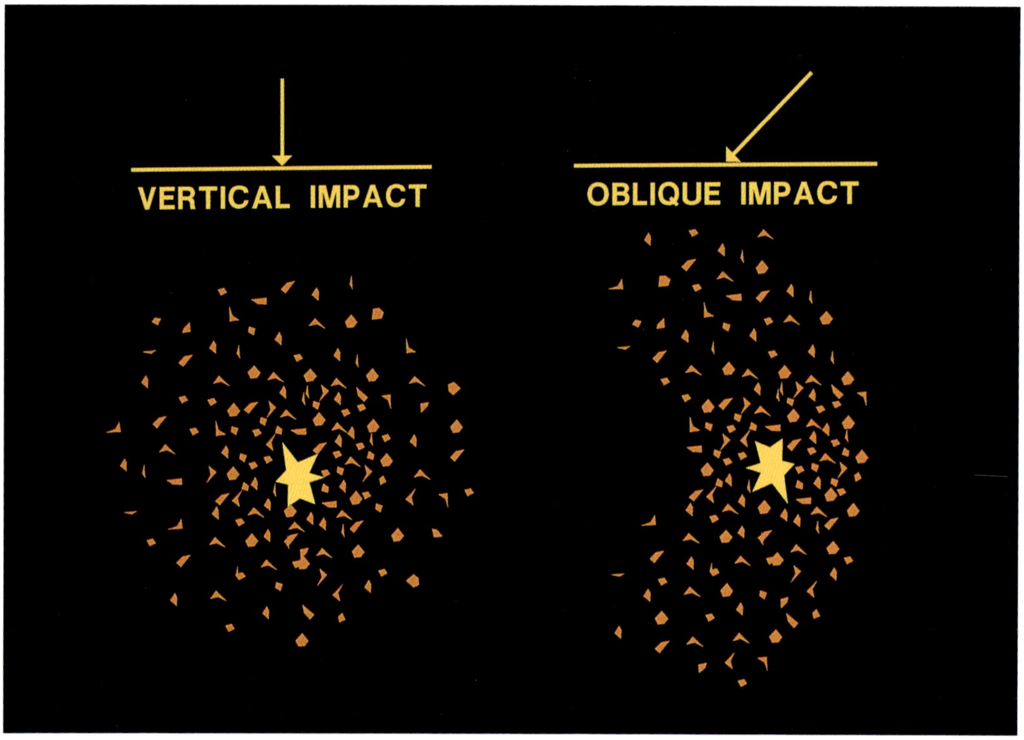

Fig. 1-48. The pattern of fragmentation produced by a random-fragmentation munition depends on the missile's trajectory at impact.

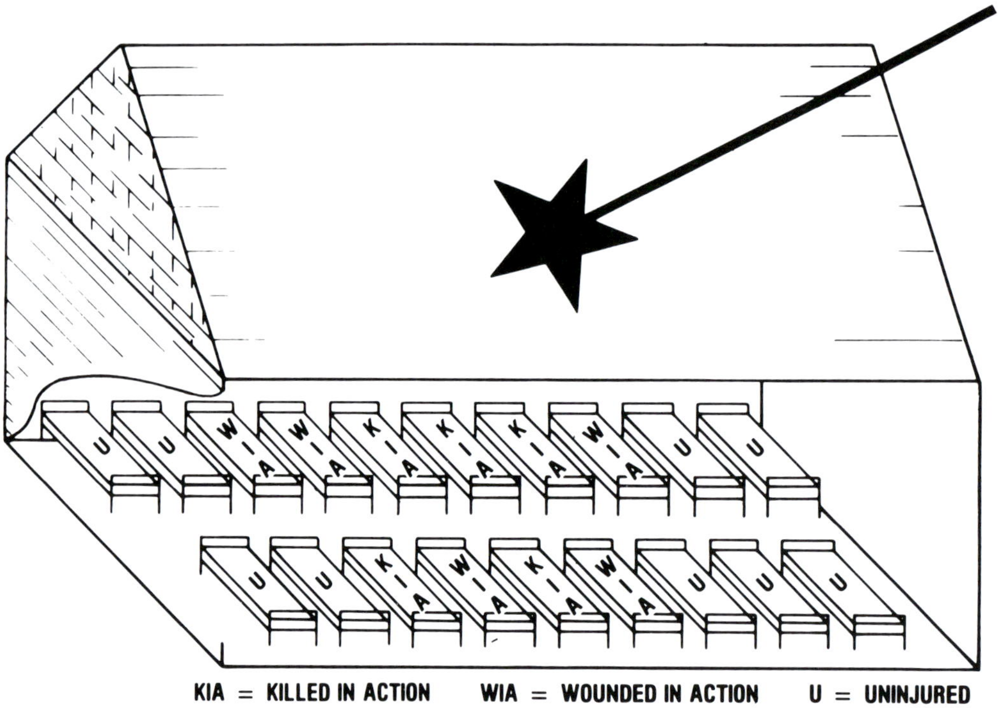

Fig. 1-49. This diagram illustrates the asymmetrical pattern of casualty generation that occurred when a 122-mm rocket struck the roof of a barracks in which soldiers were sleeping. The soldier who was immediately behind the detonation site sustained a nonlethal wound, as did the two soldiers directly in front of the rocket. However, several soldiers who were perpendicular to the rocket's impact trajectory on either side were killed.
Source: Wound Data and Munitions Effectiveness Team

pound FAE) to 150 feet (from a 2,000-pound FAE). The cloud flows around objects, such as trees and rocks, and into structures or field-fortification ventilation systems before it is detonated (Figures 1-51, 1-52, and 1-53).

Next, a second small charge ignites the fuel-air mixture (Figure 1-54). Given the appropriate complex conditions, the resulting detonation creates a lethal blast overpressure of 250–300 pounds/square inch (psi) throughout the cloud.

The vast dimensions of the FAE cloud ensure that the blast effects will occur over a much wider area than that affected by any conventional explosive munition. Since the Vietnam War, FAE weapons (such as the American-made BLU 96 guided glide bomb, which contains the tremendous load of 635 kg of propylene oxide fuel) have been improved so that their blast effects may now rival that of a small tactical nuclear warhead.[16]

Unlike fragments, which move only on a linear trajectory, the FAE's blast wave can go around corners, penetrating the apertures in bunkers, the open hatches in armored fighting vehicles, and the hollows of trenches and foxholes. As this munition is used more frequently in conflict, blast lung and ruptured tympanic membranes will become more common; in Afghanistan, for example, FAE munitions (called *volume bombs* or *vacuum bombs)* made up a significant percentage of all the bombs that were dropped from Soviet aircraft.[17]

Grenades. Grenades have been called the infantry's pocket artillery. These small explosive munitions are *(a)* thrown by hand, *(b)* fired from rifles, or *(c)* shot from specialized grenade launchers.

Hand grenades (the oldest of the three designs) have evolved in the way their fragments were generated. The earliest versions looked like small cast-iron or steel pineapples. The grooves cut into their casings were supposed to determine the size and shape of the casing fragments that would be produced upon detonation. In actual practice, however, fragmentation tended to be much more random. Most modern hand grenades have improved-fragmentation designs (Figure 1-55). The preformed fragments usually consist of several thousand small steel spheres held together in a plastic matrix. Like all explosive munitions, hand grenades have a fuse, but they also are designed with a delay of 4–5 seconds so that the thrower is not killed by the

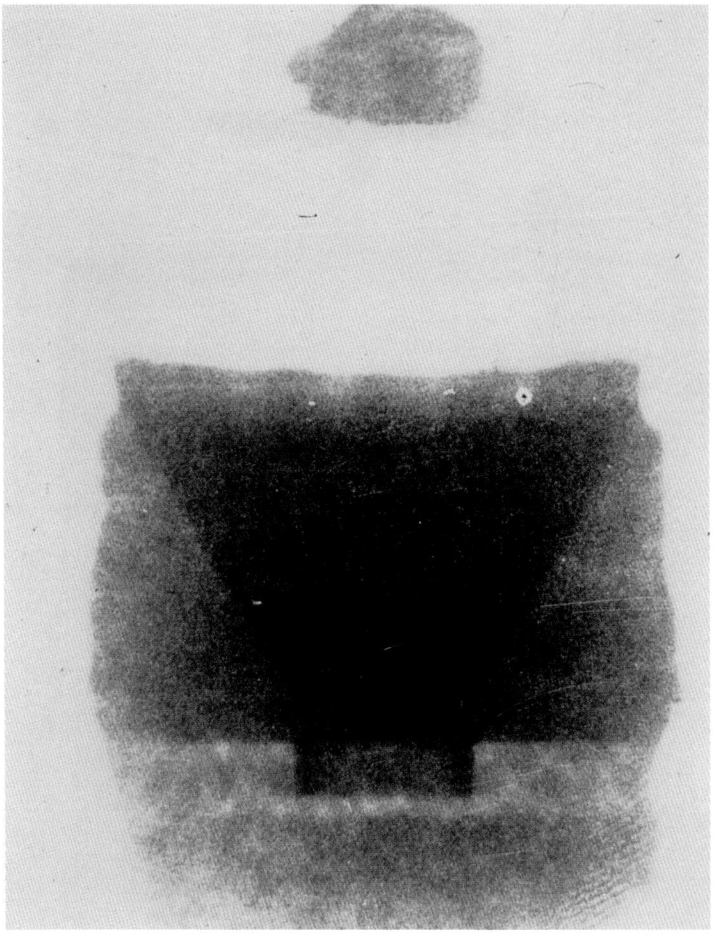

Fig. 1-50. The dual-purpose submunition shown in this roentgenogram measures about 4 cm in diameter and 8 cm in length. It contains about 30 g of explosive. The characteristic funnel shape of the shaped-charge warhead can be clearly seen. It not only can penetrate 80 mm of armor, but also can generate many antipersonnel fragments.
Source: Explosive Ordnance Disposal Group, Quantico Marine Corps Base

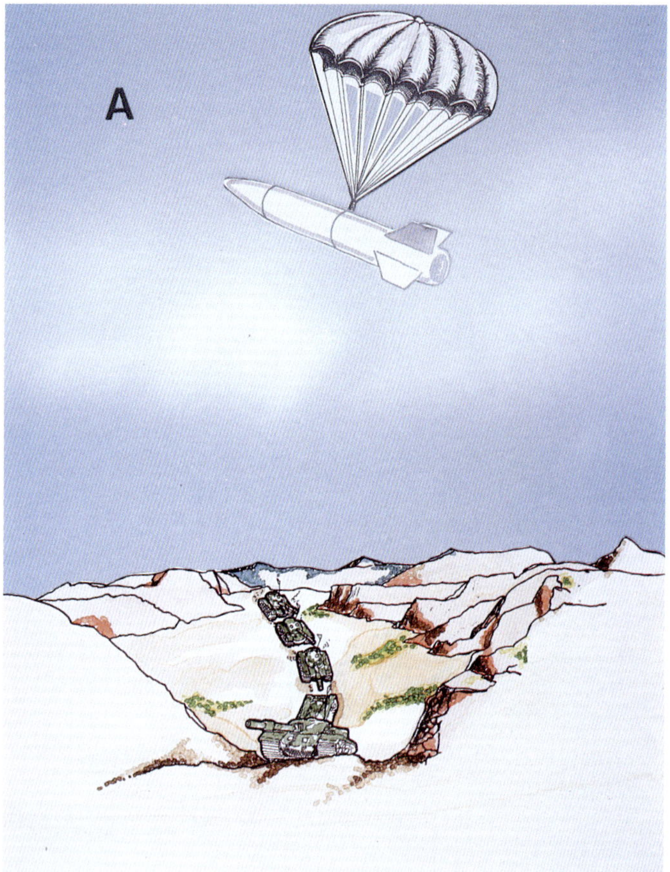

Fig. 1-51. The FAE container is dropped over the target. A parachute slows the bomb's descent and carries the charge for the second detonation.

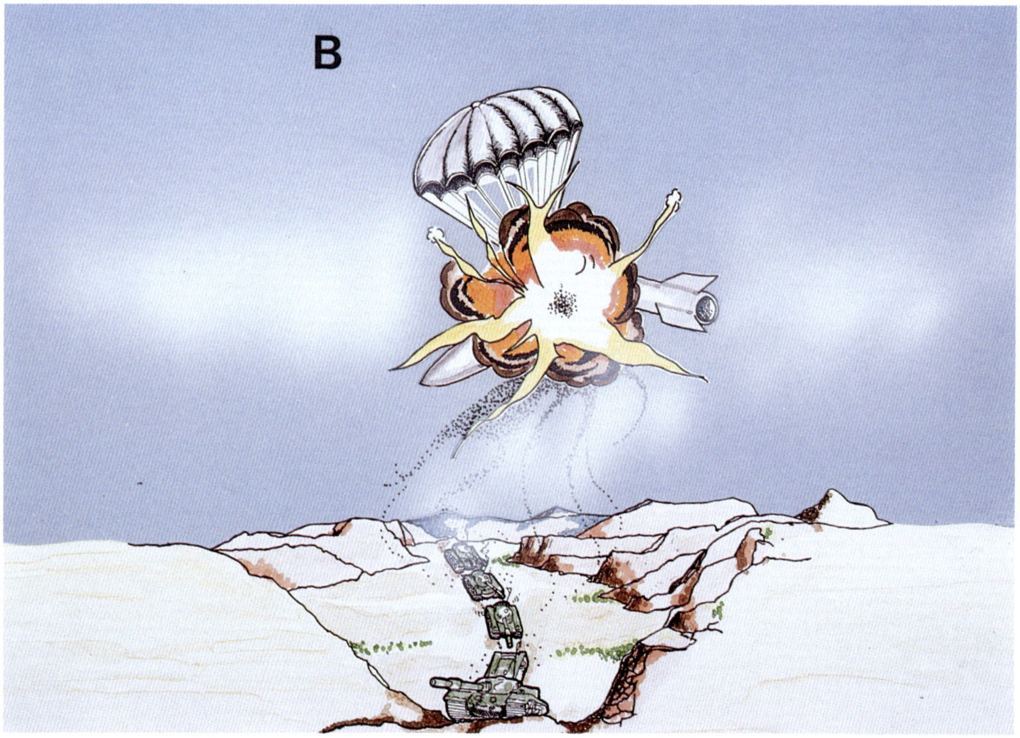

Fig. 1-52. The burster charge detonates, breaking open the FAE container and disseminating its fuel, which may be a highly flammable gas or liquid, through the atmosphere.

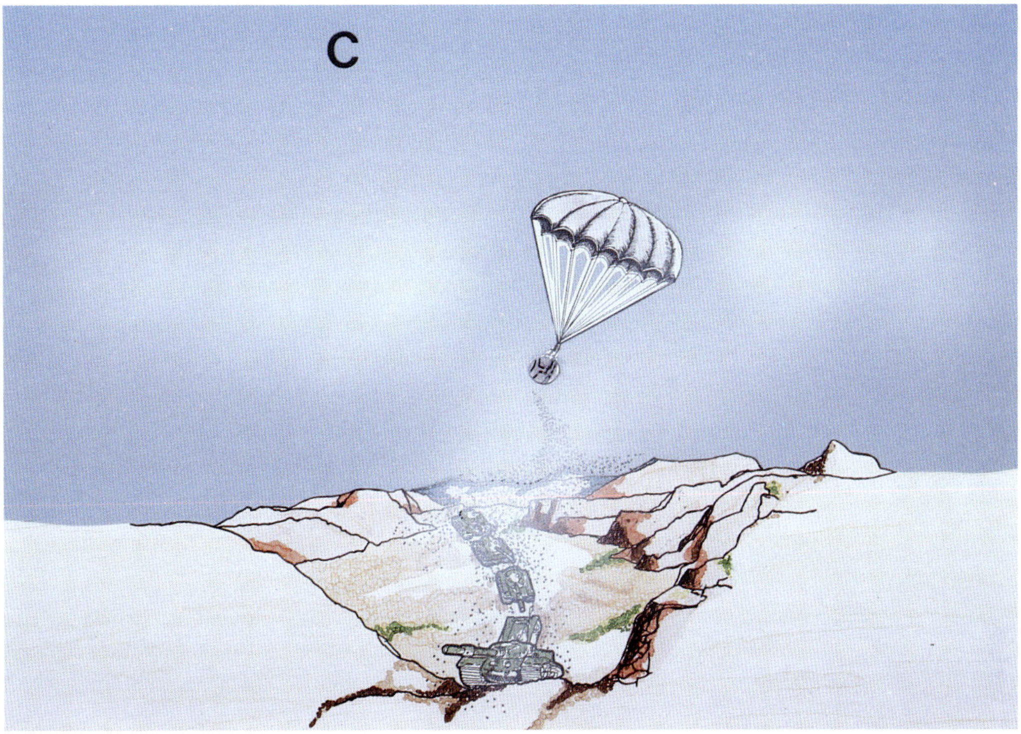

Fig. 1-53. The fuel mixes with the ambient air, forming an aerosol.

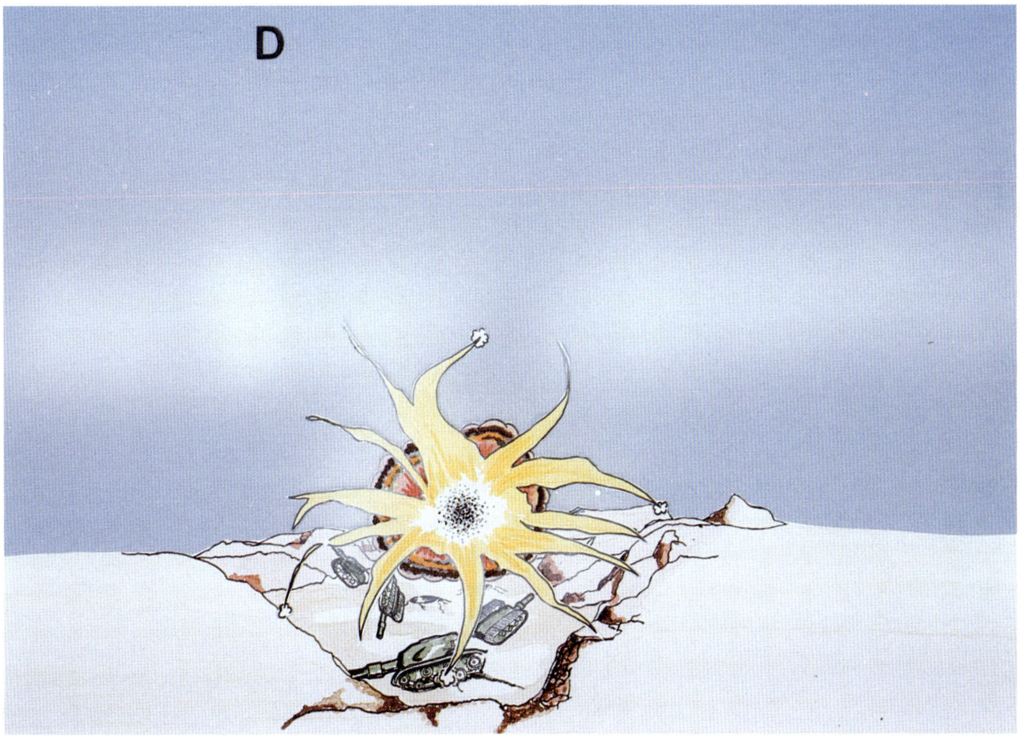

Fig. 1-54. The fuel-air mixture is detonated by the second explosive charge, which is still attached to the parachute. The delay times between the dispersion of the cloud and its detonation would be about 0.1 second (for an 80-pound FAE) and 2.0 seconds (for a 2,000-pound FAE). Pressures of about 250 psi extend out to the periphery of the cloud, which, for an 80-pound FAE, is about 20–25 feet. At that distance, the pressure from an equivalent weight of TNT would be just over 30 psi.

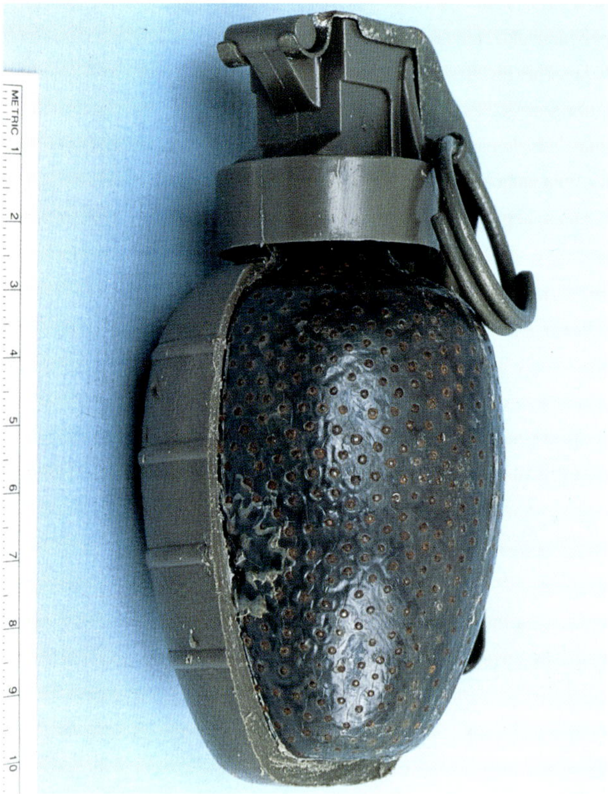

Fig. 1-55. This modern defensive hand grenade has had its plastic jacket removed to reveal its contents: 4,000 50-mg steel balls embedded in an explosive matrix. Compare this improved-fragmentation design with the Soviet-made POMZ-2 stake mine (Figure 1-66), which resembles an older pineapple-like hand grenade, to see the different thicknesses of the casings.
Source: Explosive Ordnance Disposal Group, Quantico Marine Corps Base

explosion. All hand-grenade designs have had firing pins of some sort, but not all have a safety lever that pops off when the thrower releases it.

Hand grenades have traditionally been classified as either *offensive* or *defensive*. An offensive hand grenade has a thin fragmenting wall, and the fragments tend to be less significant than those produced by a defensive grenade. The effective radius of an offensive grenade is quite localized—usually less than the distance that the weapon can be thrown—and its purpose is to create transient incapacitation in a few enemy troops, creating a subsequent opportunity to fire upon the opponents. For example, when making a forced entry in a rescue attempt, an antiterrorist squad may use *concussion grenades* (offensive grenades that produce blast effects without fragments) to disorient and startle hostage-holders. The transient incapacitation produced by the blast is enhanced in an enclosed space. Although the blast of a concussion grenade is normally not powerful enough to cause injury, a person who is extremely close to the grenade might be vulnerable to *primary blast injury* (PBI).

Defensive hand grenades are bigger and more powerful than offensive grenades. They also have a thicker wall, and rely upon its fragmentation to do their damage.

Because it is undesirable for the soldier to have to carry both types of grenades into combat, some hand grenades are designed to convert from offensive to defensive modes. The West German-made DM51, for example, is an offensive (or blast) grenade when its cylinder of explosive is used alone. It can be converted into a defensive (or fragmentation) grenade, however, by sliding it into a cylindrical sleeve that is made of spheres embedded in plastic.

Rifle grenades are explosive munitions that are designed to be fired from an adapter fitted onto the barrel of an assault rifle (Figure 1-56), and so will have a much greater range of action than hand grenades will. Gas pressure from a blank round fired by the rifle propels the grenade for several hundred meters. Either antiarmor shaped-charge grenade warheads or antipersonnel fragmentation grenade warheads can be used with this design.

Grenade launchers (such as the M79) can be used alone to fire an explosive munition that consists of a grenade-like warhead plus its own propellant-filled cartridge. The M79 can also be mounted onto an M16, just as a bayonet can be mounted onto a rifle. The two weapons are independent and give the soldier the option to use one or the other in a given tactical situation.

The effective range of the M79 launcher (about 300 m) is greater than that of the rifle grenade. The M79 and its successor, the M203, can fire a variety of grenades with different warheads (Figure 1-57); the casualty-generating radius around the warhead's detonation point is about 30 m.

The M79 and M203 are single-shot grenade launchers, but several modern weapons can fire munitions automatically. The U.S. Navy's Mark 19 40-mm automatic grenade launcher, for example, is similar in size to a general-purpose machine gun and can, in just a few seconds, saturate several hundred square meters with fragmentation grenades from more than 1,000 m away. The Soviets have developed a similar 30-mm grenade launcher (Figure 1-58) that fires an improved-fragmentation munition (Figure 1-59). The fragments from this warhead (Figure 1-60), which have an average weight of about 200 mg, have a velocity of 3,200 fps at the point of detonation.[18] In future conventional conflicts, the automatic grenade launcher or the grenade

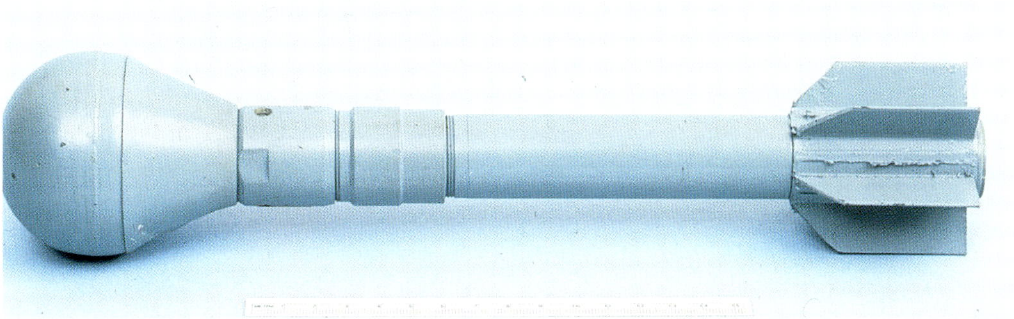

Fig. 1-56. A modern high-explosive rifle grenade
Source: Explosive Ordnance Disposal Group, Quantico Marine Corps Base

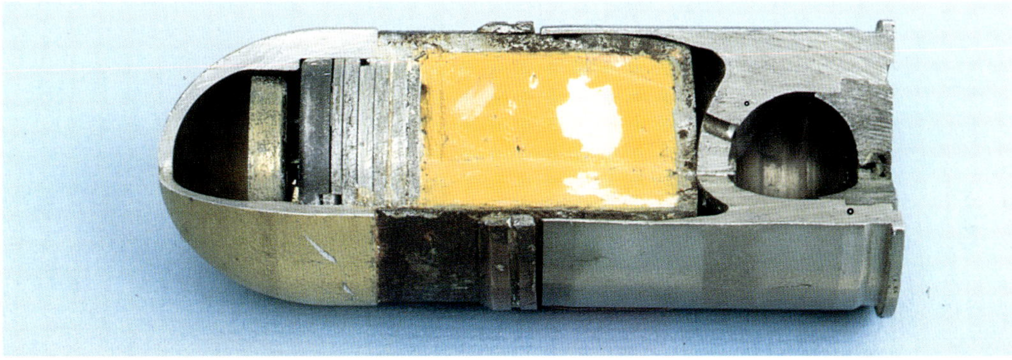

Fig. 1-57. The M79 grenade launcher fires this round, which has been cut open to show the yellow explosive charge, the fuse in the warhead's tip, and the cartridge's propellant charge in the lower third of the munition.
Source: U.S. Army Armament Research, Development, and Engineering Center, Picatinny Arsenal, NJ

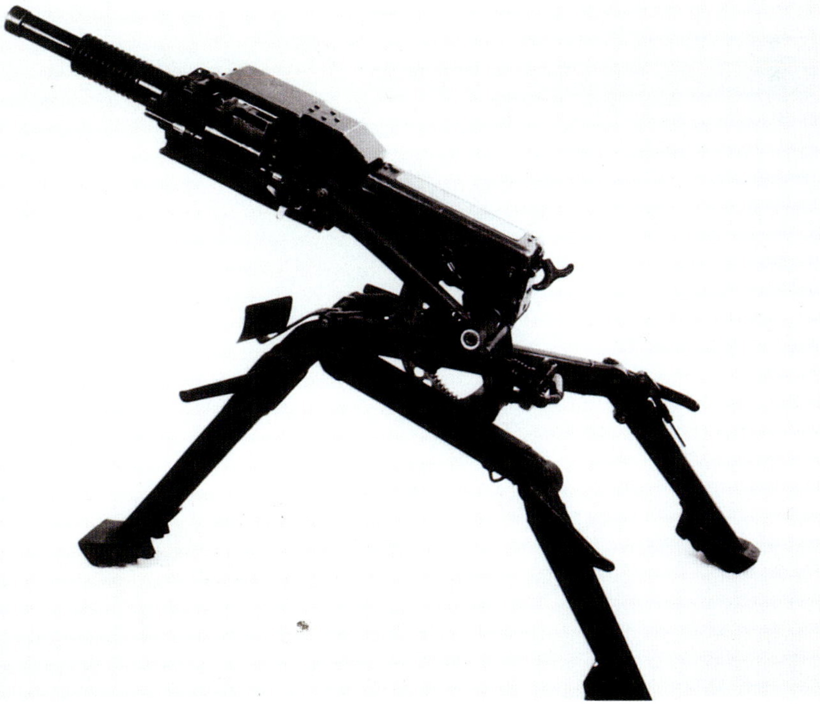

Fig. 1-58. A Soviet-made 30-mm grenade launcher (AGS-17), code-named *Flame* by the NATO forces
Source: Foreign Science and Technology Center, Charlottesville, VA

Fig. 1-59. This roentgenogram shows one of the rounds (the VOG-17) that the AGS-17 can fire, including its coil of notched wire, which is the source of the fragments. Note that the coiled wire and the explosive charge occupy about 75% of the round's total volume.
Source: Foreign Science and Technology Center

machine gun may be as predominant a source of casualties as the machine gun was in World War I.

A warhead shot from a grenade launcher may result in an unusual injury that will be described here in some detail to illustrate why medical officers need to understand how certain weapons work.

In the Vietnam War and in subsequent training accidents, soldiers were occasionally hit by M406 warheads that were fired by grenade launchers only 5–10 meters away. At that short distance, the projectile had just enough velocity to bury itself in the casualty's soft tissue, but the warhead did not detonate (Figure 1-61). Medical personnel may have believed that the warhead's failure to explode when it hit the casualty meant that it was a dud, but the benign behavior was actually a function of the design of the warhead's M551 fuse.

All fuses must do two things perfectly: *(a)* detonate the munition when it is supposed to explode and *(b)* prevent the munition from exploding when it is not supposed to explode. The M406 warheads were designed to explode only after the grenade launcher had propelled them farther than their effective fragmentation radius, and their sophisticated mechanical fuses ensured not only that they would not explode before they passed that point, but also that they would be

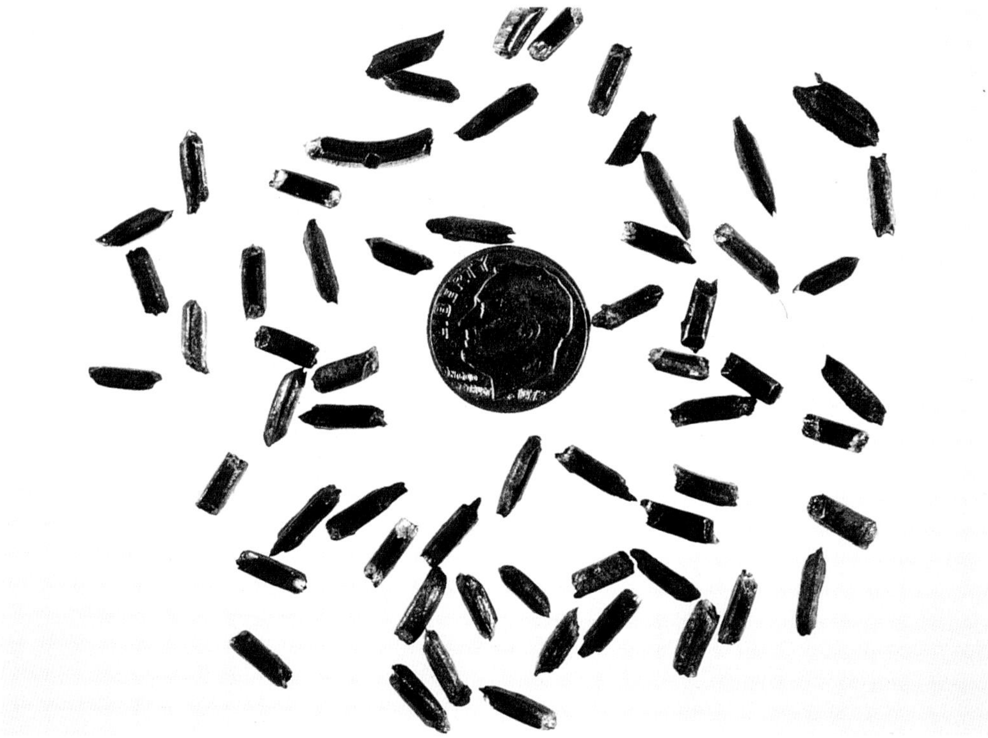

Fig. 1-60. Some of the fragments that are formed from the notched wire in the VOG-17 round after it has been detonated are compared in size to a dime.
Source: Foreign Science and Technology Center

certain to explode after.

Because both the firing pin and the fuse detonator in this warhead must interact precisely, the machinery must follow a carefully designed sequence of events in order to detonate:

(*a*) The fuse detonator (which contains a small amount of very sensitive explosive) is located in a rotor that is held in place by both a set-back pin and the firing pin. The set-back pin must retract so that the fuse detonator can rotate 180° from its original position to align with the firing pin (Figure 1-62). At the precise moment that the warhead is fired, the set-back pin is dislodged from the rotor.

(*b*) As the warhead travels through the rifled launcher barrel, it gains centrifugal force. If the centrifugal force can continue over the time that it takes to travel about 14 m, the firing pin will be dislodged, thus completely freeing the rotor. (If the warhead does not cover this minimum distance before it hits a target, it will not have rotated enough to allow centrifugal force to dislodge the firing pin, and the warhead will remain unarmed.)

(*c*) The rotor rotates so that the fuse detonator on it lines up with the firing pin (Figure 1-63).

(*d*) If there is any sudden deceleration of the warhead, the firing pin will strike the fuse detonator, which ignites the explosive.

(*e*) This small explosion ignites a larger amount of explosive in the lead charge, which, in turn,

(*f*) detonates a booster charge.

(*g*) Finally, the main high-explosive bursting charge explodes, fragmenting the warhead casing.

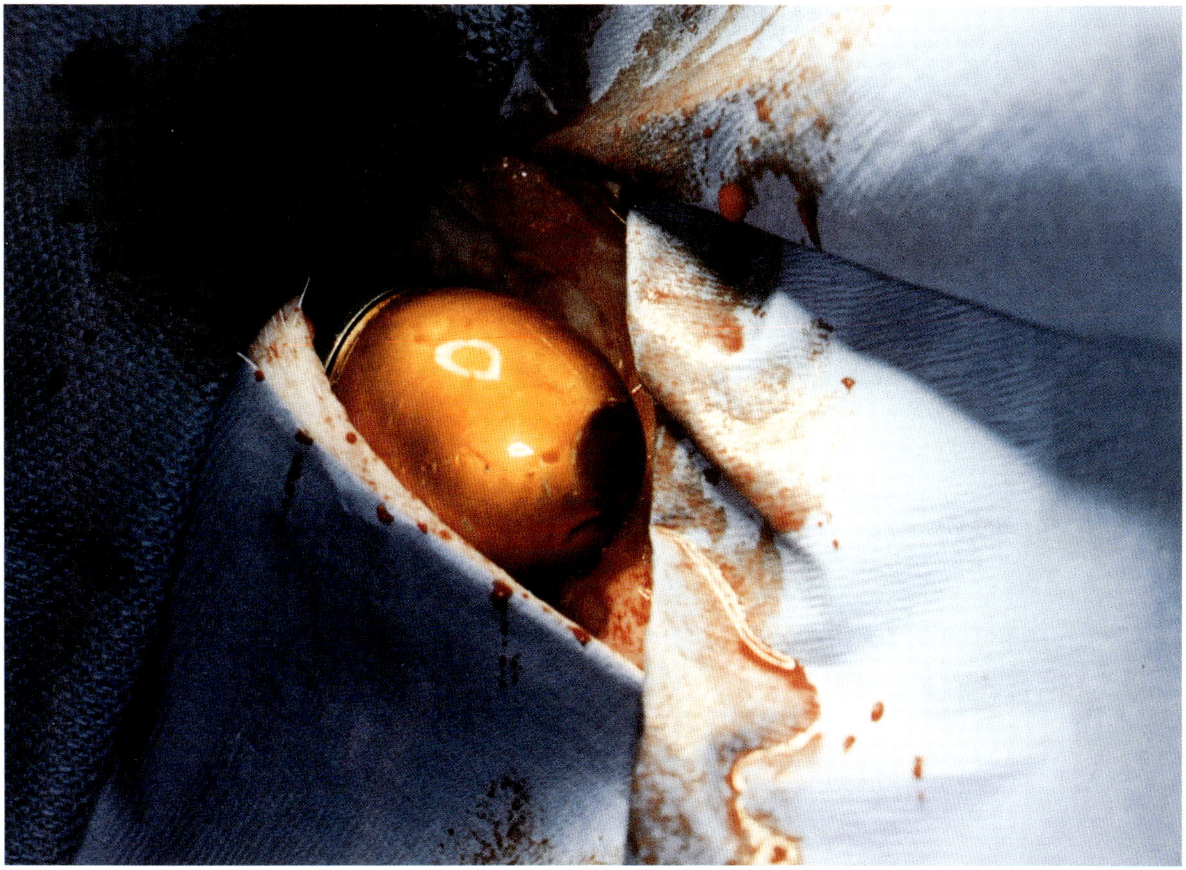

Fig. 1-61. This gaping soft-tissue wound contains an M406 grenade. Of all the munitions used in Vietnam, this was the type most likely to be found embedded and unexploded in tissue. The fuse is located at the tip of the warhead, and is activated and will detonate on contact only after the warhead has rotated 10–12 times, the equivalent of traveling a distance of about 45 feet. This characteristic of the fuse made the removal of the unexploded munition relatively safe for medical personnel.
Source: U.S. Army Armament Research, Development, and Engineering Center, Picatinny Arsenal

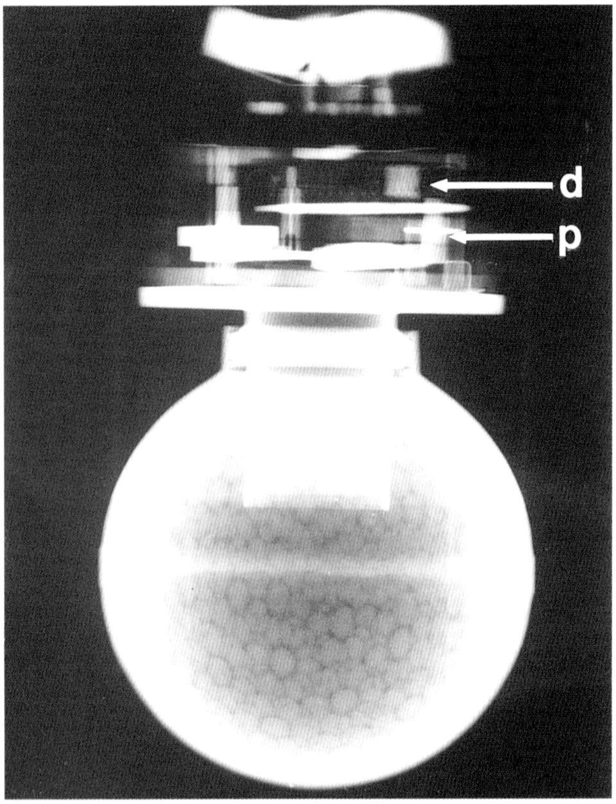

Fig. 1-62. The M551 fuse before the set-back pin (p) has withdrawn from the rotor upon which is mounted the fuse detonator (d). The warhead is in the unarmed position.
Source: U.S. Army Armament Research, Development, and Engineering Center, Picatinny Arsenal

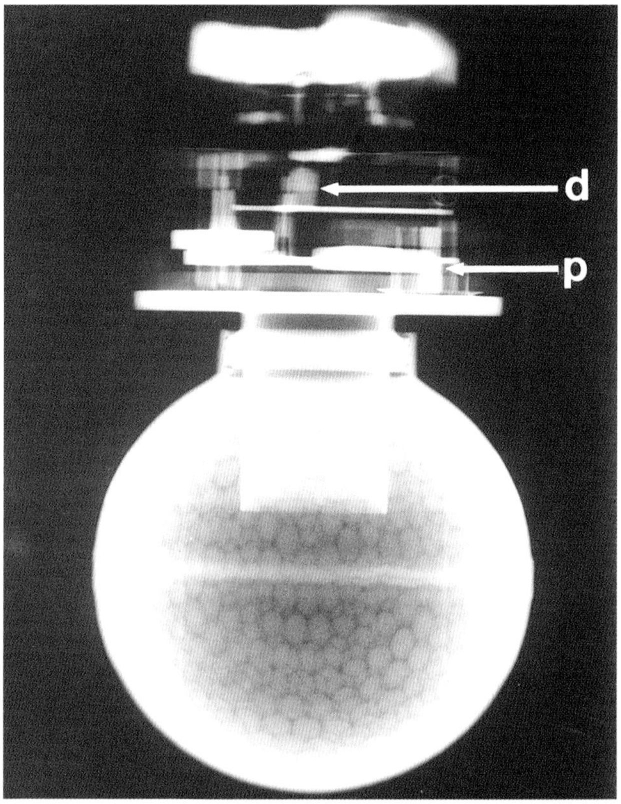

Fig. 1-63. The M551 fuse after the set-back pin and the firing pin (p) have moved and the fuse detonator (d) on the rotor is in line with the firing pin. The warhead is now armed and can explode.
Source: U.S. Army Armament Research, Development, and Engineering Center, Picatinny Arsenal

The critical point in the sequence is *(c);* before this step, the warhead is unarmed, but as soon as this step occurs, the warhead needs only sufficient deceleration to explode. Thus, when an unexploded warhead of this type has become embedded in a casualty's soft tissues, it usually has not traveled far enough (and thus has not made enough rotations) for centrifugal force to disengage the firing pin from the rotor.

Medical personnel facing this situation have to make a quick decision, upon which depends not only the safety of the casualty but also their own. Is the warhead indeed a dud, or is it a warhead with a fuse—like that of the M406—that has not traveled far enough before impact to be activated? Although it may not be reasonable to expect that medical officers become experts on fuses, an elementary understanding of the weapon's design would reassure the medical team that they probably could, in the absence of other evidence, safely remove the warhead.

Mines. In a narrow sense, a *mine* is defined as an explosive ordnance designed to be buried in the ground. In the broader sense, a mine is any hidden explosive ordnance that lies in wait for its target. As such, it may be equally dangerous to friendly or enemy forces. Depending on the size and design of their fuses, mines can be used against matériel or personnel.

Antimatériel mines are designed to damage armored fighting vehicles, especially tanks. Conventional antitank mines contain 10–20 pounds of explosive and have a fuse that is activated when it is compressed by 300–500 pounds of weight (Figure 1-64). Thus, the weight of one person who happened to step on a buried antitank mine would probably not be enough to detonate it. Antitank mines usually damage the tank's track or suspension, although lighter vehicles (such as armored personnel carriers) may sustain more severe structural damage. Personnel inside the vehicle, however, would be susceptible to the same kinds of rapid acceleration-deceleration injuries and other blunt trauma that they might receive in a car wreck. Newer antitank mines use shaped-charge warheads to penetrate the tank's belly armor; more frag-

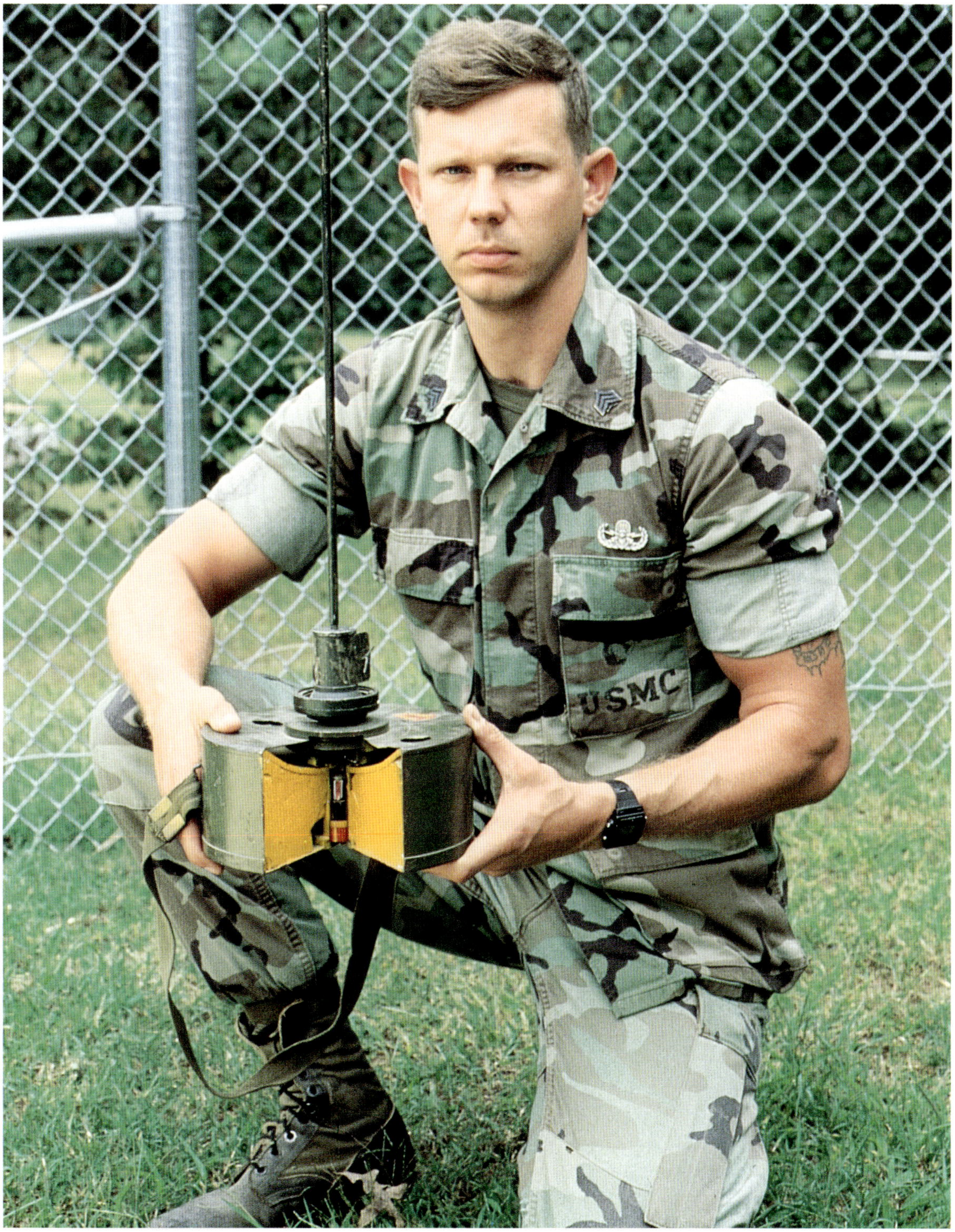

Fig. 1-64. This cutaway shows a portion of the 11-pound explosive charge (painted yellow) of an M21 antitank mine. The function of the thick concave melt plate that forms the upper margin of the explosive charge is similar in some respects to the melt sheet of a shaped-charge warhead. When the charge explodes, the metal plate breaks up into many high-velocity fragments that penetrate the tank and create far more damage than the blast alone would have done. The mine can be detonated either by a conventional pressure fuse that is activated by weight or a sophisticated tilt-rod extension fuse that is activated when the target vehicle's underside brushes it.
Source: Explosive Ordnance Disposal Group, Quantico Marine Corps Base

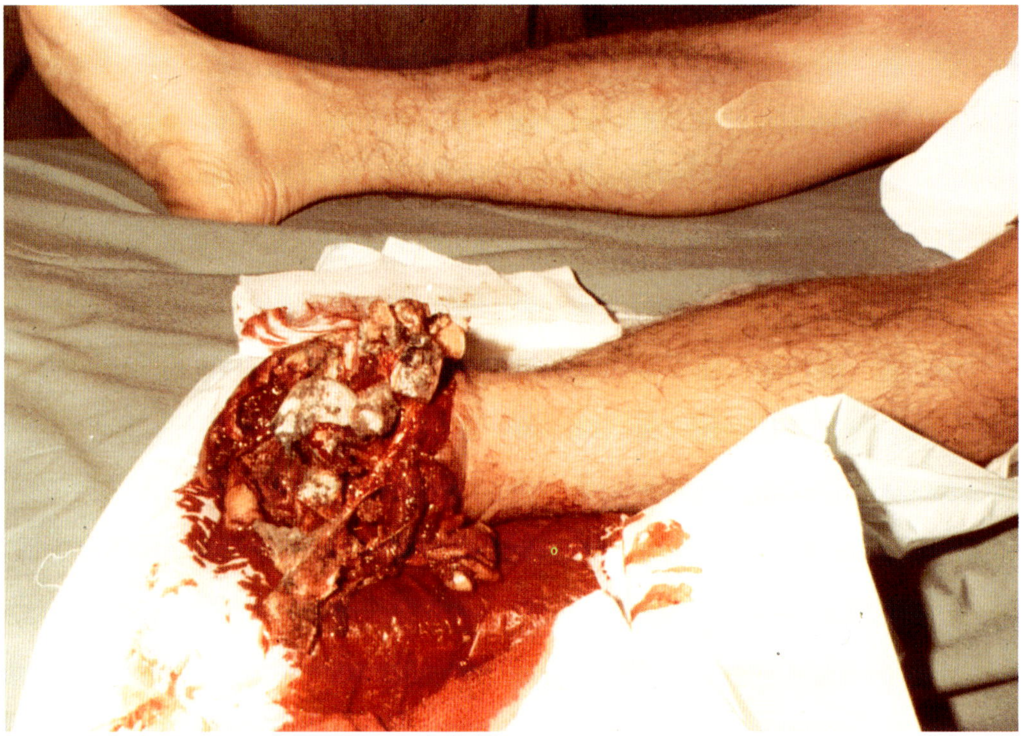

Fig. 1-65. The casualty has suffered a traumatic amputation of the distal portion of his foot, typical of the injuries caused by a buried antipersonnel mine.
Source: Wound Data and Munitions Effectiveness Team

mentation and thermal injuries may result.

The buried antipersonnel mine is designed to maim rather than to kill. It can be made in a variety of sizes and shapes, but commonly resembles a shoe-polish can. About one-half pound of explosive in a buried mine can blow off a victim's foot (Figure 1-65). In addition, when the mine explodes, the particles of dirt in which it was buried become secondary missiles that grossly contaminate any resulting wounds. Although a traumatic amputation certainly incapacitates the individual soldier, the fact that only the soldier who actually steps on the mine is likely to be injured limits the mine's usefulness.

To increase the casualty-generation radius, buried mines with improved-fragmentation designs have been developed. The M16A2 *bounding* or *pop-up mine* (commonly called a *Bouncing Betty*) is an example. When activated by being stepped on, a small explosive charge blows a 4-inch wide steel case about 2–4 feet into the air. This steel case is packed with about one pound of explosive. It immediately detonates and sprays fragments as far as 35 m from the site.

Until recently, surface or fixed antipersonnel mines have been somewhat primitive. The Soviet-made POMZ-2 stake mine (Figure 1-66) was used in World

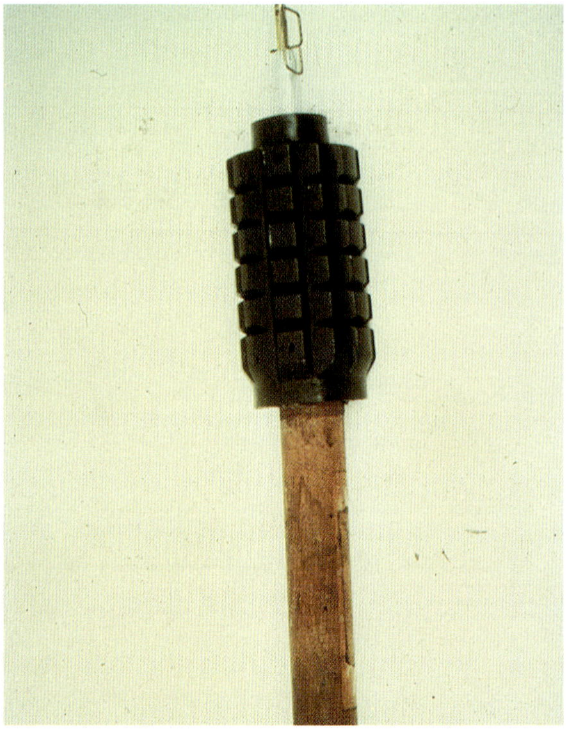

Fig. 1-66. A POMZ-2 stake mine
Source: Letterman Army Institute of Research

War II and resembled older hand grenades. Its explosive charge splintered its thick cast-iron or steel jacket into fragments, the size of which were supposedly determined by deep external grooves. However, the jacket tended to break apart into much larger chunks, similar to those formed by a random-fragmentation shell. Four or five of these 2-kg munitions were connected by a trip wire that, when yanked, detonated the entire line. Fragmentation injuries would occur up to 25 m from each mine.

Modern designs are both more destructive and more easily deployed. Whereas older designs fragmented in all directions upon detonation, newer designs—such as the M18 antipersonnel mine and the M21 antitank mine (Figure 1-64)—focus their fragmentation effects in one direction. The metal plate of the M21 breaks up into fragments when it is blown against the tank's underside. In the M18 (called the *Claymore,* after the sword used by the Scottish highlanders), this metal sheet has been replaced by a layer of 700 ballbearing-like steel spheres, each weighing 0.75 gram. A 670-gram explosive charge blows the spheres outward over a 60° arc for distances up to 250 meters. Lethal injuries occur within 50 meters, and gross mutilation is common. The Claymore mine is primarily used to defend an area's perimeter, and may be detonated *(a)* electrically, *(b)* by a timed fuse, or *(c)* by a trip wire. Its effects were devastating in Vietnam.

Booby Traps. A *booby trap* is a concealed device that explodes when a nearby harmless-looking object is touched. Although the explosive device may be any commercially available grenade, mine, or shell, booby traps will often be improvised, especially when they are used in terrorist and counterinsurgency operations. A pipe bomb, for example, is a length of steel pipe filled with TNT and fused with a length of detonating cord. Improvised booby traps often contain preformed fragments such as nails, small pieces of wire, or chunks of metal or glass. Such weapons can cause devastating injuries (Figure 1-67).

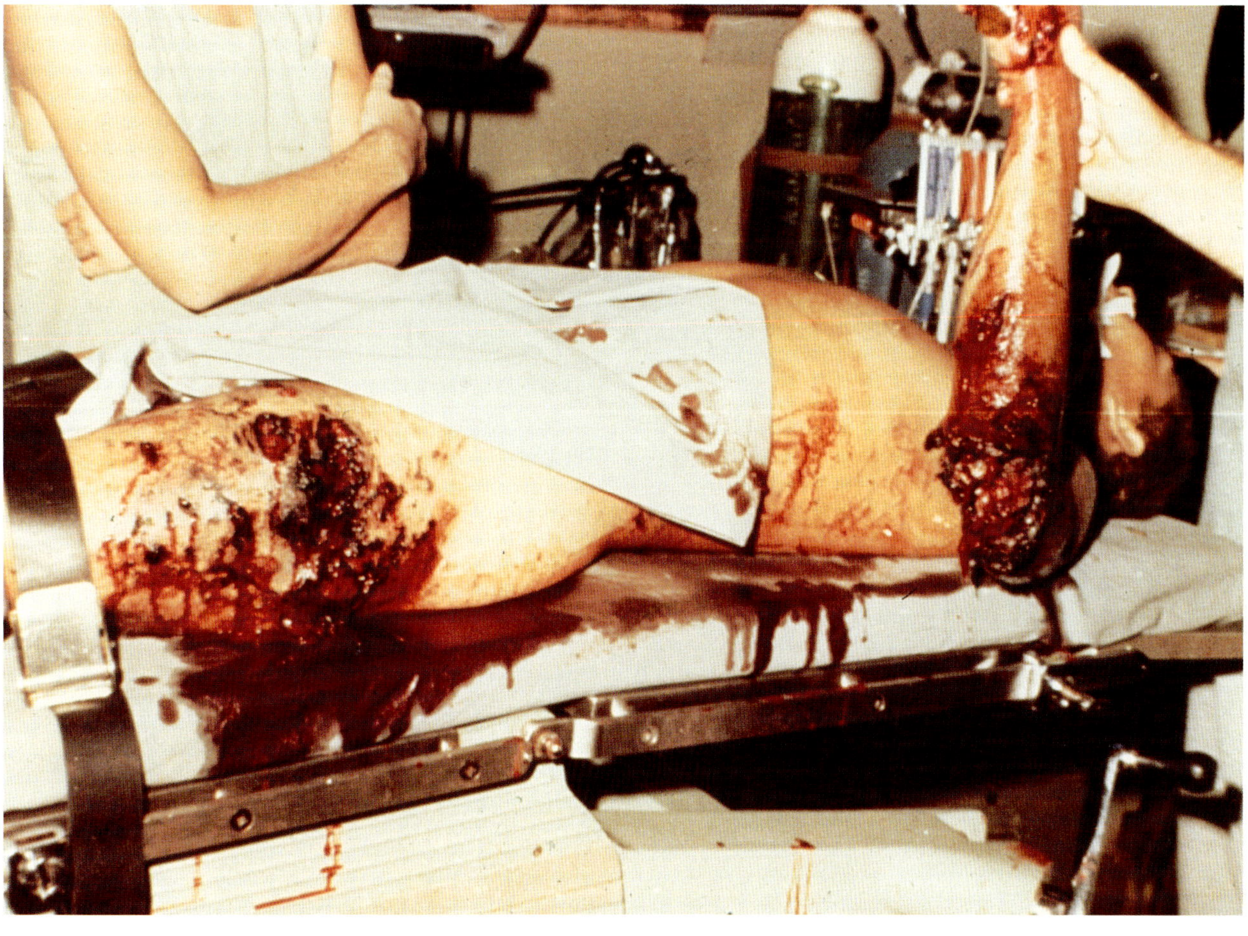

Fig. 1-67. This casualty has a massive soft-tissue injury that was caused by a booby trap made from several hand grenades and assorted pieces of scrap metal.
Source: Wound Data and Munitions Effectiveness Team

FLAME AND INCENDIARY MUNITIONS

Although *flame* and *incendiary munitions* theoretically constitute separate classes of weapons, they both use fire to expel the enemy from fortified or concealed positions. Flame weapons deliver the combustible materials to the target, and it is this combustible material—not the target itself—that initially burns. Incendiary weapons also contain a combustible material but use it to set a combustible target on fire, the way a match would ignite a pile of papers. The care of combat casualties who have been injured by flame and incendiary weapons does not differ from the care of burn casualties in general. However, because phosphorus-containing munitions may have the effects of both flame and incendiary munitions (that is, the phosphorus itself can cause a chemical burn as well as ignite the victim's clothes), the injuries that result do raise special treatment concerns.

Flame Munitions

Flame munitions are designed to expel people from strongholds or hidden positions. Because burns are such painful, disfiguring injuries, the fear of being burned—perhaps more than the actual burns themselves—may be the crucial incapacitating factor in the effectiveness of these weapons.

The combustible used in all modern flame weapons is a hydrocarbon fuel (such as gasoline) with a thickening agent added to make the mixture viscous. The thickening agent was originally prepared by combining aluminum hydroxide with naphthenic and palmic acids. The combustible is now known by the generic name *napalm,* even though the original thickener has long been superseded by substances based on soaps of aluminum and a more suitable fatty acid, such as isooctanoic acid. The original napalm formula of 91%–98% gasoline and 2%–9% thickener has been replaced by more sophisticated preparations; the U.S. Air Force's Napalm B, for example, consists of 25% gasoline, 25% benzene, and 50% polystyrene. This adhesive, slow-burning, jelly-like liquid will cling to the victim long enough for deep burns to occur. Gasoline-filled bottles (known as Molotov cocktails) and other improvised flame munitions lack these characteristics, and so, although they might be effective in starting localized fires, they are relatively ineffective against personnel.

Flame munitions can be delivered by *(a)* air-dropped bombs, *(b)* flame throwers, or *(c)* warheads fired from rocket launchers.

Air-dropped bombs, such as the MK79 (Model 1) 1,000-pound fire bomb, are by far the most common flame munitions. The extensive use of these napalm bombs during the Vietnam War generated considerable notoriety. Compared with many other weapons, however, they were able to hit targets more precisely, leaving surrounding structures untouched and thus producing relatively little collateral damage. Nor was the workload of medical personnel burdened by napalm injuries; an equivalent weight of high-explosive or cluster munitions would have been likely to create many more casualties. About 100 casualties in the Wound Data and Munitions Effectiveness Team (WDMET) study, for example, were known to have been inadvertently engulfed by napalm fireballs in Vietnam. Six of them died, which was one-fifth the mortality rate that would be expected in an equal number of casualties suffering from rifle wounds.[19] Death from asphyxia or carbon monoxide poisoning was not a likely consequence of being engulfed by napalm fire.

Flame throwers, which eject a burning combustible through a nozzle, may be carried into battle by individuals or mounted in armored fighting vehicles. As originally designed, the hand-held flame thrower had dubious practical value: Its effective range was only 20–40 m, and the operator needed to stand up to use it. Any soldier who carried a pressurized air-tank flame thrower and managed to stick its nozzle through the gunport of an enemy bunker, Hollywood-style, would have been extremely vulnerable; such attacks would have succeeded only if the defenders of the enemy position had been previously incapacitated.

Flame throwers mounted on tanks and armored personnel carriers are much less vulnerable, can carry far more combustible material, and can squirt a jet of flame for 300–400 m.

The rocket launcher has been developed because both American and Soviet weapons designers have been reluctant to abandon completely the concept of a soldier-carried flame thrower. They have tried to overcome the flame thrower's deficiencies by designing weapons that have longer ranges. The American-made M202A1 (*Flash*) incendiary rocket launcher and the Soviet-made RPO-A recoilless flame thrower are shoulder-borne weapons that fire incendiary warheads, each one of which holds several liters of napalm. The

Soviet-made weapon can fire two napalm warheads per minute with a range of 400 m. The new warheads burst on contact with the target, unlike an earlier version in which combustion began as soon as the warhead left the launcher, its trail of fire extending from the weapon to the target.

Incendiary Weapons

Unlike weapons that use napalm, incendiary bombs and grenades are used almost exclusively to set matériel on fire. The casualty-generating potential of these weapons is not unique, and is incidental to their use as antimatériel weapons. Incendiary bombs were used extensively in World War II (for example, to create the firestorms over Tokyo), but since then, they have become curiosities.

Magnesium metal or *thermite* (that is, ferric oxide and aluminum in a 3:1 ratio) are the common constituents of incendiary weapons. Thermite is a stable, inert powder that must be purposely ignited. Whereas napalm burns at about 1,000° C, thermite burns at 2,000°–3,000° C, and therefore it can be used to damage metal. For example, thermite grenades can destroy gun barrels.

Casualties who have been burned by these materials should receive standard burn care.

Phosphorus-Containing Munitions

Phosphorus-containing grenades, shells, or bombs can cause severe thermal and chemical burns. Phosphorus ignites spontaneously in air at 44° C and produces a temperature of about 800° C. In hot climates, the storage of phosphorus-containing munitions is difficult; phosphorus tends to liquefy in warm weather and may leak, causing fires.

Liquefied phosphorus is particularly dangerous to personnel; its continued presence on the skin results in dermal penetration and tissue necrosis. Phosphorus-containing munitions (such as the M34 hand grenade) are designed to fragment, and tissues deep under the skin may be impregnated by both metal and phosphorus fragments. Whereas metal fragments from most other weapons do not need to be surgically removed, any metal fragments that are covered with liquid phosphorus—as well as any embedded pieces of white phosphorus—must be excised (Figure 1-68).

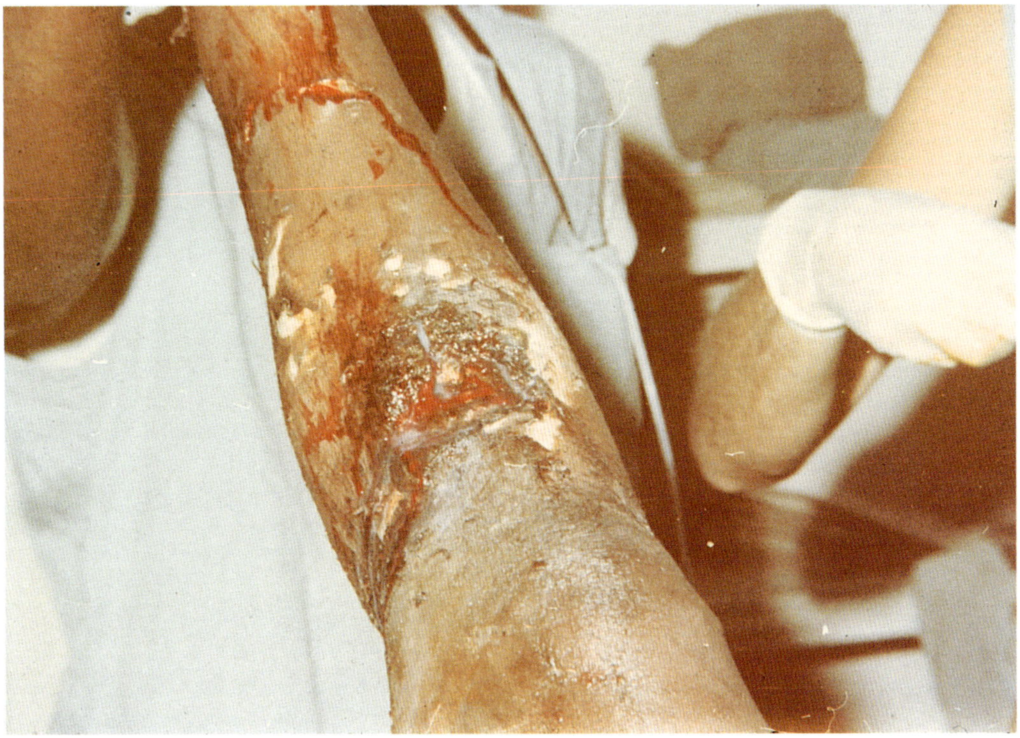

Fig. 1-68. This casualty suffered a mutilating injury of the lower leg that was caused by an M34 white phosphorus grenade. Most of the tissue damage was caused by the grenade's fragmentation, but treatment was complicated by the white phosphorus (which appears as the yellowish-white material in the illustration) that impregnated the wound.
Source: Wound Data and Munitions Effectiveness Team

The usefulness of flame and incendiary munitions on the battlefield is limited, despite their hellish effects. Compared to the number of American casualties burned by fires in armored fighting vehicles and aircraft, very few were wounded by flame, incendiary, or phosphorus-containing munitions. Data from the Korean War indicate that there were only 312 American casualties with burns from white phosphorus during the entire war.[20] In the Vietnam War, only eight out of almost 8,000 casualties had white phosphorus burns, and seven of those were accidental wounds caused by M34 white phosphorus grenades.[21]

MEDICAL IMPLICATIONS

The weapons of conventional land warfare are designed to inflict physical harm on opponents by wounding them with bullets or fragments, damaging their internal organs with blast effects, or burning them. Even though some of the weapons that cause such injuries have become extremely sophisticated in modern times, most armed aggression through the centuries has been based on these three injuring mechanisms. The military physician must be prepared to treat the effects of them all.

Most casualties in modern conventional wars are injured by weapons that cause ballistic wounds. These weapons either fire projectiles at a target or explode into fragments. Although the severity of the wound depends to some extent upon the nature of the projectile or fragment, the most important factor in ballistic injury is the anatomical site that is hit: A small, jagged fragment from a primitive booby trap can be lethal if it hits the heart, whereas a high-velocity bullet from a sophisticated assault rifle might be only mildly incapacitating if it hits a finger.

Blast injuries may not at first be obvious to medical personnel. As weapons increasingly take advantage of the physical properties of blast waves (particularly in enclosed spaces, such as tanks, or in conjunction with body armor), medical officers should be aware that a blast injury may also be present in a casualty whose only overt injuries are the more immediately threatening blunt, penetrating, or thermal trauma.

Burns cause relatively few casualties in conventional warfare. Because they can be so disfiguring and painful, however, these injuries have serious psychological implications for both combat and medical personnel, as well as intensive medical-resource allocation requirements.

The following sections of this textbook are devoted to detailed discussions of ballistic, blast, and burn injuries.

REFERENCES

1. Parkinson, R. 1979. *Clausewitz.* New York: Stein and Day.

2. *Sierra bullets rifle reloading manual.* 1985. 2d ed. Santa Fe Springs, CA: Leisure Group, Inc.

3. Greenwood, C. 1980. The political factor. In *The Gun Digest.* 34th ed., 161–168. Northfield, IL: DBI Books, Inc.

4. Dupuy, T. N. 1980. *The evolution of weapons and warfare.* Indianapolis, IN: The Bobbs-Merrill Company, Inc.

5. Ezell, E. C. 1984. *The great rifle controversy.* Harrisburg, PA: Stackpole Books.

6. Farrar, C. L., and Leeming, D. W. 1983. *Military ballistics—A basic manual.* Vol. 10 of *Battlefield weapons systems & technology.* New York: Brassey's Publishers Ltd.

7. Lee, R. G. 1981. *Introduction to battlefield weapons systems.* Vol. 1 of *Battlefield weapons systems & technology.* New York: Brassey's Publishers Ltd.

8. Heaton, L. D.; Coates, J. B.; and Beyer, J. C., eds. 1962. *Wound ballistics.* Washington, DC: Office of the Surgeon General, Department of the Army.

9. Hogg, I. V. 1985. *The illustrated history of ammunition.* Secaucus, NJ: Chartwell Books, Inc.

10. Reches, M. 1976. *Improved ballistic eye protection* [Interim Note No. 1]. Aberdeen Proving Ground, MD: U.S. Army Materiel Systems Analysis Activity.

11. Wound Data and Munitions Effectiveness Team. 1970. *Evaluation of wound data and munitions effectiveness in Vietnam* [Final Report]. In Vol. 3, Table D.10-6, p. 2. Alexandria, VA: Defense Documentation Center.

12. Carell, P. 1967. *Der Russland Krieg*. Frankfurt: Ullstein GmbH.

13. Palmer, A. 1962. Bomb incident: A controlled study. In reference 8, 827–841.

14. Kennedy D. R. 1983. Improving combat crew survivability. *Armor* 92 (4):16–20.

15. Lucas, J. 1982. *War on the eastern front.* New York: Bonanza Books.

16. Geisenheyner, S. 1987. FAE development: Disturbing trends. *Jane's Defense Weekly* 7: 280–282.

17. Central Intelligence Agency. Personal communication, 1987.

18. Kittrick, J. Foreign Science and Technology Center, Charlottesville, VA. Personal communication, 1990.

19. Wound Data and Munitions Effectiveness Team. 1970. Vol. 2 of reference 11. Classified. Access to original data is controlled by Uniformed Services University of the Health Sciences, Bethesda, MD.

20. Reister, F. A. 1974. *Battle casualties and medical statistics.* Washington, DC: Office of the Surgeon General, Department of the Army.

21. Wound Data and Munitions Effectiveness Team. 1970. In reference 11, Table 4, p. C-7.

RECOMMENDED READING AND RESOURCES

The definitive sources for weapons data are the technical manuals and field manuals that are published by the armed forces. The primary source of official documents on weapons effectiveness, both classified and unclassified, is available from:

Joint Technological Coordinating Group for Munitions Effectiveness
Ballistics Research Laboratory
Aberdeen Proving Ground, MD 21005

The single most useful database describing weapons effects is the Wound Data and Munitions Effectiveness Team (WDMET) study prepared by the Army Materiel Command. These data are stored at the National Naval Medical Center, Bethesda, MD, and access is controlled by:

Uniformed Services University of the Health Sciences
Bethesda, MD 20814-4799
Telephone: (301) 295-6262

Three summary volumes contain extensive abstracts of the statistical data, and can be obtained from:

Defense Documentation Center
Cameron Station
Alexandria, VA 22304-6145
Telephone: (703) 545-6700 and (703) 274-7633

Association of the U.S. Army. *The Army green book.* Published annually as the October issue of *Army.*

Beebe, G. W., and De Bakey, M. E. 1952. *Battle casualties: Incidence, mortality, and logistic considerations.* Springfield, IL: Charles Thomas.

Chant, C. 1980. *How weapons work.* Secaucus, NJ: Chartwell Books, Inc.

Farrar, C. L., and Leeming, D. W. 1983. *Military ballistics.* Vol. 10, *Battlefield weapons systems & technology,* edited by R. G. Lee. Oxford: Brassey's Publishers.

Foss, C., and Hogg, I. V. 1986. *Battlefield—The weapons of modern land warfare.* London: Orbis Publishing Corporation.

Heaton, L. D.; Coates, J. B.; and Beyer, J. C., eds. 1962. *Wound ballistics.* Washington, D.C.: Office of the Surgeon General, Department of the Army. This is the standard text in the open literature describing the wounding effects of weapons.

Hogg, I. V., and Weeks, J. 1985. *Military small arms.* 5th edition. Northfield, IL: DBI Books.

Hogg, I. V. 1985. *Illustrated encyclopedia of ammunition.* Secaucus, NJ: Chartwell Books, Inc.

Jane's Infantry Weapons. New York: Jane's Publishing, Inc. Jane's publications deal with the entire spectrum of weapons systems and are published annually.

Lee, R. G. 1981. *Introduction to battlefield weapons systems.* Vol. 1, *Battlefield weapons systems & technology.* Oxford: Brassey's Publishers.

Reister, F. A. 1973. *Battle casualties—The American experience in Korea.* Washington, DC: Office of the Surgeon General, Department of the Army.

The military medical officer can readily obtain information on weapons systems from the ordnance personnel assigned to many military installations.

Chapter 2

ASSESSING THE EFFECTIVENESS OF CONVENTIONAL WEAPONS

RONALD F. BELLAMY, M.D., FACS* AND RUSS ZAJTCHUK, M.D., FACS**

*Colonel, United States Army; Acting Chief, Department of Surgery, Walter Reed Army Medical Center, Washington, D.C. 20307-5001
**Colonel, United States Army; Deputy Commander, Walter Reed Army Medical Center, Washington, D.C. 20307-5001

INTRODUCTION

Karl von Clausewitz observed that "war is an act of violence intended to compel our opponent to fulfill our will."[1] Historically, compelling opponents "to fulfill our will" has meant that one group of people uses weapons and physical force to injure or kill another group of people, and therefore intimidates the survivors into compliance. While the specific mechanisms of ballistic, blast, and burn injuries and their medical and surgical treatments are considered in the following sections of this textbook, this chapter considers (in the broadest sense) the ability of the weapons that are used violently in conventional land warfare to inflict physical harm. Describing the outcome when weapons are employed—weapons effectiveness in the broadest sense—utilizes concepts including: *(a) lethality* (that is, the observed probability that a casualty will die if injured by a given weapon; *(b) casualty generation* (which has two definitions: the observed fraction of the total at-risk population that was injured by a given weapons system, or alternatively, the probability that a weapon's single use will generate casualties); *(c) incapacitation* (that is, the probability that an injury resulting from a weapon's single use will prevent the casualty from performing a soldier's duties); and *(d) injury severity* (that is, the observed probability that a weapon's single use will produce a certain degree of morbidity in a casualty).

Several features of these definitions require elaboration. First, they deal with probabilities. Unlike physicians who treat individual patients, medical officers who seek to understand weapons effectiveness and to predict (for planning purposes) the number of casualties that are probable need to become familiar with the concept of *conditional probability*, which can be defined as the probability (P) that a given outcome (O) will result from a specific event (E), and which can be expressed as $P(O|E)$. For example, the probability that a casualty will die given an injury made by a weapon's single use is a conditional probability. Probability is usually expressed as a ratio: the observed number of specified outcomes divided by the population at risk of that outcome. Thus, there is a need to precisely define not only those outcomes but also, even more importantly, the at-risk population.

Second, the apparent precision and simplicity of the definitions above are deceptive. For example, all four include the concept of a *casualty*. But what exactly must happen before a soldier is classified as a casualty? Officially, the U.S. Army defines a casualty as "any person lost to his organization because he is killed, wounded, missing, captured, or interned if such a loss is incurred in action."[2] From the perspective of assessing weapons effectiveness, only the casualties who are killed and wounded are relevant, but here too, precise definitions are required. What must happen for a soldier to be classified as wounded? The official definition is: "Battle casualties who require admission to a Medical Treatment Facility (MTF) or who die of their wounds after reaching any MTF are reported as Wounded in Action."[2] However, many soldiers sustain such minor injuries that they do not require admission to an MTF. During the Vietnam War, the largest group of officially recognized casualties were soldiers who were not admitted to MTFs but were *carded for record only* (that is, even though the soldiers' injuries were trivial and they did not require admission, their names were recorded on cards for record-keeping purposes), and therefore they were not casualties at all according to the official definition.[3] Including these soldiers—who were carded for record only—in data used to assess weapons effectiveness has led to misleading conclusions.

And third, military surgeons recognize *wounds* as a category of *injuries* (that is, a wound is specifically a penetrating injury caused by a projectile) and distinguish wounds from other injuries such as those caused by blasts and burns. Note that the official definition of a casualty uses the word "wound" in the sense that this textbook uses "injury."

Such seemingly minor semantic problems may limit the validity of some of the conclusions that can be drawn from some of the data presented in this chapter. Not only do some of the original sources use some of these terms interchangeably, but their definitions may also vary from war to war, from army to army, and even from one data collector to another.

Casualty generation and lethality will be discussed at great length, but medical commanders and staff officers will find other indices of weapons effectiveness to be useful, also. The concept of injury severity as an index of weapons effectiveness should be immediately appealing to medical officers. This approach is limited, however; little data exist that directly relate injury severity to specific weapons, and the assessment of severity is almost always made in purely qualitative terms (trivial, medium, serious) that are incompletely defined.

Certainly from the military standpoint, the probability that a casualty will be *incapacitated* (that is, unable to perform his or her soldierly duties) if a weapon is used has great practical importance. Precise definitions exist delineating a soldier's duties. Thus it is possible to state what a weapon must do to prevent a soldier from functioning; that is, it is possible to quantitate the violence required to cause a casualty to become incapacitated. In fact, some weapons designers during the second half of the twentieth century have predicated their work upon the goal of incapacitating—not killing—the enemy.

METHODOLOGY: DISTINGUISHING BETWEEN LETHALITY AND CASUALTY GENERATION

Death is an outcome that is recognized by all, and lethality—the probability that a casualty will be killed if injured by a specific weapon—should be one of the most commonly used indices of weapons effectiveness. Thus, lethality should be a good discriminator among weapons: The probability that a casualty will be killed if wounded by a bullet fired by an assault rifle should differ from the probability of being killed if wounded by a pellet from a BB gun. Unfortunately, however, weapons designers frequently refer to the ability to generate casualties as a weapon's "lethality." This usage is misleading. A weapon that is very likely to kill may not normally cause many casualties, and a relatively inefficient weapon may generate many nonfatally wounded casualties.

Rarely, sources can be found that document the number of casualties that a single use of a weapon will make.[4,5,6] These allow one to contrast lethality defined as casualty generation (the weapons designers' sense of the term) with lethality defined as the probability that a casualty will be killed if injured by that weapon's single use (this textbook's definition, because it is the more medically relevant). Three weapons and their effects illustrate the shortcomings of using the terms "casualty generation" and "lethality" as if they were synonyms: *(a)* the Japanese model M 97 hand grenade that was used in the Bougainville Campaign during World War II, *(b)* the 12-kiloton (kt) atomic bomb that was used at Hiroshima during World War II, and *(c)* the sword as Homer described its use in his *Iliad* and Virgil in his *Aeneid* (Table 2-1). Obviously, a properly used sword can be very lethal, but no one would suggest that a battlefield dominated by cutting weapons is a more lethal place than a city under nuclear attack. Furthermore, the relatively inefficient hand grenade is militarily more useful than the very deadly sword, because a hand grenade's single use can wound more soldiers. A weapon such as a 12-kt atomic bomb can injure vast numbers (its casualty generation) even though the fraction of the total number of injured who were actually killed (its lethality) is less than that of a weapon such as the sword, which has a very high lethality but injures only one at a time. While both definitions of lethality may have their uses, for purposes of this textbook, medical officers must carefully distinguish lethality—the fraction of the total number injured who have a fatal outcome—from casualty generation—the number of individuals in the target population who are injured by a single use of the weapon.

Lethality

Data on the lethality of historical weapons are not readily available. To calculate a weapon's lethality (that is, the probability that the casualty will die after being injured by the weapon in question), one needs to know the number of casualties produced by the weapon

TABLE 2-1

THE TWO DEFINITIONS OF LETHALITY

Weapon	Number Injured by a Single Use of the Weapon	Probability of Being Killed if Injured by the Weapon
Grenade	6–8	0.06
Atomic bomb	~144,000	~0.5
Sword	1	0.95

Source: References 4, 5, and 6

and, of these, how many died.

Two major sources of error cloud lethality assessments: missing data and the effect of medical care. Inadequate sampling and inaccurate data are common for the category "killed in action." Even during this century, only a small fraction of those killed in action have been accurately diagnosed at autopsy, with an accurate assessment of the wounding agent made by an ordnance expert. Even when this has been attempted, the difficulty of deciding which weapon made the wound is frequently so great that even an ordnance officer (to say nothing of field medical personnel, who are expected to fill out a field medical tag specifying the weapon) cannot make an accurate determination. Explosive munitions make the problem of identifying the wounding weapon especially difficult. For example, wounds made by a mortar bomb may not be distinguishable from wounds made by an artillery shell. Frequently all the data collector can do is to indicate that the wound was made by an explosive munition and not by a bullet. And complicating the matter, some casualties will have wounds made by both bullets and fragments, or combined injuries from burn, blast, and ballistic weapons.

Medical care can change the likelihood that a casualty will die from a wound and therefore can decrease the weapon's lethality. For example, during the Civil War, the hospital mortality rate for open comminuted femoral-shaft fractures caused by bullets was more than 50%.[7] The same injury in the Vietnam War was associated with a hospital mortality rate of 1.4%.[8] But one would be quite wrong to conclude that this dramatic fall in mortality resulted from less-lethal bullets being used in Vietnam.

There are several ways to avoid the errors that the effect of medical care can introduce. First, lethality should be calculated only for those casualties who are actually killed in action (that is, those who die before they receive any medical care). Unfortunately, this is not always possible; original source material may list only the total mortality and not distinguish between the categories "killed in action" and "died of wounds." Second, if only total mortality data are available, one should attempt to compare lethalities only for wars of the same era, which will minimize the effect of greatly differing medical capabilities.

Casualty Generation

The Requirement for an Operational Definition. The index of a weapon's effectiveness that a soldier thinks of first—the weapon's ability to kill or injure—is, unfortunately, not usable for several reasons. First, the number of casualties generated by the single use of a weapon will depend not only on the characteristics of the weapon, but also on the number of potential casualties (the at-risk population) that are available. Second, in order to generate casualties, the weapon must be used effectively. (Firing into the ground is less likely to cause casualties than firing into a crowded room.) Third, almost no data exist that tell how many times a weapon was used to generate the observed number of casualties. Nuclear weapons are an exception (only one atomic bomb was used at Hiroshima), but for most weapons these data are not known. For example, the conventional wisdom is that at least 10,000 rounds were fired from small arms for every casualty wounded by a bullet in World War II. But little understanding would be gained by referring to the casualty generation of military small arms as 1/10,000. (Snipers can achieve better results with bullets; data from the Vietnam War indicate that one casualty was caused by every 1.5 bullets fired by snipers.[9]) Given these limitations, an alternative definition of casualty generation is required. This textbook defines casualty generation as that fraction of the total casualty population produced by a given type of weapon. Ample data do exist from a variety of wars, campaigns, and battles that allow this definition to be used.

Changes in the Distribution of Casualties by Weapon. Although penetrating trauma caused by fragmentation munitions and especially explosive shells have been the major source of casualties on the modern battlefield, this is a rather recent development. During most of the nineteenth century, infantry weapons dominated battlefields, first smooth-bore muskets and then rifles. The predominance of small arms is quite apparent in casualty data from the

TABLE 2-2

SOURCES OF UNION CASUALTIES IN THE CIVIL WAR

Weapon or Missile	Casualties
Rifle or smooth-bore musket	124,000
Fragments from shells	12,500
Cannonball or grapeshot	359
Cutting weapons	7,002

Source: Reference 5

American Civil War (Table 2-2).[5]

The casualties in the Franco-Prussian War of 1870–1871 were similarly distributed: Rifles were responsible for 92% of German wounded and 91% of German killed.[10] But by the end of the century, technological changes (such as smokeless powder and mechanisms for controlling recoil, which made the artillery that dominated World War I battlefields possible) had occurred. The proportion of the World War I casualty population that was caused by fragmentation weapons had changed dramatically since the late nineteenth century (Table 2-3).[10]

While small arms were the source of 39%–51% of German casualties, they were responsible for only 8%–14% of American casualties. Such major differences raise important questions that illustrate some of the limitations of analyzing historical sources. Either the validity of one or both sets of data must be questioned, or the two sides fought with fundamentally different tactics. Perhaps the German commanders utilized artillery in both attacking and defending, or the Americans depended more upon infantry weapons. Regardless of the reason for these differences, these data suggest that the proportion of the total casualty population that is generated by a given weapon can be quite variable.

Methodological problems that result from data-collecting protocols must also be considered. Published data on the sources of casualties by weapon frequently fail to state whether the data pertain to the total casualty population (that is, those killed outright, plus those who died later of their wounds, plus those who were wounded but survived) or only to those casualties who were hospitalized. Uncertainty in assessing the data also arises from the data collectors' inability *(a)* to count all the dead and *(b)* to accurately identify the weapons that were the cause of death. Assessments of the causes of death are sometimes based upon surprisingly small samples. The German history of World War I upon which Table 2-3 is based states that 39% of German casualties who were killed were victims of bullets, based upon the analysis of 14,486 casualties.[10] Although an impressively large number, it is less than 1% of the total German battle deaths in World War I.

That errors in counting are responsible for some of the variation from war to war seems certain, but comparing German and American data from World War I almost certainly reveals two more important factors: *(a)* the technological state of weapons design and construction, which determines the weapons that are available, and *(b)* the tactics and the military operational situation, which determine the weapons that are used and how they are deployed.

ASSESSING WEAPONS EFFECTIVENESS IN MODERN WARS

Of the modern sources pertaining to weapons effectiveness in recent wars, ten contain information that was gathered with enough precision to be considered here. Although they will be used to assess weapons effectiveness, only two of them—the Bougainville and Wound Data and Munitions Effectiveness Team (WDMET) studies—were specifically designed for that purpose. The others must be considered in light of the constraints (misleading definitions, missing data, effects of medical care on the casualties, and so forth) that were discussed above. In all cases, the lethalities, based on information contained in the

TABLE 2-3

SOURCES OF ARMY CASUALTIES IN WORLD WAR I

Missile	German 1914–1917		English (no dates given)	American 1918		French 1918
	wounded	killed	wounded	wounded	killed	wounded
Bullet	51%	39%	39%	14%	8%	30%
Fragments*	46%	56%	61%	85%	92%	58%

*Shells, grenades, and mortar bombs

Source: Reference 10

tables or their original source material, were calculated especially for this chapter.

The German-Russian Front, 1944

German data, analyzed at the German Central Archives for Military Medicine in Berlin, include clinical records, roentgenograms, and hospital and field sick-report books that were collected during World War II. Little is known about the methods used in the field to obtain the original data. Apparently, statisticians at the Central Archives in 1944 took random samples known as spot-checks but "unfortunately, the exact figures for these spot-checks, which were made on a very wide scale, are no longer available."[11] Although the data were compiled in 1944, they almost certainly pertain to actions fought on the eastern front during the preceding 3 years (Table 2-4).

These data are valuable insofar as they are categorized by weapon. Since the absolute number of casualties is not known, however, a calculation of the casualty generation is impossible, although some of the entries such as wounds caused by bayonets, blows from rifle butts, and being run over by a tank must describe rather unusual events. Some weapons are more lethal than others. Antitank shells are very likely to kill; therefore, they cause few minor wounds. Hand grenades and mortar bombs cause few deaths but proportionately many casualties who need medical care. The most important fact is that wounds made by explosive projectile munitions used against personnel (not against tanks) were fatal 8% of the time for mortar shells and 19% of the time for artillery shells. Their calculated lethalities were 0.08 and 0.19. Bullets were fatal 30% of the time; their lethality was 0.30.

The Bougainville Campaign, February-April 1944

American data collected during the Bougainville Campaign constitute a unique study valuable for its essentially prospective organization, comprehensive

TABLE 2-4

GERMAN CASUALTIES ON THE RUSSIAN FRONT

Wounding Weapon	Percentage of Casualties		
	Killed in Action	Seriously Wounded	Slightly Wounded
Armor-piercing and antitank shells	69	22	9
Bayonet	64	14	22
Blow from rifle butt	62	31	7
Run over by tank	34	33	33
Infantry projectiles (rifles, machine guns, submachine guns, and pistols)	30	31	39
Land mine	22	40	38
Aircraft bomb	20	37	43
Artillery shell	19	29	52
Hand grenade	17	18	65
Mortar shell	8	31	61

Source: Reference 11

coverage, and depth of detail. For example, the data collectors took great care to assure that the casualty's *disposition* was known (that is, they determined whether the casualty returned to duty and, if so, from what echelon of care). Their depth of detail included using ordnance officers to identify weapons and requiring that complete autopsies be performed on the dead. Unfortunately, the original data probably no longer exist, but the study contains detailed descriptions of the methods that were used to organize and collect the data.[4] Although absolutely authoritative in its description of low-intensity, light-infantry actions, this study has little applicability to high-intensity warfare, in which the battlefield is dominated by artillery, aircraft, and armor (Table 2-5).

The term "dead" as it is used in this study applies both to casualties who were killed in action and those who died later of their wounds. The extent to which medical care altered the lethality is probably very small, since the study reports that over 90% of the mortality was killed in action.

Data were collected separately for casualties wounded by bullets from rifles and machine guns, and bullet wounds were tallied separately from fragment wounds. The calculated lethality of a wound made by a rifle bullet was 0.32 and for machine guns, 0.58. The higher lethality for machine guns probably indicates multiple bullet wounds. Bullets from both sources caused 34% of the total number of casualties, but because bullets are likely to kill, they caused a disproportionately greater number of those fatally wounded (62%). Only 25% of the casualties who required treatment were wounded by bullets, but 72% were wounded by fragments.

Mortars alone caused about 38% of the total casualties, but their lethality was only 0.12. The lethality of fragments from all explosive munitions (that is, mortars, grenades, artillery, and mines) averaged 0.11. In view of the difficulty in deploying conventional artillery in an overgrown, triple-canopy jungle island like

TABLE 2-5

AMERICAN CASUALTIES IN THE BOUGAINVILLE CAMPAIGN: CASUALTY GENERATION AND LETHALITY BY WEAPON

Weapon	Total Casualties	Living	Dead	Lethality of Weapon
Mortar	693	611 (43%)	82 (22%)	0.12
Rifle	445	302 (21%)	143 (38%)	0.32
Grenade	224	210 (15%)	14 (4%)	0.05
Artillery	193	172 (12%)	21 (6%)	0.11
Machine gun	152	64 (4%)	88 (24%)	0.58
Mine	34	21 (2%)	13 (3%)	0.38
Miscellaneous*	47	35 (3%)	12 (3%)	0.26
Totals	1,799	1,415	373	
			Average Lethality:	0.21

*Aerial bombs, pistols, bayonets, and similar weapons

Source: Reference 4

Bougainville, it is interesting to note the important casualty-generating role that mortars played. In this tactical milieu, bullets did most of the killing, but fragment wounds constituted most of the military surgeons' work, similar to the situation that was occurring at the same time in the European theater.

Although this study is far and away the most authoritative on weapons effects, the tactical situation that existed in Bougainville does not describe tank-heavy mechanized operations such as those that have occurred in Europe and the Middle East.

British Data from the Invasion of Normandy, June-July 1944

One of the British operational research groups who studied the Normandy invasion obtained these data retrospectively by analyzing field, medical, and hospital records. Since the data are based upon 3,609 of the approximately 50,000 casualties sustained by the British over the 6-week Normandy campaign, the sampling methodology is a variable that might limit the data's usefulness (Table 2-6).[12]

Although the invasion of Normandy was discrete in time and place, these data were collected from a heterogeneous assortment of tactical deployments including an amphibious invasion, several urban battles, and an enormous armor engagement (Operation Goodwood). About two-thirds of the hospitalized casualties had fragment wounds and one-third had bullet wounds. The percentage of bullet wounds shown in Table 2-6 is about 50% greater than the overall American rate in Europe, but a direct comparison of the two rates is not appropriate; the American experience in all European theaters was even less homogeneous than the British experience was at Normandy. Interestingly, Table 2-6 shows a distribution of casualties by type of projectile (bullet versus fragment), but not by weapon, that is similar to the distribution observed for hospitalized casualties in Bougainville (Table 2-5).

As the German data collectors had done (Table 2-4), the British data collectors made an effort to stratify

TABLE 2-6

BRITISH CASUALTIES IN THE NORMANDY INVASION

Weapon	Percentage of Total Casualties	Severity of Injuries: Trivial	Medium	Severe	Lethal	Calculated Lethality
Mine	4	34	42	33	25	0.19
Bomb	4	64	22	26	35	0.24
Shell	39	450	303	281	356	0.27
Mortar	21	184	228	199	134	0.18
Grenade	1	13	10	8	5	0.14
Gunshot	31	177	235	284	439	0.39
Bayonet	—	3	4	2	4	0.31
Multiple	—	—	3	6	—	—
	Total Wounded	925	847	839	998	

Source: Reference 12

the casualties by the degree of severity of their injuries. Injuries classified as *minor* probably did not require admission to a medical treatment facility; those classified as *medium* may have been incapacitating (like fractures), but were unlikely to cause death; those classified as *severe* were probably critical life-threatening injuries (like penetrating head wounds); and *lethal* refers to the total mortality (that is, both the casualties who were killed outright and those who died later of their wounds). This study's potential weakness lies in its using the total mortality, because the effect of medical care cannot be gauged. The error, however, is likely to be small, because about 83% of the total British combat mortality during the campaign were killed outright.

Casualties wounded by shells appear to be distributed bimodally, with peaks occurring at both ends of the injury-severity curve. The distributions of gunshot and mortar wounds each show a single peak, skewed toward less-serious injuries for mortar wounds and more-serious injuries for bullet wounds. The data clearly show that a gunshot wound was more likely to be serious than a wound made by any other weapon.

Grenades played a limited role at Normandy. The overall lethality for fragmentation weapons is calculated to be 0.23, which is significantly less than the 0.39 lethality associated with bullets. A grenade's range was determined then solely by the distance that a soldier could throw it—obviously much less than the ranges of guns.

TABLE 2-7

ESTIMATED LETHALITY OF WEAPONS USED AGAINST THE U.S. ARMY DURING WORLD WAR II

	Lethality	
Wounding Weapon	Killed	Killed and Died
Small arms	0.34	0.38
Explosive projectile shells	0.22	0.26
Rockets and bombs	0.22	0.26
Grenades	0.05	0.08
Mines	0.18	0.22

Source: Reference 13

U.S. Army Casualties in World War II

Nearly 25 years were spent analyzing statistical samples obtained from medical field cards, unit operational records, and hospital records of the nearly one million American casualties of World War II. Of the problems inherent in analyzing such an enormous mass of raw data, the most serious potential threat to the accuracy of these data is the questionable validity of the original records that were entered in the field, especially those casualties in the "killed" category (Table 2-7).[13] The unfortunate need to pool together data from differing campaigns, battles, time frames, and even different services (that is, the army's land forces and air corps) created another weakness in the database.

These data suffer from two serious potential defects. First, the diagnosis of the cause of death and the identification of the ordnance responsible for those casualties who were killed in action depended upon the accuracy of the field medical tag or the death certificate. A recent analysis of the WDMET database of casualties from the Vietnam War suggests that the weapons were misidentified in at least 25% of the cases; it is safe to assume that these determinations were made no more accurately during World War II than they were during the Vietnam War.[8]

The second potential source of error stems from the manipulation of the data that needs to be performed in order to obtain the figures shown in Table 2-7. Published data give the percentages of casualties who were wounded by weapons of various types and who were classified as *(a)* killed in action, *(b)* died of wounds, and *(c)* wounded in action but survived. To calculate the percentage of casualties wounded by a given weapon, statisticians must necessarily weight the outcome categories by their observed frequencies. The required data in this instance are the percentages of the total casualty population in each of the outcome categories. These data for the U.S. Army in all theaters of World War II are: 24.5% killed in action, 3.4% died of wounds, and 72.1% wounded but survived.[13] Bearing in mind that multiplying two sets of data—each of which is subject to error—will compound the error, the calculated lethalities of 0.34 for small-arm wounds and 0.21 for fragment wounds are, surprisingly, quite similar to those observed in the British study of Normandy casualties (Table 2-6). The database also treats the fatal (killed in action) and nonfatal (hospitalized) wounds suffered by U.S. Army casualties separately (Tables 2-8 and 2-9).

Overall, the U.S. Army in World War II sustained about one-third of its battle deaths and about one-fifth

TABLE 2-8

U.S. ARMY CASUALTIES KILLED IN ACTION IN WORLD WAR II, BY MUNITION

Casualty	Total	EUR	MED	SWP	POA
		Theater of Action*			
		Numbers and Percentages of Known Killed**			
Killed	192,220	120,043	35,185	19,426	12,361
Killed by known munition	90,975	53,553	18,809	11,940	4,278
Bombs	1%	1%	2%	2%	2%
Shells***	50%	52%	65%	28%	40%
Bullets	32%	33%	20%	52%	44%
Mines	2%	2%	4%	2%	2%
Grenades	—	—	—	1%	1%

*EUR: European Theater
MED: Mediterranean Theater
SWP: Southwest Pacific
POA: Pacific Ocean Area

**Sums are less than 100% because combat losses sustained in aircraft and armored fighting vehicles were excluded

***Shell: artillery and mortar

Source: Reference 13

of its hospitalized wounded from bullet wounds. The great majority of the remainder in both categories sustained fragment wounds. When viewed theater-by-theater, the only significant deviation from this pattern is the higher proportion of casualties with bullet wounds in the Southwest Pacific Theater; this no doubt reflects the tactical realities of jungle warfare. Comparing the relative importance of small arms as a source of casualties in Europe in the two world wars (Tables 2-3 and 2-9) reveals the unexpected finding that small arms were more significant during World War II. One might have expected that the highly mechanized campaigns in Europe during 1944–1945 would have deemphasized the importance of the infantryman and his rifle. Apparently this did not happen, perhaps because much of the actual fighting was done by mechanized or motorized infantry. Of course, the logic of speculating about the impact of American tactics by studying American casualties is flawed; we need to know the sources of casualties in the German army in France and Germany but, unfortunately, such data no longer exist.

U.S. Army Casualties in the Korean War, 1950–1953

The official U.S. Army medical historian of the American experience in Korea required nearly 15 years to analyze the data obtained from the more than 100,000 American army casualties of the Korean War. This database is considerably more valuable to medical officers seeking to understand the nature of combat injury and field medical care in general than the same author's World War II medical-statistics volume.[14] Not only was the database from Korea a more manageable size than the World War II database, but the statisticians also recognized that lumping together data from diverse time frames and tactical postures was unsatisfactory. Once again, the accuracy of data recorded in the field must not be taken for granted, and an independent source did not specify the proportion of casu-

TABLE 2-9

U.S. ARMY CASUALTIES HOSPITALIZED IN WORLD WAR II, BY MUNITION

Casualty	Total	EUR	MED	SWP	POA
		Theater of Action*			
	Numbers and Percentages of Total Hospitalized Population**				
Hospitalized	599,724	393,987	107,323	59,646	33,556
Munitions involved					
Bombs	2%	1%	2%	3%	3%
Shells***	57%	59%	62%	41%	49%
Bullets	20%	19%	14%	32%	29%
Mines	4%	4%	5%	2%	1%
Grenades	2%	2%	2%	7%	2%

*EUR: European Theater
MED: Mediterranean Theater
SWP: Southwest Pacific
POA: Pacific Ocean Area

**Sums are less than 100% because combat losses sustained in aircraft and armored fighting vehicles were excluded
***Shell: artillery and mortar

Source: Reference 13

alties in each outcome category. Nevertheless, the lethalities of the weapons employed (Table 2-10) can be computed. The sample population contained about 42% of the total American soldiers killed in action in Korea; 19.7% were killed in action, 2.1% died of their wounds, and 78.2% were wounded but survived. The lethality of small arms during the Korean War (0.26) is about one-third below that calculated for all previous wars, but the overall lethality for fragmentation weapons (0.22) is similar.

Table 2-11 presents the actual numbers of U.S. Army soldiers who were wounded during the Korean War. When the data are examined by weapon, the large number of soldiers whose deaths could not be definitely attributed to a specific weapon makes the implausibly low lethality calculated from the crude data suspect (for example, for grenades, 0.01 and for bullets, 0.11). However, if we assume that the sample of those killed for whom the causative weapon has been assigned accurately reflects the whole, then bullets killed 33% and fragments 62%.

We are on more solid analytic ground when examining the data for those casualties who were wounded: Bullets wounded 28% and fragments wounded 66%. One of the most valuable aspects of this database is its description of how the tactical situation alters the mix of wounding weapons. The data (available for wounded only) indicate that small arms caused almost one-half the wounding in operations such as pursuits and withdrawals. When soldiers were engaged in static defensive operations from fixed lines, however, bullets accounted for only about 15% of the casualties. These differences undoubtedly arise from the fact that concealment and cover are much more difficult for soldiers to obtain when they are either advancing or retreating. Furthermore, since whole campaigns can be so characterized, it is not surprising to find that during the period July-November 1950, when the front rapidly shifted back and forth, small arms accounted for 37% of the casualties. Conversely, only 11% of them

TABLE 2-10

ESTIMATED LETHALITY OF WEAPONS IN KOREA

	Lethality	
Wounding Weapon	Killed in Action	Total Killed in Action and Died of Wounds
Small arms	0.23	0.26
Explosive projectile	0.20	0.22
Shells, rockets, and bombs	0.17	0.34
Grenades	0.03	0.04
Land mines	0.22	0.25
Other fragmentation munitions	0.50	0.54

Source: Reference 14

sustained bullet wounds during the period October 1951-July 1953. During this time, as truce talks proceeded, the tactical situation was defensive and conducted behind well prepared fortified lines, reminiscent of World War I trench warfare.

TABLE 2-11

AMERICAN SOLDIERS KILLED AND WOUNDED IN KOREA, BY WEAPON

Missile	Killed	Wounded
Bullet	2,584	19,833
Shell	3,859	36,379
Mine	305	2,401
Grenade	97	6,557
Unknown	10,643	1,377

Source: Reference 14

U.S. Army and Marine Corps Casualties in Vietnam, 1965–1970

Although the official medical statistical history of the Vietnam War has not yet been published, information exists on weapons effects.[15, 16] The most authoritative and useful database on the nature of combat injury extant was compiled by WDMET in Vietnam. It consists of detailed descriptions (written records and photos) of *(a)* the tactical posture, *(b)* the nature of the wound (including autopsy results for those killed), *(c)* the wounding weapon, *(d)* the field care, and *(e)* the hospital care for nearly 8,000 U.S. Army and Marine Corps casualties during 1967–1969. Ironically, the WDMET database describes the same type of warfare—low-intensity, light-infantry jungle operations—that the Bougainville study covered. No database that specifically applies to understanding the nature of combat injuries in high-intensity warfare with its abundance of armor, aircraft, and artillery exists.

The analysis of the wounded in Vietnam shown in Table 2-12 shares the problems that analyses of other databases have—the accuracy of the field data and the need to specify the proportion of casualties in the outcome categories—with the added difficulty that the actual number of American casualties in the Viet-

TABLE 2-12

U.S. ARMY CASUALTIES IN VIETNAM: OUTCOME BY TYPE OF WEAPON

Wounding Weapon	Outcome		Lethality Assumptions	
	Deaths	Survivors	A*	B**
Small arms	51%	16%	0.49	0.30
Fragmentation munitions	36%	65%	0.14	0.07
Mines and booby traps	11%	15%	0.15	0.08

*Assumption A: excluding those carded for record only, 23% were fatally wounded
**Assumption B: including those carded for record only, 12% were fatally wounded
Source: Reference 15

nam War is still disputed. Data shown under Assumption A excluded those casualties who were carded for record only, while Assumption B included them.[3]

It is intriguing to compare the American experiences in France in 1918 with those in Vietnam 1965–1970. If the wounding weapon were the sole criterion, surgeons might have difficulty telling the two wars apart. Yet, a comparison of the casualties who did not leave the battlefield alive tells a different story. In Vietnam, 51% of those killed (Table 2-12) sustained bullet wounds, while in France in 1918, fewer than 10% of those who were killed were hit by bullets (Table 2-3). The tactics and weapons employed in both wars must be incorporated into a plausible explanation of both the similarities and dissimilarities. Small-unit actions with frequent, deadly firefights characterized the action in Vietnam. When the enemy used fragmentation weapons, they did not employ conventional artillery of the type that made the massive barrages that occurred in World War I possible, but rather they used mortars and grenades: low-lethality but high-casualty-generating weapons. Most soldiers and marines were killed by assault rifles during firefights, while most casualties were wounded by mortars and rocket-propelled grenade attacks on base camps (Table 2-13).[15] These data are perhaps the best twentieth-century examples showing that the tactical situation determines the casualty proportions that various kinds of weapons cause. During the search-and-destroy missions that were conducted in 1966, assault rifles were the weapons most likely to be used against American troops. By 1970, American forces were confined to base camps, and the only way the enemy could attack them was to employ rockets and mortars.

TABLE 2-13

U.S. ARMY CASUALTIES IN VIETNAM: TACTICAL POSTURE AND TYPE OF MISSILE

Projectile	Casualties* per Tactical Posture	
	Search and Destroy (1966)	Base Defense (1970)
Bullets	42%	16%
Fragments	50%	80%

*Wounded in action only
Source: Reference 15

In the particular sample of the WDMET database from which these data were gleaned (Table 2-14), the data collectors were nearly certain whether individual wounds were inflicted by bullets or by fragments from explosive munitions. Fifteen percent of the total group wounded by bullets and 29% of those killed by bullets had multiple wounds. About 75% of those with fragmentation wounds had multiple injuries. Since the 290 casualties sustained a total of 426 bullet wounds, the probability that a casualty would be fatally wounded

TABLE 2-14

U.S. ARMY CASUALTIES IN VIETNAM: OUTCOME BY TYPE OF PENETRATING MISSILE

Missile	Fatal	Nonfatal	Lethality
Bullets	124 (36*)	166 (7*)	0.43
Fragments	56	320	0.15
Both bullets and fragments	4	7	

*Multiple wounds

Source: Reference 8

by a single bullet can be calculated to be about 0.30.[8,16]

The data contained in Table 2-15 are drawn from two WDMET sources: *(a)* one that lists 7,964 casualties (essentially all of the WDMET casualties) both killed and wounded, caused by nineteen different types of weapons;[17] Table 2-15 records only the seven most common (which caused 91% of the total injuries); and *(b)* another that lists 5,329 wounded casualties.[18] Although the difference between these two casualty totals should equal those killed in action, the two sources of data comprising Table 2-15 do not exactly correspond. The second source lists more than thirty wounding-weapon categories; therefore, calculating lethality in this instance is inappropriate.

The WDMET database reflects the overall American casualty rate in the Vietnam War. Forty-six percent of those killed and 27% of those who survived long enough to be evacuated from the battlefield sustained bullet wounds. This distribution of casualties by weapon represents low-intensity or counterinsurgency actions in general. Most of those killed had been hit by small-arms fire and most of the surviving wounded had been injured by fragments produced by lower-lethality weapons including mortars, booby traps, and hand grenades. (An unknown fraction of the total casualty population, but almost certainly more than 10%, were victims of friendly fire.) Among those casualties not injured by bullets, the proportion of those fatally wounded may increase in the future, if weapons using shaped-charge warheads

TABLE 2-15

U.S. ARMY IN VIETNAM: CASUALTY GENERATION BY WEAPON

Weapon	Killed	Wounded	Percentage of Total
Bullets*	926	1,455	30
Mortars	187	1,299	19
Booby traps	388	734	14
RPG series**	396	561	12
Hand grenades***	115	786	11
Antipersonnel mines	30	239	3
Artillery	59	180	3

*About one-half were caused by AK47s; M16s caused 10% of the killed and 12% of the wounded.

**Shaped-charge warhead weapon of Soviet design, of which the RPG 2 and RPG 7 were the most common, used against both matériel and personnel

***Excluding rifle grenades and grenades that were used as booby traps

Source: References 17 and 18

TABLE 2-16

BRITISH CASUALTIES IN NORTHERN IRELAND

	Outcome		
Wounding Weapon	Fatal	Nonfatal	Lethality
Low-velocity bullets*	35	430	0.08
High-velocity bullets**	152	261	0.37
Fragmentation munitions	5	33	0.13
Homemade bombs	10	164	0.06
High-explosive devices	79	281	0.22
Hand-thrown missiles	0	304	—

*Of the 465 casualties with low-velocity bullet wounds, ninety were known to have wounds made by 0.22-inch, 0.38-inch, 0.45-inch, or 9-mm bullets. Lethality in this subgroup was 0.24.

**Of the 413 casualties with high-velocity bullet wounds, 169 casualties were known to have wounds made by 0.303-inch, 0.30-inch, M1 Garrand, 5.56-mm, or 7.62-mm bullets. Lethality in this subgroup was 0.46.

Source: Reference 19

such as dual-purpose submunitions become more widespread.

Of course, we do not know the distribution of casualties by type of wounding weapon for the Viet Cong and North Vietnamese. The percentages of both those killed and those who survived their bullet wounds were probably quite low. The great majority of their casualties probably sustained fragmentation wounds from both conventional artillery and from rockets and bombs delivered by tactical air strikes.[8]

British Casualties in Northern Ireland, 1969-Present

Using computerized data-entry forms, the British in Northern Ireland have compiled a state-of-the-art databank, and the information it contains is probably typical of the weapons effects seen in urban terrorist incidents (Table 2-16).[19] The data clearly show that small arms of military design killed by far the most casualties (54%). Overall, bullets caused a much higher proportion of the total wounded population than is commonly found on battlefields. This study is especially valuable because it permits comparison between the lethalities of typically military (0.37, the high-velocity bullets) and typically civilian (0.075, the low-velocity bullets) small arms. Furthermore, while 9% of the survivors of the low-velocity bullet wounds were found to be unfit for duty, 21% of survivors of high-velocity bullet wounds were considered unfit. The blast effects from high-explosive devices were second only to bullets as a cause of death.

Israeli Casualties in the Israeli-Lebanon War, 1982

While no official study applying to weapons effects and the nature of combat injuries in the Israeli-Lebanon War has yet been published by the government of Israel, two sources of information do exist. First, an entire issue of *Israeli Journal of Medical Science* was devoted to medical problems encountered in Lebanon.[20] The method of collecting data was rather interesting: Medical students on active reserve military status were assigned the task of preparing the data-collection forms, which frequently included interviewing surviving casualties (Table 2-17). And second, an Israeli medical officer collected data comparing the nature of combat injuries by weapon (Table 2-18) and in two distinctly different tactical postures: urban fighting and rural armor operations (Table 2-19).[21]

TABLE 2-17

WEAPONS EFFECTS IN THE 1982 ISRAELI-LEBANON WAR: I

Wounding Weapon	Percentage of Total Wounded	Hospitalized (N)	Killed (N)	Lethality
Shells (mortars, cannons, rockets)	77	827	80	0.11
Bullets	23	181	86	0.31

Source: Reference 20

These two sources probably include some of the same casualties; thus, information from the two databases cannot be added together.

Whether or not the data in Table 2-17 includes those casualties who died of their wounds is not specified, but the data in Table 2-18 definitely excludes this category. The data in the "hospitalized" and "killed" categories in Table 2-17 are from different researchers and may not be samples from the same original population of casualties. Table 2-17 indicates that only 11% of casualties wounded by fragmentation weapons were killed, but in Table 2-18, 25% of all casualties who were injured by fragments were killed. This large discrepancy seems unlikely to be an artifact of the data-collecting methodologies. About 20% of the data included in Table 2-17 pertains to casualties killed by antitank weapons, but whether their deaths were directly due to the weapons or to indirect causes such as secondary explosions cannot be determined.

Additional data apply to the effects that tactical posture and terrain have on the distribution of injuries caused by specific types of weapons (Table 2-19). The Israeli medical officer who collected these data sought to determine if differences existed between the distribution of wounds by weapon (the "epidemiology" of combat casualties) in urban and nonurban (open-terrain) warfare. Data were collected from two groups of Israeli casualties: *(a)* those injured while fighting in Beirut and several other cities and towns and *(b)* those injured while fighting in armor and mechanized operations in the field (especially the Bekka valley), which has characterized previous Israeli wars. Surprisingly, the Israeli findings do not conform to the picture of urban warfare that developed from the World War II experience. In Stalingrad, for example, small groups of assault troops, armed with grenades and automatic weapons, engaged in savage room-to-room and building-by-building fighting, interspersed with one side or the other calling in artillery or air strikes to demolish an enemy's position. Rather than showing the expected high incidence of casualties with wounds made by small arms, these data actually show the opposite. The major differences seen between the two groups are *(a)* the higher incidence of fragmentation injuries caused by explosive projectiles from artillery and mortars found in urban fighting and *(b)* the higher incidence of casualties injured by aerial bombs and antitank guns found in nonurban fighting. Rocket-propelled grenades (RPGs), the ubiquitous shaped-charge warheads, were commonly used in both tactical postures.

TABLE 2-18

WEAPONS EFFECTS IN THE 1982 ISRAELI-LEBANON WAR: II

Wounding Weapon	Wounded (N)	Killed (N)	Calculated Lethality
Artillery*	264	69	0.21
Small arms	198	77	0.28
Bombs	83	24	0.22
Rockets	77	25	0.24
Grenades	62	10	0.14
Mines	52	6	0.12

*Includes mortars

Source: Reference 21

TABLE 2-19

DISTRIBUTION OF ISRAELI CASUALTIES IN THE 1982 ISRAELI-LEBANON WAR BY WEAPON AND TERRAIN

	Terrain	
	Urban (N) = 580*	Nonurban (N) = 820*
Wounding Weapon	Percentage of Total Casualties	
Artillery and mortars	33	17
Small arms	18	21
Rocket-propelled grenades (RPGs)	19	10
Antitank weapons	3	10
Bombs	2	12
Rockets	5	9
Grenades	6	4
Mines	4	4
Booby traps	2	1
Miscellaneous	9	12

*Casualty count includes both killed and nonfatally wounded.

Source: Reference 21

ASSESSING LETHALITY

All sources agree that the probability that a bullet wound will have a fatal outcome is about one in three, except for the notably different findings from the Korean War. It is probably safe to say that this means that a bullet striking the human body at random will kill about one-third of the time. The lethality of multiple bullet wounds (assuming that the individual wounds are randomly distributed) should approximately equal $1 - (1 - p_1)(1 - p_2) \ldots (1 - p_n)$, where p is the lethality of the *nth* hit. Thus the probability of being fatally wounded by two gunshot wounds, either one of which has a lethality of one-third, should be 0.55. For three wounds, the probability should be 0.70.

Aimed fire by snipers should be more lethal because the head and chest are the usual targets. However, recent data compiled by the British army in Northern Ireland, against whom sniping is common, do not indicate a significant increase in lethality for bullets. Death occurred in 152 of 413 (37%) soldiers hit by high-velocity bullets (mostly 5.56-mm and 7.62-mm), not greatly different from the lethality calculated from other databases.[19]

The databases that permit calculations of lethality to be made indicate that the lethality of fragmentation munitions appears to range between 0.10 for mortar bombs and grenades to about 0.20 for conventional artillery shells. It is unclear to what extent, if any, data reported from the Vietnam and Israeli-Lebanon wars reflect the lethality of improved-fragmentation munitions (Tables 2-12 through 2-15 and 2-17 through 2-19). A recent analysis of the WDMET data suggests that the lethality of 105-mm random-fragmentation shells (0.21) is slightly, but not significantly, higher than the lethality of 105-mm improved-fragmentation shells (0.16).[8] Injuries that antitank and antiaircraft weapons make on crews of armored fighting vehicles, ground-support aircraft, and helicopters are generally more lethal than injuries that result from small arms and fragmentation munitions (their lethalities range between 0.4 and 0.8), but since these crews normally constitute only a small fraction of the total force, the infantry ground casualties dominate the overall mortality.

It is possible that a useful measure of the lethality of a battlefield (but not the number of casualties) could be obtained by appropriately weighting the established lethalities of the deployed weapons by the observed number of casualties generated by type of weapon. For example, the probability of being killed if wounded on a battlefield in which only small arms are used should approach one in three. At the other extreme, a battlefield on which only hand grenades were used would perhaps yield one out of ten of those wounded being killed. For any historical battle, the probability of being killed if injured should fall between these two (or similar) limits, and would depend upon the mix of weapons. This approach, if valid, suggests that, in the sense of the probability of being killed if injured, Vietnam was the most lethal battlefield for Americans.

Future developments will probably not alter these conclusions. If anything, ordnance design is evolving toward *(a)* assault rifles that fire even more rapidly and *(b)* improved fragmentation munitions that create more numerous—but less lethal—fragments, which will increase the tendency for small arms to be the most lethal weapons on conventional battlefields.

ASSESSING CASUALTY GENERATION

The proportion of combat casualties caused by specific types or classes of military weapons has varied widely in the wars of this century. Even if the analysis is confined to the population of those who are killed, the observed proportion of casualties with bullet wounds to casualties with fragment wounds has varied from 1:10 to 1:1. Although the primary determinants of casualty generation are no doubt *(a)* the tactics that are employed and *(b)* the state of weapons technology, simple formulations seem unlikely to explain the observed variations in the distribution of wounds by their causative weapon. The best that can be said is that fragmentation munitions—whether artillery shells, mortar bombs, or grenades—account for most of the living wounded and those who are killed. Bullets are more lethal than fragments, but fragments injure—and kill—more casualties.

Attackers are likely to sustain a higher proportion of casualties from small arms when they assault a fortified position or move across terrain that offers poor concealment. For example (although the actual data do not exist), it would not be surprising to find that the great majority of the German parachutists killed during their airborne assault on Crete in 1941 were hit by small-arms fire. Defenders are likely to be subjected to artillery and rocket bombardment, as well as to airstrikes made with explosive munitions in preparation for an assault. Thus the proportion of fragment wounds will be greater relative to bullet wounds, at least in the early stage of the battle. (Verdun is a case in point. Estimates of French casualties during the first German attack, in February 1916, indicate that artillery caused 80% or more of the wounding.)

But this assessment is too simplistic if it fails to consider other relevant variables. If, as is likely, most German battle casualties in Crete were caused by small arms, it is also likely that the reason why is complex. While the attacking Germans were very exposed as they jumped from their aircraft, the fact that their opponents had only small arms with which to defend their positions is equally important. Comprehending the observed distribution of casualties by weapon requires knowing both the tactical posture and the nature of the deployed weaponry on both sides. The data (both for casualties and weapons) included in this chapter almost exclusively describe the winners of the battles. But understanding why the Israelis observed the types of casualties that they did in Beirut, for example, requires more than a superficial knowledge of how their enemies fought. Perhaps the generally accepted view of them as aggressive street fighters armed with a plentiful supply of AK47s is inaccurate. If so, then the observed percentage of Israeli urban-warfare casualties who were wounded by small arms might not be so unexpected.

MEDICAL CRITERIA FOR ASSESSING WEAPONS EFFECTIVENESS

Quantifying the expenditure of medical resources per casualty by class of weapon is an attractive but little-used operational definition of weapons effectiveness. Theoretically, the use of medical resources can be quantitated by counting the man-days spent caring for each casualty, the number of surgical operations performed per casualty, the money expended, and so forth, but except in isolated instances, such data do not exist. Surrogate measurements such as the average time a soldier spends in a noneffective status per class of weapon, changes in a soldier's physical condition, and the probability that the soldier will be discharged for a medical reason following a combat injury made by a specific class of weapon are both useful and practicable, however.

Data on *(a)* man-days lost and *(b)* the percentage of soldiers discharged, both as functions of the class of injuring weapon, were collected during World War II (Table 2-20).[13] Judging from the days soldiers were noneffective and the probability that they would require separation from the army for medical reasons, injuries caused by land mines and bullets have consumed more medical resources per casualty than injuries that were caused by any other weapon system. About 30% of those who were shot received disability discharges. If we remember that about one-third of those who were shot were fatally wounded, then it becomes apparent that shooting a soldier will effectively remove him as a combatant. Clearly, however, within the entire casualty population, those with fragmentation wounds from explosive shells utilize medical resources more than casualties from any other weapon category do.

One of the uniquely valuable aspects of the Bougainville study is its detailed determination of the echelon of the medical system that casualties reached before they returned to duty (Table 2-21). Because Bougainville is a small island and the combat zone included most of it, all casualties requiring more than a few weeks of care were evacuated to safe offshore islands. Furthermore, because the logistics of supporting extensive medical facilities in so isolated an area proved difficult, casualties whose recoveries would require months were promptly evacuated to the continental United States (CONUS). The Bougainville study recognized three levels of care, which modern terminology designates: *(a)* the combat zone, *(b)* the communication zone, and *(c)* CONUS. Bullets were much more likely to cause a wound requiring evacuation to CONUS (implying a serious wound). Conversely, most survivors of fragmentation-munition wounds returned to duty from the combat zone (implying that their wounds, particularly those made by grenades, were of modest severity).

TABLE 2-20

U.S. ARMY, ALL THEATERS IN WORLD WAR II: DISCHARGE AND NONEFFECTIVE DAYS AS FUNCTIONS OF WOUNDING WEAPONS

Weapon or Missile	Total Wounded	Disability Discharge	Percentage of Wounded Discharged	Days Non-effective
Shell	340,651	73,158	21	123
Bullet	120,455	36,240	30	158
Land mine	25,529	8,267	32	174
Grenade	14,929	3,063	21	105
Bomb	10,484	1,704	16	94

Source: Reference 13

TABLE 2-21

U.S. ARMY, BOUGAINVILLE CAMPAIGN: DISPOSITION OF SURVIVING WOUNDED BY CAUSATIVE WEAPON

Weapon	Casualties (N)	Returned to Duty From		
		Combat Zone	Communication Zone	CONUS
Rifle	306	37%	31%	32%
Machine gun	64	34%	17%	49%
Mortar	611	53%	28%	19%
Artillery	150	56%	26%	18%
Grenade	210	63%	14%	18%

Source: Reference 4

Data from the Korean War tell a similar story: 37% of survivors with land-mine injuries were evacuated to CONUS, and about one-half of those evacuated were given disability separations. One-third of casualties with wounds made by small arms required evacuation, and one-third of these evacuees were separated. As in World War II, the greatest claim on medical resources came from the large population who had been wounded by shell fragments.[14] No data analyzing noneffective days by class of weapon exist from the Korean War.

INDICES OF INCAPACITATION

For more than 100 years, weapons designers and military medical scientists have striven to develop concepts of weapons effectiveness that go beyond such simple outcomes as death and wounding. Their goal has been to find a projectile's measurable property that can be correlated with the probability that it will cause a measurable, functional, militarily relevant disability. More often than not, the projectile's ability to incapacitate has been related to mechanical properties such as the projectile's mass, velocity, and such derived parameters as its momentum or kinetic energy, but contemporary computer-simulation techniques allow a more sophisticated approach.

Historical Attempts to Quantify Incapacitation

One of the first attempts to quantify a projectile's ability to incapacitate occurred during the nineteenth century and concluded that delivering 58 foot-pounds (equivalent to 83 joules in today's nomenclature) of kinetic energy would probably put a soldier out of action. This figure's origin is shrouded in mystery, and its validity is dubious. Thought by some to have originated in Germany, it is said to have been derived from experiments in which one-ounce lead balls were shot at horses. Others say that the experiments were done in France, with half-inch balls shot at cadavers.[22]

Whatever its derivation, this approach's obvious weakness lies in the fact that the damage done by 58 foot-pounds depends upon the body part that is hit. (To put 58 foot-pounds of kinetic energy in perspective, a beanball thrown by a major-league pitcher will deliver about 90 foot-pounds, an uppercut by a heavyweight boxer several hundred foot-pounds, most rifle rounds more than 1,000 foot-pounds, and a typical kinetic energy antitank projectile over 1 million foot-pounds.) Obviously, the outcomes when 58 foot-pounds are delivered to a finger and to the brain stem will be quite different. This conceptual deficiency, and the need for a more functional test that recognized the different vulnerability of body parts to injury, has been recognized by several authorities, including the American military surgeon Louis A. La Garde, whose textbook *Gunshot Injuries* was the standard on ballistics and war surgery for many years.[23]

La Garde's involvement in assessing weapons effectiveness dated back to the Spanish-American War and the ensuing Philippine insurrection. Then as now, some ballisticians believed that a bullet striking almost anywhere on the body could cause immediate incapacitation due to shock. The shock itself was thought to make the victim fall down and stop fighting. The pathophysiology of this mysterious phenomenon was believed to be related to an indirect effect of the bullet on the nervous system, and this attribute was referred to as the bullet's stopping power or its knockdown power. Military handguns then in use were found to have inadequate stopping power, since the enemy did not fall down unless the bullet fractured a leg bone or hit a vital organ such as the heart.[24]

La Garde and members of the U.S. Army Ordnance Corps were assigned the task of testing existing pistol ammunition and finding a pistol round with the desired stopping power. Working in the Chicago stockyards in 1904, they shot unanesthetized cattle with various weapons, assessing incapacitation by recording the number of bullets required to knock the animal down. Recognizing that a shot into the heart would have similar stopping power regardless of the ammunition they used, they tried to hit only body parts that would not cause immediate death. In a typical experiment, they shot one animal for each type of ammunition tested and reported:

> .45 Colt 220-grain lead bullet with small flat on [*sic*] point
> 720 fps, 288 foot-pounds
> 7th animal: Bull, 10 years old, 1,300 lbs
>
> Shot through lungs. At 1 minute, shot again through lungs. At 2 minutes 35 seconds, shot through abdomen and fell. At 2 minutes 45 seconds, shot again through abdomen, got up, then fell again—tried to regain his feet for 70 seconds—and was killed by hammer blows to the head.[24]

The sad truth about wound-ballistics research is that much information that could be relevant and important is gathered under conditions that are barbarous as well as scientifically unsound, and information that is more esthetically pleasing and scientifically elegant often consists of esoterica that are meaningful in a laboratory but irrelevant to battlefield conditions. While La Garde's Chicago-stockyard experiments fall into the relevant-but-barbarous category, they showed that no shock, stopping-, or knockdown power was observable beyond that directly attributable to the effect of the bullet at the site of wound. His official report stated the only reasonable conclusion regarding handguns: "[They] offer no hope of stopping an adversary by shock."[24] Inexplicably, not only did La Garde not restate this firm conclusion in *Gunshot Injuries,* he also misquoted his own official report, and suggested that he had actually observed shock. Because of this misinformation, for the past 70 years ballisticians have continued to search for a mathematical explanation of the shock that La Garde said he observed in bullet wounds made by handguns.

Wounds made by military rifles and machine guns are frequently incapacitating, however. One of the specific goals of the WDMET study was to collect information on the behavior of soldiers after they were wounded. The database also includes the soldiers' (and their buddies') recollections of their behavior just before they were wounded. Almost every casualty who was shot—whether in the head, trunk, legs, or arms—immediately stopped his pre-wounding behavior. In fact, most casualties fell to the ground and lay there, suggesting that assault rifles and machine guns do indeed have stopping power.[8]

Modern Concepts of Personnel Vulnerability: Computer Man

The U.S. Army has led efforts to find a scientific basis for predicting the effects of ballistic injury on a soldier's performance. The effort is distinguished by: *(a)* emphasizing fragments rather than bullets, *(b)* recognizing that some body regions are more vulnerable to ballistic injury than others, *(c)* establishing concrete criteria for incapacitation, based on well-defined soldier tasks required to complete a given mission, *(d)* quantitating the wounding effects of missiles by their mass, velocity, and shape, *(e)* expressing results in terms of probability, and *(f)* using sophisticated computer technology.

The need to optimize the wounding potential of preformed fragments has driven the emphasis on fragmentation injury. What is the combination of mass and velocity most likely to wound? A random-fragmentation munition such as an 81-mm mortar bomb breaks into a wide range of different-sized fragments, but only the heaviest—those weighing 1–10 g and constituting about 10% of the total number of fragments—are likely to retain sufficient velocity beyond 50 m to wound. The smallest fragments—those weighing less than 100 mg—will not even travel 50 m, although their initial velocities may be 4,000–5,000 fps. So fragments ranging in weight from several hundred milligrams to one gram (the median fragment mass in the WDMET study is 200 mg) and with velocities of several thousand feet per second seem to be reasonable values for the desired mass and velocity.[8]

But how can this conjecture be tested short of war? Modern mathematical modeling can address such problems. Researchers "shoot" a fragment of specified mass, velocity, and shape at a random target on a "Computer Man."[25]

The fragment's mass, velocity, and shape determine the depth and lateral extent of the wound tract. For any given hypothetical wound, these parameters are known from a well-documented body of knowledge derived from experimentation on animals and the tissue-simulant gelatin. (This is discussed at length in Chapter Four of this textbook.) The researchers select a computerized simulation of the external projection of the human body as the target. Next, they superimpose the depth of the fragment's penetration and the lateral extent of damage (the width of the permanent cavity plus several millimeters around the permanent tract) caused by the fragment's passage on an axial section of the computerized target. Then, the researchers medically assess how the injured structures lying along the wound tract might affect the performance of the limbs "[b]ecause of the intimate dependence of perfomance on the behavior of the limbs."[25] This prediction of incapacitation assumes that no medical care is given. The level of incapacitation is then related to four tactical roles (assault, defense, supply, and reserve) at six post-wounding times (30 seconds to 24 hours). The researchers then repeat the procedure for many different fragment masses, velocities, and trajectories through the Computer Man. Although this was not part of the original methodology, the effects of fragments with oblique trajectories (that is, trajectories that traverse two or more axial cross sections) can now be studied.

The computer generates a diagram similar to the one shown in Figure 2-1. The probability of incapacitation can be understood as an expected value. For example, a 75% probability of incapacitation means that there is a 100% probability that a soldier will be unable to perform 75% of the tasks required to carry out a given mission. It does *not* mean that there is a 75% probability that 100% of the tasks cannot be performed. One limitation of the original Computer-Man methodology is that the computer is not programmed to include a medical reason for the soldier's incapacitation. For example, we are not told whether a soldier who is incapacitated because he cannot move his arm has a soft-tissue wound of the arm, a fractured humerus, a transected brachial plexus, or some other injury.

Incapacitation is predicted to be a function of not only the fragment's mass (M), but also its velocity (V) raised to the 3/2 power. Thus incapacitation is not directly related to either kinetic energy ($1/2\ MV^2$) or momentum (MV). While the biophysical explanation for this function seems intuitively obvious to some ballisticians, others disagree. This line of reasoning holds that, other factors being unchanged, the greater the fragment's mass, the larger the fragment will be, and therefore, the larger the hole that it makes as it penetrates will be. Similarly, other factors being equal, the greater the fragment's velocity, the greater its depth of penetration, and the greater the probability that it will strike a body part whose function is necessary for performing a soldier's tasks. Finally, we might expect other than a linear function because biological phenomena are notoriously complex. The point in Figure 2-1 indicated by the X is satisfied by such combinations of fragment mass and velocity as 2 g and 1,000 fps, 693 mg and 2,000 fps, and 377 mg and 3,000 fps. Since the corresponding calculated kinetic-energy values for these combinations of mass and velocity are 69, 95, and 117 foot-pounds, respectively, the historical value of 58 foot-pounds for incapacitation may not be all that dubious.

The subtlety, sophistication, and complexity of this methodology has only been suggested in this chapter's introductory treatment, and interested readers should consult the primary source for a detailed discussion of Computer Man.[25] Medical commanders and staff officers should also be aware that similar analyses have been performed for blast and blunt traumas and for burns.

The ability to predict the magnitude of the treatment problem that results from a combat casualty's missile wound will probably interest medical officers more than predictions of soldier-incapacitation will. The Computer-Man methodology is also well-suited for this purpose.[26] An extensive body of experimental data exists showing that kinetic-energy expenditure along a missile's trajectory through the tissue simulant gelatin correlates with the permanent tract's cross-sectional area or volume made by the same missile in living soft tissue. After researchers determine the kinetic energy that will be expended along the trajectory of a fragment of specific mass, velocity, and shape, they superimpose the resulting energy-deposit contour along the missile's trajectory onto a randomly selected axial cross section of the computer-simulated body. Then they assess the severity of the injury, based upon the interaction of the missile and the organs in its path.

This approach recognizes two degrees of injury severity: lethal and serious. *Lethal* wounds are those

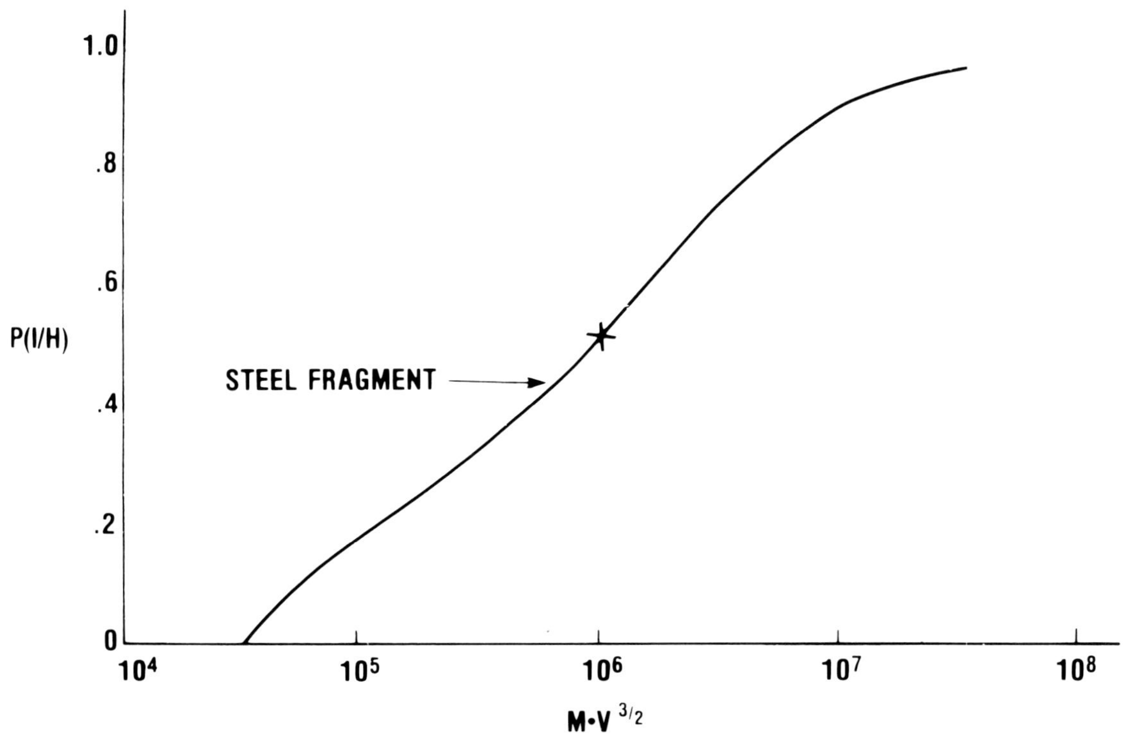

Fig. 2-1. The probability that a steel fragment will incapacitate a soldier. P(I|H) represents the probability of incapacitation if the soldier is wounded; M, the fragment's mass in grains; and V, its velocity in fps. Notice that the relationship is semilogarithmic: The point labelled X can be interpreted to mean that an irregular steel fragment with mass and velocity such that $M \times V^{3/2} = 1 \times 10^6$ striking a soldier at random will prevent him from performing 50% of his duties in an assault that began 5 minutes after he was wounded.
Source: Redrawn from reference 25

of the heart, large blood vessels, lung hilum, the midline central nervous system, and certain abdominal structures such as the hepatic hilum. In this computer program, lethal does not necessarily mean that death is certain, only that it is probable even with optimal care. *Serious* wounds, those that make it unlikely that a soldier will return to duty, are those of the cranial, pleural, or peritoneal cavities in general (excluding wound tracts that involve organs whose injuries would be lethal), large muscular wounds, and bony and neurovascular wounds of the extremities. While modern computer technology makes the study of multiple trajectories produced by many missiles of different masses, shapes, and velocities possible (Figure 2-2), the computer does not tell us anything about the pathophysiology of the casualty's hypothetical injury. For example, judging from the missile's trajectory and the computer's assessment of the degree of injury severity, the simulated casualty described in Figure 2-2 might have a tension pneumothorax, a massive hemothorax, or an open sucking chest wound.

Of course, a computer's predictions are only as good as its program. Although there can be little doubt that this technological approach is the correct one to solve the physical aspect of this biophysical problem, the same is not necessarily true of its medical aspect. As proponents of Computer Man frankly admit:

> [o]f crucial significance to the study are the judgments made by the medical assessors on the relationships between behavior of the limbs and the ability of the wounded "enemy" soldier to carry out his assigned task.[25]

A similar concern applies to the injury-severity assessment. Nevertheless, evidence strongly suggests that the Computer-Man methodology may have validity. A recent analysis of the WDMET database found that 382 casualties with penetrating wounds of the thorax had an observed mortality of 65%.[8] About two-thirds of these casualties had been wounded by 7.62 x 39-mm rounds, for which $M \times V^{3/2}$ equals about 1.0×10^7. According to the Computer-Man predictions, this bullet's lethality is about 0.70 (Figure 2-2).

The casualty's behavioral or psychological status, especially immediately after being wounded, remains

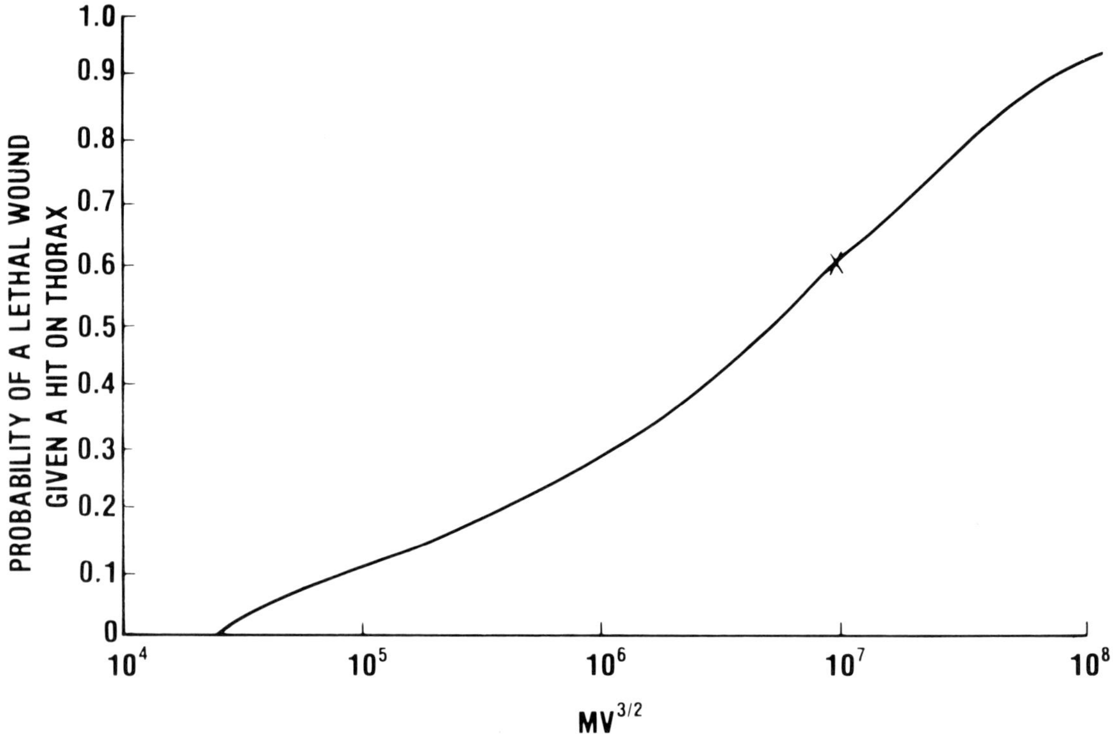

Fig. 2-2. This graph shows a predicted relationship between the probability that a projectile will create a lethal wound in the thorax and its physical parameters (that is, the product of mass and velocity raised to the 3/2 power). When $M \times V^{3/2} = 1 \times 10^7$, which corresponds to a typical M43 ball (marked X on the graph), the probability that a thoracic wound will be lethal approaches two out of three.
Source: Redrawn from reference 26

inscrutable. The WDMET data clearly demonstrate that the great majority (about 90%) of casualties who were wounded by exploding munitions immediately fell to the ground and frequently remained lying there for some minutes. Whether this behavior resulted from their sudden absorption of some critical number of foot-pounds of kinetic energy, a self-preserving reflex induced by a bright flash and a loud noise, or the fact that there was no need to move is not so clear. Of course, incapacitation that begins, or continues for, hours after wounding is a different matter, not being so subject to intangibles.

An important related problem is how to predict the effect of multiple wounds. How should the potential synergistic interaction of many wounds in a casualty be assessed? This problem remains to be solved. Thus, even though Computer Man in its present state has great practical use and considerable heuristic value, it needs further refinement.

Relative Incapacitation Index

Although it uses much of the same methodology that Computer Man does, the Relative Incapacitation Index (RII) has a different focus and emphasizes a different aspect of the projectile-target interaction.[27] The focus has come from civilian law-enforcement agencies such as the Federal Bureau of Investigation (FBI), who want to arm their agents with weapons capable of immediately stopping a felon who is committing a crime. There must also be little risk to bystanders. This proviso precludes the FBI from using military weapons such as submachine guns or hand grenades; their only practical alternative weapon is the handgun. Thus, the FBI's need for optimal performance from its ammunition and weapons has allowed the old question of stopping power to be reassessed with the entire armamentarium of modern computer-oriented ballistic modeling.

The aspect of the projectile-target interaction that RII emphasizes is temporary cavitation. As a projectile passes through a target with viscoelastic properties—such as the human body—energy transfer is manifested in two ways: *(a)* laceration of tissue along the projectile's pathway, which usually is the major determinant of the size of the *permanent wound tract*, and *(b)* radial displacement, with stretching and tearing of the tissue surrounding the projectile's pathway, which

TABLE 2-22

STOPPING POWER OF PISTOL AMMUNITION

	Pistol Ammunition	
Result of Firing	Sheriff RII = 13.3	Police RII = 6.4
Felons shot	28	32
Felons killed	14	18
Felons killed instantly	4	5
Rounds fired per officer	1.6	1.7
Number of organs hit per felon	3.1	3.2

Source: Reference 28

creates the *temporary cavity*. (These phenomena are discussed in great detail in Chapter Four.) RII assumes that temporary cavitation is the major wounding mechanism.

To assess RII, researchers first shoot potentially useful bullets into gelatin blocks to determine the physical characteristics of the temporary cavity that the bullet creates. Next, they determine the contour of the maximum instantaneous temporary cavity for that bullet. In simulated handgun shootouts, they select the body sites most likely to be hit by experienced law-enforcement officers. Then they superimpose the contour of the maximum temporary cavity onto those selected axial cross sections of Computer Man and medically assess the degree of incapacitation likely to result from damage done at each increment of the projectile's path through the tissue. After the incremental incapacitations have been added together, they repeat the process until all cross sections corresponding to likely hits have been studied. The individual results are averaged and the final product is a number, the RII, specific for each type of ammunition. The higher the RII, the likelier the ammunition should be to cause a felon's immediate incapacitation. Relative Incapacitation Indices range between 1.2 (for the .38 special lead round-nose bullet) to 67.3 (for the .44 magnum jacketed hollow-point bullet). RIIs for common military rounds are 11 for the 9-mm parabellum fired by the Beretta M9 and 3.6 for the .45 ACP (better known as the Colt .45).

Fortuitously, actual field testing of RII predictions regarding handgun ammunition—and in a sense, the validity of the mathematical approach to assessing weapons effects—occurred. During 1978–1979, the Los Angeles Police Department and the Los Angeles County Sheriff's Office used 0.38-caliber pistol ammunition of different designs. The police used 150-grain Winchester round-nose bullets and the sheriff's office used 110-grain Federal jacketed hard-point bullets, with the sheriff's bullets having a much higher RII.[28] All other factors being equal, one might predict that to achieve their goal, the sheriff's officers fired fewer rounds per felon or, alternatively, killed more felons. The actual results are shown in Table 2-22.

Clearly, the superiority that the RII methodology predicted for the sheriff's ammunition was not seen. Whether or not this indicates a fallacy that might invalidate the entire mathematical-modeling approach is unclear, but readers should not forget that RII differs from the military applications of Computer Man in two ways: *(a)* the civilian sector requires immediate incapacitation, while the military modelers have emphasized both immediate and delayed incapacitation (that is, from 5 seconds to 24 hours) and *(b)* the RII methodology's assumption that temporary cavitation determines the outcome. What this field test clearly demonstrates, however, is that computer predictions need to be subjected to realistic tests.

PREDICTING THE EFFECTS OF FOREIGN WEAPONS

Predicting the nature of the next major war is a problem of compelling importance for military leaders. Modern computer technology holds the promise that the diverse factors that determine events at the tactical and operational levels can be successfully modeled. Medical commanders will be especially interested in two such simulations: *(a)* predicting casualty rates and *(b)* stratifying combat injuries by their anatomical location and severity. Computer-Man methodology can supply the information on stratification, and, together with an approach that couples a knowledge of weapons effects with the likelihood of their employment, will make a comprehensive prediction of the medical workload probable. Organizations such as the Armed Forces Medical Intelligence Center, the Army Materiel Systems Analysis Activity, and the Foreign Science Technology Center have adopted this approach.

Given a knowledge of the following factors, it is theoretically possible to predict the maximum number of casualties that will result from a given weapon's use:

- the weapons effects, including *(a)* the munition's characteristics such as the size, shape, and velocity of fragments; *(b)* the rate of fire; *(c)* the range required to hit the target, and the angle of impact for explosive munitions; and *(d)* the weapon's reliability
- the target's vulnerability, including *(a)* the tactical posture (for example, defending from a prepared position); *(b)* the terrain and the weather (for example, the forest in winter); and *(c)* the protective equipment available, individual (for example, helmets) and collective (for example, bunkers)

Calculating the mean area of effectiveness (also known as the lethal area) presents the results of com-

TABLE 2-23

CALCULATED MEAN AREA OF EFFECTIVENESS FOR SOVIET 160-mm HIGH-EXPLOSIVE HOWITZER SHELLS

P(CC | H) = 0.9

Environment: Open Burst Height: 3 m Burst Velocity: 400 m/s Angle of Impact: 50°		Troop Posture and Area of Effectiveness (m^2)		
		Standing	Prone	Foxhole
Casualty categories (CC) are assessed in terms of the probability of 90% incapacitation:				
Defense	30 sec	600	350	70
Assault	5 min	900	600	80
Supply	12 hr	1,100	600	90
Casualty categories (CC) are assessed in terms of medical consequences:				
Lethal		450	350	40
Both serious and lethal		1,200	800	60
All wounds		1,500	1,000	100

Source: Reference 21

puter simulations in a conceptually useful way. The mean area of effectiveness is defined as the area in which a given munition has a specific probability (P) of causing a given casualty outcome or casualty category (CC), for example, a serious wound, given that the weapon actually causes an injury or hit (H). These factors can be expressed mathematically as P(CC|H), and can yield the information, for example, that there is a 90% probability that a serious wound will result if a casualty is injured by a given weapon. The source document detailing the mean areas of effectiveness and their associated medical implications for foreign weapons is classified.[29] However, in order to acquaint potential users with the methodology, an unclassified example describing a *notational* weapon (that is, one that is feasible but presently nonexistent), has been prepared (Table 2-23).

The methodology used to generate Table 2-23 predicts, among other outcomes, that a soldier standing in an open field devoid of any cover has a very high probability of being fatally wounded if a shell with the specified characteristics bursts within 12 m of his position. A foxhole would appear to offer substantial protection: The lethal radius is reduced to 3.6 m. Clearly, if a medical commander knew all the relevant factors describing the troop concentration—including the total number present in the target area—a prediction of the medical workload could be made for a given action. By adding all the individual actions for a given battle, commanders or their staff officers could theoretically estimate both the total number of casualties and their requirements for medical care.

What should the military medical officer's attitude be towards this grand synthesis? There seems to be little doubt that accurate predictions of the wounding characteristics of a given munition can be made. Facts such as the number of fragments produced by a shell, their velocity and the distance they will travel, and the probability that they will hit a soldier are readily available. What a given hit will do to a soldier is perhaps less well established, but predictions of injury severity based on Computer-Man simulations may nevertheless be taken as a useful first approximation. The aspect of this approach that is most questioned (and most suspect) is that it requires a detailed knowledge of how the deployed weapons will be used in battle. This is no small problem. For example, operational research during World War II found that only one rifleman in ten was likely to fire his weapon in battle. Predicting the number of casualties on the basis of the number of rifles present will overestimate the number of casualties by a factor of ten.[30]

The probability that the weapon will hit its target is even harder to predict. Predicting what will happen if a munition hits within a certain distance of a target is one thing. It is much more difficult to accurately predict the number of times the weapon will have to be employed to hit within the selected distance from the target (Table 2-24).[31] (These data might apply to the performance of the notational munition described in

TABLE 2-24

EXPECTED FRACTION OF CASUALTIES FOR SOVIET 152-mm HOWITZERS FIRING HIGH-EXPLOSIVE MUNITIONS*

Radius of Target (m)	Number of Volleys/Shells	Expected Fractional Incapacitation for Assault Posture		
		Standing	Prone	Foxhole
100	1/18	0	0	0
	10/180	0.34	0.26	0.04
	20/360	0.48	0.39	0.08
200	20/360	0.43	0.36	0.07
350	20/360	0.26	0.21	0.04

*12-km range, proximity fuse, indirect fire by map coordinates
Source: Reference 31

Table 2-23.)

The following extreme example may help both to interpret Table 2-24 and to suggest the considerable difficulty inherent in predicting casualty rates. Assume that a single soldier stands at the center of a circle with a radius of 100 m, which is the target for a battery of 152-mm howitzers that are 12 km away. To be 100% certain to cause a 48% reduction in that soldier's ability to assume an assault posture, the howitzers would have to fire no fewer than 360 shells! This datum reflects artillery's well-known lack of pinpoint accuracy when used indirectly, and especially when firing conventional munitions. As the diagram in Figure 1-34 (in Chapter One) clearly shows, using cluster munitions greatly increases the probability that a hit will be made. These highly probabilistic assessments, together with the degradation of weapons effectiveness caused by the vagaries of human performance in battle (a factor that is more than a little refractory to computer modeling), requires that predicted casualty rates be assessed cautiously.

SUMMARY

Once casualty generation and lethality are defined so they can be applied to the data that are available, two generalizations emerge that apply to the wars of this century: Bullets kill people more effectively, but fragment wounds predominate on modern battlefields.

Incapacitation and injury severity, both logical endpoints of descriptions of weapons effectiveness, can certainly be rigorously defined. Mathematical models that relate incapacitation and injury severity to measurable properties of the wounding agent can also be developed. Military medical officers need to be conversant with this modern approach toward estimating personnel vulnerability on the battlefield—typified by the Computer-Man methodology—if for no other reason than to avail themselves of its considerable heuristic power. Furthermore, because it focuses attention on developing—and by implication, using—munitions that are designed to incapacitate rather than to kill, the Computer-Man methodology unexpectedly introduces ethical considerations that the military needs to ponder. Unfortunately, no evidence suggests that contemporary designers of small-arms ammunition have also been motivated by similar humanitarian considerations.

All too often, modern munitions are used in the spirit of the celebrated Confederate General Nathan Bedford Forrest's reputed declaration: "Fightin's fer killin'."

REFERENCES

1. Parkinson, R. 1979. *Clausewitz.* New York: Stein and Day.

2. Headquarters Department of the Army. 1985. *Planning for Health Service Support* [FM 8–55, 15 February 1985]. Washington, DC: Department of the Army.

3. Bzik, K. D., and Bellamy, R. F. 1984. A note on combat casualty statistics. *Milit. Med.* 149:229–230.

4. Oughterson, A. W.; Hull, H. C.; Sutherland, F. A.; and Greiner, D. J. 1962. Study on wound ballistics—Bougainville campaign. Chapt. 5 of *Wound Ballistics,* edited by J. C. Beyer, 281–436. Washington, DC: Office of the Surgeon General, Department of the Army.

5. Dupuy, T. N. 1982. *The evolution of weapons and warfare.* Indianapolis: The Bobbs-Merrill Company, Inc.

6. Adamson, P. B. 1977. A comparison of ancient and modern weapons in the effectiveness of producing battle casualties. *J. Roy. Army Med. Cps.* 123:93–103.

7. Wangensteen, O. H., and Wangensteen, S. D. 1967. Military surgeons and surgery, old and new: An instructive chapter in the management of contaminated wounds. *Surgery* 62:1102–1124.

8. Bellamy, R. F. 1987. The author's analysis of the Wound Data and Munitions Effectiveness Team data, which will be published in the TMM volume *The Casualty.* Access to the original classified data is controlled by the Uniformed Services University of the Health Sciences University, Bethesda, Maryland.

9. Fackler, M. L. Personal communication, 1988.

10. Heeres Sanitätsinspektion des Reichswehrministeriums. 1934. *Die Krankenbewegung bei dem Deutschen Feld und Besassungsheer im Weltkriege 1914–1918.* Vol. 3 of *Sanitätsbericht über das Deutsche Heer.* In German. Berlin: E. S. Mittler & Sohn.

11. Mueller-Hillebrand, B. 1949. *Statistisches system.* United States Army Historical Division Study No. PC 011 [Koenigstein Ts. 1949]. The unpublished data are stored at the National Archives, Washington, DC.

12. Crews, F. A. E. 1962. *Campaigns: North-west Europe.* Vol. 4 of *The Army Medical Services.* London: Her Majesty's Stationery Office.

13. Reister, F. A. 1975. *Medical statistics in World War II.* Washington, DC: Office of The Surgeon General, Department of Army.

14. Reister, F. A. 1973. *Battle casualties and medical statistics: U.S. Army experience in the Korean War.* Washington, DC: The Surgeon General, Department of the Army.

15. Neel, S. 1973. *Medical support of the U.S. Army in Vietnam 1965–1970.* Washington, DC: Department of the Army, U.S. Government Printing Office.

16. Joint Technical Coordinating Group for Munitions Effectiveness. 1970. *Evaluation of wound data and munitions effectiveness in Vietnam.* Vols. 1 and 3. Alexandria, VA: Defense Documentation Center of the Defense Logistics Agency.

17. Wound Data and Munitions Effectiveness Team. 1970. *Evaluation of wound data and munitions effectiveness in Vietnam* [Final Report]. In Vol. 3, Table 4, p. C–7. Alexandria, VA: Defense Documentation Center of the Defense Logistics Agency.

18. Wound Data and Munitions Effectiveness Team. 1970. In reference 17, Table D.10–3, p. D–19.

19. Owen-Smith, M. S. 1981. A computerized data retrieval system for the wounds of war—The Northern Ireland casualties. Hunterian lecture 1980. *J. Roy. Army Med. Cps.* 127:31–54.

20. Rogov, M. 1982. Pathological evaluation of trauma in fatal casualties of the Lebanon War. *Israeli J. Med. Scien.* 20:367–372.

21. Besser, Y. 1985. Military operations in urbanized terrain (MOUT). Thesis submitted in partial fullfillment of the requirements for the degree of MPH. Uniformed Services University of the Health Sciences, Bethesda, Maryland.

22. Rohne, H. 1898. *Schiesslehre für Infanterie.* Berlin: Ernst Siegfried Mittler und Sohn.

23. La Garde, L. A. 1916. *Gunshot injuries.* 2d rev. ed. New York: William Wood and Company.

24. Day, L. 1982. The hole in stopping power theory. In *The Gun Digest.* 37th anniversary ed. Northfield, IL: DBI Books, Inc.

25. Kokinakis, W., and Sperrazza, J. 1965. *Criteria for incapacitating soldiers with fragments and flechettes* [Report No. 1269]. Aberdeen Proving Ground, MD: Ballistic Research Laboratories, U.S. Army Materiel Command.

26. Waldon, D. J., and Kokinakis, W. 1969. *A parametric analysis of body armor for ground troops* [Technical Report 2]. Aberdeen Proving Ground, MD: Ballistic Research Laboratories, U.S. Army Materiel Command.

27. Bruchey, W. J., Jr., and Frank, D. E. 1983. Police handgun ammunition: Incapacitation effects [NIJ Report 100–83]. Vol. 1, *Evaluation.* Vol. 2, *Experimental Data.* Washington, DC: National Institute of Justice, U.S. Department of Justice.

28. Stolinsky, D. C. 1986. Stopping power—A physician's report. In *Guns and Ammo Annual*, edited by E. G. Bell. Los Angeles: Peterson Publishing Company.

29. Defense Intelligence Agency. n.d. Compilation and assessment of wounding characteristics and potential of foreign weapons. Part 2 of *Medical planning factors.* DIA DST 1810(S):243–81. Classified.

30. Rowland, D. 1986. Assessment of combat degradation. *Roy. Uni. Serv. Inst. J.* (June):33–43.

31. Joint Technical Coordinating Group for Munitions Effectiveness. 1980. *Handbook of effects and lethality of selected U.S. and Soviet weapons.* Vol. 1. 61 JTCG/ME-80–7–1. [Publication FO8635–79-C-0255]. Tinker Air Force Base, Oklahoma 73145

Chapter 3

THE EVOLUTION OF WOUND BALLISTICS: A BRIEF HISTORY

RONALD F. BELLAMY, M.D., FACS* AND RUSS ZAJTCHUK, M.D., FACS**

*Colonel, United States Army; Acting Chief, Department of Surgery, Walter Reed Army Medical Center, Washington, D.C. 20307-5001
**Colonel, United States Army; Deputy Commander, Walter Reed Army Medical Center, Washington, D.C. 20307-5001

INTRODUCTION

Some think that wound ballistics is uncomplicated. After all, what could be simpler than the study of a little hole? Yet, if wound ballistics is straightforward, why, both now and in the past, have there been controversies regarding the wounding done by high-velocity versus low-velocity projectiles, incision versus excision of wounds, primary closure versus delayed primary closure, among many examples? If wound ballistics and its practical application, military surgery, are uncomplicated, why has one of the recurrent themes of military history been the lament that the surgical lessons of past wars—lessons based on an understanding of wound ballistics—have been forgotten by the beginning of the next war, with dire consequences for the first casualties? Fortunately—and in marked contrast to other types of military trauma (biological, nuclear, and chemical), in which actual experience with medical management is limited or even nonexistent—there is a rich store of knowledge dating back almost five centuries that can be used to understand the nature of ballistic injuries and the management of battlefield wounds.

The fact is that the simplicity of wound ballistics is deceptive. One need only look at the history of military surgery with its attendant confusion, disarray, and controversy, to see its true complexity. The nature of wounds changes with the new weapons that are introduced in each succeeding war, and the evolution of wound ballistics is mirrored in the response of military surgeons to the injuries caused by these newer, more destructive weapons. The new weapons—higher-velocity bullets, deforming bullets, fragmenting munitions, and so forth—not only cause new problems for military surgeons, they also provide new insights into the nature of ballistic injuries. These developments in the types of wounds that occur and the medical response to them are tantamount to the experimental variables that scientists introduce in their laboratories. Thus, considerable understanding of wound ballistics is possible by reviewing the history of military surgery. To ignore the past and to base an appreciation of wound ballistics on narrow personal experience risks repeating the mistakes of the past.

In this volume, wound ballistics is treated in three chapters, which are designed as a unit. First, important concepts of wound ballistics are developed in the context of the history of military surgery, and, to a lesser extent, as a result of the successes of experimental and theoretical wound-ballistics research. Second, the basic physics and biophysics of wound ballistics are synthesized with modern experience. And third, the medical aspects of wound ballistics as they apply to managing soft-tissue wounds are considered. The specific aspects of penetrating injuries of the viscera are the subjects of other volumes of this series of textbooks.

WOUND BALLISTICS: THE MANAGEMENT OF PENETRATING INJURIES

Wound ballistics began as an empirical rather than an experimental study. During combat, military physicians have never had a dearth of wounds to observe and treat, and the relationship between certain kinds of munitions and the wounds they caused was often readily apparent, even if not always understood. Until the twentieth century, gunshot wounds to the head or trunk were usually fatal; only since the last decade of the nineteenth century have the wound ballistics of specific organs been investigated. The observations in the historical anecdotes that follow were based primarily on wounds of the extremities.

Penetrating wounds made by projectiles called *shot* that were fired from small arms were first described in the fourteenth century. These wounds contained tissue that was torn or lacerated rather than cut (such as wounds from swords or spears) or crushed (such as the massive mutilating blunt wounds made by cannonballs). They also usually contained a large foreign body (the shot) and were much more likely to become inflamed and to suppurate than other penetrating wounds were.

The prevention and treatment of sepsis have always been dominant issues in wound ballistics. Medieval physicians believed that infection resulted from a poisoned projectile or from the contamination of the wound path with gunpowder, and treated the wound not only by aggressively removing the projectile but also by destroying the tissues surrounding the wound path with boiling oil or a hot cautery. Unfortunately, these treatments traumatized and contaminated what was already a dirty wound, further lowering the casualty's ability to resist infection.

Pioneers Who Advanced the Management of Ballistic Injuries

Ambroise Paré. The poisoned-wound theory was not disproved until the sixteenth century, when the French surgeon Ambroise Paré found himself improvising a treatment during his first military campaign. He knew that the standard surgical practice involved pouring a scalding mixture of oil and treacle into the wound as the first dressing. As he went on his rounds, Paré ran out of boiling oil and had to resort to a *digestive*, a substance that promoted suppuration and the discharge of *laudable pus*. Physicians at that time encouraged these processes, believing that unhealthy humors or fluids were eliminated from the injured body along with the laudable pus. Paré wrote:

> At last my supply of oil ran out, and I was obliged to use in its place a digestive made of yolk of egg, oil of roses, and turpentine. That night I could not sleep well, thinking that I might find the wounded, who had been deprived of the oil, dead from poisoning through the lack of proper cauterization. It made me get up very early to go to see them. Beyond all my hopes, I found that those who had received the application of the digestive on their wounds were feeling little pain, they were without inflammation or swelling, and they had rested quite well during the night. The others, to whom application of the oil had been made, I found had a fever, with great suffering, and with swelling and inflammation around the wounds. And then I resolved never again so cruelly to burn poor men wounded with gunshot.[1]

By the early eighteenth century, empirical observations of gunshot wounds began to take on a modern tone:

> [The] opening of entrance was described as dark, torn, and depressed, tending to be associated with ecchymosis; the opening of exit was often wider and less crushed. If the wound involved the soft parts alone and was superficial, the bullet path was split open; if deep, incisions in the long axis of the extremity were made on both sides. When the wound had been laid open, it was scarified [abraded]. . . . If [the bullet] could not be easily drawn out after the tubular crushed wound had been converted by a broad incision into a gaping, crater-like structure, it was left in place. . . . If the bones were splintered, any loose pieces were extracted.[2]

The creation of this "gaping, crater-like structure," which was intended to allow laudable pus to drain out of the wound and therefore aid the natural healing process, was itself, though unintentionally, suppurative. Eighteenth-century surgeons continued to use digestives in local wound treatment, and began to emphasize emetics and other internal treatments as well.

John Hunter. By this time, the most common small arm on the battlefield was a smooth-bore musket that fired a round lead ball (Figure 3-1). The English surgeon John Hunter (the "founder of modern surgery") was one of the first to recognize that the velocity of the projectile was a determinant of the nature of the wound:

> Gun-shot wounds . . . are in general contused wounds, from which contusion there is most commonly a part of the soluds [*sic*] surrounding the wound deadens . . . which is afterwards thrown off in form of a slough, and which prevents such wounds from healing by the first intention. . . . When the velocity is small, the deadened part of the slough is always less . . . while when the velocity is great, the contrary must happen. . . . Velocity in the ball makes parts less capable of healing, than when it moves with a small velocity.[3]

Hunter, of course, could not measure the velocity of the projectile. What he called "great" velocity was only about 180 meters per second (m/s), lower than the velocity of a modern pistol bullet. (In modern usage, *high velocity* is defined as faster than 700 m/s.)

Finding the projectile and other foreign material that was embedded in wounded tissue was not often easy. Hunter tended to be less willing than most of his contemporaries were to search and further traumatize the tissue:

> It has been hitherto recommended, and universally practiced by almost every surgeon, to open immediately upon being received . . . the external orifice of all gun-shot wounds . . . [because] there was an immediate necessity to search for after [*sic*] those extraneous bodies [such as the ball, clothing, and body parts] . . . [but] the impossibility of finding them. . . . without dilatation gave the first idea of opening the mouths of the wounds. . . . [I]t was oftener impossible to find [the foreign bodies] than

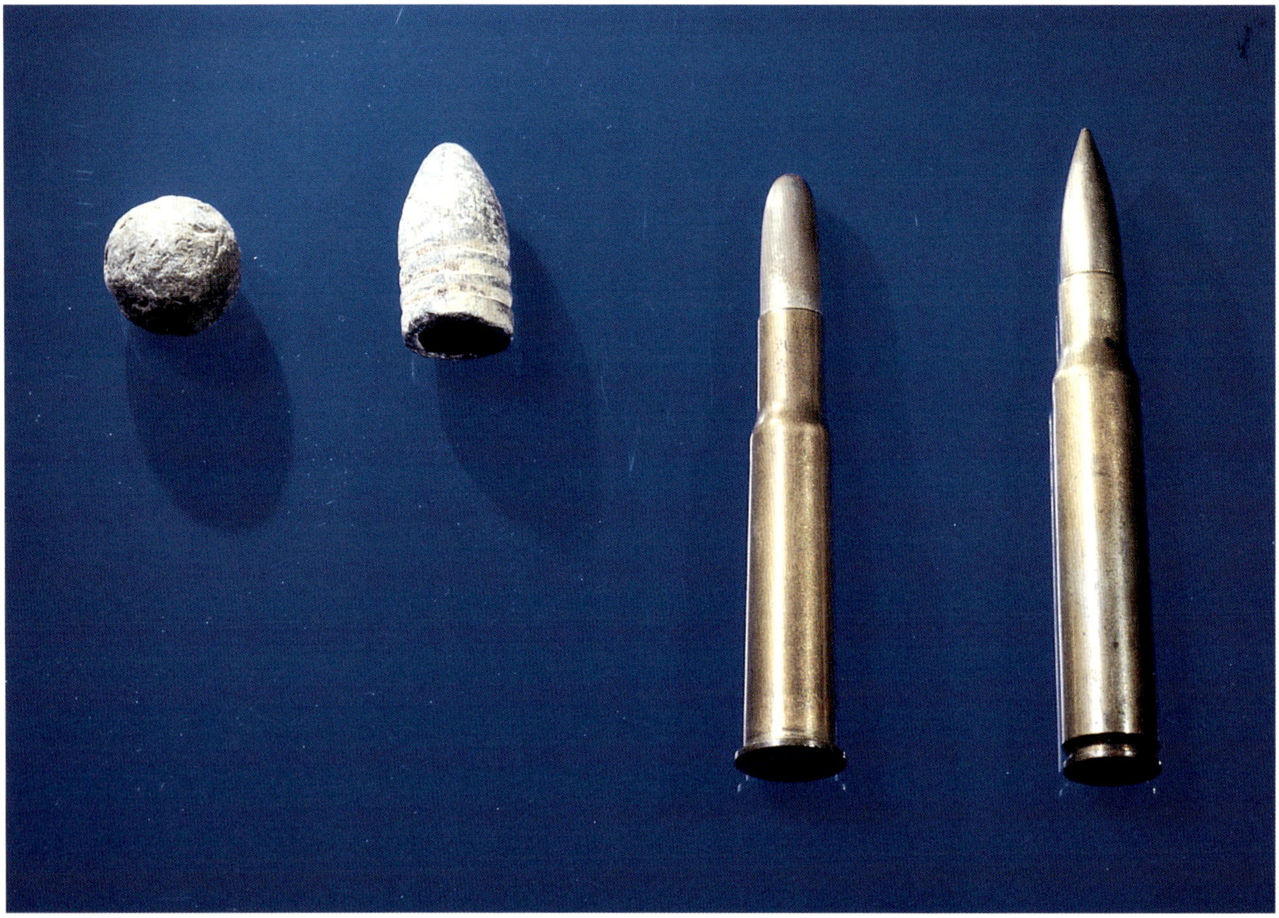

Fig. 3-1. Some bullets of historical importance are, from left to right: musket ball, 69-caliber smooth bore, dating from about 1840; Minié bullet, 58-caliber, dating from about 1855; blunt-nose, 30–40 Krag-Jorgensen, dating from about 1892; spitzer, 1903 Springfield, dating from about 1906.
Source: Division of Armed Forces History, National Museum of American History, Smithsonian Institution, Washington, D.C.

> could at first have been imagined, and when found that it was not possible to extract them.... [Y]ou can gain nothing by opening immediately, but will only increase the inflammation . . . [which] may be too much for the patient.[3]

If the foreign material were not expelled by the body in its slough, Hunter recommended making a later incision *(a)* if "a ball, or broken bone [were] pressing upon a large artery, nerve or vital part," *(b)* if "an artery [were] wounded," *(c)* "in a wound of the head," or *(d)* "where there are fractured bones in any parts of the body that can be immediately extracted."[3] Hunter also noted that gunshot wounds may contain dead tissue and that they commonly become inflamed. The treatment of such wounds, he urged, should be individualized.

Pierre Joseph Desault and Dominic Jean Larrey. The great French military surgeons Pierre Desault and Dominic Larrey made important contributions, both to the management of individual wounds and to the organization of the medical service to care for the mass casualties that characterized the wars of the Napoleonic era. Desault and Larrey are historically associated with the surgical procedure known as *débridement* (from the French, meaning "to unbridle"), which they defined as an incision "[to] relieve tissue tension and [to] establish free wound drainage."[4] Debridement had been introduced several centuries before, but because of Desault's and Larrey's great prestige, this process of wound incision became the predominant surgical intervention used to manage penetrating wounds.

It is to Larrey more than to anyone else that we owe the concept that a penetrating missile wound is a *dynamic entity* (that is, the condition of the wound changes over time). For example, when confronted with a badly injured extremity, Larrey believed that it was far better to amputate immediately through uninjured tissue than to wait until suppuration or gangrene had developed, which made amputation mandatory. The need to care for large numbers of casualties as soon as possible after they were wounded dictated that surgeons opt for standard, aggressive wound management rather than take the time to develop individualized treatment plans. Immediately amputating a badly injured extremity would not only allow surgeons to treat more casualties, but would also allow them to treat a wound definitively before the otherwise healthy soldier's condition had deteriorated. This philosophy of active intervention differed from Hunter's conservative approach.

The Nineteenth Century

Conoidal Bullets. By 1850, smooth-bore muskets and their soft lead balls had begun to be displaced in favor of muzzle-loading rifles that fired small-caliber, high-velocity, cylindro-conoidal projectiles known as Minié bullets (Figure 3-1). Armies also began to use shrapnel-filled explosive shells. As a result, military surgery and the study of wound ballistics began to change dramatically. The wounding effects at longer ranges of the new conoidal bullets were compared with those of lead musket balls:

> [T]he opinion being generally expressed by surgeons [is] that wounds caused by the elongated missile [conoidal bullet] are more severe and dangerous than those resulting from the spherical ball. ... [I]t opposes less frontage to the resistance of the air and its velocity suffers less retardation. . . . [R]otation upon its long axis tends to give it a steadier flight. . . . [I]ts pointed apex enables it to pierce more easily. . . . [A]dding the factor of velocity, we have a missile deadly in its effects.[5]

At close range, however, quite the opposite effect occurred:

> It is probable that the effects produced by round bullets (musket balls) at very close quarters are equally if not more destructive than those produced by elongated missiles; the initial velocity in the two cases does not vary greatly, and, in short distance, the advantage of form as a destructive element is on the side of the round ball.[5]

The guidelines of wound management that Hunter had established continued to be the standard of care:

> [B]alls and foreign bodies were extracted, bleeding vessels secured, and splinters of bone removed. ... [I]t was not unusual to enlarge the wound.[6]

Civil War casualties sometimes had the benefit of anesthesia, but no procedures were done under sterile conditions. The surgeon's bare finger was considered to be the "surest and most intelligent probe" for finding foreign bodies. Wound dressings were examined every 2–3 hours for maggots and surgeons continued to worry about "hospital gangrene, traumatic erysipelas, and pyemia."[6]

Artists who visited Civil War hospitals painted pictures of wounds (color photography had not yet been invented), which give us an idea of the actual appearance of the wounds of entrance and exit made by musket balls and conoidal bullets (Figures 3-2 and 3-3). Surgeons also compared the wounds that the two types of projectiles made:

> [T]he track of a small conoidal ball passing swiftly through a muscle is generally more cleanly cut than

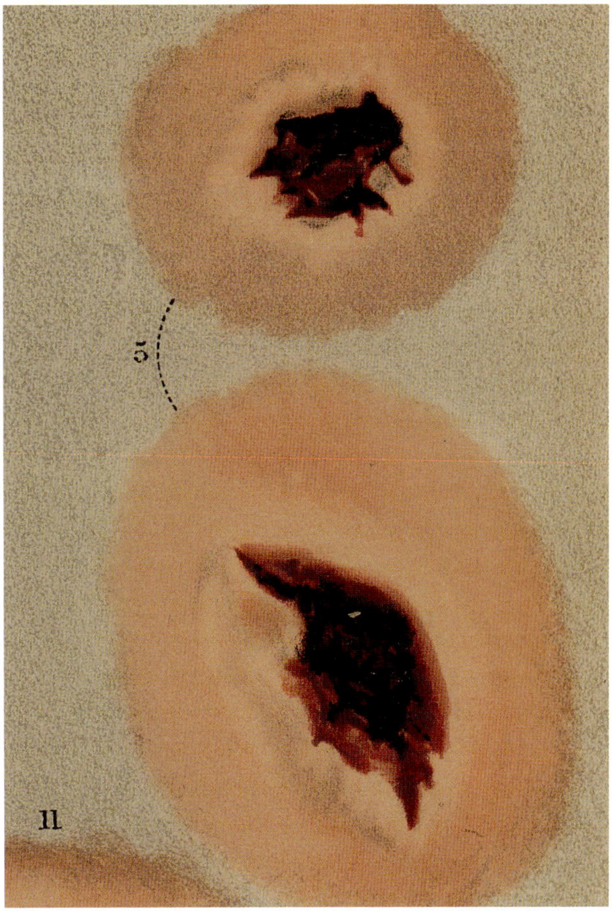

Fig. 3-2. Paintings of wounds made by a spherical ball in a Civil War casualty. Upper: wound of entrance; lower: wound of exit. The wound of entrance is quite large compared to those made by modern bullets. The even larger wound of exit suggests that the bullet deformed during its trajectory through the casualty's soft tissue.
Source: Plate 39, reference 6

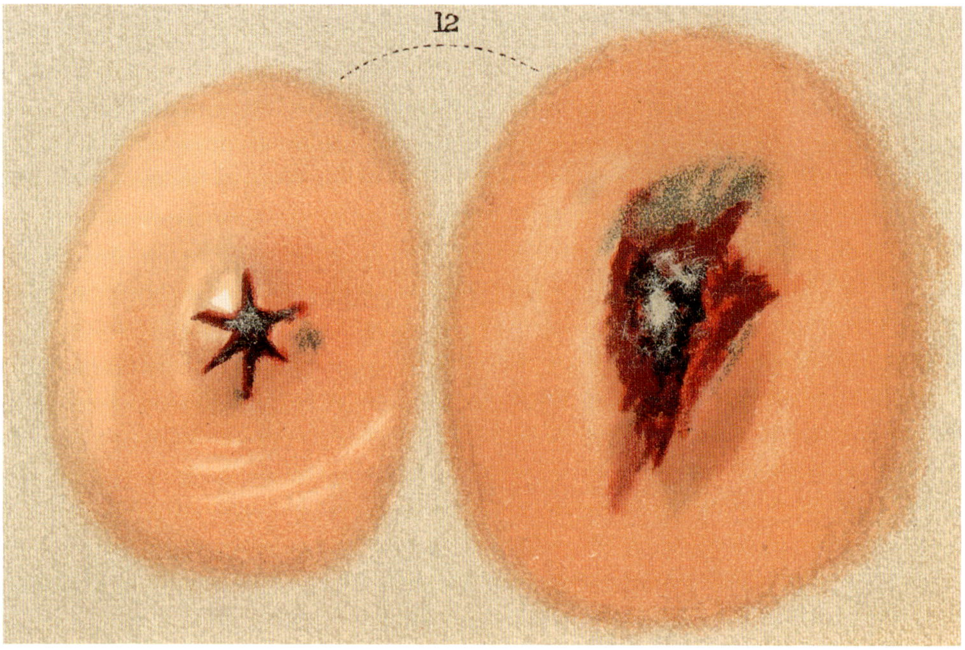

Fig. 3-3. Paintings of wounds made by a conoidal bullet in a Civil War casualty. The source contains the following legend: "Shot flesh wound made by conoidal ball—entrance wound to left, exit to right—typical representation of the effect of a conoidal ball of high velocity." The small wounds of entrance and the large (almost explosive) wounds of exit appear similar to twentieth-century wounds.
Source: Plate 40, reference 6

> that made by a large or round ball; but in all shot wounds there is usually found an irregular channel with contused and lacerated walls, more or less devitalized by contact with the missile, the area of injury gradually shading off by concentric layers until lost in healthy tissues.[6]

When conoidal bullets were first used, not much was known about the effects that bullet deformation and fragmentation had on tissue. Because both the musket ball and the conoidal bullet sometimes deformed upon impact (Figures 3-4 and 3-5), a distinction between the two in this regard was not immediately obvious. Civil War surgeons observed that whether or not a projectile deformed determined the kind of wound it might cause. This question of bullet deformation was one of the first that the new experimental science of wound ballistics addressed. Writing in the 1890s about the wounds caused by projectiles that had been used during the Civil War, the American military surgeon Louis La Garde noted that "the [round] bullet was capable of causing extensive damage, though less than that observed from conoidal rifle bullets." This was especially apparent in wounds in which bone was hit:

> Wounds produced in soft parts were not attended with so much contusion and laceration as with the use of old spherical balls. The amount of devitalized tissue surrounding the bone wounds, however, resembled the effects of an explosion.[7]

Conoidal bullet wounds were the first to demonstrate *explosive effects* in tissue. They were described as

> characteristic lesions . . . notably seen in the proximal ranges—from the muzzle up to about 350 yards. . . . [T]he wound of entrance presented no special features. . . . The point of impact against resistant bone showed loss of substance . . . larger spicules of bone were driven into the soft parts. . . . Pulpification of soft parts was noticed at some distance from the tract of the bullet. . . . The wound of exit was irregular, and measured as much as 3 and 4 inches in its longest diameter.[7]

Jacketed Bullets. After the Civil War, weapons designers developed military bullets that were *jacketed* (that is, the lead core was surrounded by a layer of hard metal, such as steel or a copper alloy) in order to increase the muzzle velocity—and thus the range—of small-arms projectiles (Figure 3-1). Surgeons during the Russo-Japanese and the Spanish-American wars had found that the faster, jacketed bullets were frequently not as destructive to human tissues as the slower, softer bullets were. La Garde, writing from his historical perspective in the early 1900s, observed that "Injuries inflicted outside the zone of explosive effects

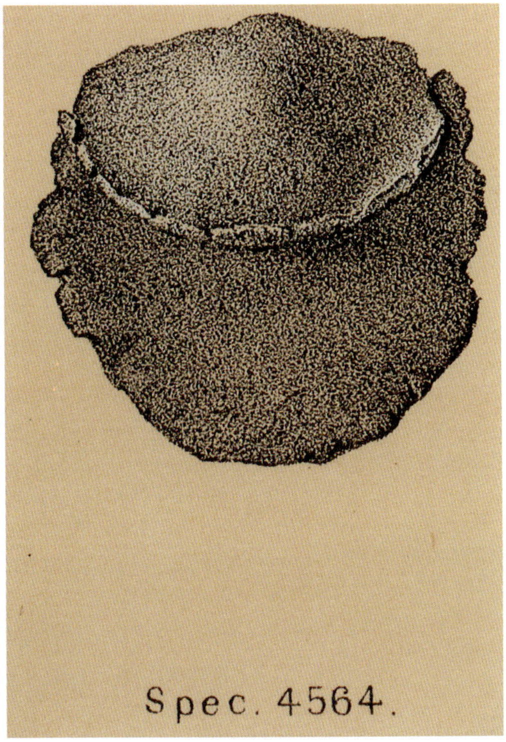

Fig. 3-4. A deformed spherical ball found in the soft tissue of a casualty's upperarm
Source: Plate 78, reference 6

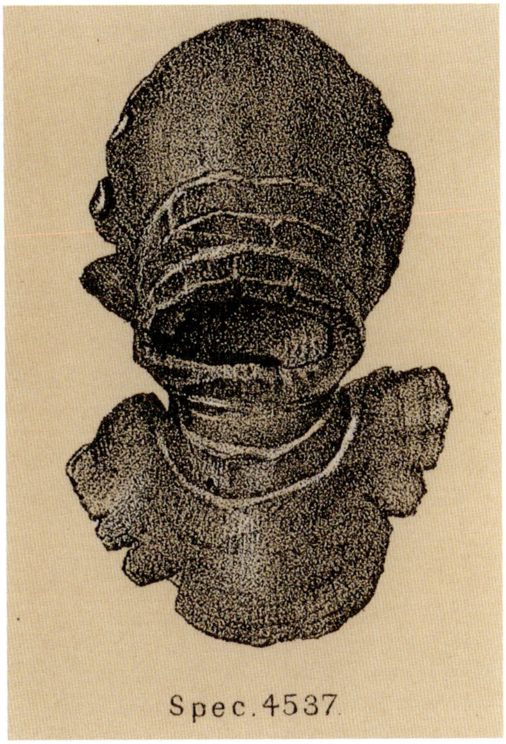

Fig. 3-5. A deformed conoidal bullet found in the soft tissue of a casualty's cheek
Source: Plate 78, reference 6

upon the shafts of long bones always show less comminution with the small bullet of hard exterior."[7] There were also characteristic differences in the behavior in tissue between the older projectiles and the new jacketed bullets:

> [T]he leaden bullet [round ball or conoidal bullet] was so soft that it often separated into a number of fragments.... [T]he steel-jacketed bullet... seldom encounters resistance enough in the human body to disintegrate it....
>
> [T]he small frontage of the jacketed bullets cause them to inflict injuries resembling subcutaneous wounds when the soft parts alone are traversed, and ... the small wounds of entrance and exit and the narrow tract of the missiles were favorable circumstances to rapid healing.[7]

Dumdum Bullets. From a military perspective, however, the unexpectedly humane features of the jacketed bullets were less desirable because the wounds to nonvital areas were less severe. In the early 1890s, at their military arsenal in Dum-Dum, near Calcutta, the British experimented with ways to take advantage of the effects of both the old, soft bullets (that is, their tendency to deform or fragment, causing destructive wounds) and the new higher-velocity, jacketed bullets (that is, their greater range). Making ad-hoc modifications in the field, they simply removed about 1 mm of the jacket at the tip of the bullet and exposed the soft lead in its core. These soft-point bullets became known as *dumdums*.[8] Responding to the soldiers' need for a more lethal bullet, the British armament industry created hollow-point bullets, which also were known as dumdums (Figure 3-6).

Verbal charges and countercharges, particularly between Germany and Great Britain, alleging that dumdum bullets caused unusually devastating wounds, created a heated political climate among the fifteen governments represented at the Hague Convention of 1899. The Third Declaration of that convention agreed to ban the use of deforming bullets in wars between signatories. Although the ban did not apply to countries that had not signed the declaration, the practical result was that all military bullets were expected to have full metal jackets.

Antisepsis. Civil War surgeons used general anesthesia, but sterile techniques—antisepsis and asepsis—were not introduced until after the war. Joseph Lister's first paper describing the use of carbolic acid to achieve antisepsis appeared in 1867, but his principles were not generally accepted for another 20 years.

In 1881, the Russian surgeon Carl Reyher reported the first well documented use of antisepsis in the management of penetrating trauma sustained on the

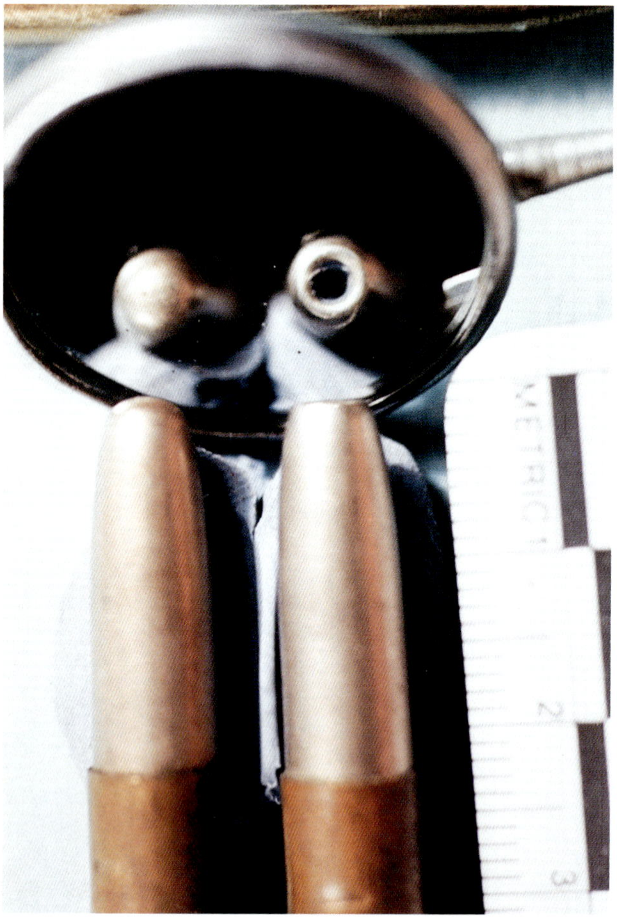

Fig. 3-6. The Mark II bullet, left, which British soldiers modified in the field at Dum-Dum, India, by cutting away about 1 mm of its jacket to expose the tip of the bullet's soft lead core, and the Mark V bullet, right, which was the British armament industry's response to the soldiers' need for a manufactured deforming bullet. Its copper and nickel jacket is folded back at the bullet's nose, exposing a 0.35 x 0.1-in lead-lined cavity.
Source: P. M. Dougherty

battlefield. He found that when antisepsis technique was applied to very fresh wounds, the mortality rate among his patients fell to 50% of that when conventional treatment was applied to day-old wounds. Reyher was said to have also performed wound excision on those casualties whom he treated with antiseptic techniques, so it is not clear what antisepsis alone accomplished to reduce mortality from infection. However, he was one of the first to recognize that battlefield wound sepsis has an iatrogenic component, and he divided casualties into two groups: those whose wounds had been "fingered" and those whose wounds were "unfingered."[9] His observation implies that at least some of the problems of wound sepsis are caused not by bullets but surgeons probing the wounds with their unsterile fingers.

By the end of the nineteenth century, the medical community thought that antiseptic techniques had resolved the problems of wound sepsis. They were rudely awakened at the onset of World War I to find that their approach was ineffective.[10]

World War I

Spitzer Bullets. After the turn of the century, weapons designers turned their attention to increasing the effective range of jacketed projectiles by making them more streamlined. They developed bullets that had a *spitzer* (or pointed) shape, which has continued to be the basis for all subsequent bullet designs (Figure 3-1). This seemingly minor modification also caused the bullet to behave differently in tissue. After examining the wounds made by this new bullet in World War I, a British surgeon compared them to those made by the old blunt-nosed bullets:

> The so-called "normal" bullet wound [made by blunt-nose, cylindrical, jacketed bullets] . . . that was characterized by a tiny aperture which might have been made by a gimlet or a trocar, is in this war quite rare, and even if the entry is of this nature, the exit [of a wound made by a spitzer bullet] is almost always ragged and large. In many of the cases bullets tear the soft tissue to rags, and blow out the muscles and fascia through great rents in the skin. . . . [S]uch injuries as these are always due to the discharge of the rifle at close quarters, and generally within fifty yards. When a large bone is struck, the damage is yet greater.[11]

Although they may not have intended to do more than improve the projectile's aerodynamic properties, weapons designers were now becoming aware of the important relationship between bullet stability and wound severity. For example, the explosive effects of the spitzer bullet occurred because its center of mass was located further back than it would have been in a blunt-nose bullet, which increased its tendency to "turn over within the body."[11] Surgeons noted that these explosive effects occurred at some distance from the projectile's path through tissue:

> [T]he main injury is done by a force of a divulsive or expanding nature, so that the tissues are torn asunder from within instead of being crushed slowly from without. . . . [T]he injury, instead of being limited to the tissues on either side of the bullet track—as it would be if the wound were not made by a bullet but by a trocar—is diffuse in every direction, and radiates through all the surrounding structures. . . . [I]n the case of the brain enclosed in

> the skull, or the liver enclosed in a strong capsule, explosive effects are typical. . . . [T]hese same effects are produced in every other part of the body and limbs also. . . . [T]he missile has not only shattered the tissue in the line of its flight, but the divulsive force has separated the fascia from the skin, and split the muscles from each other along their intermuscular plane. . . . [T]he effect of the injury may, indeed, spread up and down a great part of the length of the limb, and vessels may be burst and extravasation of blood may be found far from the obvious tract of the missile.[11]

The fragmentation of explosive shells also caused devastating injuries and their treatment, at least at the beginning of the war, was frequently unsatisfactory:

> The wounds caused by high-explosive shell fragments . . . are so infinitely various. . . . [A]ll shell fragments being rough and jagged, they tear away parts of the clothing and carry the latter into the extreme depths of the wound. . . . [L]arge fragments tear away portions of skin and muscle from the limbs or trunk . . . the whole of the calf or thigh may be destroyed . . . tissues are crushed and lacerated . . . vessels are pulped, and extensive areas die. Nothing is more striking than the immense amount of destruction wrought by even quite small pieces of a shell burst . . . for the wound in the tissues may be ten times as large as the missile. . . . [B]ombs and grenades are especially likely to cause multiple wounds. . . . At very close quarters, quite small, sharp-edged strips of metal may penetrate very deeply. . . . These wounds are especially liable to be infected.[11]

Developing protocols for the optimal management of penetrating missile wounds is a goal of wound-ballistics theory. Conversely, the failure to obtain adequate results in treatment may provide useful insights into the deficiencies of the theory.

During World War I, surgeons found that when they applied not only the current civilian concepts of wound management but also the experiences of prior small wars (which had been fought with different weapons under different conditions), their efforts in the first months of the war met with dismal failure. Foremost among the factors leading to these failures was their lack of understanding that the battlefield milieu was an important determinant of the surgical treatment of penetrating wounds.

Environmental Factors in Wound Contamination. When dirt and other foreign matter entered the wounds that were seen in World War I, serious infections were almost certain to develop. Battlefields are filthy places, but the soil at the western front seemed to be particularly so:

> [M]ud and dirt pervade everything; and bacteriological investigations of the soil, of the clothing, and of the skin demonstrated the presence of the most dangerous pathogenic organisms in all three.[11]

Sepsis, including gas gangrene, was common. Surgeons came to realize that there was a relationship between local environmental conditions and the nature of wound management. One surgeon compared

> the fields of war in South Africa and in France. . . . In the former . . . the soil was almost entirely free from all pyogenic bacteria. . . . At the present seat of war [France] . . . [the soil] is more heavily manured with the excrements of man and animals than almost any other land. . . . [E]very form of microorganism flourishes . . . [and] spore-bearing pathogenic organisms abound.[11]

Surgical Treatment of Penetrating Wounds. Most wounds seen at the beginning of World War I were massively contaminated, and the majority were clinically infected when they were first seen at a surgical facility. For these casualties, surgical care consisted of opening the wound to allow the free drainage of pus, a practice that was combined frequently with irrigating the wound with an antiseptic solution in an effort to sterilize it. As the war progressed and hospitals filled with septic casualties, surgeons became increasingly dissatisfied with this passive approach. Some sought to mechanically sterilize the wound before it became septic:

> [N]o antiseptic lotion can possibly, by its mere application to the soiled tissue, ensure healing without suppuration. In a contused and lacerated wound, such as we get from bombs, high explosive shells, and often from shrapnel, nothing short of complete excision of the soiled and devitalized tissues can be relied on to secure the healing by first intention that should always be regarded as our ideal.[12]

The French termed this excision of damaged or devitalized and contaminated tissue *épluchage,* (that is, "to pare" or "to trim"). This type of surgery was quite different from debridement, in which the emphasis was upon opening the wound by incision. During World War I, the term "debridement" gradually came to be interpreted by Americans to include both of these formerly distinct meanings.

The official U.S. Army history of medicine in World War I described the evolution of these wound-care concepts:

> Following the disastrous practice in the early months of the war of abstention from surgical inter-

> vention, it was for a time considered sufficient to remove projectiles and superficially clean the wound channel. Experience soon showed the inefficiency of these procedures. This tentative period lasted nearly two years, 1914 and 1915. In 1915 the method of debridement was initiated; in 1916 it was practiced, and in 1917 and 1918 it was elaborated and improved. This practice was dependent upon careful observation of the pathological factors involved in wounds produced by projectiles.[13]

The word "debridement" is used definitively in this history, establishing it in the American medical lexicon:

> debridement of tissue—that is, . . . [the] free incision and excision of injured and contaminated tissue and . . . [the] removal of the foreign material carried by the missile into the wound.[13]

By the end of World War I, American surgeons recognized debridement as the most important single step in the management of penetrating injuries:

> Physical disinfection consists of ablation of necrotic tissue and removal of foreign bodies. This method, known as debridement, constitutes the greatest advance from a surgical standpoint in the recent war.[13]

Regardless of the nature of the initial surgery, the surgeon's goal was to obtain healing of an open wound. With the gaping, infected wounds that most casualties had, wound closure involved *(a)* the formation of granulation tissue, *(b)* fibrosis, *(c)* contracture, and *(d)* epithelization. This process usually took many months and resulted in a nonpliable and grossly deformed wound. Spontaneous closure of this sort, known as healing by *secondary intent*, prolonged the period that a wounded soldier was unavailable for duty, and therefore was not appropriate in a war of attrition.

Many surgeons attempted to accelerate the healing process after several weeks by closing the wound with sutures. This procedure was known as *secondary closure*. Unfortunately, wound breakdown due to persistent sepsis, while uncommon, was an occasional complication.

A few surgeons employed wound excision and immediate closure as an alternative method. If a wound could be mechanically sterilized before sepsis developed, then perhaps it could be safely closed immediately. This procedure, called *primary closure,* was successfully employed by only a few surgeons in World War I, who obtained healing in more than 90% of their patients.[13] Successful primary closure depended upon satisfying the following strict criteria: *(a)* the wound was less than 12 hours old, *(b)* the wound could be completely excised, *(c)* the casualty could be kept at complete bed rest, and *(d)* the casualty could be observed until healing was complete. When surgeons attempted primary closure without satisfying these criteria, the procedure failed in two-thirds or more of the casualties, and severe wound sepsis frequently developed.

The success of primary closure depended upon adequate wound excision. During the initial surgery, the surgeon had to be sure that most (if not all) of the contaminated and injured tissue around the wound tract was excised. A technique that developed late in World War I involved leaving the wound open after the initial surgery and then reinspecting it within 4–6 days, which was enough time for sepsis to appear but not enough time for the wound to become indurated with granulation tissue. If there was no evidence of sepsis, the wound was closed with sutures. This approach, called *delayed primary closure,* was widely utilized by the end of World War I, and remains the standard method by which the military surgeon closes penetrating soft-tissue injuries.[13]

While penetrating injuries to the gut, the chest, and the brain tend to be far more serious than injuries to the soft tissues (skin, fat, and muscle), the wounds that caused the greatest mortality and morbidity—before antibiotic drugs were available—were *open comminuted fractures of the extremities* (that is, open wounds that involve both splintered bone and bony penetration of the soft tissues). In World War I, the standard treatment for these ballistic wounds was to splint the limb and irrigate the open wound with antiseptic solutions. This treatment resulted in a high incidence of osteomyelitis and nonunion of the fractured bone. The military medical system needed simpler, more effective procedures to care for mass casualties with open comminuted fractures. During the Spanish Civil War in the 1930s, the surgeon Raspall José Trueta developed a closed-plaster technique for treating these casualties:

- *(a)* thoroughly wash the wound,
- *(b)* incise and excise the devitalized tissue,
- *(c)* allow the wound to close by secondary intention rather than by suturing it,
- *(d)* establish dependent (downward) drainage of the wound, and
- *(e)* immobilize the limb by plaster cast until the soft-tissue wound and the bone heal.[14]

With the exception of step *(c)*, which some might (in retrospect) consider retrogressive, Trueta's regimen was used successfully to treat thousands of open comminuted fractures in the early years of World War II.

Trueta himself, who performed more than 1,000 of these procedures, believed that step *(b)* was the most important:

> The excision of all devitalized tissue is the basic factor in the treatment of war wounds. The patient's progress, good or bad, bears a direct relation to the skill and thoroughness of this excision. . . . [T]he chief cause of the many surgical disasters of the War of 1914–1918 . . . was that the technique of excision was not properly understood.[15]

World War II

Surgical Wound Management. Soft-tissue wound management as practiced by the British in the first years of World War II strongly depended upon their World War I experience. The British maintained the semantic distinction between épluchage (which they called *primary wound excision* if it was performed soon after wounding) and debridement:

> Debridement is the very antithesis of primary wound excision. Wound excision is a meticulous process, often time-consuming, and only to be carried out soon after wounding. Debridement simply implies enlargement of the wound in order to effect free drainage combined with rapid removal of foreign bodies and obviously dead tissue. The latter is the only local treatment permissible when more than eighteen hours have elapsed since the infliction of the wound.[16]

Nevertheless, the British still performed thorough surgical excision

> if the muscle in any part of the wall of the wound shows evidence of altered color or consistence, fails to bleed when it is cut, or does not contract when it is pinched with the forceps.[16]

These criteria, which date back to at least World War I, have become known as the *four Cs:*

- *Color*—the tissue is darkish
- *Consistency*—the tissue is mushy
- *Contractility*—the tissue fails to contract
- *Circulation*—the tissue fails to bleed[13]

The dynamic nature of the wound—as Larrey had noted over a century earlier—was a crucial consideration to these British surgeons:

> Primary excision is the treatment of election for recent wounds, but unless the surgeon is quite sure that the wound is recent (signs of inflammation have not [yet] developed) he should not even contemplate carrying out this procedure.[17]

The likelihood that initial wound surgery will be performed to drain an infected wound, rather than to prevent infection from occurring, increases with the time that elapses between wounding and surgery. The British emphasis on the management of infected wounds was understandable given their disastrous Dunkirk retreat, with its prolonged and difficult evacuation of casualties. Just as the battlefield milieu influences the nature of wound care, so also do the combat conditions and the tactical posture (for example, slow evacuation during a retreat versus more rapid evacuation during victorious advances).

The techniques that had been developed during World War I and the Spanish Civil War to obtain soft-tissue wound closure (that is, secondary closure and especially delayed primary closure) might have been expected to have been applied immediately in World War II. The need for wound closure was especially great with open comminuted fractures. The major drawback of Trueta's five-step regimen was that the required immobilization of casualties with these injuries frequently was not possible. The plaster casts usually disintegrated and the soft tissue commonly failed to heal. The alternative approach—skeletal traction in the presence of an open wound—was impracticable during evacuation and undesirable in a combat-zone hospital. The World War I wound closure techniques appear to have been downplayed by American military medical authorities during the initial stages of World War II. In fact, Edward Churchill, the surgical consultant to the North African theater, found shortly after his arrival there early in 1943 that

> steps were underway to FORBID this procedure [secondary closure and, by implication, delayed primary closure] from being undertaken.[18]

Wounds were expected to heal by secondary intention. The origin of this attitude is unclear, but within a few months both secondary and delayed primary closures were widely performed.[18]

The theoretical basis for wound closure changed significantly between the two world wars. In World War I, the wound was not considered to be ready for closure until bacteriological studies showed that contamination had been reduced below an arbitrary minimum. In World War II, the wound was closed if it appeared clinically clean. In essence, the policy in World War I was to sterilize the wound so that it could be closed; in World War II, the wound was closed so that it would not become infected.[18]

Antibiotics. World War II saw the introduction of antimicrobial drugs—the sulfonamides and penicillin. Medical personnel hoped that these miracle drugs would bring about revolutionary changes in wound management.

Sulfa drugs were used extensively in the treatment of casualties at Pearl Harbor. Doctrine soon mandated that sulfa be applied to all wounds. Initial reports suggested that infection could be prevented by simply applying sulfa topically to the wound, but by 1943 the wisdom of this intervention was being questioned:

> The extensive application of sulfa to wounds was certainly one aspect of wound management that contributed to infection and suppuration.[18]

In retrospect, it is clear that sulfa is not a good antibiotic; it is merely *bacteriostatic* (that is, it arrests or retards the growth of bacteria) and does not sterilize the wound. Opening the wound to apply the sulfa topically could have contaminated it further, and packing sulfa powder into a contaminated wound could have aided, not prevented, suppuration.

The introduction of penicillin in 1943 raised hopes that the extent of wound excision could now be decreased. However, controlled studies are nearly impossible to conduct on the battlefield. Clinical trials with what are now recognized as inadequate doses of penicillin (15,000–150,000 units daily) demonstrated inconclusive benefits, except in those instances when penicillin was used successfully *(a)* as an adjunct in secondary closure by suture, and *(b)* prophylactically, and was shown to prevent gas gangrene in severe wounds.[19] The official doctrine about 1944 concerning soft-tissue wound care stated:

> Chemotherapy has been recommended: (1) as a substitute for adequate wound surgery, seeking to delay and minimize operative procedures; (2) as an adjunct to established and progressive surgical measures designed to achieve better results with an increased margin of safety. The latter has been and will continue to be the policy governing the management of the wounded in this theater. . . . The use of penicillin as an adjunct to surgery outlined in this circular is defined as therapy rather than prophylaxis. . . . [P]enicillin does not sterilize dead, devitalized or avascular tissue, nor does it prevent the septic decomposition of contaminated blood clots. . . . These limitations demand that surgical wound management retain the principles of excision of devitalized tissue, dependent drainage of residual dead space, evacuation of pus and delayed or staged closure of contaminated wounds.[19]

As the war proceeded, the need to excise tissue was emphasized repeatedly, and was illustrated in the slogans "When in doubt cut it out" and "If a little bit is good, a lot will be a lot better." And therein lay the problem that faced the battlefield surgeons: the potential that too much tissue would be removed. Since surgeons were not able to follow their patients and to know the results of their surgical procedures (because most casualties are evacuated to the next echelon of care as soon as they are able to be moved) most surgeons probably tended to err, in retrospect, on the side of excessive excision. By the end of World War II, excessive surgery was condemned:

> The unnecessary method of excision *en bloc* ([that is, the] aseptic excision of the whole wound tract from outside without cutting into it) was again repeatedly described during the period 1939–1945. Excision of living tissue caused needless mutilation.[14]

By 1944, some categories of gunshot wounds were thought not to require any surgery. For example, the incision and excision of *en seton* bullet wounds of the extremities (that is, perforating wounds not involving neurovascular structures or bone, and with little external evidence of tissue damage) were considered to be "cardinal sins of war surgery."[21]

There is general agreement that soft-tissue and orthopedic wound management in World War II was better than it had been in World War I. The mortality rate for soft-tissue wounds of the lower extremities in World War II was 0%–0.3% for the Fifth U.S. Army in Italy, much lower than the overall rate of 6.1% for mortality from soft-tissue wounds during World War I.[22] Prevention of wound sepsis was probably an important factor in making this advance possible:

> [U]p to that time [June 1944] at least 25,000 soft-tissue wounds [had] been closed by delayed primary closure. . . . In at least 95% . . . healing occurred with no loss of life or limb and without serious complications. The most usual explanation in the 5% [who had] unsuccessful closure was failure to remove dead tissue.[20]

The German Army during World War II, however, continued to rely on older methods and did not have such successful results:

> [T]he Germans assumed . . . that all penetrating wounds received in combat would become infected and that pus was anticipated. . . . [Wound] surgery consisted of no more than incision of skin and fascial planes, the removal of gross debris and devitalized tissue, and usually trimming of devitalized edges of the skin wound. The careful wound excision practiced by Allied surgeons was done in German hospitals only in rare instances.[23]

It is not clear whether the better treatment results that Allied surgeons obtained in World War II were due to *(a)* more complete mechanical cleansing of the wound at the time of initial surgery, *(b)* the use of penicillin and sulfa drugs, *(c)* the conditions of the battlefield (that is, less mud and dirt), *(d)* more rapid evacuation from the battlefield (thus, fewer casualties would have had gross wound sepsis when they were first seen by physicians), *(e)* the less severe nature of the wounds, *(f)* the overall health of the troops (as the World War II history suggests), *(g)* the fact that, unlike World War I, World War II was not "fought during a pandemic of hemolytic streptococcus"[18] or, *(h)* some combination of these factors. These variables interact in a manner that makes analysis difficult, and wound-ballistics experimentation is needed to separate and analyze them.

The first efforts to collect data on wounds in a systematic fashion were made in World War II. The U.S. Army's leading wound-ballistics expert, Brigadier General George Callender, deplored the "startling lack of information" concerning the actual nature of combat wounds in a paper that provided much of the impetus for this data-collection effort.[24] The classic "Study on Wound Ballistics—Bougainville Campaign," a chapter in the standard text *Wound Ballistics*, was a result of Callender's concerns. The Wound Data and Munitions Effectiveness Team (WDMET) continued this effort during the Vietnam War.

Post–World War II

Our understanding of the nature and treatment of ballistic injuries has been extended only marginally since World War II. The surgical doctrine that was followed in the Vietnam and Middle-East conflicts has emphasized thorough wound excision combined with delayed primary closure. The preamble of the instructional document prepared for U.S. Army surgeons in Vietnam clearly states that

> [d]ebridement is the surgical technique of excising devitalized tissue. The experience of several wars has demonstrated that proper debridement is the key to surgical treatment of soft-tissue wounds and provides the best means of reducing morbidity and mortality.[25]

Some think that this approach has resulted in excessive excision of tissue, but its success can be seen in the very low incidence of soft-tissue wound sepsis during that war. Among American forces in Vietnam, the early infection rate of extremity wounds (that is, those infections that developed within the first week after wounding) was only 4%–5%.[26] During the Yom Kippur War, the total soft-tissue wound-infection rate among Israeli casualties was only 6%.[27]

The role of antimicrobial drugs as adjuncts to the surgical management of soft-tissue ballistic injuries sustained on the battlefield has not been clarified significantly. Most casualties in Vietnam who had penetrating trauma received penicillin or tetracycline, so the effect of surgery alone could therefore not be determined. An Israeli study of casualties wounded in the Yom Kippur War found that, while all casualties had received prophylactic antibiotics, the antibiotic used was effective against the offending pathogen in only one-third of the 6% who developed wound infections. Since penicillin was the most commonly used prophylactic antibiotic, Gram-negative organisms, not unexpectedly, were commonly encountered in infected wounds. The researchers concluded that

> the practice of antibiotic wound prophylaxis may contribute to the incidence and nature of infection in battlefield wounds. . . . The temptation to "sterilize" the wound with massive doses of antibiotics . . . favors a false security with less reliance on good surgical technique.[28]

Weapons development since World War II has been characterized by two design trends: firearms that shoot small-caliber, high-velocity bullets, and explosive munitions that produce large numbers of small, fast-moving fragments. Both developments are predicated on *(a)* the assumption that wound severity is determined by kinetic energy, which some believe is an oversimplification, and *(b)* the fact that greater kinetic energy can be more readily obtained by using high-velocity, small-size projectiles rather than massive, low-velocity projectiles. Wound management has been influenced by the corollary assumptions, which also may be oversimplified, that *(a)* kinetic energy kills tissue, and *(b)* all dead tissue must be removed in the optimal treatment of penetrating wounds.

The wounds produced by bullets fired by the M16 assault rifle in the Vietnam War are frequently used to illustrate the relationship between kinetic energy and wound severity. This cause-and-effect relationship is flawed, however: The kinetic energy of the bullet fired by the M16 rifle (that is, 1,650 joules) is nearly identical to that of the conoidal bullet fired by the muzzle-loading rifle of the 1850s (that is, 1,665 joules), and has lower kinetic energy than any bullet fired by a military rifle fielded since then. The wounding potential of the bullet fired by the M16 rifle depends upon its fragmentation in tissue and not on its kinetic energy and velocity. This information appears in the WDMET data that were published but not publicized during the 1960s: "In almost all cases in the series involving 5.56 x 45 mm bullets, the projectile fragmented after striking the body."[29] In a very real sense, M16 ammunition is the contemporary equivalent of a nineteenth-century dumdum.

WOUND BALLISTICS: THE THEORETICAL AND EXPERIMENTAL SCIENCE

The problems encountered by battlefield surgeons in their treatment of ballistic wounds have always driven the scientific advances made in wound ballistics laboratories. The Swiss surgeon Emile Theodor Kocher (who is regarded as the founder of wound ballistics as an experimental science), the German pathologist Paul L. Frederich, the American physician Charles Woodruff, and the American military surgeon Louis La Garde were among the first researchers to investigate systematically the individual projectile variables that determine the nature of ballistic wounds, as well as the special treatment problems these wounds present. Contemporary wound ballistics has become a rigorous and specialized field; it studies an array of projectile effects on tissue, and uses the most sophisticated scientific technologies to support its findings.

Early Research

Emile Theodor Kocher. Although no doubt others had observed the effects of military projectiles in tests involving animate and inanimate objects, Theodor Kocher appears to be the first who systematically investigated the individual variables that are the determinants of wounding. Kocher is well known in the history of medicine for his contributions to orthopedics and surgery: He was the first surgeon to win the Nobel Prize in medicine (in 1909, for his work on the thyroid gland). He is less well known for his accomplishments in experimental wound ballistics, which were performed during 1874–1879 in Thun, Switzerland.[30, 31] Much of our understanding of Kocher's contributions to wound ballistics comes from the research of Dr. Paul J. Dougherty.[32]

Though Kocher, who was a member of the Swiss militia, never saw a war wound until he was invited to tour a German military hospital early in World War I, he knew about the "explosive" injuries that conoidal bullets made. He sought both to *(a)* systematically determine the mechanisms that caused ballistic wounds and *(b)* provide a rational treatment for explosive gunshot wounds. An explanation then current was that a bullet's rotation—imparted by a rifle barrel's grooves—caused centrifugal forces that ripped apart the tissue. Kocher disproved this, showing that the wounding effect was no different from that of a conoidal bullet fired from a smooth-bore barrel. Kocher also obtained the equivalent of the explosive wounds that he had previously observed in cadaver skulls—small wounds of entrance, enormous wounds of exit, and separated cranial sutures—by shooting into water-filled metal cans. The cans had small entry holes, very large exit holes, and the inelastic seams of the cans were ruptured.[33] He fired equivalent shots into empty metal cans and demonstrated the resulting small entry and slightly larger exit holes and intact seams. This indicated to Kocher that hydraulic or hydrodynamic factors, which subsequently came to be known as *cavitation*, were responsible for the explosive effects in tissue. He noted that muscle seemed to act like a fluid; it stretched, transmitting the energy of a bullet rather than rupturing, as did inelastic tissues such as bone.[32] In soft-tissue injuries where a bone was not struck, however,

> a different effect was observed. In the shots to the extremities small entry and exit holes were observed if a bone was not struck. The exit holes tended to have split skin, which was along the axis of least resistance, along fascial planes. Skeletal muscle showed this same effect when it was dissected out.[33]

Kocher emphasized the importance of projectile deformation as a major determinant of wounding potential, and was able to separate the variables of velocity and deformation. In his experimental design, he isolated the variables of linear and rotational velocity, bullet composition, and target media. He changed only one variable at a time, and noted its effect on both the target and the projectile. He reported only what he observed and did not speculate about his observations.[32] In his 1879 studies he *(a)* compared bullets of varying degrees of hardness; *(b)* obtained (from the arsenal at Thun) early chronograph-measurements of muzzle velocities; *(c)* introduced the technique of "reduced-power loading," which is still used in ballistics laboratories today to simulate varying target distances by reducing bullet velocity in measured steps; and *(d)* caught his projectiles in water-filled tanks and compared their deformation and fragmentation.[34]

Kocher was the first researcher to study the effects that varying a projectile's velocity had on a target. He demonstrated that the destructive effects seen in water-filled cans seemed to depend upon the projectile's velocity. He predicted that less severe wounds would be made with solid, nondeforming bullets (made of metal harder than lead), regardless of their velocities.

Kocher was also the first to suggest that, in order to reduce their wounding potential, the core of military bullets should be made of metal so hard that they would not deform in tissue. In 1875, he wrote that "the goal of weapons designers should be to design a firearm that would incapacitate rather than cause inhumane destruction."[33] In a speech delivered at the Eleventh International Medical Congress in Rome, Kocher recommended that "from the standpoint of humanity,"[35] a projectile should have *(a)* a 5–6-mm diameter, *(b)* a hard steel point to prevent deformation, and *(c)* a tapered point to moderate the damage as the bullet passed through tissue.

Another of Kocher's contributions to wound ballistics was his modification of the gelatin tissue simulant, which was used in lieu of living animal tissue. He devised a gelatin and concrete "sandwich"—a 3-cm concrete block covered on both sides with 3-cm gelatin plates—that he thought was analogous to soft tissue and bone. After he fired into it, he found a small entry hole through the first layer of gelatin, a large (10–15-cm diameter) defect through the concrete, and an exit hole through the gelatin that was somewhat larger than the entry, with pulverized concrete throughout the exit canal. He described these experimental findings as being similar to a compound fracture.[34]

Political Influences on Science. The flurry of ballistic experiments that occurred in the last quarter of the nineteenth century were stimulated by the controversy over deforming bullets, such as the British dumdums, that had just been developed. Some of these early experiments were marred by extremely emotional political considerations. Hostilities between Germany and Great Britain were intensifying, and the Germans conducted experiments to show that deforming bullets fired into long-dead cadavers caused especially massive wounds, and should therefore be banned. However, the bullets that the Germans used in these experiments had higher velocities and much more lead core exposed at the tip than the dumdum bullets did. British and American investigators countered by citing anecdotes to show that the then-new jacketed bullets caused just as much damage as the deforming bullets did.[8] Because both sides used evidence to support their desired conclusions, science was lost to political controversy, and important methodological standards—such as comparing bullets of like velocities and designs and using similar tissue simulants in comparable experiments—were ignored.

Paul L. Frederich. One study of permanent worth was conducted during this period, however: The German pathologist Paul L. Frederich investigated the temporal relationship between wound contamination and invasive sepsis. This study provided the scientific basis for the concept that a penetrating wound is a dynamic entity, which Larrey had introduced 70 years before. (Frederich did not refer to Larrey's concept in his paper; it is possible, due to the political enmity between France and Germany, that Frederich was unaware of Larrey's work.) In his landmark study, Frederich contaminated an experimental wound in a rat triceps with soil, and sutured the wound closed. He then periodically examined biopsies removed from more proximally situated muscle for microorganisms. None were apparent before 6 hours had elapsed. He concluded that surgical manipulation of the contaminated area might be curative for up to (but not later than) 6 hours after wounding. Frederich demonstrated that excision of 1–2 mm of the contaminated wound lining within 6 hours prevented invasive sepsis and death (Figure 3-7). In his historic paper, which has been translated and interpreted extensively (but not always accurately) since its publication, Frederich concluded:

> [I]n each so-called "spontaneous infected" wound, the infection process is very nearly a localized one. It is important for arriving at a therapeutic and diagnostic judgement to keep in mind that in the great majority of instances this process will remain so until at least the sixth hour after wounding, and often longer. This span of time represents, to a certain extent, the germination time of the infection (the infection's latency period and incubation time).
>
> The most reliable means of attaining an infection-free healing process through medical treatment is to apply at this time [during the first 6 hours] a precise freshening [in the original, *anfrischung*] in addition to a complete distension or opening up of the wound area.
>
> Where the circumstances forbid or do not indicate this treatment method (due to time, wound size, [or the] lack of assistance, skillful anesthesia, or aseptic instruments and equipment), a more-or-less open management is the best prevention of a serious infection.
>
> The use of antiseptics is only sensible if the wounded area is by-and-large accessible to them, if they are used within the indicated germination period, or if the infection is produced as a result of bacteriological agents and not chemical substances. In the case of progressive or generalized infections, antiseptics are futile and often detrimental. The sum total of their effect is little more than to prevent the use of open management.[36]

Frederich's most important conclusions are that *(a)* wound contamination is not synonymous with wound infection and *(b)* if the contaminants can be removed during their latency period, infection will not occur. This latency period, approximately 6 hours, was subsequently called by others, but not by Frederich himself, the *golden period*. Although the word he used to describe his infection-prevention process was *freshening*, Figure 3-7 shows quite clearly that he actually practiced wound excision. By World War I, Frederich's concept of freshening had been exaggerated: His experiments were commonly thought to demonstrate that one approach to managing a contaminated war wound was to completely excise it during the golden period "as though it were a neoplasm." This is the origin of the concept of Frederich's *totaler Wundexzision*,[37] that is, Frederich's complete wound excision (and the equivalent expression in French and English, *wound excision en bloc*).

Frederich's own conclusions were sound and reasonable. Complete wound excision, however, is rarely, if ever, either a practical possibility or sound medical practice in treating combat casualties. Fortunately, a lesser degree of excision may accomplish the same result. Even more importantly, he also recognized that if excision were not possible, simply leaving the wound open was therapeutically sound.

Charles Woodruff. Two seminal communications that appeared in English in 1894 and 1898 advanced the understanding of explosive wounds and supported the observations that Kocher had made in the 1870s. Victor Horsley published evidence that hydrodynamic effects are the origin of explosive wounds of the skull.[38] Charles Woodruff was the first to suggest that it is the transfer of kinetic energy from the projectile to the tissue—and not the projectile's amount of energy (or velocity) on impact—that determines the nature of the ballistic injury. He studied the wounding ability of fully jacketed bullets, and inferred the behavior of the older, larger lead balls:

> The energy or ability to do work is proportional to the mass and the square of the velocity [MV^2]; hence the new bullet, though smaller, has much greater energy than the old, and can do more work, though it rarely gives up all its energy, because it passes entirely through the body.... The slow, large bullet ... has less energy than the new ... [and] is so large [that] it can not plow its way through the tissues like a small bullet.... [I]t is therefore stopped, gives up all its energy, and delivers a far greater blow than the new bullet.[39]

Woodruff noted that bullets that transfer more of their kinetic energy are more likely to cause explosive effects, as though the bullet itself had exploded within the tissue. He suggested that the interaction of bullet and tissue can be understood

> almost exclusively by the capability or incapability of the tissues to take up and transmit vibration or wave motions, [and explained that] tissue may be set into such violent vibrations that, like a pane of glass, it may be strained beyond its limit of elasticity, and may fly to pieces.... The particles of tissue moving away from the bullet track, even after the bullet has passed, must then form a vacuum or cavity. This cavitation is the basis of the explosive effects. . . . The enormous extent of the cavity or vacuum thus formed depends solely upon the velocity of the particles [of tissue] moving outwards from the track of the bullet. As soon as the particles are brought to rest [that is, as soon as the cavity reaches its maximum expansion] they are acted upon by the forces driving them back, for they now surround a vacuum. They rush back again to the track of the bullet, and come together with great force.... They [the particles of tissue] thus vibrate back and forth until their energy is dissipated.[39]

Woodruff compared a fast-moving projectile's passage through tissue with the cavity that would be seen in water around the rapidly rotating propeller of a ship.[39] He suggested that this phenomenon, cavitation, is possible only in an incompressible (that is, liquid) medium. It is the hydrodynamic effect (that is, the moving fluid)—rather than the hydrostatic pressure (that is, the pressure wave moving through a fluid at rest)—that causes the tissue damage.

Another of Woodruff's insights was that the collapse of the cavity itself causes damage. Contemporary Swedish ballistics experts suggest that this phenomenon (implosion contrasted to explosion) is a major source of the tissue damage associated with cavitation.

Louis A. La Garde. Louis A. La Garde dominated American wound ballistics in the two decades before World War I. He wrote *Gunshot Injuries* (Figure 3-8), a comprehensive survey of clinical, experimental, and theoretical wound ballistics that remained the best-known treatise in English on that subject until Beyer's *Wound Ballistics* was published in 1962. One of his experimental contributions was to challenge the notion that bullets (and, by implication, fragments from explosive munitions) were sterilized by being shot out of a gun barrel. La Garde disproved this belief by shooting bullets that had been contaminated with anthrax bacilli into animals, who later developed the disease.[40]

La Garde's research using animals, cadavers, and tissue simulants allowed accurate predictions to be made regarding the nature of the wounds made by both the round-nose jacketed bullet (the Spanish-American War) and the pointed jacketed bullet (World War I).[41] It is doubtful that any of La Garde's experi-

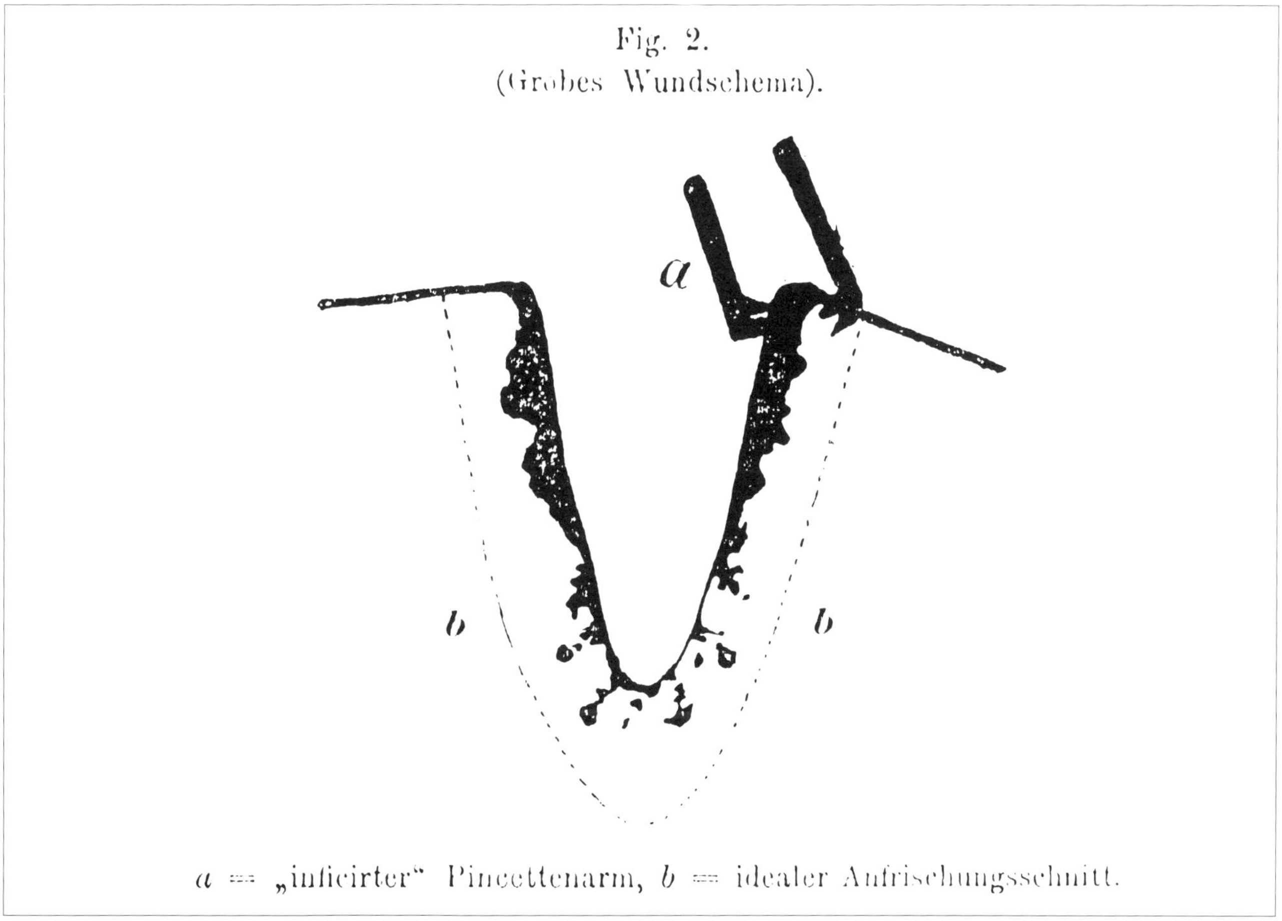

Fig. 3-7. This is a reproduction of Figure 2 in Frederich's paper. The original caption, translated from German, reads: "Drawing of a Wound *a* = 'nonsterile' forceps; *b* = idealized wound-freshening." His drawing clearly shows that the procedure Frederich called "freshening" is equivalent to the procedure we call "excision" today.
Source: Reference 36

mental findings were used by military surgeons in those wars, however, and there has been little interaction between weapons designers and medical officers since that time.

Modern Research

Louis Wilson. Ballistics researchers were ready for the vast amounts of wound data that became available as a result of World War I. They began to describe the injuries they saw in terms of physics as well as simply those of pathology. An American medical officer, Louis Wilson, proposed that a ballistic wound could best be understood in terms of energy transfer. He wrote:

> The wounding effect of a bullet depends upon *(a)* the amount of energy it transmits to the tissues, *(b)* the velocity of the transmission, *(c)* the direction of the transmitted energy, and *(d)* the density of the tissues. The first three of these factors depend almost entirely on the energy, velocity and shape of the bullet. . . . The proportion of the energy transmitted [of the total available on impact] depends on the [cross-]sectional area of the bullet, the shape of its head, the character of its surface, and the relative densities of the tissues struck.[42]

Whether Wilson actually had the experimental data to justify these conclusions is unknown, but his ideas led to the development of the lightweight high-velocity projectiles that are common today.

George Callender and Ralph French. In the 1930s, the U.S. Army began conducting wound-ballistics research at Aberdeen Proving Ground in Maryland. George Callender and Ralph French built upon Wilson's energy-transfer hypothesis, measuring both impact and exit velocities of projectiles and, thus, calculating an amount of energy transfer that they could qualitatively correlate with aspects of tissue destruction.[41]

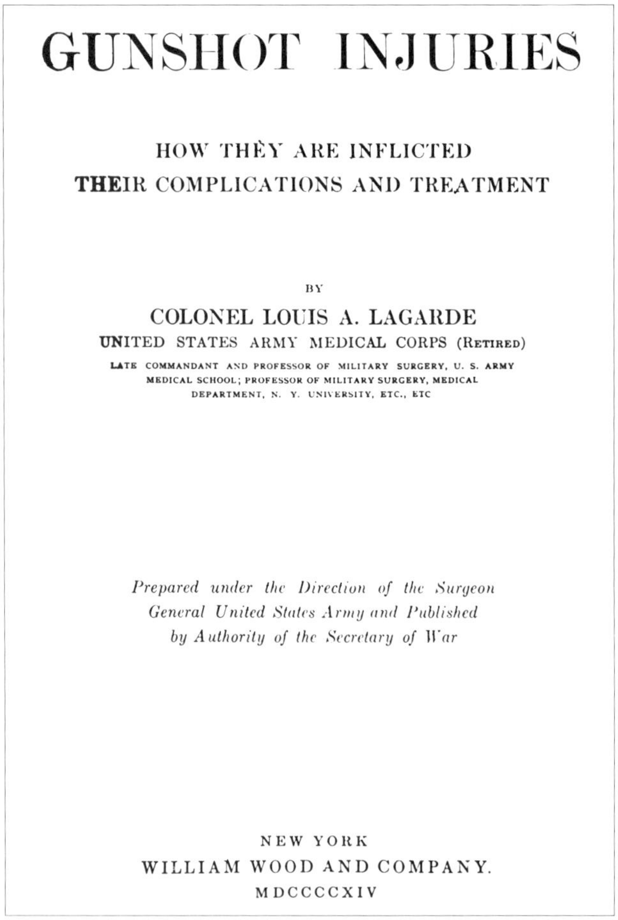

GUNSHOT INJURIES

HOW THEY ARE INFLICTED
THEIR COMPLICATIONS AND TREATMENT

BY

COLONEL LOUIS A. LAGARDE
UNITED STATES ARMY MEDICAL CORPS (RETIRED)
LATE COMMANDANT AND PROFESSOR OF MILITARY SURGERY, U. S. ARMY MEDICAL SCHOOL; PROFESSOR OF MILITARY SURGERY, MEDICAL DEPARTMENT, N. Y. UNIVERSITY, ETC., ETC

Prepared under the Direction of the Surgeon General United States Army and Published by Authority of the Secretary of War

NEW YORK
WILLIAM WOOD AND COMPANY.
MDCCCCXIV

Fig. 3-8. The title page of the second edition of Colonel Louis A. La Garde's famous book. Note that he was commandant of the U.S. Army Medical School.
Source: Reference 7

The aspect of projectile-target interaction that is probably of greatest interest in contemporary wound ballistics—cavitation, the putative source of the mysterious explosive effect that was first described in the nineteenth century—was not even mentioned by Callender and French in their early writings. This might have been because neither they nor anyone else had yet visualized the cavity that Woodruff (and others) hypothesized followed a high-velocity missile as it passed through tissue. In fact, it was not until 1941 that a group of English investigators led by Solly Zuckerman conclusively demonstrated the phenomenon, using sophisticated photographic techniques for that era. That paper begins:

> The fact that the amount of tissue destruction caused by small high-velocity bomb splinters may be out of all proportion to their size has been recognized for some time.[43]

After reproducing photographs showing large cavities in gelatin blocks that occurred "with explosive violence" several hundred microseconds after a rapidly moving missile (700–1,000 m/s) passed through, the paper concludes:

> As the missile passes through the block it imparts motion to the particles in its track, and these fly off radially, imparting their momentum in turn to further particles (and so on).[43]

The term by which this phenomenon is now known, *temporary cavitation*, was not used by these researchers.

E. Newton Harvey. Like other research efforts in World War II (such as those that led to the development of radar and the atomic bomb), certain wound-ballistics studies that had been started in wartime England were continued in the United States. The National Research Council held a conference on wound ballistics in late 1943, which resulted in support for several ballistics-research contracts. One of these studies, conducted by E. Newton Harvey, is still an important source of information on the physical aspects of projectile-target interaction; Harvey's group wanted "to predict exactly what damage may be expected from the impact of a known mass moving with any known velocity."[44] To do so, they would need to *(a)* relate injury to the physical characteristics of the projectile, and *(b)* study the nature of the damage to tissue. Some of their conclusions were:

- A sonic shock wave precedes the passage of a projectile, and (depending on the physical characteristic of the tissue) may or may not cause injury.
- A wound consists of a permanent cavity (the hollow path left by the projectile as it cuts through the target), as well as the surrounding tissue that was stretched by a temporary cavity. And, most importantly,
- The size of the temporary cavity is determined by energy transfer (that is, if other factors are the same, the higher the projectile's velocity, the larger the temporary cavity will be).

Not all contemporary ballisticians view Harvey's work as the scientific foundation of modern wound ballistics. Some believe that his interpretation of the damage done by temporary cavitation is exaggerated.[45]

Harvey's group published some of the first studies of animal survival following soft-tissue gunshot wounding; they noted "the absence of dead tissue in the wound" and that many of the wounds healed naturally without any care being given. Ironically, they wanted to understand the nature of wounding not so much to improve the care of the wounded, but rather to

> predict the degree of incapacitation [that] may result from a hit by a missile . . . [so] as to test the casualty-producing effectiveness of [American] weapons.[44]

Much of the wound-ballistics research since World War II at Aberdeen Proving Ground and the nearby Edgewood Arsenal has had the improvement of weapons effectiveness as its goal.

An important post–World War II study done at Edgewood investigated why penetrating wounds sustained on the battlefield were *(a)* likely to be contaminated, and *(b)* at risk to become septic.[46] Dziemian and Herget showed (with gelatin tissue-simulants) that temporary cavitation was frequently associated with the aspiration of foreign material into the wound tract. This was especially likely to happen if the cavity (with its subatmospheric pressure) was connected to the outside through the wounds of entrance or exit. These researchers concluded that, because *(a)* high-velocity projectiles capable of causing large temporary cavities are common on a battlefield, and *(b)* the battlefield environment has a ready source of material capable of being aspirated into the cavities and contaminating those wounds, then *(c)* the likelihood of increased sepsis in war wounds is understandable.

D. Lindsey and J. A. Mendelson. Many of the researchers at the Aberdeen-Edgewood complex used animal experimentation and mathematical models to predict the wounding effects of various projectiles. During the decade before the Vietnam War, D. Lindsey and J. A. Mendelson attempted to determine the natural history of untreated penetrating missile wounds. Building upon the work that Harvey began, they investigated how the natural course of healing might be altered by various therapeutic interventions such as using antibiotics and debridement. These studies concluded that

- undebrided missile wounds of nonvital areas may indeed lead to a fatal result, and
- many of the high velocity missile wounds healed quite uneventfully and extensive soft tissue necrosis was not an inevitable accompaniment of them.[47,48]

The same investigators also made exhaustive measurements of bacteriological, histopathological, and biophysical phenomena. From their measurements of the biophysical interactions, they prepared a series of elegant diagrams correlating the absorption of energy and tissue damage as functions of the depth of the wound tract. But none of these studies appears to have had any influence on wound management in the war then going on in Vietnam. Some military medical officers considered experimental wound-ballistics research to be too esoteric, and the same attitude exists today.

Contemporary Wound-Ballistics Research

Since World War II, strong but short-lived research efforts have appeared in several countries. British clinical researchers in the 1960s, for example, showed that, in sheep, penicillin (used as the sole therapeutic intervention) could prevent death from experimental gas gangrene.[49]

Returning to the work that Harvey's group had done in the 1940s, reseachers at Aberdeen in the early 1970s performed a flurry of wound-ballistics experiments to investigate their possible clinical importance. They studied organ-specific aspects of temporary cavitation, especially as they apply to the lungs and large arteries. Joseph Amato demonstrated, using X rays with a pulse of less than 0.1 microsecond, the formation of a temporary cavity within a goat's thorax.[50] Amato and Norman Rich, in another study, shot the femoral arteries of mongrel dogs with high-velocity projectiles to demonstrate *(a)* the shearing effect on the artery and *(b)* the

> significant additional injury. . . caused by the crushing effect of the temporary cavitation. . . [and the] rapid acceleration of the tissue [which is] proportional to the transfer of energy expended in the formation of the temporary cavity.[51]

Confirming Harvey's earlier observations, Rich also found that the temporary cavity caused by a high-velocity bullet can *(a)* be many times larger than the permanent wound tract, and *(b)* cause arterial thrombosis or fracture a bone without the bullet's actually having hit these structures.[52]

Swedish researchers in the 1970s and early 1980s attempted to determine—as Kocher had done a century ago—the modifications that might make bullets less destructive. Going beyond researchers of the Callender-and-French discipline, who concentrated on the qualitative relationship between energy and tissue damage, Swedish investigators have striven to find an exact quantitative relationship between the two, using the amount of debrided tissue as an index of tissue damage.[53] Some researchers dispute this assessment, saying that it has no practical clinical application; others agree that the quantitative approach has considerable value.

Six international wound-ballistics symposia have been organized as a result of the Swedish research, and hundreds of papers have been added to the literature.[54, 55, 56] The most recent International Wound Ballistics Symposium was held in China in 1988. China currently has the most active research programs, perhaps because the animal-rights movement is not as strong there as it is in western countries.

Finally, American wound-ballistics research has undergone a resurgence due to the efforts of Colonel Martin Fackler. His contribution has been to emphasize observables such as bullet deformation and fragmentation rather than intangibles such as energy and temporary cavitation, and he has sought to make complicated aspects of projectile-target interaction understandable.[57]

SUMMARY

Military surgeons over the past 500 years have observed certain common problems as they have managed ballistic injuries. The evolution of the surgical management of these injuries has included these observations, which valid theories of wound ballistics must incorporate:

- Untreated penetrating wounds sustained on the battlefield are likely to develop sepsis.
- The likelihood that sepsis will develop seems to be related to *(a)* the condition of the battlefield, *(b)* the ability to provide timely care, *(c)* the presence of foreign material in the wound, *(d)* the presence of dead tissue in the wound tract, and *(e)* the ballistic characteristics of the projectile.
- Surgical removal of foreign material and dead tissue seems to decrease the likelihood of sepsis.
- Primary closure of war wounds is usually unsatisfactory.
- The more a projectile deforms or fragments in tissue, the more damage it will do.
- Projectiles with higher velocities tend to cause more tissue damage than slower-moving projectiles.
- The more unstable a projectile is in tissue, the greater the tissue damage will be.
- Projectiles of irregular shapes, such as fragments from an explosive munition, may cause torn, jagged wounds.
- These factors may interact and modify the observed tissue damage.
- Under certain conditions, tissue damage is out of proportion to what would be expected from direct physical contact with the projectile, and has been likened to the effects of an explosion.

Although wound-ballistics researchers at first tried only to replicate battlefield wounds in controlled environments, the field soon expanded to include laboratory studies of the physical mechanisms that determine the way projectiles behave in tissue. Before long, laboratory evidence showed that a projectile's velocity, deformation, and stability combine to determine the severity of the wound that it caused.

Measuring physical parameters, such as the projectile's velocity, could obviously not be done during a battle, but was ideally suited to the laboratory and could result in a unifying physical concept (such as transfer of energy) that might explain the projectile's behavior in tissue. The history of wound ballistics has been dominated by the study of these physical parameters, sometimes to the exclusion of more practical clinical questions.

One of the most valuable contributions that wound-ballistics researchers have made is their provision of a clearer understanding of the explosive effects of projectiles in tissue, which had been observed by military surgeons for more than a century. This phenomenon of temporary cavitation could only have been demonstrated in the laboratory.

Questions of wound management have been more difficult to study, although wound-ballistics researchers have not ignored them. Tissue simulants, or even conscious but chronically instrumented laboratory animals, do not provide completely accurate models of wounding effects and their treatments. Therapeutic questions are probably best answered during actual combat conditions, but military surgeons should not ignore the contributions that have been made in wound-ballistics laboratories.

REFERENCES

1. Billroth, T. 1859. *Historical studies on the nature and treatment of gunshot wounds from the fifteenth century to the present time.* Translated by C. P. Rhoads. 1933 edition. New Haven, CT: The Nathan Smith Medical Club.

2. Le Dran, H. F. 1736. *Traité ou reflexions tirées de la protique sur les playes d'armes a feu.* In reference 1.

3. Hunter, J. 1794. *A treatise on the blood, inflammation, and gunshot wounds.* London: John Richardson. 1982 edition. Birmingham, AL: Classics of Medicine Library, Division of Gryphon Editions, Ltd.

4. Fackler, M. L. 1989. Misinterpretations concerning Larrey's methods of wound treatment. *Surg. Gynecol. Obstet.* 168:280–282.

5. Otis, G. A., and Huntington, D. L. 1883. Weapons. Chapt. 11 of vol. 2, part 3, *Surgical history* of the series *Medical and Surgical History of the War of the Rebellion.* Washington, DC: Government Printing Office.

6. Otis, G. A., and Huntington, D. L. 1883. Wounds and complications. Chapt. 12 of reference 5.

7. La Garde, L. A. 1916. *Gunshot injuries.* New York: William Wood and Company.

8. Greenwood, C. 1980. The political factors. In *The gun digest.* 34th ed., ed. K. Warner. Northfield IL: DBI Books, Inc.

9. Reichert, R. L. 1928. The historical treatment of the procedure termed debridement. *Bulletin of The Johns Hopkins Hospital* 42:93–104.

10. Wangensteen, O. H., and Wangensteen, S. H. 1967. Military surgeons and surgery, old and new: An instructive chapter in the management of contaminated wounds. *Surgery* 62:1102–1124.

11. Bowlby, A. A. 1915. *Wounds in war: The Bradshaw lecture.* Bristol, Eng.: John Wright and Sons Ltd.

12. Morlay, J. 1915. Surgery on the Gallipoli peninsula. *BMJ* (Sept. 25) 461–483.

13. Pool, E. H. 1927. Wounds of soft parts. Chapt. 12 of *Surgery.* Vol. 11 of *The Medical Department of the United States Army in the World War.* Washington, DC: Government Printing Office.

14. Scott, J. C. 1953. Closed plaster treatment of wounds. Part 3 of Chapt. 6, Orthopaedic surgery, in *Surgery,* edited by Zachary Cope. London: Her Majesty's Stationery Office.

15. Trueta, R. J. 1943. *The principles and practice of war surgery.* St. Louis: The C. V. Mosby Company.

16. Barling, S. 1942. Local treatment of infected war wounds, with special reference to debridement. Chapt. 11 of *Surgery of modern warfare,* edited by H. Bailey. Baltimore: The Williams and Wilkins Company.

17. Samson, H. H. 1942. Primary wound excision. Chapt. 10 of reference 16.

18. Churchill, E. D. 1972. *Surgeon to soldiers.* Philadelphia: J. B. Lippincott Company.

19. Fisher, G. H.; Florey, M. E.; Grimson, T. A.; and Williams, P. M. de C. 1945. Penicillin in clostridial infections June 8 to July 24, 1944. *Lancet* (March 31) 395–399.

20. Hampton, O. P. 1957. *Orthopedic surgery in the Mediterranean theater of operation.* In the unnumbered 30-vol. series *Surgery in World War II.* Washington, DC: Office of the Surgeon General, Department of the Army.

21. Ogilvie, W. H. 1944. *The bulletin of the U.S. Army Medical Department.* 76(1):35.

22. Beebe, G. W., and DeBakey, M. E. 1952. *Battle casualties.* Springfield, IL: Charles C. Thomas.

23. Wiltse, C. M. 1965. *The Medical Department: Medical service in the Mediterranean and minor theaters.* Washington, DC: Department of the Army, Office of the Chief of Military History.

24. Callender, G. R. 1944. Data on the distribution of missile wounds. *Bull. U.S. Army Medical Department* (March) 74: 19–22.

25. Commander in Chief, Pacific. 1970. Proceedings of the Fourth Conference on War Surgery (16–19 February). Tokyo. Washington, DC: Department of Defense and the Pacific Command.

26. Hardaway, R. M. 1978. Vietnam wound analysis. *J. Trauma* 18:635–643.

27. Simchen, E., and Sacks, T. 1975. Infection in war wounds. *Ann. Surg.* 182:754–761.

28. Klein, R. S.; Berger, S. A.; and Yekutiel, P. 1975. Wound infection during the Yom Kippur War. *Ann. Surg.* 182:15–20.

29. Wound Data and Munitions Effectiveness Team. 1970. *Evaluation of Wound Data and Munitions Effectiveness in Vietnam.* [Final Report]. In Vol. 1. Alexandria, VA: Defense Documentation Center.

30. McGreevy, P. S., and Miller, F. A. 1969. Biography of Theodor Kocher. *Surgery* 65:990–999.

31. Weise, E. R., and Gilbert, J. E. 1931. Theodor Kocher. *Ann. Med. Hist.* 3:521–529.

32. Dougherty, P. J. 1987. Theodor Kocher and the foundation of scientific wound ballistics. Paper presented at Surgical Associates Day, Uniformed Services University of the Health Sciences, Bethesda, Maryland.

33. Kocher, E. T. 1912. Über die Sprengwirkung der modernen Kleingewehr-Beschosse. *Corresp. Blt. Schweiz. Arz.* In reference 31.

34. Kocher, E. T. 1879. Neue Beltrage zur Kenntnis der Wirkungsweise der Modernen Kleingewehr Geschosse. *Corresp. Blt. Schwz. Arz.* In reference 31.

35. Kocher, E. T. 1894. Die Verbesserung der Geschosse von Standpunkte der Humanität. *Atti. D. XI Cong. Med. Internaz.* In reference 31.

36. Frederich, P. L. 1898. Die Aseptische Versorgung frischer Wunden. *Archiv für Klinische Chirurgie* 57:288–310. Translated (unpublished) for TMM by R. Miller, 1990.

37. Kaffer, H., ed. 1944. *Feldchirurgie.* Dresden: Verlag von Theodor Steinkopff.

38. Horsley, V. 1894. The destructive effects of small projectiles. *Nature* vol. 50(1283):104–108.

39. Woodruff, C. E. 1898. The causes of the explosive effects of modern small caliber bullets. *N. Y. Med. J.* 67:593–601.

40. La Garde, L. A. 1903. Infected bullets. *JAMA* 40:984–987.

41. Callender, G. R., and French, R. W. 1935. Wound ballistics—Studies in the mechanism of wound production by rifle bullets. *Milit. Surg.* 77:177–201.

42. Wilson, L. B. 1927. Firearms and projectiles; their bearing on wound production. Chapt. 2 of reference 13.

43. Black, A. N.; Burns, B. D.; and Zuckerman, S. 1941. An experimental study of the wounding mechanism of high-velocity missiles. *BMJ* 2: 872–874.

44. Harvey, E. N.; McMillen, J. H.; Butler, E. G.; and Puckett, W. O. 1962. Mechanism of wounding. Chapt. 3 of *Wound Ballistics,* edited by J. C. Beyer. Washington, DC: Office of the Surgeon General, Department of the Army.

45. Peters, C. E. 1990. Common misconceptions about the physical mechanisms in wound ballistics. *J. Trauma* (China) 6(2) suppl.:319–326.

46. Dziemian, A. J., and Herget, C. M. 1950. Physical aspects of the primary contamination of bullet wounds. *Milit. Surg.* 106:294–299.

47. Dziemian, A. J.; Mendelson, J. A.; and Lindsey, D. 1961. Comparison of the wounding characteristics of some commonly encountered bullets. *J. Trauma* 1:341–353.

48. Mendelson, J. A., and Glover, J. L. 1967. Sphere and shell fragment wounds of soft tissues: Experimental study. *J. Trauma* 7:889–914.

49. Owen-Smith, M. S., and Matheson, J. M. 1968. Successful prophylaxis of gas gangrene in the high velocity missile wound in sheep. *Br. J. Surg.* 55:36–39.

50. Amato, J. J.; Billy, L. J.; Gruber, R. P.; and Rich, N. M. 1974. Temporary cavitation in high velocity pulmonary missile injuries. *Ann. Thorac. Surg.* 18:565–570.

51. Amato, J. J.; Rich, N. M.; Billy, L. J.; Gruber, R. P.; and Lawson, N. S. 1971. High velocity arterial injury: A study of the mechanism of injury. *J. Trauma* 11:412–416.

52. Rich, N. M. 1978. Military surgery: Bullets and blood vessels. *Surg. Clin. North Am.* 58:996–1003.

53. Janzon, B. 1983. *High-energy missile trauma: A study of the mechanisms of wounding of muscle tissue.* Göteborg, Sweden: University of Göteborg. Doctoral dissertation.

54. Seeman, T., ed. 1979. Proceedings of the Symposium on Wound Ballistics, 1977. *Acta Chir. Scand.* (Suppl. 489).

55. Seeman, T., ed. 1982. Proceedings of the Fourth Symposium on Wound Ballistics, 1981. *Acta Chir. Scand.* (Suppl. 508).

56. Proceedings of the Fifth International Symposium on Wound Ballistics, 1988. *J. Trauma* 28 (Suppl.).

57. Fackler, M. L., and Malinowski, J. A. 1985. The wound profile: A visual method for quantifying gunshot components. *J. Trauma* 25:522–529.

Chapter 4

THE PHYSICS AND BIOPHYSICS OF WOUND BALLISTICS

RONALD F. BELLAMY, M.D., FACS* AND RUSS ZAJTCHUK, M.D., FACS**

*Colonel, United States Army; Acting Chief, Department of Surgery, Walter Reed Army Medical Center, Washington, D.C. 20307-5001

**Colonel, United States Army; Deputy Commander, Walter Reed Army Medical Center, Washington, D.C. 20307-5001

INTRODUCTION

Ballistics is the science that studies the motion and impact of *projectiles* (that is, objects that are designed to be hurled or shot forward). Thus, ballistics pertains only to inert, not to self-propelled, objects.

When the behavior of bullets is studied, ballistics is usually considered in three parts: *(a) internal,* which seeks to understand what happens to the projectile while it is still within the gun barrel, where enormous pressures act for an instant upon it; *(b) external,* which seeks to describe the factors (air resistance and gravity being the most important) that determine the projectile's trajectory between the muzzle and the target; and *(c) terminal,* which seeks to describe the interaction of the projectile and the target. *Wound ballistics* is the study of the terminal ballistics of both fragments and bullets in living human tissue, and *ballistic wounds* are penetrating injuries caused by projectiles.

While the nature of ballistic wounds would seem to depend upon *(a)* the physical characteristics of the projectile, *(b)* the biophysical properties of the target tissue, and *(c)* the interaction between the projectile and the tissue, this seemingly rational classification is difficult to apply. Important physical properties of the projectile, such as its construction, become apparent only during the interaction of the projectile with the target tissue. Thus, projectile construction as a determinant of wounding is best considered as a manifestation of the projectile-tissue interaction. Also, because little is known about the material strength and viscoelastic properties of human tissue, integrating their biophysical properties into a meaningful theory of wound ballistics is difficult.

Because of these limitations, this chapter discusses *(a)* the physical characteristics of projectiles, which culminate in their ability to penetrate the target, *(b)* the biophysics of the projectile-target interaction, and *(c)* ballistic tissue damage. For the medical officer, however, the problems of ballistic wounds are inseparable from the problems of wound management, especially the treatment of wounds of soft tissue. More than 90% of battlefield casualties sustain soft-tissue wounds. Because of this incidence, the clinically relevant aspects of wound ballistics, especially the management of soft-tissue wounds, constitute a separate chapter.

THE PHYSICAL CHARACTERISTICS OF PROJECTILES

Mass

While physicists consider mass and weight to be quite different, for the purposes of practical ballistics the mass of a projectile is numerically identical to its weight, and is usually conceptualized as being *(a)* located at a point within the projectile and *(b)* usually located near its geometric center—its *center of mass.* The forward motion of the center of mass defines the projectile's *trajectory* (that is, its line of flight).

Most bullets that modern military small arms fire weigh 3.5–12.0 g; typical nineteenth-century bullets commonly weighed 20–30 g (Table 4-1). Cannonballs and the largest fragments from older, random-fragmentation shells weighed many kilograms, but the projectiles from the explosive, improved-fragmentation munitions used today weigh 50 mg to several grams (Table 4-2).

Density is the ratio of the mass of an object to its volume. Bullets usually contain lead, which has a density of 11.4 g/cm^3, and are disproportionately smaller than fragments, which are usually made of steel, which has a density of 7.9 g/cm^3. Lightweight metals such as aluminum, which has a density of 2.7 g/cm^3, have been used as part of a bullet's core, and are the constituents of the fragments that are formed from the outer walls of certain modern explosive munitions. Tungsten, at the other end of the density spectrum with a density of 19.4 g/cm^3, is used as the core penetrator in small-caliber bullets of advanced design.

Shape

A projectile's shape, in addition to its mass, determines how the projectile will behave not only on its trajectory through air but also as it strikes and penetrates its target. Shapes of projectiles vary from arrow-like fléchettes to the irregular chunks of random fragments. The shape of a chunky fragment is difficult to quantify, but the pointed, curved shape of a bullet's nose, its *ogive,* and the cross-sectional area of projectiles can be described.

Ogive. The ogive measures the number of projectile calibers that would constitute the radius of a hypo-

TABLE 4-1

CHARACTERISTICS OF IMPORTANT MILITARY SMALL-ARM PROJECTILES

Weapon	Era	Construction of Projectile	Diameter (mm)	Weight (g)	Muzzle Velocity (m/s)	Kinetic Energy (muzzle) (J)	Important Features
Smooth-bore musket*	1700	Soft lead round ball	18	33	180	530	Deformation
Muzzle-loading rifle*	1850	Soft lead conoidal bullet	17	37	300	1,655	Deformation
Breech-loading rifle*	1870	Hard lead cylindro-conoidal bullet	11	25	430	2,300	Deformation
Breech-loading magazine rifle*	1890	Blunt nose lead core, steel jacket	7.9	14	600	2,650	Good stability
Single-shot bolt action rifle*	1910	Pointed nose lead core, steel jacket	7.9	9	830	3,100	Poor stability
Vickers Mk 7 machine gun (GB)**	WWI	Aluminum cap lead core, copper jacket	7.7	11	750	3,060	Poor stability
Karabiner Model 1898 single shot, bolt action rifle (GER)**		Lead core steel jacket	7.9	11	740	3,000	Poor stability
ACP M1911 automatic pistol (USA)**		Lead core copper jacket	11.7	15	265	527	Good stability
PPSh machine pistol (USSR)**	WWII	Lead core steel jacket	7.62	4.8	490	560	Multiple hits possible
Garand M1 semiautomatic rifle (USA)**		Lead core copper jacket	7.62	10.5	830	3,600	Poor stability
MG 42 machine gun (GER)**		Lead core steel jacket	7.92	11	800	3,600	Poor stability
AK47 assault rifle (USSR)**	post–WWII	Steel and lead core steel jacket, M43 ball	7.62	7.6	730	2,000	Poor stability multiple hits
M16 assault rifle (USA)**		Lead core copper jacket, M193	5.56	3.5	980	1,650	Fragmentation multiple hits

Note: Representative values are shown; numerical quantities are rounded; the bullets from WWI and post–WWI periods are spitzers except those fired by the ACP M1911 and the PPSh, which have the characteristic round-nose design of pistol ammunition.

*La Garde, L. A. 1916. *Gunshot Injuries*. 2d revised edition. New York: William Wood and Company.

** Hogg, I. V. and Weeks, J. 1985. *Military Small Arms of the 20th Century*. 5th ed. Northfield, IL: DBI Books, Inc.

TABLE 4-2

CHARACTERISTICS OF PROJECTILES FROM EXPLOSIVE MUNITIONS

Weapons and Projectiles	Projectile Characteristics Mass*** (g)	Velocity † (m/s)	Kinetic Energy (J)	Important Features
Muzzle-loading cannon; French 12-pounder cannonball; solid lead*	5,450	~300	260,000	Massive crush
Spherical case shot; lead ball shrapnel**	60	~200 at100 m	400	Deformation
High-explosive shell projectile; irregular iron or steel fragments with different mass	30	~1,100 at 200 ft	18,000	Catastrophic injury
	4	~500 at 200 ft	550	
	0.3	~690 at 30 ft	70	Most common size
Fléchettes	1.5	~400 at 200 m	140	Multiple hits
Modern Claymore mines; steel ball shrapnel**	0.6	~700 at 50 m	150	Multiple hits

*Not an explosive munition, but included for purposes of comparison.

**Strictly defined, shrapnel means preformed fragments (the fragments exist already made within the explosive munition). Thus, fragments from a random-fragmentation shell are not shrapnel. Also note that by strict definition, fléchettes are shrapnel.

***Representative values.

†Velocity of the fragments at the time of detonation from the explosive munition at a defined distance from the weapon. The values represent velocity at stated distance, if given, or maximum velocity of the projectile.

Sources:

Douglas, H. 1860. *A treatise on naval gunnery*. 5th rev. ed. London: John Murray, Albemarle Street. (cannonball)

Beyer, J. C., ed. 1962. *Wound ballistics*. Washington, D.C.: Office of the Surgeon General, Department of the Army. (spherical case shot and high-explosive)

Explosive Ordnance Disposal Group, Quantico Marine Corps Base, VA. (Claymore mines; fléchettes)

thetical circle that includes the ogive as an arc. Thus, when a bullet has an ogive of 7, the curved portion of its nose forms an arc of a circle with a radius seven times the projectile's caliber (Figure 4-1). The round-nosed jacketed bullets that were introduced at the end of the nineteenth century had ogives of 1.5–2.0. The spitzer bullets that followed had ogives of 6–7.

Cross-Sectional Area. Another index of shape is the projectile's maximum cross-sectional area perpendicular to its line of flight (A). Complicating the role of shape as a physical parameter, a projectile not symmetrical in the three dimensions of space will present differing cross-sectional areas as it wobbles around its asymmetric axes. A sphere, since it has perfect sym-

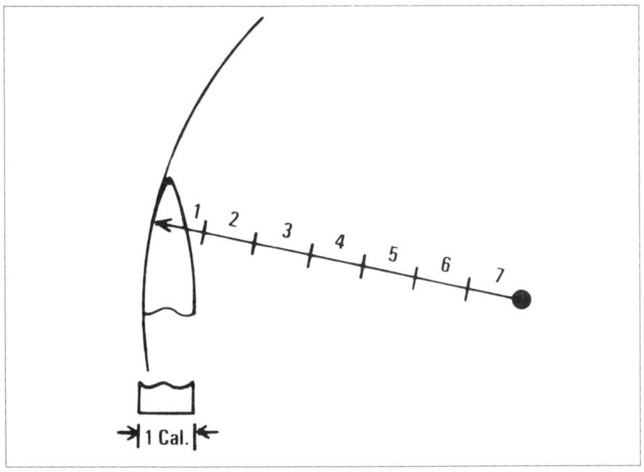

Fig. 4-1. Calculation of ogive. The nose of the bullet forms an arc of a circle. The radius of this circle is expressed as the number of calibers (in this example, 7) that equal the absolute length of the radius.

metry, and chunky fragments that are nearly symmetrical cannot present different cross-sectional areas as they move along their trajectories. But an elongated cylinder such as a bullet, which is symmetrical only around its long axis, can *tumble* (that is, flip end-over-end) around its center of mass. Its cross-sectional area will not be constant because, at least part of the time, a tumbling bullet's side (rather than its nose or base) will be perpendicular to the line of flight.

Sectional Density. Dividing a projectile's mass by its cross-sectional area (that is, M/A) yields a parameter known as the sectional (or frontal) density. A long, narrow fléchette, because it has a tiny cross-sectional area, has a high sectional density compared to a sphere or an irregular chunky fragment.

Velocity

Velocity is usually considered to be the single most important property of a projectile. This may be true in theory. In practice, however, the velocity of a projectile as it hits its target is usually not known because its velocity decreases as a projectile travels along its trajectory. Because a bullet's impact velocity usually is estimated from the small arm's published muzzle velocity, the estimate requires knowledge of the distance from the weapon to the target. The impact velocity of a projectile from an explosive munition is even more difficult to quantify. While accurate measurements of a bullet's velocity—as a function of downrange distance—can be made in the laboratory using electronic timers (chronometers), measuring a fragment's velocity requires sophisticated photo-optic techniques, which are available in only a few weapons-research institutes.

Most impact velocities range between 80 m/s (about 250 fps), the minimum velocity required for a round or pointed projectile to penetrate human skin, and 1,500 m/s (about 4,900 fps), the highest velocity at which a projectile from an explosive munition is likely to wound a casualty who will not have been killed by proximity to the blast.

Projectiles are customarily described as "low-" or "high-velocity," but the actual corresponding speeds have not been well defined. This textbook arbitrarily defines *low velocity* as slower than the speed of sound in air (that is, 334 m/s or 1,100 fps) and *ultrahigh velocity* as the speed of sound in soft tissue (that is, 1,500 m/s or 4,900 fps). (Projectiles with ultrahigh velocities are uncommon on a battlefield.) Since the first observations of "explosive" wounds occurred when "high-velocity" bullets were fielded in the mid-nineteenth century, it seems reasonable to connect the two. Therefore, this textbook defines *high velocity* as that at which explosive effects begin to be commonly seen (that is, 600–700 m/s, or 2,000–2,300 fps). Velocities between 1,100 fps and 2,000 fps are known as *intermediate* or *medium*. The velocity of a typical musket ball that Hunter described in the eighteenth century as "great" (that is, 180 m/s) was actually low velocity by our definition (Table 4-1). Rifles firing high-velocity bullets have been the norm since the end of the nineteenth century, and velocity has barely increased since the early twentieth century. The velocity of the M193 ball fired by the M16 rifle of 1965 is only about 10% greater than that of the 1910 spitzer bullets.

Table 4-1 lists the muzzle velocities of some common bullets. Because bullets are streamlined, they maintain their velocities far better than projectiles from explosive munitions do, with the exception of fléchettes (Figure 4-2).

Kinetic Energy

Energy is the ability to do work, and any physical body that moves has an ability to exert force and to do work—simply by virtue of its motion—called *kinetic energy* (KE). This derived parameter, measured now in *joules* (J) but formerly in foot-pounds, can be calculated when the projectile's properties of mass and velocity are known:

$$KE = \frac{MV^2}{2}$$

Since velocity V enters the equation raised to the second power, changes in a projectile's velocity cause greater changes in its kinetic energy than do changes in the projectile's mass M. The dominant features of military small arms bullet-design during the past two

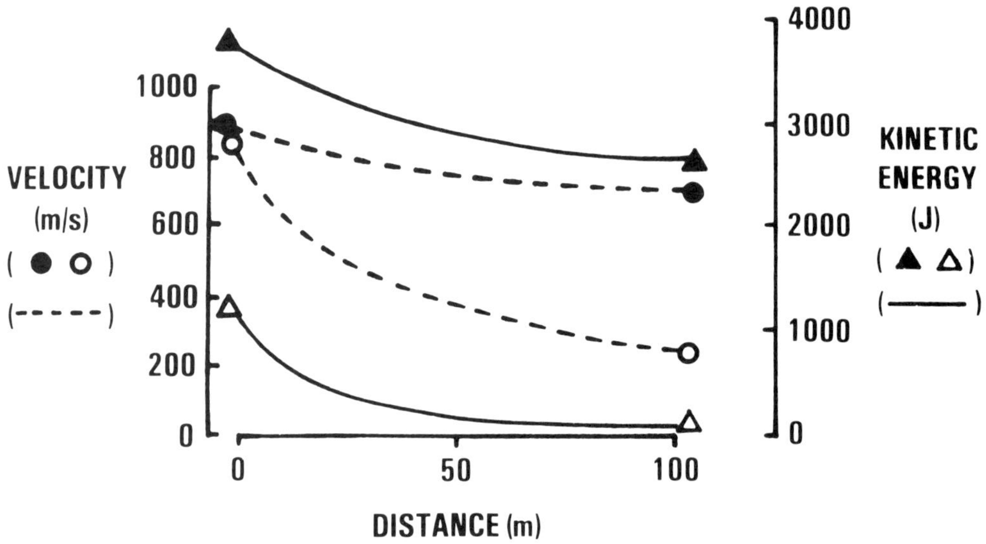

Fig. 4-2. The decrements in velocity (broken lines) and kinetic energy (solid lines) for a typical "chunky" fragment (open circle and triangle) and a 7.62-mm bullet (closed circle and triangle) in air. The fragment is assumed to weigh 3 g and the mass of the bullet is 9.75 g. For purposes of illustration, the initial velocities of both projectiles is taken as 862 m/s. The decrements in velocity and kinetic energy are much greater in the unstreamlined fragment than in the streamlined bullet.
Source: Reference 7.

centuries were *(a)* reducing the bullet's mass and *(b)* increasing its velocity, which consequently increased its kinetic energy. For example, a typical musket ball used in 1850 had a kinetic energy of about 1,665 J, while one of the most important rifles used in World War II, the American M1, fired a bullet that had a muzzle–kinetic energy of 3,600 J. Only since World War II has reducing projectile mass outstripped increasing velocity, resulting in a consequent fall in kinetic energy: The M193 ball fired by the M16A1 rifle had a muzzle–kinetic energy of only 1,650 J.

As with high velocity, we can speak of high kinetic energy. As was true of velocity, a projectile's kinetic energy at impact depends upon the target's distance from the muzzle or the site of detonation. The kinetic energy of an irregularly shaped fragment degrades faster than does the kinetic energy of a streamlined bullet (Figure 4-2).

Drag

A medium, whether air, water, or human tissue, hinders or resists a projectile as it passes through. This resistance is called *drag,* which degrades both velocity and kinetic energy (Figure 4-2), and is an important determinant of the magnitude of ballistic injury.

Drag depends upon the properties of both the projectile and the medium it passes through. As a projectile penetrates, the medium in its path is split apart and displaced to the side. The medium's splitting and displacement both create drag, and their net effect slows and may ultimately stop the projectile.

Displacement of the medium is the most important source of drag as a projectile moves through air. As the gas molecules in air are displaced, drag arises from three sources (the sources of drag are much more complicated when a projectile passes through tissue):

- Air is compressed at the tip of the projectile, forming a region of high pressure. This is by far the most important source of drag for a projectile moving through air at velocities greater than the speed of sound.
- Turbulence occurs at the base of the projectile as the displaced air returns to its original position.
- Friction occurs as air slides around the body of the projectile. This is the least important source of drag.

The mathematical expression for the drag that occurs when a projectile passes through a fluid is:

$$\text{Drag} = 1/2\,[(CD)\,(d)\,(A)\,(V^2)]$$

where *CD* is the proportionality constant known as the coefficient of drag, *d* is the density of the target medium, *A* is the projectile's cross-sectional area, and *V* its velocity.

The drag equation indicates that, if all other factors remain the same, changing the density of the medium from that of air (0.001 g/cm^3) to that of water (1.00 g/cm^3) will result in a thousandfold increase in drag. Similarly, increasing the cross-sectional area of the projectile (for example, as when a deforming bullet such as a dumdum hits a solid target, or when a bullet tumbles) will increase drag. Because velocity is raised to the second power in the equation, doubling the projectile's velocity increases drag fourfold.

All other factors, such as the coefficient of drag and the shape, being the same, drag is much greater with high- than with low-velocity projectiles. For example, high-velocity rifle bullets slow more rapidly than do similarly shaped pistol bullets.

The drag equation omits a factor for the splitting of the medium, a phenomenon that depends upon the medium's material strength. Because of this omission, the increase in drag that occurs when a projectile passes from air into human soft tissue will be much greater than a prediction based simply on the change in density (from 0.001 g/cm^3 in air to 1.05 g/cm^3 in muscle). This factor is unknown and is one of the areas that requires the attention of sophisticated ballistics researchers.

When drag is treated mathematically as the force of retardation, it is usually normalized for projectile mass (that is, drag/mass) and can be expressed:

$$[(CD)\,(d)\,(V^2)\,(A/M)]$$

or, by transposition:

$$\frac{(CD)\,(d)\,(V^2)}{M/A}$$

However, a projectile's sectional density (M / A) is an important determinant of drag: the higher the sectional density, the lower the drag. The velocity of a heavy, narrow projectile (such as a long penetrator rod made of tungsten) will degrade less rapidly than the velocity of a lightweight, large projectile (such as an artillery rocket) will.

Projectiles undergo an enormous force of retardation when they cause ballistic injuries. When traveling point-forward through air, a bullet with a velocity of about 2,000 fps will be retarded by a force of about one *newton* (N, the force that imparts to a mass of 1 kg an acceleration of 1 m/s^2), which is equivalent to about 3 psi. Forces measuring tens of thousands of newtons develop during maximum retardation in a tissue simulant such as gelatin or in soft tissue.[1, 2]

Coefficient of Drag

The coefficient of drag (CD) depends upon a combination of *(a)* the ratio of the projectile's velocity to the speed of sound in the medium through which the projectile is traveling, *(b)* the shape of the projectile, and *(c)* the viscoelastic properties of that medium.

While a projectile's shape is the most important determinant of the coefficient of drag, for the data to be interpreted correctly, the velocity at the time the measurement was made must also be known. A projectile's CD is not constant for a given shape, because it depends upon the ratio of the velocity of the projectile (Vp) to the velocity of sound in the medium (Vs), that is, Vp/Vs. This ratio is known as the Mach number. By definition, a Mach number less than 1 is *subsonic*, and greater than 1 is *supersonic*. When the Mach number is 0.6–0.7 or less, CD is relatively constant, but as the Mach number increases from 0.8–1.2 (the *transonic* region), a three- to fourfold increase in CD, and therefore in drag, occurs. As the Mach number approaches 2.0, CD falls again, but is always higher than it was in the subsonic region. At very low velocity (that is, less than 100 m/s), the coefficient of drag increases greatly, but because the velocity is so low, the increase in the absolute magnitude of drag is probably of little consequence.[3] Although projectiles may travel at supersonic speeds through air, they rarely exceed the speed of sound characteristic of the target tissue (except lung) while they are penetrating it.

Irregular fragments have very high CDs (that is, a value greater than 2.0). A round-nose bullet of the type that was introduced in the 1890s has a CD (in air, in the subsonic region) of about 0.9. The spitzer bullet that was introduced 10 years later had a CD (in air, in the subsonic region) of 0.4. The difference between the two CD values appears to be small, but the superior aerodynamic property of a pointed bullet compared to a round-nose bullet is that a spitzer's CD increases less rapidly in the supersonic and transonic regions.

The viscoelastic properties of the medium are the third (and least important) determinant of CD. When balls are fired into various media at subsonic speeds (that is, the velocity of sound in the medium is greater than the velocity of the projectile through the medium), although the CDs of the media do vary,[4] the variance is not great: in water, the CD is 0.30; in gelatin (20%) at 20° C, 0.35; in swine skeletal muscle, 0.45; and in swine skin, the CD is 0.53. While precise CDs for human tissue have not been determined, they probably do not differ significantly from these.

The CD is difficult to measure. Until recently, a bullet's *aerodynamic performance* (that is, its deceleration as a function of its velocity) was estimated by dividing the experimentally determined drag of a bullet of standardized shape by a constant known as the *ballistic coefficient,* which is directly related to both that bullet's sectional density and its ogive. Thus, a heavy, narrow, spitzer bullet has a high ballistic coefficient and therefore low drag compared to the standardized bullet. Currently, the ballistic coefficient is most frequently used to evaluate handgun bullets. The ballistic coefficient and the coefficient of drag give information that appears to be similar, but the parameters are quite different and should not be confused.[5]

Stability

A projectile that maintains a constant cross-sectional area perpendicular to its line of flight is said to be stable. It has minimal drag compared to a projectile that is unstable and therefore *tumbling* (that is, it flips over in the plane parallel to its line of flight). Unstable projectiles lack both range and accuracy and have little military value. An elongated cylindrical projectile like a bullet is inherently unstable, but it can be stabilized by being spun around its long axis, which imparts *gyroscopic stability.* The factors that render an unspun bullet unstable demonstrate this phenomenon.

The Center of Pressure. The hypothetical unspun bullet in Figure 4-3 is shown with its line of flight and long axis exactly coinciding. As air resists the forward motion of the bullet, an area of high pressure develops near the bullet's nose. The airflow from the nose back around the bullet is symmetrical because *(a)* the bullet is symmetrical and *(b)* the bullet's line of flight and its long axis coincide. The force retarding the bullet's forward motion (that is, drag) therefore acts symmetrically on the bullet, and can be imagined to be located at a site known as the *center of pressure* (CP). In the hypothetical example shown in Figure 4-3, the center of pressure lies on both the line of flight and the long axis. In this instance, the sole effect of the center of pressure is to retard the forward motion of the bullet.

Tumbling. An unspun bullet is unstable because the slightest separation of its line of flight and its long axis—as a gust of wind might cause—will cause the area of high pressure at the bullet's nose to move to one side. The airflow will no longer be symmetrical around the long axis, creating unequal air pressures above and below the bullet, generating lift. The force acting at the center of pressure will separate into two vectors (Figure 4-4): *(a)* drag, which continues to retard the forward motion of the bullet and *(b)* the new lift force, which attempts to flip the bullet over around its center of mass. A perpetuating cycle develops: the greater the separation of the long axis and the line of flight, the greater the lift force; the greater the lift force, the more the long axis and the line of flight will be separated, until the bullet turns over or tumbles. Theoretically, once tumbling begins it will continue because the center of pressure, which remains near the projectile's leading edge, will always be located ahead of the center of mass. More commonly, though, as a bullet slows in tissue, it only tumbles once, then progresses base-forward.

Gyroscopic Stabilization. Even a minor disturbance can cause any unspun projectile to tumble if its center of pressure is located ahead of its center of mass. But a minor disturbance affects a spinning projectile differently. The separation of the projectile's long axis and line of flight generates lift, but rather than causing the projectile to tumble, the lift force interacts with the spin to produce an angular force or *torque,* which displaces the long axis of the projectile perpendicular to the line of flight. Because the long axis and line of flight are separated, lift continues to be generated as the projectile moves forward through air. Lift and spin continue to act together to produce a torque that effects a continuous displacement of the projectile's long axis in the plane perpendicular to its line of flight. Thus, the projectile's long axis rotates around the line of flight, describing a cone. Viewed head-on (Figure 4-5), the projectile's nose rotates around its center of mass, in the same direction as the spin.

Precession and Yaw. This rotation around its center of mass is known as *precession*; the angle that the long axis deviates from the line of flight is known as the *angle of yaw* (Figure 4-6). In a spinning bullet, precession is the response to a disturbance that in an unspun bullet would cause tumbling. But gyroscopic stabilization does more than simply prevent tumbling. If precession occurs over a long enough time, the angle of yaw will nearly disappear (that is, the bullet's long axis and its line of flight will again converge). This aspect of gyroscopic stabilization depends upon the fact that air resistance acting near the bullet's base creates a torque that pushes the portion of the bullet behind the center of mass back toward the line of flight. As precession is damped by air resistance, the angle of yaw becomes smaller. Since a bullet's drag is approximately proportional to the square of its angle of yaw,

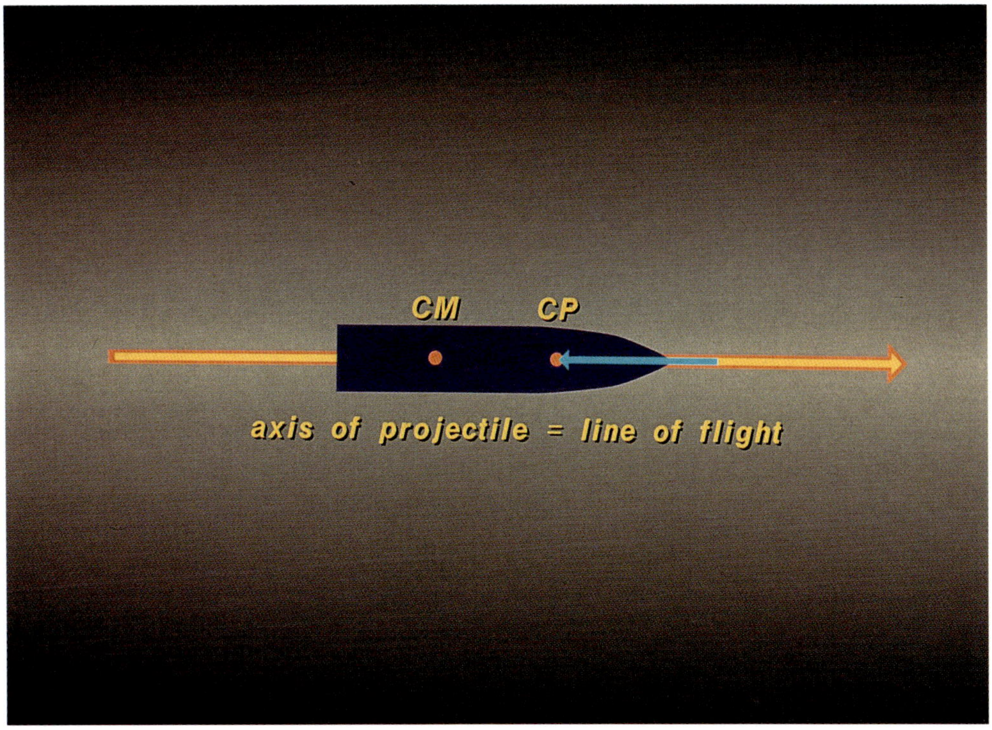

Fig. 4-3. The forces that act on a projectile moving with both its long axis and line of flight coinciding (yellow lines). Air resistance creates a force (light blue line) that acts through the center of pressure (CP) to retard the forward motion of the center of mass (CM). Since this force acts along both the line of flight and the long axis, its sole effect is to create drag.

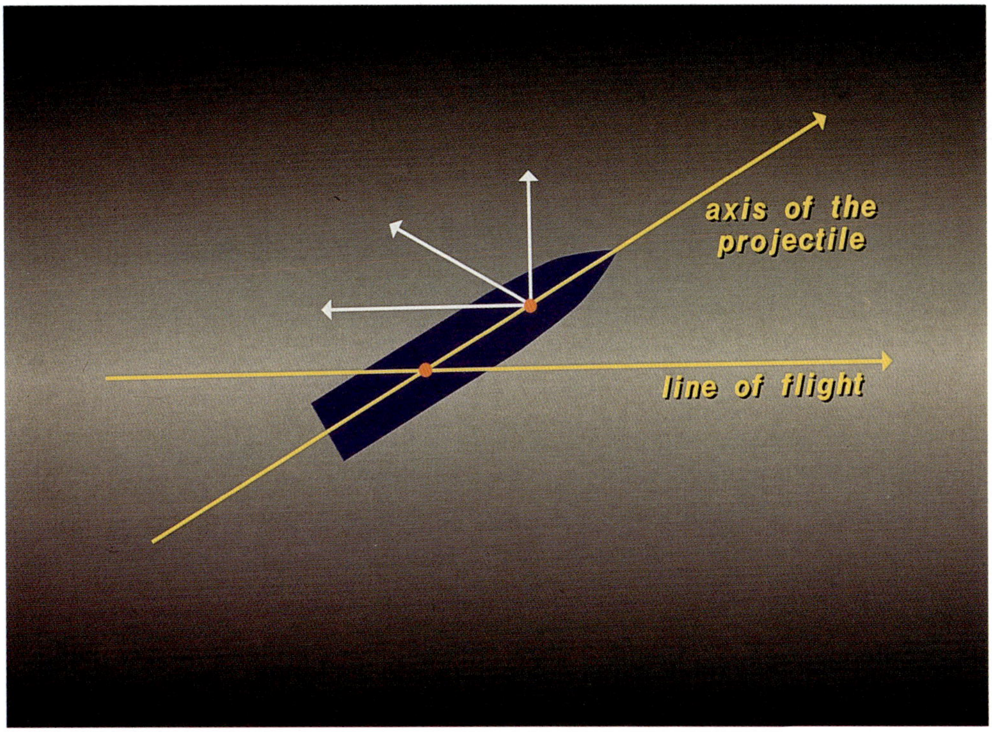

Fig. 4-4. The forces acting on an unspun, moving projectile that has been disturbed. The long axis no longer coincides with the line of flight (yellow lines). The force arising from air resistance acting at the center of pressure (CP) decomposes into two force vectors. One force acts parallel to the line of flight; this force—drag—retards the forward motion of the center of mass (CM). The second force acts in the vertical direction; this force—lift—attempts to flip the projectile over around its CM.

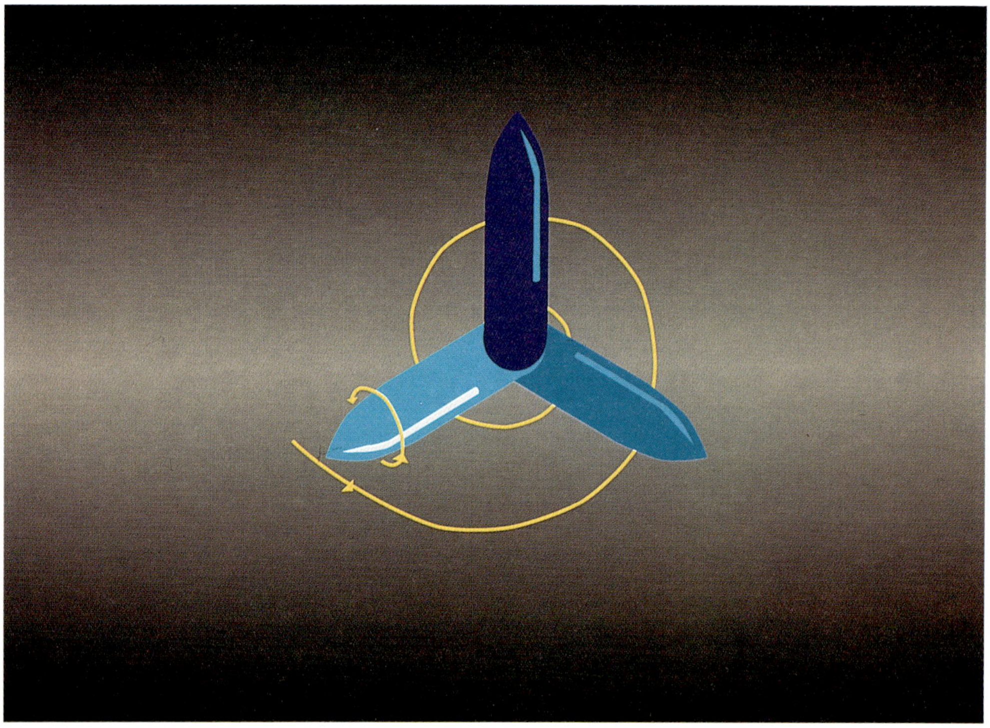

Fig. 4-5. In a spinning projectile, the forces associated with spin and lift interact to create a new force, or torque, which makes the nose of the projectile revolve around the center of mass in a plane perpendicular to the line of flight. This motion is known as precession.

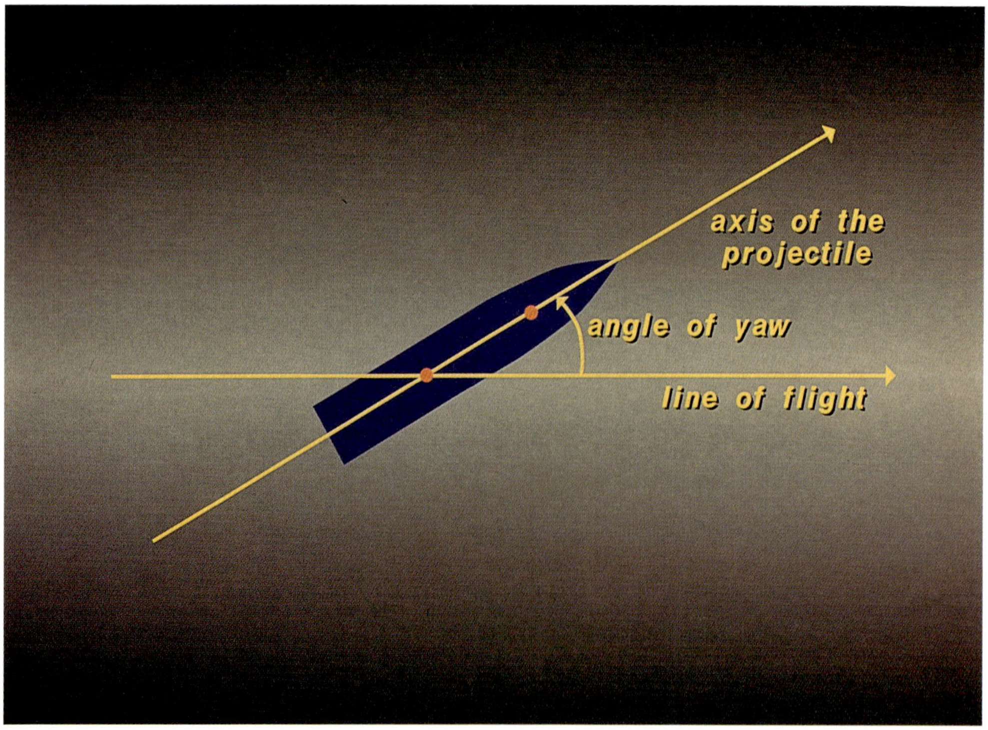

Fig. 4-6. The angle between the long axis of the projectile and the line of flight is known as the angle of yaw.

a gyroscopically stabilized bullet, since it has a smaller angle of yaw, will maintain its velocity and improve its long-distance performance. (The actual motion of a spun projectile is complex and involves more than just precession. Interested readers can find a more comprehensive treatment of the subject in manuals such as Farrar and Leeming's *Military Ballistics*.)

The Stability Equation. The factors that determine gyroscopic stabilization can be described mathematically. Stability is proportional to:

$$\frac{(\text{rate of spin})^2}{(d)\ (\text{the distance between CM and CP})\ (V^2)}$$

where d is the density of the medium and V is the projectile's velocity. For a given rate of spin, the equation indicates that the larger the factors in the denominator, the more likely a given disturbance will destabilize a projectile. The density of the medium and the distance separating the centers of mass (CM) and pressure (CP) are especially important.

Bullets have poor stability in tissue. In passing from air to soft tissue, the density of the medium increases from 0.001 g/cm^3 to 1.05 g/cm^3. Even if all other factors remained unchanged, in order to obtain the same degree of stability in soft tissue as in air, a bullet would need to be spun about thirty-two times faster—a practical impossibility.

A short distance separating the centers of mass and pressure is crucial to a bullet's stability. The pointed bullets that were introduced early in the twentieth century became more unstable than the earlier round-nose bullets, because a pointed bullet's center of mass (located toward the base near the bullet's geometric center) was much farther from its center of pressure (located in the tip) than was a round-nose bullet's. Bullets fired from handguns tend to be more stable than rifle bullets; because handgun bullets are shorter, the separation between their centers of pressure and mass is smaller.

All other factors being equal, the faster a projectile spins, the slower will be the rate of precession, the more acute will be the angle of yaw, and the quicker will its long axis and line of flight realign. Stability is relative; a sufficiently powerful disturbance will make any bullet tumble.

Rifling. The spiral grooves on the inside of a rifled barrel force a bullet to spin around its long axis as it travels the length of the barrel. The rate of spin that a rifle barrel imparts is determined by the weapon's design, and for a typical rifle bullet is several hundred thousand revolutions per minute. Although an impressive figure, the bullet's angular velocity (that is, the velocity characteristic of a rotating object) is much less than its linear velocity; a value of about 250 fps is common. The number of spirals and their *twist* (that is, the number of caliber lengths required for the bullet to make a complete revolution) are unique for each rifle and the bullet it is designed to fire. For example, the M16A1 was designed with a twist of 55 (12 inches). The newer version, the M16A2, has a twist of 32 (7 inches). The bullet that the M16A2 fires (the M855) is longer than the bullet that its predecessor fires, and therefore it requires a faster twist to obtain the same degree of stability. Because the bullet is longer, its centers of mass and pressure are farther apart, and it is more likely to become unstable. The stability equation shows that, other factors remaining the same, the longer the bullet (and thus the greater the separation between the centers of mass and pressure), the faster the spin required for a given degree of stability. Although the M16A1 rifle can fire M855 rounds, the bullets will not be optimally spin-stabilized and therefore will be unusually prone to yaw and tumble.

Internal and External Ballistic Factors That Affect a Bullet's Stability. While even wind gusts and transient encounters with leaves may disturb a bullet's trajectory so much that it precesses, bullets commonly display marked yaw as they are propelled out of the muzzle of a small arm. Factors that are likely to destabilize a bullet include:

- Imperfections in the bullet and damage it sustains as it passes down the barrel can cause the center of mass to lie outside the bullet's long axis
- The bullet can actually tilt within a badly worn barrel and already be yawing significantly when it leaves the muzzle
- The barrel can vibrate and hit the bullet as it exits, causing it to yaw
- Rapidly moving gases exiting from the muzzle can strike the base of the bullet downrange and deflect it from its line of flight[6]

Downrange 30–40 m, the interaction of the bullet's spin and air resistance will have dampened precession and markedly decreased the angle of yaw. But when a projectile passes from one medium to another of different density, (that is, from air to soft tissue), it becomes less stable. A soldier who is shot from closer than 30 m will probably be hit by a bullet that yaws significantly, and any preexisting yaw will greatly increase when the bullet penetrates tissue. Experimental evidence shows that the angle of yaw of a bullet may increase from 1°–2° in air to 180° in tissue.[7]

Fin Stabilization. Not all projectiles of military importance have to be spun to be stable. Bombs, rockets, and more recently, fléchettes, are inherently stable because they have fins. Like arrows, the tail fins of fléchettes have a huge surface area. Their center of pressure is displaced to the rear behind the center of mass, which is located near the tip. When fléchettes are propelled point-forward they cannot tumble in air, and they make tiny wounds of entrance and exit. But when they are packed fin-forward into their canisters, as some American munitions manufacturers pack them, the fléchettes must tumble—to reposition themselves so that the center of mass is near the leading edge and the center of pressure is at the rear—before they can become aerodynamically stable.

But fin-stabilized projectiles are the exceptions. Military projectiles characteristically behave like the rifle bullet shown in Figure 4-7, displaying marked precession and yaw after emerging from the muzzle. Gyroscopic stabilization gradually realigns the bullet's long axis with its line of flight; as the bullet nears its target, its angle of yaw will have decreased to only 1°–2°. When the bullet penetrates the much denser target, it destabilizes; its angle of yaw increases rapidly to 90° and the bullet tumbles.

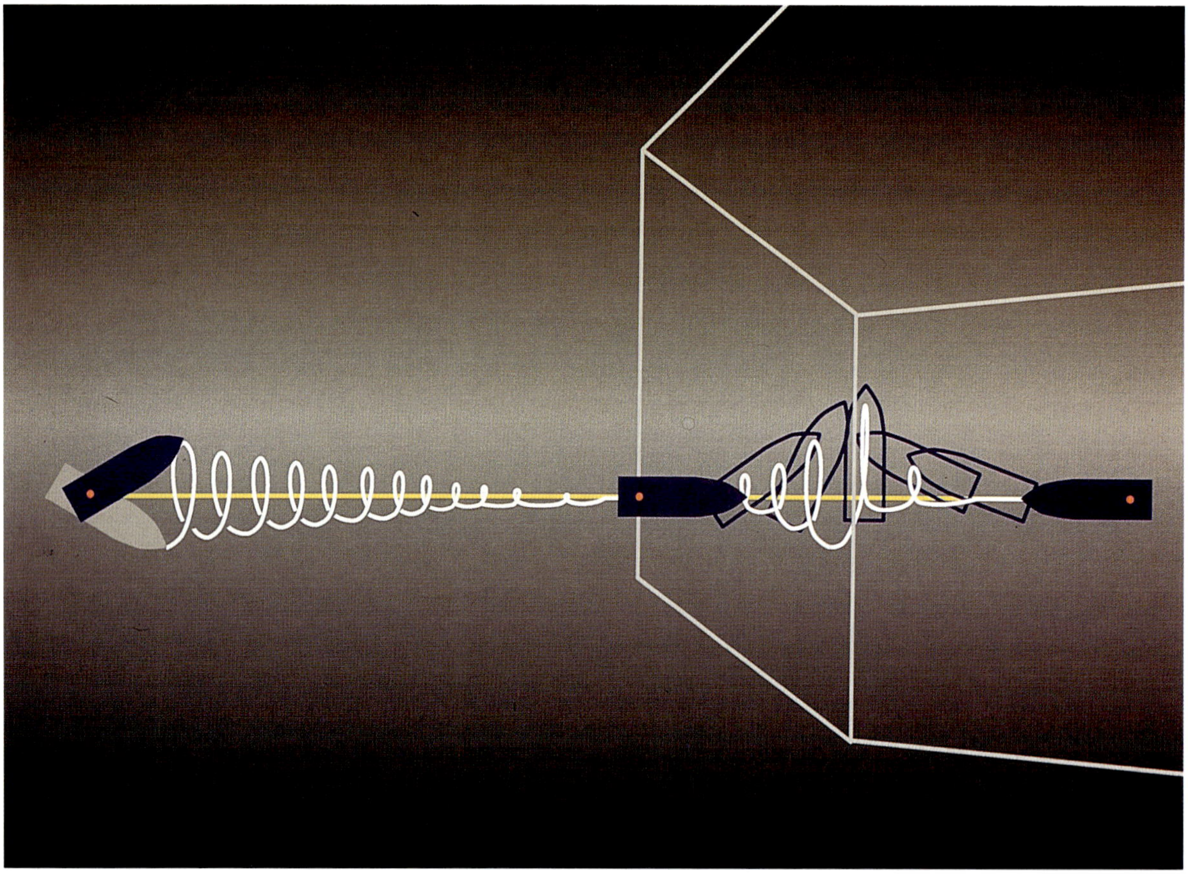

Fig. 4-7. The idealized behavior of many rifle bullets. The bullet emerges from the rifle muzzle with a significant angle of yaw. Gyroscopic stabilization gradually aligns the long axis of the bullet and the line of flight. After travelling about 100 m downrange, the angle of yaw has become very small. When the bullet enters the much more dense target tissue, it rapidly destabilizes. The angle of yaw increases until the bullet tumbles.

PENETRATION

The factors in the drag equation (that is, the coefficient of drag, the density of the medium, and the cross-sectional area and velocity of the projectile) also determine *(a)* the depth that a projectile will penetrate its target and *(b)* the velocity of the projectile at a given depth of penetration. Ideally (that is, if a stable, nondeforming projectile passes through a homogeneous, infinite solid), the depth of penetration X will be:

$$X = \frac{M}{(CD)\,(d)\,(A)} \ln \frac{V_i}{V_x}$$

and the residual velocity Vx at X will be:

$$V_x = V_i \frac{1}{e^{(X)\,(CD)\,(d)\,(A/M)}}$$

where *Vi* is the initial velocity, *CD* is the coefficient of drag for a projectile of mass *M* and cross-sectional area *A* passing through a medium of density *d*. In these equations, penetration is a logarithmic function of initial velocity, and decrement in velocity is an exponential function of penetration. The equations demonstrate that, all other factors being equal,

- the greater a projectile's mass, the greater will be its depth of penetration
- the greater a projectile's residual velocity, the greater will be its depth of penetration
- the greater a projectile's sectional density, the greater will be its depth of penetration

Conversely, a lightweight projectile with a large presenting surface, such as a chunky aluminum fragment, will penetrate shallowly. These formulae also demonstrate that, given equal initial kinetic energies, a light, fast projectile will slow more rapidly and penetrate less deeply than will a heavy, slow projectile.[8]

These penetration equations apply to a hypothetical target of infinite length. In the practical situation when the target has finite thickness, knowing the projectile's residual velocity is more useful, but the mathematical treatment is also more complicated. To perforate, a projectile must have a striking velocity above a characteristic minimum, which is determined by the target's material properties. The curve relating the striking and residual velocities of stable, nondeforming projectiles is exponential:

$$\frac{V_r}{V_s} = 1 - e^{-a\,[V_s - MIN]^b}$$

where *Vr* and *Vs* are the projectile's residual and striking velocities, *MIN* is the minimum striking velocity compatible with perforating the target, and *a* and *b* are experimentally derived constants related to the material properties of the target and the ballistic characteristics of the projectile.

Figure 4-8 illustrates the mechanics of penetration. A perforating projectile loses little velocity unless its striking velocity approaches the minimum velocity required for perforation. This explains the frequent all-or-nothing performance of protective equipment such as helmets and armored vests: The projectile is either completely stopped and does no damage, or else it perforates and loses little of its damaging potential.

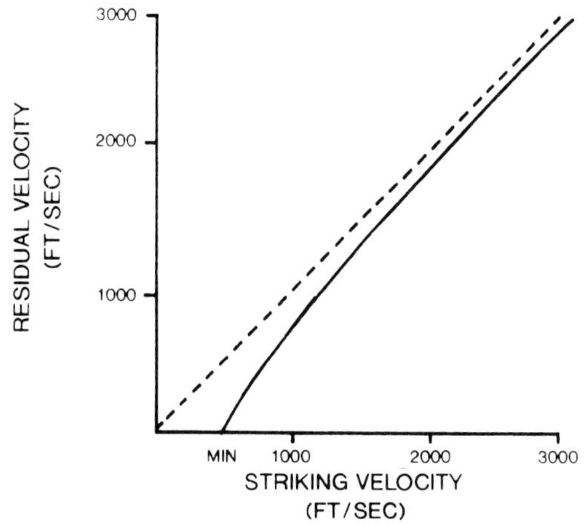

Fig. 4-8. The curved line shows the relationship between striking velocity and residual velocity after penetrating a target for an idealized, nondeforming, stable projectile. MIN is the minimal velocity that the projectile must have to perforate the target. The separation between the curved and broken lines represents the loss of velocity that the perforating projectile incurred. The residual velocity is only slightly degraded, except when the striking velocity is near the minimal velocity required for perforation.

ENERGY TRANSFER IN THE PROJECTILE-TARGET INTERACTION IN TISSUE

Drag slows a projectile as it passes through a medium. The medium also exerts an equal but opposite force on the projectile, and the medium is physically disrupted as a result. If the medium is tissue, the physical disruption is a wound. The projectile's kinetic energy *works* on the tissue (that is, the energy of the projectile's motion is transferred from the projectile to the tissue) and causes the tissue's disruption.

Kinetic energy and drag are independent descriptors of a projectile's behavior in tissue. Neither high nor low values of drag necessarily accompany high or low values of kinetic energy. But kinetic energy and drag together do determine the amount of the projectile's kinetic energy that will be transferred to the target as the projectile slows. A projectile with high kinetic energy and high drag will be associated with *high energy transfer*, and a projectile with low kinetic energy and low drag will be associated with *low energy transfer*. The concept of energy transfer clarifies the physical and biophysical aspects of the projectile-target interaction.

Total Energy Transfer

Theoretically, measuring the energy transferred from a projectile to a target tissue is easy. If a projectile perforates without either losing its substance or deforming, the formula for calculating the energy transferred is:

$$1/2\ \text{MASS}\ [(V_{et})^2 - (V_{ex})^2]$$

where V_{et} and V_{ex} are the velocities of the projectile as it enters and exits the target, respectively. If the projectile does not perforate but comes to rest within the target tissue, the formula for calculating the energy transferred is:

$$1/2\ \text{MASS}\ (V_{et})^2$$

Extensive data describe energy transfer for a variety of different bullets and fragments measured in tissue simulants such as gelatin and soap, and in living animal tissues.[2, 9, 10, 11] Among the conclusions are the following:

- Perforating, nondeforming rifle bullets transfer a small fraction (8%–19%) of their kinetic energy in traversing soft tissue. (Dr. Charles Woodruff strongly suspected this fact in the late nineteenth century.)
- Stable, perforating, nondeforming rifle bullets transfer less of their kinetic energy than do similar bullets that became unstable (11% versus 16%).
- Bullets that break up while traversing tissue transfer more of their kinetic energy than do bullets that remain intact (40% versus 23%).
- Fragments, because they usually do not perforate the target, are much more likely than bullets are to transfer their total kinetic energy.
- Projectiles with lower absolute kinetic energy sometimes transfer more kinetic energy to the target than do more energetic projectiles. In these instances, energy transfer by the less energetic projectile is more complete. For example, the M193 bullet of the M16 assault rifle frequently transferred more kinetic energy than the 7.62-mm bullet of the AK47 assault rifle did (424 J versus 153 J) even though the latter fired a much more energetic bullet (1,919 J versus 1,543 J).
- The target medium (that is, soap, gelatin, pig thigh, and so forth) affected energy transfer less than was anticipated.

The available kinetic energy of the projectiles in these studies ranged between 1,000 and 3,000 J. Both the absolute magnitude of the energy transfer and the fraction of the total kinetic energy transferred depend upon the length of the projectile's trajectory in the target, which, in turn, depends upon the size of the target. In most of these experiments, the trajectory lengths were similar to those found in wounds of human extremities.

Nonuniform Energy Transfer. Energy transfer that is calculated for the projectile's entire trajectory through tissue (that is, the *wound tract* or *permanent cavity*) may be misleading. Energy transfer usually does not occur uniformly along the trajectory because *(a)* the projectile may behave unpredictably (that is, it may yaw, deform, and so forth) and *(b)* the target substance will be nonhomogeneous (that is, it is composed of skin, fat, muscle, and bone). For these reasons, tissue damage also may not be uniform along the wound tract.

Experiments performed at the army's ballistics laboratory at Edgewood, Maryland, demonstrate nonuniform energy transfer occurring along a wound tract.[12] An ultrahigh-speed motion picture photographed a 30-caliber Ball M1 bullet as it passed through a gelatin block (Figure 4-9). Measuring frame-by-frame the distance the bullet travelled, the researchers could calculate the bullet's velocity, kinetic energy, and energy transfer. They showed that the sudden increase in energy transfer after the bullet had penetrated 14 cm was due to marked yaw. They elaborated upon these data by performing a series of experiments with the same type of bullets penetrating goat thighs. By measuring multiple cross sections of the wound tract and plotting these measurements against energy-transfer data from the gelatin blocks, they demonstrated that the wound tracts through the goats' thighs increased in size at the same point that significant yaw occurred in the gelatin blocks. The wound tracts, narrow at the wounds of entrance, broadened considerably at the wounds of exit, where bullet yaw became prominent in the goats' thighs.

A second example from the same laboratory[13] shows energy transfer both as suggested by the gross tissue disruption in sheep and as a function of depth of penetration in gelatin (Figure 4-10). The researchers shot a sphere through the hind legs of a sheep. After sacrificing the animal, they made multiple transverse cuts across the wound tract. They measured the cross-sectional area of the wound tract as they had done with the goat thighs. They also shot identical spheres into 20% gelatin blocks and recorded the spheres' passage on ultrahigh-speed motion pictures. Measuring frame-by-frame, the researchers used the changes in velocity to calculate energy transfer.

Figure 4-10 illustrates two facts that emerged. First, energy transfer (as calculated from the retardation of the sphere) was maximal at the sphere's point of impact, and the huge wound of entrance shows that tissue damage there was correspondingly massive. And second, the cross-sectional area of the wound tract was not uniform. The marked diminution in the size of the hole in the muscle of the downrange thigh signifies that the sphere's velocity falls as it penetrates the tissue. The differences in morphology along the wound tract (and the implied differences in energy transfer) may also be due to the different viscoelastic properties of skin, fat, and skeletal muscle that the sphere passed through. Such differences in energy transfer would not be apparent in the homogeneous gelatin block.

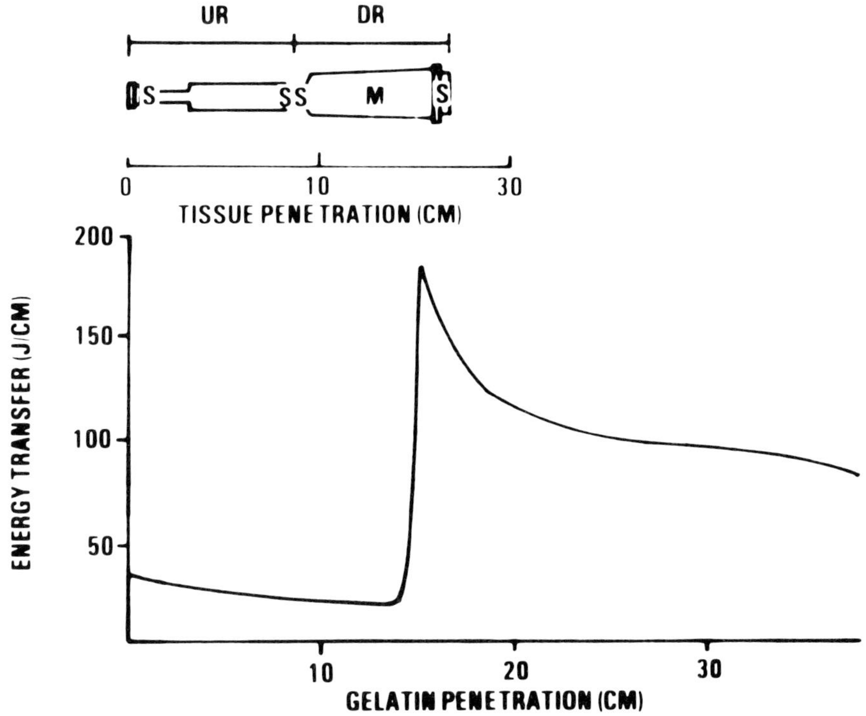

Fig. 4-9. Data pertaining to the penetration of a .30-caliber Ball military bullet: *(a)* energy transfer as a function of the depth of penetration in a block of 20% gelatin (lower diagram), and *(b)* a qualitative assessment of the width of the permanent cavity observed in the combined thighs of a goat (upper diagram). The width of the permanent cavity was larger in the downrange thigh (DR) and the wound of exit in the downrange thigh was larger than the wound of entrance in the uprange (UR) thigh. By comparing the two types of data, it can be seen that there is a rough correspondence between gelatin-block energy transfer and wound morphology. Skin: (S); muscle: (M).

Source: Redrawn from Figure 3c in reference 12

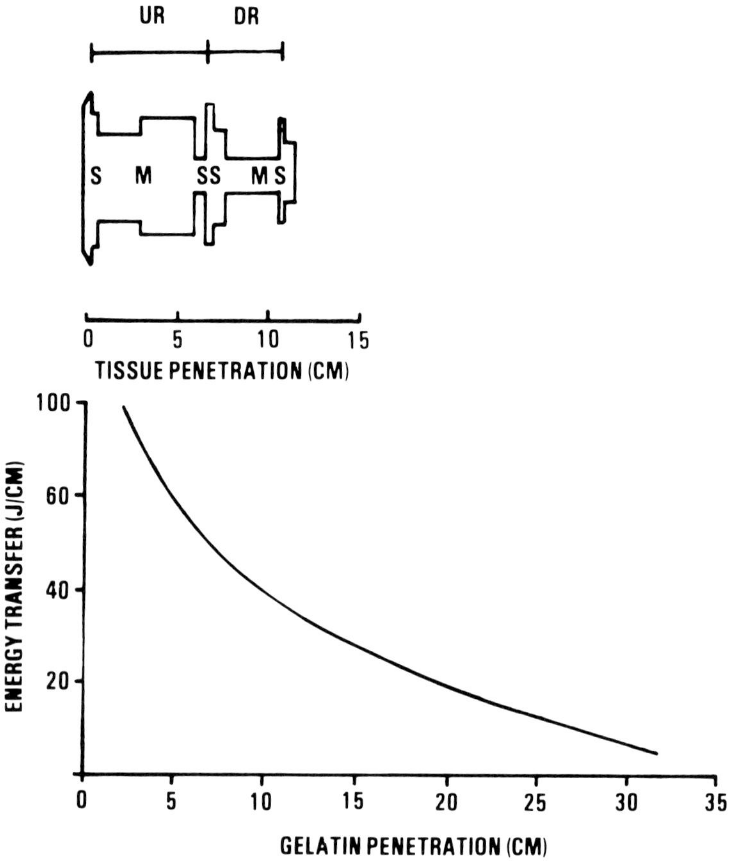

Fig. 4-10. The methodology used to obtain these data is similar to that used in Figure 4-9, except that the projectile shown here is a 2.6-g sphere and the wound morphology is the reverse: The permanent cavity is smaller in the downrange thigh and the wound of entrance is larger than the wound of exit. Energy transfer as measured in the gelatin block falls as a function of the missile's depth of penetration. The greater energy transfer in the uprange thigh appears to be associated with greater tissue disruption.
Source: Redrawn from Figure 11 in reference 13

Newer methodologies using multiple-flash roentgenography to measure velocity in tissue and tissue simulants have confirmed these findings.[14] Figure 4-11 shows energy transfer (as assessed by the force of retardation) as a function of depth of penetration for 5.56-mm bullets into both pig thighs and soap blocks. The initial trajectories (8–12 cm) of the bullets are stable and associated with little energy transfer. Then, in what can only be described as an explosion, the bullets transfer much of their kinetic energy. This methodology clearly shows that yaw, tumbling, and breakup caused the nonuniform energy transfer along the wound tract.

The Wound Profile. Idealized projectile-target interactions called *wound profiles*[15] depict hypothetical energy transfer occurring in a homogeneous target (Figures 4-12 and 4-13). A wound profile is a drawing made after a projectile has been shot through a block of 10% gelatin. This concept assumes that the radial fissures or cracks around the projectile's path through the gelatin block indicate the size of the temporary cavity created by the passage of the projectile. The size of the temporary cavity is an important factor in determining the magnitude of the energy transferred from a projectile to its target, and the length of the radial fissures, indicating the imaginary diameter of the void

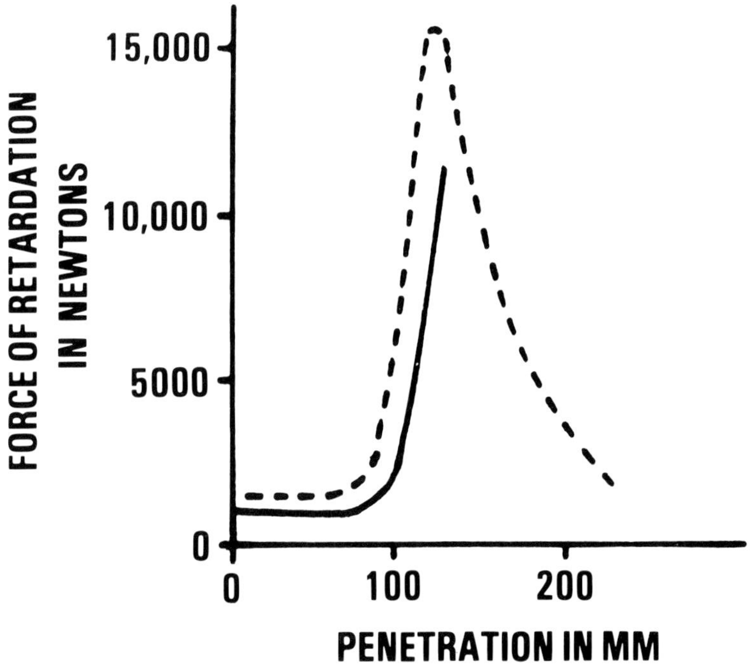

Fig. 4-11. The force of retardation calculated from the deceleration of 5.56-mm bullets as a function of the depth of penetration in a swine thigh (solid lines) and soap (broken line). In both cases, the sudden increase in retardation was associated with tumbling, which was clearly visible in high-speed roentgenograms.
Source: Redrawn from Figure 36 in reference 14

shown in the wound profile, may be taken as a qualitative index of energy transfer.

Figure 4-12 shows the presumed behavior of a stable, nondeforming bullet, with a channel of fairly uniform width extending along the entire trajectory. Energy transfer (and, by implication, tissue disruption) is fairly uniform along the line of flight.[16]

Figure 4-13 shows the more complex, as well as the more common, situation: nonuniform energy transfer.[16] Once again, the width of the disturbance created by the bullet indicates the magnitude of energy transfer. The first third of the trajectory is uneventful and consists of a narrow uniform channel. The middle third of the trajectory is very different: The actual gelatin block from which the drawing of the wound profile was made showed both a huge cavity and long fissures running perpendicular to the trajectory in this region. The final third of the trajectory resembles the first third. The vastly greater width of the trajectory in its middle third indicates that energy transfer markedly increased. For there to have been such a marked increase in energy transfer, there must have been a marked increase in projectile drag. Although the wound-profile methodology does not allow direct visualization of projectile yaw, the site of maximum disruption in the gelatin was probably also the site of the projectile's maximum yaw.

Projectile Characteristics That Determine Energy Transfer Within Tissue

Just as the characteristics of the target determine the energy that is transferred (that is, a bullet's striking a bone ensures high–energy transfer), so the physical characteristics of the projectile, which may change as it penetrates the target tissue, also must be considered separately. If a bullet (or all or most of its fragments) comes to rest within the target tissue, all (or most) of the bullet's kinetic energy will transfer to the tissue and will have the potential to produce greater wounds.

Shape at Impact. Blunt or irregular projectiles make larger wounds of entrance than smooth or pointed projectiles of the same relative size. Researchers at Letterman Army Institute of Research (LAIR) convincingly demonstrated this fact (Figure 4-14).[17] Holding all other variables constant (such as velocity, distance from the target, and projectile size and construction) and varying only the orientation of the bullets, they shot a pig in each buttock: on the left with a rifle bullet loaded point-forward, and on the right with an identi-

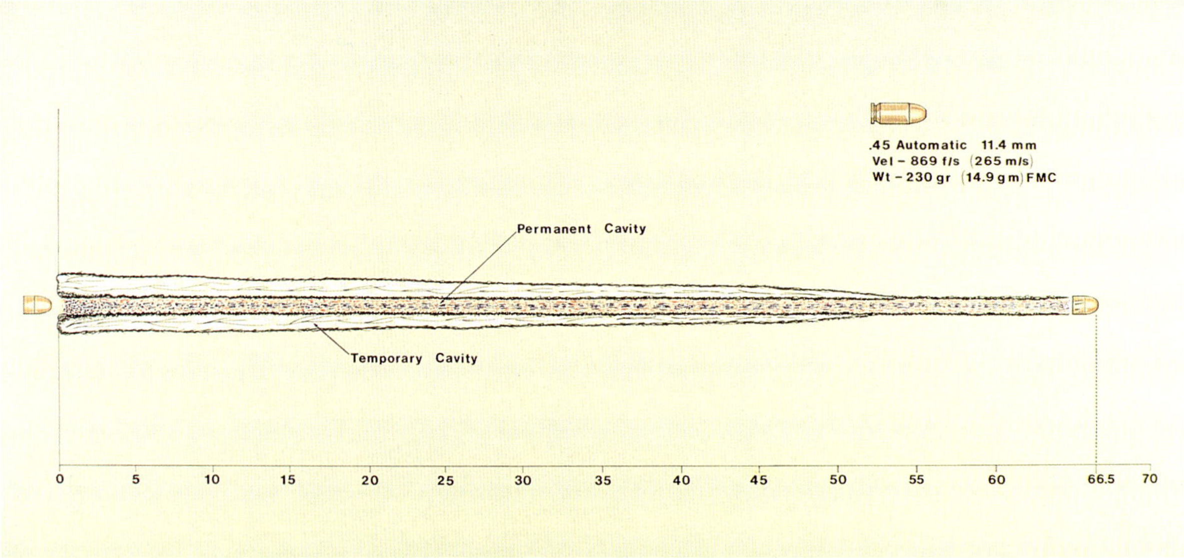

Fig. 4-12. A wound profile for an ACP M1911 .45-caliber bullet. Energy transfer, shown by the width of the idealized permanent and temporary cavities, is fairly uniform along the line of flight.
Source: Reproduced from Figure 4 in reference 16

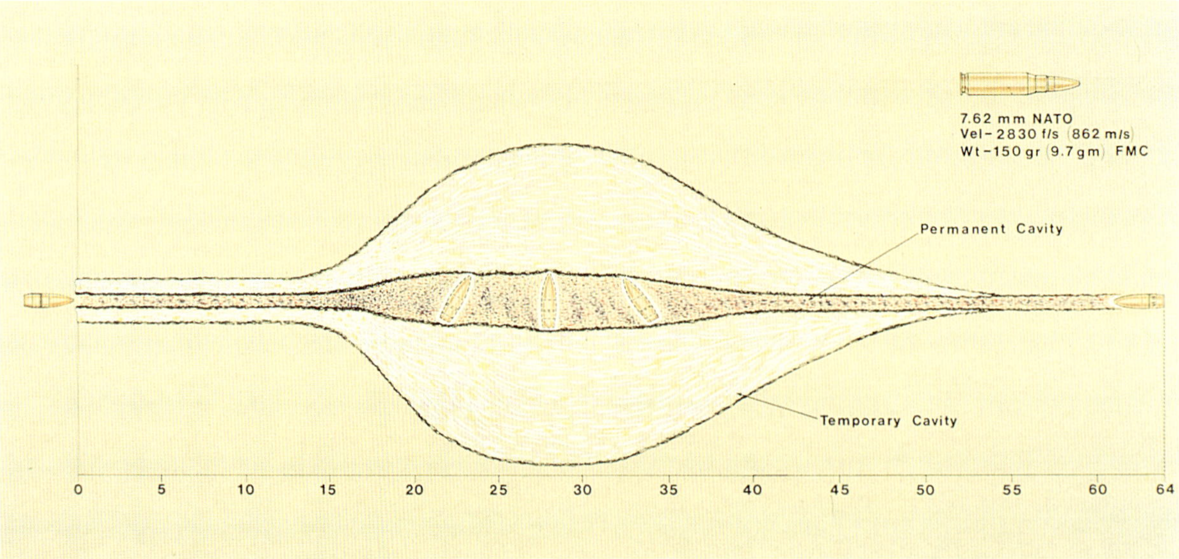

Fig. 4-13. A wound profile for a NATO 7.62-mm bullet. Energy transfer, shown by the width of the idealized permanent and temporary cavities, was greatly increased at the presumed site of the bullet's tumbling in mid-trajectory.
Source: Reproduced from Figure 7 in reference 16

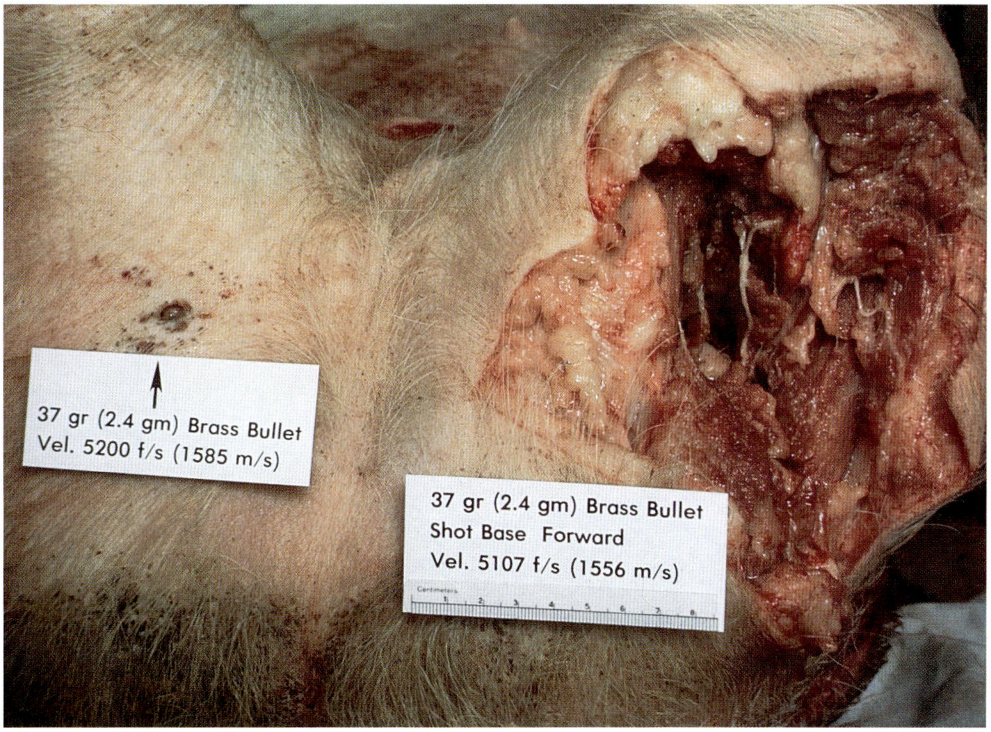

Fig. 4-14. This photograph shows the importance of the projectile's shape to a wound's morphology. The buttocks of a 100-kg swine (that had been sacrificed earlier) were struck by two solid brass 5.56-mm bullets with striking velocities greater than 5,000 fps. The wound on the left was made by a bullet traveling point-forward; the wound on the right by a bullet traveling with its flat base forward.
Source: Letterman Army Institute of Research

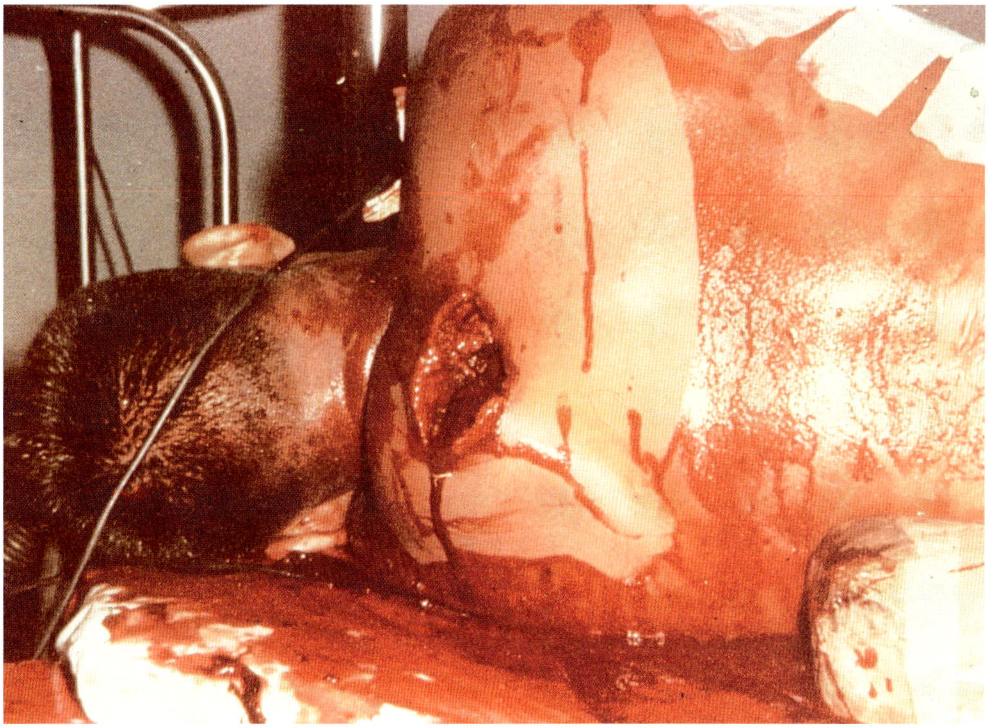

Fig. 4-15. This casualty's wound of entrance was made by a large, blunt, irregular fragment from a 105-mm shell. The permanent cavity involved the second thoracic vertebra, the left lung, and the subclavian artery. The casualty died about 3 hours after being wounded.
Source: Wound Data and Munitions Effectiveness Team

cal bullet loaded base-forward. The dramatic difference in the two wounds is due entirely to the different shapes of the two bullets at the moment of impact. Because blunt or irregular projectiles present relatively large areas of contact with the target tissue, their energy transfer is accelerated compared to that of more streamlined projectiles. Nonuniform energy transfer due to projectile shape may be further complicated by the fact that projectile velocity is not constant throughout the tissue trajectory but is greatest at the instant of penetration. Large fragments from older, explosive, random-fragmentation munitions characteristically caused huge wounds of entrance (Figure 4-15).

Fragmentation. The fact that bullets break up in tissue is an important but frequently ignored factor in projectile-target interaction.[18] Most bullets will fragment if they hit a large bone, but some bullets are notorious for breaking up even in soft tissue. Figure 4-16 shows the two basic types of bullet construction: *(a)* the NATO 7.62-mm bullet, which has a copper jacket and a lead core, and *(b)* the M43 bullet (fired by the Soviet AK47 rifle), which has a thick steel jacket, a large soft-steel core, and a small amount of lead. Because of its construction, the M43 bullet is quite strong and usually breaks up only when it strikes bone or a hard external object. Figure 4-17 shows a casualty whose skull was penetrated by a bullet fired from an AK47. The bullet broke up after hitting and fracturing the opposite occipital bone. Figure 4-18 shows the bullet after it was removed from the dead casualty's brain.

Figure 4-19 is a roentgenogram of an M43 ball fired from an AK47 that broke up within a casualty's abdomen. The bullet probably started to break up when it struck a hard object on the casualty's web gear just before it penetrated the soldier's body. The large size of the wound of entry suggests that the bullet either yawed significantly or deformed before it struck the soldier (Figure 4-20).

Although it is unusual for an AK47 bullet to break up when not associated with hitting a hard object first, such breakup commonly occurs with bullets fired by the M16. Figure 4-21 is a roentgenogram showing a fragmented bullet within the wound of entrance in a casualty's chest. Even though there is no evidence of a fractured rib, the collection of lead within the casualty's lung indicates that the bullet fragmented. Figure 4-22 is an abdominal roentgenogram showing the bullet's nose. This large fragment (the bullet's nose, a breakup characteristic of the M16 bullet) was extracted from the casualty's abdomen at autopsy (Figure 4-23).

A bullet's construction may increase its tendency to break up. Some copper-jacketed bullets with lead cores (such as the M193 fired by the M16A1) cannot stand the stress caused by angular velocity during yaw. The radial stress created when the bullet tumbles around its center of mass (as measured with multiple-flash roentgenograms) has been estimated to exceed by a factor of four the force required to fracture a bullet-sized cylinder of lead.[19] Furthermore, as the bullet slows, very high retardation forces crush the jacket, expell lead from the core, and flatten the bullet. The M16 bullet (and others with lead cores) begins to break up when lead extrudes from its base and the bullet fractures at its *cannelures* (that is, the grooves that circle the middle of its jacket).

The M193 and other bullets with copper jackets and lead cores can be expected to break up and fragment whenever the bullet's trajectory through the target is long enough for significant yaw to develop. Breakup also depends upon the bullet's striking velocity. An M193 might break up at about 600 m/s, and breakup is assured at speeds faster than 700 m/s.

Externally similar bullets may have very different tissue effects because they have been constructed differently. Breakup of the Soviet M43 bullet fired by the AK47 starts at the nose, where the jacket usually peels back and exposes the steel core (Figure 4-18), but design and construction of ammunition for the Kalashnikov assault rifle is not uniform worldwide. For instance, unlike the bullets designed and made by the Soviets, bullets that are produced by Chinese and Egyptian manufacturers of AK47 ammunition have a copper jacket and a soft, lead core. This bullet is far more likely to break up than is the M43. Unfortunately, examples of similar differences in construction are commonplace. For instance, the NATO standard 7.62-mm bullet manufactured in West Germany has a copper jacket only one-half as thick as the same bullet made in the United States (Figure 4-16). Not surprisingly, bullet breakup is much more common with the former than with the latter.[20]

Deformation. All other factors being the same, a projectile that deforms will transfer more of its kinetic energy than will a projectile that does not deform (Figure 4-24).[21] Bullets that are designed to deform, such as hollow- and soft-point bullets (forbidden for use by the military) will do so only if they strike with a velocity above a characteristic minimum. Since the bullet's velocity will be greater early in its trajectory through tissue, deformation, if it occurs, will occur shortly after the projectile strikes. Thus, maximal energy transfer will occur near the wound of entrance. Of course, a projectile that does not normally deform in soft tissue may do so if it hits bone, and maximal energy transfer will occur there.

Stability. Energy transfer will greatly increase when a projectile's angle of yaw increases from a few

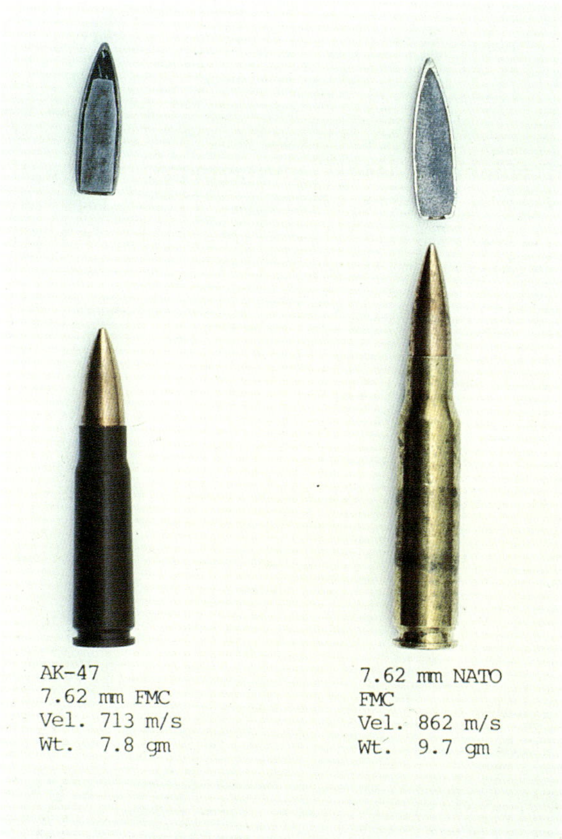

Fig. 4-16. Examples of the two most common forms of bullet construction: (left) the M43 round of the AK47 with its steel jacket and steel core penetrator and (right) the NATO 7.62 round with its copper jacket and lead core.
Source: Letterman Army Institute of Research

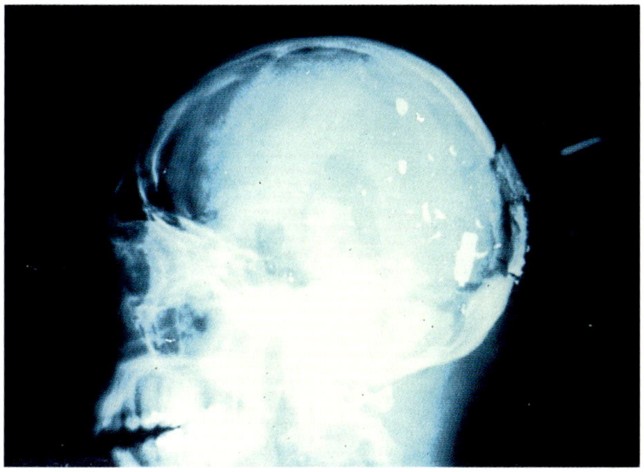

Fig. 4-17. The casualty whose skull is shown in this roentgenogram was killed by an M43 ball fired from an AK47. The bullet broke up as it perforated the temporal bone and ricochetted after fracturing the opposite occipital bone. Note that a segment of the occipital bone has been detached from its surrounding tissue.
Source: Wound Data and Munitions Effectiveness Team

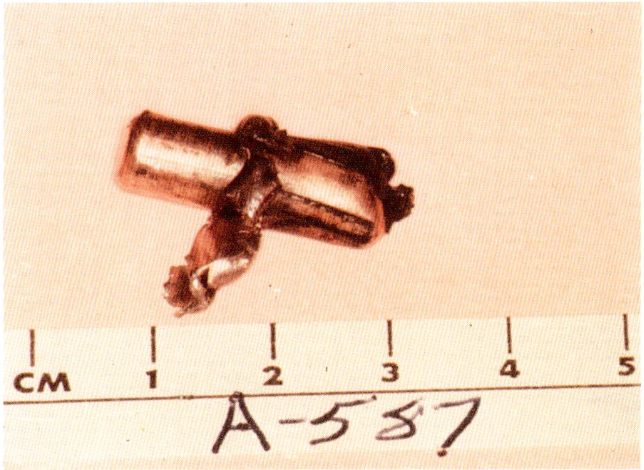

Fig. 4-18. The bullet after it had been extracted from the brain of the casualty shown in Figure 4-17. The steel jacket has peeled back, exposing the penetrator that constitutes the bullet's core. This behavior is characteristic of the breakup of the M43 bullet.
Source: Wound Data and Munitions Effectiveness Team

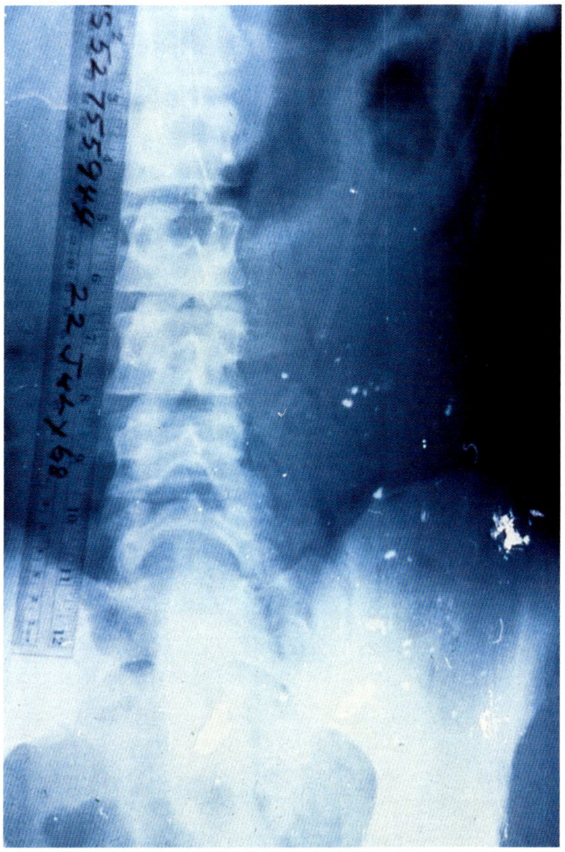

Fig. 4-19. An abdominal roentgenogram of a casualty who was wounded by an M43 ball fired from an AK47 rifle. The M43's steel core lies in the left lower quadrant of the casualty's abdomen. There was extensive damage to the small intestine and the sigmoid colon.
Source: Wound Data and Munitions Effectiveness Team

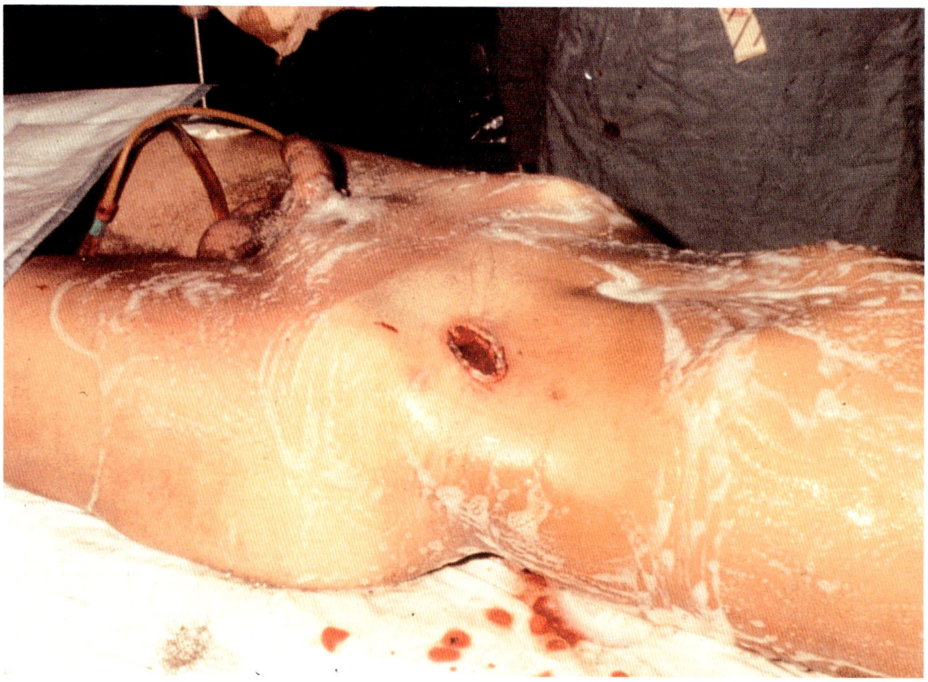

Fig. 4-20. The wound of entrance of the casualty whose roentgenogram is shown in Figure 4-19 suggests a likely explanation for the bullet's breakup. The wound's very large size indicates that the bullet had either already broken up or had a substantial angle of yaw before it penetrated the casualty's abdomen. A reasonable assumption is that the bullet initially hit an object outside the casualty, such as his web gear.
Source: Wound Data and Munitions Effectiveness Team

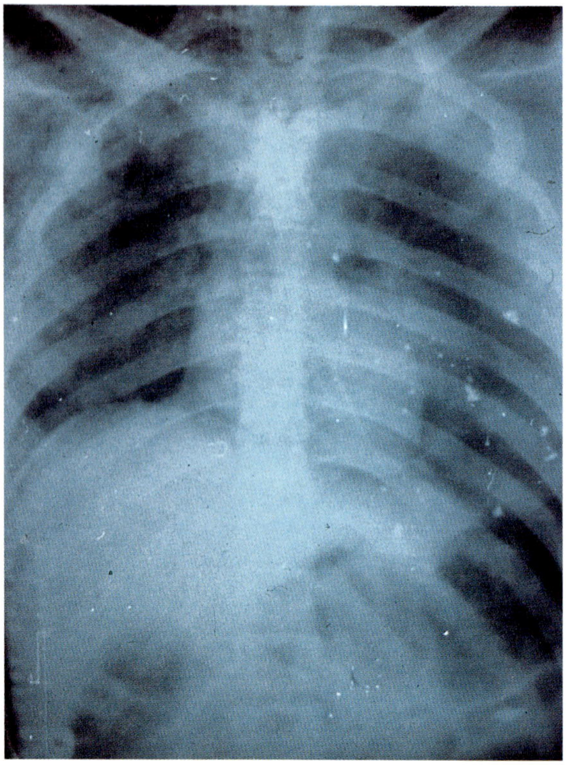

Fig. 4-21. This chest roentgenogram was taken of a casualty who was killed by an M193 ball fired by an M16. The bullet entered his chest, where the lead that constituted the bullet's core broke up into multiple metal fragments.
Source: Wound Data and Munitions Effectiveness Team

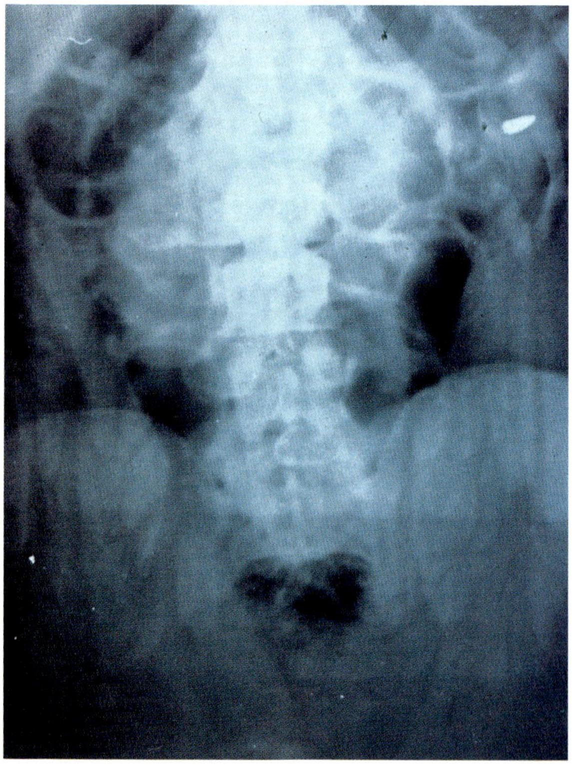

Fig. 4-22. This abdominal roentgenogram of the casualty whose chest roentgenogram was shown in Figure 4-21 shows a major fragment of the bullet.
Source: Wound Data and Munitions Effectiveness Team

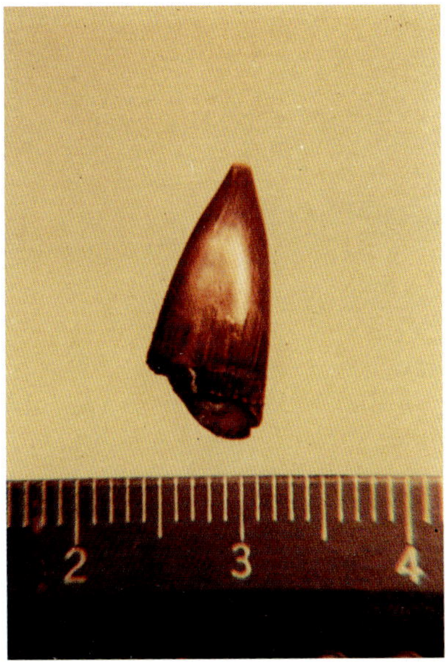

Fig. 4-23. The bullet fragment shown in Figure 4-22 after it had been extracted at autopsy. The characteristic fragment is the nose of the M193.
Source: Wound Data and Munitions Effectiveness Team

degrees to actual tumbling. In fact, projectile instability is probably the single most important cause of a bullet's nonlinear energy transfer. Yaw and tumbling may occur and increase anywhere along a trajectory, but most bullets require a characteristic minimum trajectory length within the target before they become unstable. For example, the M193 fired by the M16 requires a 6–7-cm trajectory through the target, and a bullet from the AK47 a 15–20-cm trajectory.[22] If the target trajectory is less than this critical distance, significant yaw will not occur, and energy transfer will be not only lower but also more uniform. External disturbances, such as striking foliage or pieces of the soldier's gear, may cause a bullet to yaw significantly before it hits its target. A bullet striking with a large angle of yaw ensures that accentuated yawing will also occur within the target, with correspondingly greater and earlier energy transfer and tissue damage.

The phenomenon of yaw helps to explain subtle problems in wound ballistics, such as the report that the exit wounds made by M193 bullets fired from the M16 were sixfold larger at target distances of 30 m than at 100 m. Perhaps at a distance of only 30 m from the muzzle, gyroscopic stability had not yet decreased the yaw that was present shortly after the bullet left the rifle barrel. Thus the angle of yaw—and the potential for accelerated increase in yaw on penetration—were greater at 30 m than at 100 m.[9]

Bullet design also influences stability. The apparent increased tendency of the Soviet 5.45-mm bullet to yaw very early in its trajectory through tissue may be due to its design. This bullet deforms internally on impact: Lead at the front of the bullet's steel core shifts forward, replacing a small pocket of air in the tip, thus shifting the center of mass.[23] However, if this explanation is correct, the shift must be asymmetric, because a symmetrical forward shift of the center of mass will increase stability

Velocity. The drag equation shows that the force of retardation is greater when the projectile's velocity is greater. A projectile will slow more rapidly in the early part of its target trajectory and therefore, all other factors being the same, it will transfer more of its energy at the beginning of its penetration than at the end. Even a symmetrical, nondeforming, non-yawing projectile such as a sphere normally has a nonlinear energy transfer. Energy transfer is maximal at the point of impact because projectile velocity is maximal then. The biophysical consequence of early energy transfer is greater tissue disruption near the wound of entrance (Figure 4-10).

The coefficient of drag is known to increase when the projectile's velocity exceeds the speed of sound in the medium. Since the speed of sound in soft tissue is about 1,500 m/s, much greater than the velocity of most projectiles on the battlefield, nonuniform energy transfer in tissue due to a supersonic coefficient of drag is not likely to be common. Nevertheless, some have suggested that very fast fragments cause explosive wounds of entrance for that reason.[24] A more recent study, however, found no indication that energy transfer accelerated (as measured by the size of the temporary cavity in gelatin) as striking velocity increased from subsonic to supersonic Mach numbers.[25] The

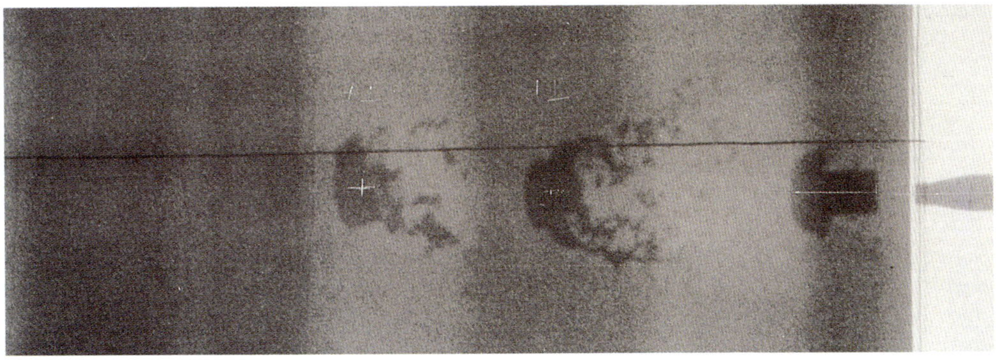

Fig. 4-24. A roentgenogram made with flash X rays of a .308 soft-point bullet as it deforms within a gelatin block, demonstrating massive increase in cross-sectional area and, by implication, drag.
Source: Reproduced from reference 21

appearance of the wound shown in Figure 4-14 provides no support for the suggestion that projectiles with very high velocities will necessarily make very large wounds of entrance: The bullet (traveling nose-forward) struck at greater than 5,000 fps, but created only a tiny wound of entrance.

MECHANISMS OF ENERGY TRANSFER WITHIN TISSUE

The energy that a projectile transfers as it penetrates tissue is associated with several direct and indirect phenomena:

- *Cutting*—the tissue that comes in direct contact with the projectile is cut.
- *Stretch and shear*—the transfer of kinetic energy from the projectile to the tissue causes low-frequency, high-displacement transverse waves (known as *shear waves*), which cause the tissues surrounding the bullet's trajectory to be thrust aside creating a temporary void. (Since the time of Woodruff, this process has been called *cavitation* in ballistics literature.)
- *Compression*—transferring kinetic energy from the projectile to the tissue also causes high-frequency, low-displacement longitudinal waves known as *stress waves*. (This mechanism is usually called the *shock wave* in ballistics literature.)
- *Heating*—some energy that is transferred from the projectile to the target is in the form of heat.

Cutting and heating are direct effects of the projectile's passage through tissue. Damage resulting from shear and stress waves is indirect, since these injuries do not depend on direct contact between the injured tissue and the projectile.

Both shear and stress waves generate pressure transients that, in theory, can propagate throughout the body and cause damage. Pressure transients arising from shear waves have been measured in the abdomen of swine that were shot in the thigh, and systemic effects due to propagation of stress waves through major blood vessels are possible.[26] A controversy exists regarding the relative importance of direct and indirect effects, but indirect effects occurring more than several centimeters from a wound tract are probably clinically insignificant except in organs such as brain, heart, and liver.

Cutting

During the several hundred microseconds that it takes for a typical rifle bullet to penetrate tissue, a region of very high pressure develops at the bullet's leading edge. The force per unit area in the direction of the line of flight (technically, a *stress*), which theoretically may approach 10^6 psi, ruptures the tissue. (Similarly great pressures are also associated with the penetration of slow-moving but very sharp objects such as knives and arrows.)

The *rupture modulus* is a biophysical parameter that can be used to quantitate the ease of cutting through a viscoelastic medium such as tissue. A modulus relates *stress* to *strain* (that is, it relates a fractional change in an object's dimension to the applied force). The rupture modulus describes the stress required to strain a tissue to the point of disruption. Unfortunately, data on rupture moduli in tissue, which would greatly advance our understanding of wound ballistics, are not available.[27]

However, certain conclusions can be drawn from the facts known about moduli in other areas of physics. Since moduli usually depend upon the rate at which the stress is applied (that is, the shorter the time over which a given force is applied, the stiffer the tissue will be), it is likely that the rupture modulus, when such data do become available in wound ballistics, will be found to depend upon the velocity of the penetrating projectile. That is to say, the faster the projectile, the greater the force required to cause a given degree of tissue disruption. This is another reason why a relatively slow but very sharp object like an arrow expends far less energy than a rifle bullet does in cutting through tissue.

Stretch and Shear

Energy transfer associated with shear waves is almost always discussed in the context of cavitation in ballistics literature. Cavitation is a poorly understood process; its essence is its dynamic nature—the duration is measured in milliseconds—and the process and its result are usually called *temporary* cavitation and the *temporary* cavity. (The observed wound is called the *permanent* cavity.)

Temporary Cavitation. Ordinary experience provides no clue to the mechanism of temporary cavitation; it is not apparent in everyday life that the viscoelastic properties of tissue depend upon the time-course of an applied force. The more rapidly a force acts upon viscoelastic tissue, the stiffer the tissue becomes. Tissues that might behave like marshmallows when a force is gradually applied over seconds behave more like marbles when the same force is applied over milliseconds. In fact, the process of temporary cavitation can be compared with striking a heap of marbles with a hammer. A void is created as the marbles in the middle move outward and strike peripheral marbles that, in turn, move outward and strike even more-peripheral marbles. The important difference is that the marbles fly off unrestrained, while tissues moving away from a projectile snap back to their original location. The elasticity and weight of the surrounding tissues not only arrest the cavity's expansion but also cause its ultimate collapse.

Energetics of Cavity Formation. Forming a temporary cavity requires considerable kinetic energy. Calculations based on data that Harvey and his group gathered in the mid-1940s (Callender and French published equations derived from Harvey's data in *Wound Ballistics*) demonstrate that, in this instance, forming a temporary cavity required approximately 83% of the kinetic energy transferred during projectile-target interaction (Table 4-3).[28] Harvey's original data are no longer available, but assuming that they are approximately correct, these calculations show that the size of the temporary cavity increases by 0.7 ml for each joule of kinetic energy transferred. Most of the kinetic energy transferred from a high-velocity projectile is probably expended on cavitation.

Temporary cavitation and its consequent tissue damage have important organ-specific aspects: The physical properties of the target tissue determine the dimensions of the temporary cavity. For example, the cavity may be small in lung but large in liver. In lung, the cavity's expansion as tissue is flung aside is presumably arrested as air is compressed in the alveolar spaces, but no such containment occurs in liver once the capsule has been ruptured.

Gross Characteristics. The low-frequency, high-displacement transverse wave that follows a rifle bullet through a tissue simulant and generates the temporary cavity has been visualized (Figure 4-25). Formation of the temporary cavity follows the passage of the projectile by about 1 msec; thus, the projectile has already left the target before the cavity begins to form. The shape of the cavity in this instance is that of an axially symmetrical ellipse, but it is not unusual to find a more irregular cavity, reflecting both the heterogeneity of most body parts and the irregular shape and trajectory of the projectile. Cyclic expansion and collapse of the cavity may occur in gelatin (nine times

TABLE 4-3

ENERGY REQUIREMENTS IN WOUND CAVITATION

Components of the Wound	Transferred Energy* (x 10^{-3} ft-lb)	Volumes Found in a Typical Wound** (in^3)	Total Energy† (ft-lb)
Temporary cavity	66.247	132.49	8.8
Zone of Extravasation	30.105	60.21	1.8
Permanent Cavity	2.547	5.09	0.013

*Transferred energy required to form a 1.0 in^3 cavity in tissue

**Measured cavitation volumes from a projectile with a striking energy of 2,000 ft-lbs. These are volumes of a wound that Callender and French considered "typical."
Source: Reference 7

†Source: Authors' calculations from data in columns 2 and 3

CAVITATION PHENOMENON

Fig. 4-25. Frames from a high-speed movie showing cavitation (opposite page)
Source: Letterman Army Institute of Research, Department of Audio-Visual Resources

---

25–*a*. A 5.45-mm bullet fired from an AK74 has just struck the left side of a 7-inch-thick block of 10% gelatin (note that the ruler is calibrated in centimeters). The striking velocity is about 2,900 fps. A small amount of the gelatin—the tail splash—is being extruded from the site of impact.

25–*b*. The bullet has exited from the right face of the block and is followed by a small amount of expelled gelatin. Although not visible on the motion picture, it is likely that the bullet tumbled before it exited from the target.

25–*c*. The earliest stage in the development of the temporary cavity. At this stage, the cavity lacks perfect axial symmetry.

25–*d*. The cavity's explosive expansion is apparent.

25–*e*. Note the extensive amount of gelatin displaced—the head cone—at the wound of exit as the cavity continues to expand.

25–*f*. The cavity has reached its maximum size.

25–*g*. The cavity begins to collapse.

25–*h*. The negative pressure within the cavity has aspirated the previously expelled gelatin.

25–*i*. The cavity has completely collapsed. The total elapsed time (Figures 4-25–*a* through 4-25–*i*) is about 4 msec.

25–*j*. The peak cavity size of the second oscillation

25–*k*. The peak cavity size of the fifth oscillation. Note the distortion of the block as a whole and the displacement of the attached ruler.

25–*l*. Cavitation is complete. The gelatin block has a permanent deformity at the site of the bullet's exit, and the gelatin that was displaced by the cavity shows multiple air-filled fissure fractures. Note that in this example, the radial fissures underestimate the maximum size of the temporary cavity.

Figure 4-25

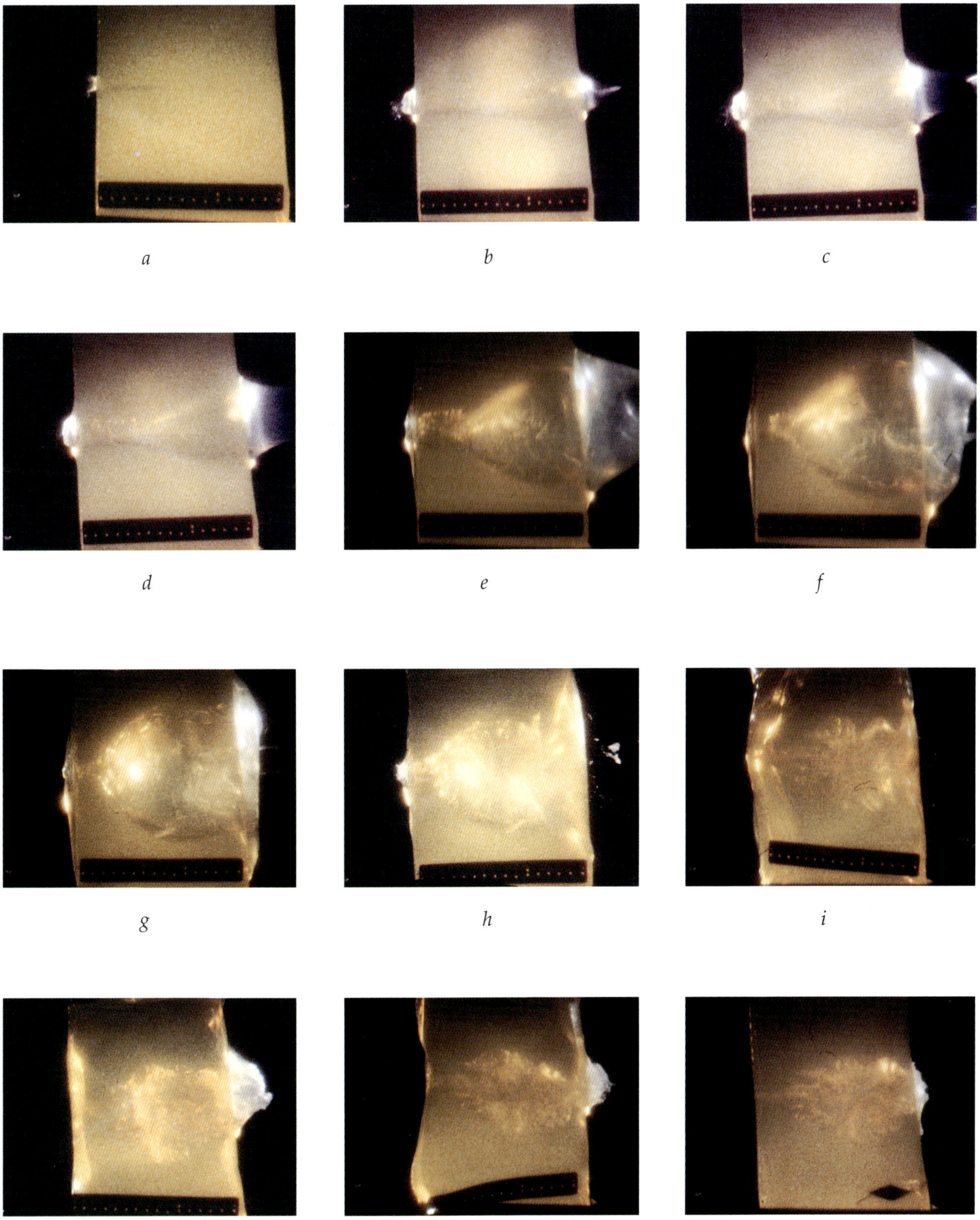

a *b* *c* *d* *e* *f* *g* *h* *i* *j* *k* *l*

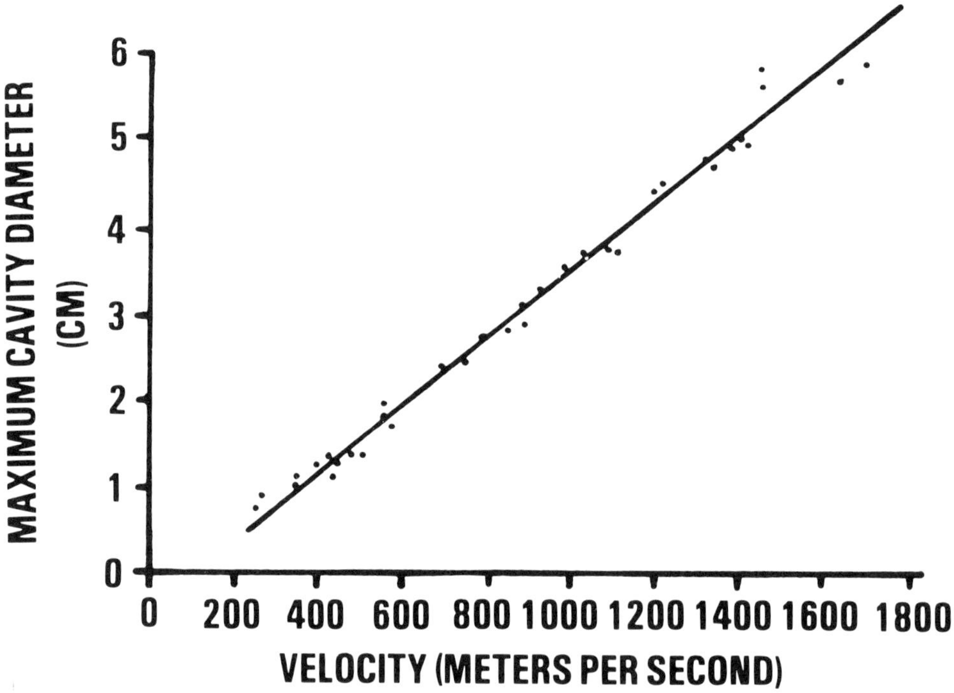

Fig. 4-26. Maximum diameter of temporary cavities in soap blocks struck by steel spheres, plotted as a function of impact velocity
Source: Redrawn from Figure 5 in reference 30

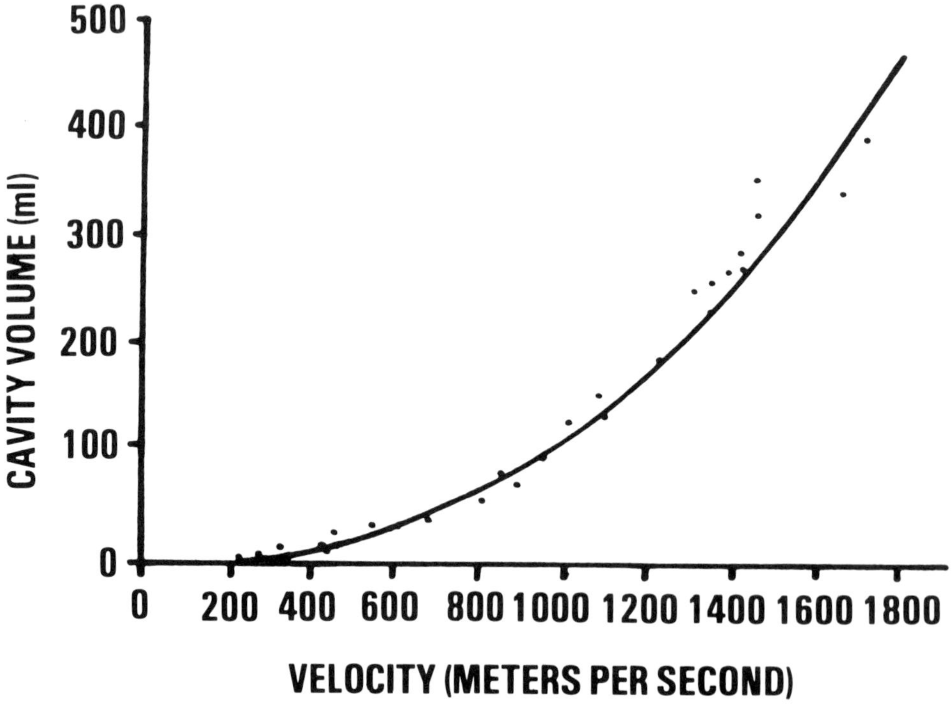

Fig. 4-27. Maximum volume of temporary cavities in soap blocks struck by steel spheres, plotted as a function of impact velocity
Source: Redrawn from Figure 4 in reference 30

over 40 msec in Figure 4-25), although one cycle is the rule in body parts such as the abdomen. The speed at which maximal expansion of the cavity occurs is much lower than the speed of the missile that made it (that is, several hundred feet per second, or about 10% of the projectile's impact velocity.)

The permanent cavity often contains foreign material.[29] Part of the target that had been expelled as the projectile perforated (Figure 4-25, frames *b* and *c*) was sucked back into the cavity along with air (frame *h*). For this to occur, pressure within the fully developed cavity must be subatmospheric, and the cavity must communicate with the outside through either the wound of entrance or exit.

Determinants of Cavity Dimensions. Cavity size can be impressive: The maximum cavity diameter shown in Figure 4-13 is 20-fold larger than the diameter of the bullet that made it, and the cavity's cross-sectional area is more than 400-fold larger. The quantitative relationship between cavity dimensions and projectile parameters—such as velocity and energy transfer—is best determined in homogeneous solids using spherical projectiles, so that extraneous factors like projectile stability and deformation are unlikely to interfere. Figure 4-26, showing cavity diameter, and Figure 4-27, showing cavity volume, both as functions of impact velocity, are from experiments that studied steel sphere projectiles being shot into soap blocks.[30]

The linear relationship between the cavity's diameter and the projectile's velocity is unexpected. The curvilinear relationship between cavity volume and projectile velocity seems intuitively more reasonable, since one does not expect a simple linear relationship to exist in so complicated a process as projectile penetration. Since none of the projectiles in either experiment perforated their targets, the abscissas in both figures are directly proportional to the kinetic energy and energy that was transferred. The researchers found no threshold velocity beyond which cavitation appeared. Nor was there any evidence that projectiles striking at velocities above the speed of sound in the target transferred their energy by a different process than did the subsonic projectiles.

The exact relationship of cavity volume and energy transfer in tissue is not known, but, contrary to Harvey's opinion,[28] it is unlikely to be linear. No doubt boundary effects are prominent. Target size is one determinant of maximum cavity volume (that is, for a given energy transfer, the smaller the target, the larger the cavity). This is known as a *scaling effect* and is an important methodological consideration influencing the design of wound ballistics experiments.[31]

In general, the more energy that is transferred, the larger the temporary cavity will be. A large cavity requires substantial energy transfer. In practice, however, cavitation is not usually significant when the striking velocity is less than 1,000 fps unless *(a)* the projectile is massive, with great striking kinetic energy, or *(b)* the projectile's tumbling, fragmenting, or deforming maximizes its energy transfer.

Pressure Transients Around the Temporary Cavity

In a series of ingenious experiments, Harvey's group investigated pressure transients in target material lying outside the temporary cavity. They shot spheres into water tanks containing many tiny air-filled balloons, and correlated changes in the balloons' dimensions with the phases of the temporary cavity. The balloons expanded and contracted with the cavity, indicating that pressure around the cavity fell as the cavity expanded, and increased as the cavity retracted. In some experiments, the air bubbles expanded so greatly that the balloons ruptured. In subsequent experiments, the researchers observed air bubbles expanding in intestinal segments. Harvey suggested that intestinal rupture might occur when gas within the bowel expands in response to subatmospheric pressure around an expanding temporary cavity.

"[T]his decreased pressure . . . in part [is] due to Bernoulli lowering of pressure as a result of the high radial velocity of water around the expanding cavity."[32] If this is why pressure falls around an expanding temporary cavity, the explanation must apply only to cavitation occurring in a nonrigid structure like the abdomen, because bulk movement of the target's material must occur. The rigid skull does not meet this condition. Since an intact skull would prevent the radial thrust of brain tissue that temporary cavitation requires, positive-pressure transients should be prominent in the early phase of a penetrating head wound. This aspect of the projectile-target interaction is poorly understood. Harvey's mid–1940s experimentation needs to be reinvestigated with modern technology.

Stress Waves

Stress waves are elusive and poorly understood phenomena that occur when a projectile hits its target tissue. They probably cause less tissue damage than the other methods of energy transfer (except heating) do. Stress waves propagate through tissue from the point of impact with that tissue's characteristic speed of sound (usually about 1,500 m/s). Therefore, stress waves precede the projectile and appear as a pressure transient much earlier than the pressure transients associated with the expansion and contraction of the temporary cavity. Do not confuse the two pressure transients. Overpressures as high as 100 atmospheres have been measured in water and homogeneous solids such as gelatin, but the duration of an individual wave is very short (20–30 µsec is typical). Bursts of stress waves of much longer duration (about 1 msec) have been recorded in tissue. This exceptional duration, which approaches that of stress waves associated with blast overpressure in air, probably results from the reflection and diffusion of stress waves by heterogeneous body parts.[33]

Harvey and his group demonstrated (somewhat artificially—they suspended still-beating frog hearts in water and injected air into some of them) that stress waves probably do not cause any tissue damage.[28] However, this conclusion obscures the fact that the air-filled frog hearts *were* damaged. Since blast overpressure waves (which are known to damage air-containing organs such as the lungs) are also stress waves, the possibility that stress waves from a penetrating projectile might also cause tissue damage cannot be completely ruled out. Interpreting these results leaves room for doubt, because Harvey's experimental design did not totally suppress temporary-cavity formation; thus damage from the explosive expansion of air in the region of subatmospheric pressure around the temporary cavity cannot be excluded. Furthermore, even given the existence of stress waves of considerable amplitude and duration, bulk movements of tissue—caused by the temporary cavity and not pressure transients alone—are likely to be the major source of indirect tissue injury.

Heating

Heating is the energy-transfer method least likely to kill or damage tissue. For example, assume than an M193 ball with an energy transfer of 400 J makes a soft-tissue wound containing 60 g of damaged tissue. The specific heat of an adult human male is 0.8 (that is, 0.8 calorie will raise the temperature of 1 g of tissue by 1° C). Let us assume that the specific heat of skeletal muscle is also 0.8. If all the transferred energy were instantaneously absorbed as heat, the temperature of the 60-g core of tissue around the bullet's path would increase by only 2.0° C (400 J equals 95 cal).

The friction that occurs as a bullet passes through a gun barrel does produce heat, but not enough to increase tissue damage.

THE PERMANENT CAVITY

The mechanisms of energy transfer are usually discussed only in the contexts of *(a)* the visible hole—the permanent cavity—which is the most impressive aspect of the wound and *(b)* the transient hole caused by shear waves—the temporary cavity—which can be seen only when special techniques are used to make it visible. Many believe that the projectile's cutting through the target tissue is the only determinant of the permanent cavity; therefore, the diameter of the permanent cavity should approximate the diameter of the projectile. This view oversimplifies the wounding process and ignores the actual determinants of the permanent-cavity's dimensions:

- The permanent cavity is completely defined only after temporary cavitation has occurred. In organs such as liver, the temporary cavity itself is an important determinant of the size of the permanent cavity.
- The presenting area of the projectile may change due to yaw, deformation, or fragmentation as it cuts through tissue.
- The elastic recoil of the severed tissues and the weight of the overlying surrounding tissues may alter the dimensions of the permanent cavity.

A permanent cavity has an entrance wound and, if the projectile perforates the tissue, an exit wound. A wound made by a nonperforating fragment is said to be *blind*.

Much of our understanding of permanent cavities comes from experimental studies rather than from battlefield observations. Many experimental studies contain quantitative data on the dimensions of the wounds of entrance and exit and on the volumes of permanent cavities; few studies, however, report the simultaneous measurement of the maximum volume of the temporary cavity. In a study performed on excised goat skeletal muscle and liver (Table 4-4), researchers fired 30-caliber (7.62-mm) armor-piercing bullets at well-defined velocities.[34] They filled the permanent cavities with plastic and determined their volumes from the weights, and they measured the temporary cavities using X rays. This study has several significant limitations: *(a)* the skin had been excised, *(b)* the tissues were not only dead but were studied *ex situ*, and *(c)* the wound tracts were extremely short (average 4 cm). Nevertheless, two concepts emerge:

- As velocity increased, the dimensions of both

TABLE 4-4

WOUND DIMENSIONS IN SKELETAL MUSCLE AND LIVER*

	Permanent Cavity (midtrack)		Temporary Cavity	
Velocity (m/s)	Diameter (cm)	Volume (cm³)	Diameter (cm)	Volume (cm³)
Skeletal Muscle N = 10 (for each velocity group)				
419.0	0.6 ± 0.07	0.7 ± 0.23	3.0 ± 13.0	30.0 ± 13.0
857.0	1.0 ± 0.13	2.7 ± 0.65	4.9 ± 0.32	116.0 ± 34.0
1,291.0	2.2 ± 0.44	14.0 ± 4.8	6.8 ± 0.75	320.0 ± 54.0
Liver N = 5 (for each velocity group)				
419.0	1.0 ± 0.35	3.4 ± 0.98	4.0 ± 0.68	52.0 ± 9.9
857.0	2.6 ± 0.63	30.0 ± 9.0	6.1 ± 0.63	198.0 ± 69.0
1,291.0	4.8 ± 0.43	65.0 ± 16.0	9.6 ± 0.48	708.0 ± 106.0

*Mean ± 1.0 standard deviation
Source: Reference 34

the temporary and the permanent cavities also increased, and were (in all groups but one) substantially larger than the diameter of the bullet. Since the researchers did not detect yaw in the roentgenograms and since they used nondeforming-nonfragmenting bullets, it is hard to escape the conclusion that temporary cavitation associated with high velocity increased the size of the permanent cavity.

- Liver is more sensitive than muscle is to cavitation. The permanent cavity in skeletal muscle was about 3% of the maximum volume of the temporary cavity; in liver, it was about 10%.

In another study from the same laboratory, researchers measured wound dimensions at autopsy 4 days after wounding. They found that average permanent-cavity dimensions in goat thighs were slightly smaller along the entire wound tract than they had expected from the bullet dimensions alone. There was one exception: "[T]he permanent wound tract was larger in the wounds from higher velocity missiles and in areas where bullets had tumbled."[12]

Studies in which measurements are made in living animal tissue give especially useful information concerning the morphology of the permanent cavity. Researchers shot dogs with two commonly used military assault-rifle bullets (Table 4-5). To obtain a wide spectrum of data, they *(a)* varied the amount of propellent to adjust bullet velocity and *(b)* measured impact and exit velocities. The dogs were positioned so the bullets traversed only the soft-tissue of both thighs, yielding wound lengths of 11–12 cm. They measured the wound dimensions 6 hours after wounding.[10]

In this study, the wounds of entrance were little different than the size of the bullets that made them. The wounds of exit, however, were larger than the bullets, and were dramatically larger when, as happened with the M193 fired by the M16, the bullet fragmented before it exited. Fragmenting bullets also created the largest permanent cavities. Thus, the volume of the permanent cavity can be much larger than the projectile that created it.

Another laboratory obtained similar results (Table 4-6). In this study,[9] 30-kg anesthetized swine were shot at 30 or 100 m through the soft tissue of one thigh with bullets from either the M16 or the AK47. Researchers examined the wounds 6 hours later. The wounds of entrance were the same size as the projectile, while the wounds of exit made by the M193 were very large, no doubt reflecting the propensity of the M193 ball to fragment in soft tissue. The wounds of exit made by the M43 ball fired by the AK47, however, were little different from the wounds of entrance. Longer experimental wound tracts (about 15 cm, the average length of wounds through human extremities) would have allowed the bullets time to develop sufficient yaw before they exited, perhaps producing bigger exit wounds.

Several studies have investigated the permanent cavities of experimental fragment wounds (Table 4-7). Researchers fired square steel fragments weighing 0.35 g into the thighs of anesthetized dogs.[35] This study

TABLE 4-5

MEASUREMENTS OF PERMANENT CAVITIES IN BULLET WOUNDS IN DOGS*

Bullet	Impact Velocity (m/s)	Energy Transfer (J)	Wound Dimensions (maximum diameter in cm) Entrance	Exit	Volume of Permanent Cavity (cm^3)	Number of Animals
7.62	956 ± 4	42.6 ± 10.3	0.7 ± 0.1	3.6 ± 2.7	21	10
7.62	514 ± 12	20.2 ± 9.3	0.3 ± 0.1	1.1 ± 1.0	11	8
5.56	929 ± 8					
Intact		25.1 ± 5.8	0.2 ± 0.1	4.4 ± 3.8	13	12
Broken		51.3 ± 18.9	0.3 ± 0.03	19.7 ± 13.9	42	5

*Mean ±1.0 standard deviation

Source: Reference 10

TABLE 4-6

MEASUREMENTS OF PERMANENT CAVITIES IN BULLET WOUNDS IN SWINE*

Weapon	Impact Velocity (m/s)	Wound Areas (mm^2) Entrance	Exit	Length (mm)
AK47-M43 ball:				
30 m	693 ± 2	41 ± 13	20 ± 12	87 ± 20
100 m	641 ± 12	25 ± 8	30 ± 13	86 ± 24
M16-M193 ball:				
30 m	926 ± 9	27 ± 12	2152 ± 2841	91 ± 15
100 m	846 ± 19	26 ± 5	345 ± 533	100 ± 25

*Mean ± 1.0 standard deviation

Source: Reference 9

TABLE 4-7

THE PERMANENT CAVITY IN EXPERIMENTAL FRAGMENT WOUNDS IN DOGS*

Impact Velocity (m/s)	Area of Entrance (cm^2)	Description
716 ± 119	1.52 ± 0.71	Blind, square and regular, cylindrical
1015 ± 159	2.49 ± 1.29	Blind, elliptical and irregular, cone-shaped
1506 ± 99	6.85 ± 4.35	Blind, tissue blown out, funnel-shaped

*All fragments have diameters of approximately 4 mm; data expressed as mean ± 1.0 standard deviation.
Source: Reference 35

demonstrates that permanent-cavity formation frequently involves more than the projectile's direct cutting action. Clearly, temporary cavitation contributed to the size of the wounds of entrance seen in these experiments. The unfavorable aerodynamic shape of the projectile caused maximum energy transfer and temporary cavitation at the wound of entrance. The gigantic wound of entrance shown in Figure 4-14 was made by a bullet striking blunt-end forward. The dimensions of the wound vastly exceed the dimensions of the projectile, and can only be understood as a consequence of temporary cavitation's having ripped the tissue apart.

SOFT-TISSUE BALLISTIC WOUNDS

Damage to soft tissue (that is, skin, fat, and skeletal muscle) and to specific organs (that is, the viscera, bones, and so forth) are of course not separate, since an injury to a viscus will necessarily have a soft-tissue component. But because *(a)* experimental wound ballistics has focused upon soft-tissue injury, *(b)* ballistic injuries involving skin, fat, and skeletal muscle form the bulk of the combat surgeon's practice, and *(c)* the major controversies in wound ballistics arise from managing soft-tissue injuries, these two groups can logically be separated.

The concepts of kinetic energy and energy transfer that have been useful in understanding the physical aspects of wound ballistics are much less useful in understanding the medical aspects. There certainly can be no tissue damage if there is no energy transfer, but rigorously defining tissue damage is difficult. Can tissue damage be measured quantitatively? If it cannot, then correlating tissue damage with a measured quantity of energy transfer is futile. Furthermore, the main threat to many casualties arises not from the mechanical disruption sustained by the soft tissue but from sepsis in the contaminated wound tract, which is poorly understood in relation to energy transfer. Thus, medical officers will find that concepts such as energy transfer may be less relevant to the purely medical aspects of wound ballistics than they are to the study of wound ballistics as a branch of physics.

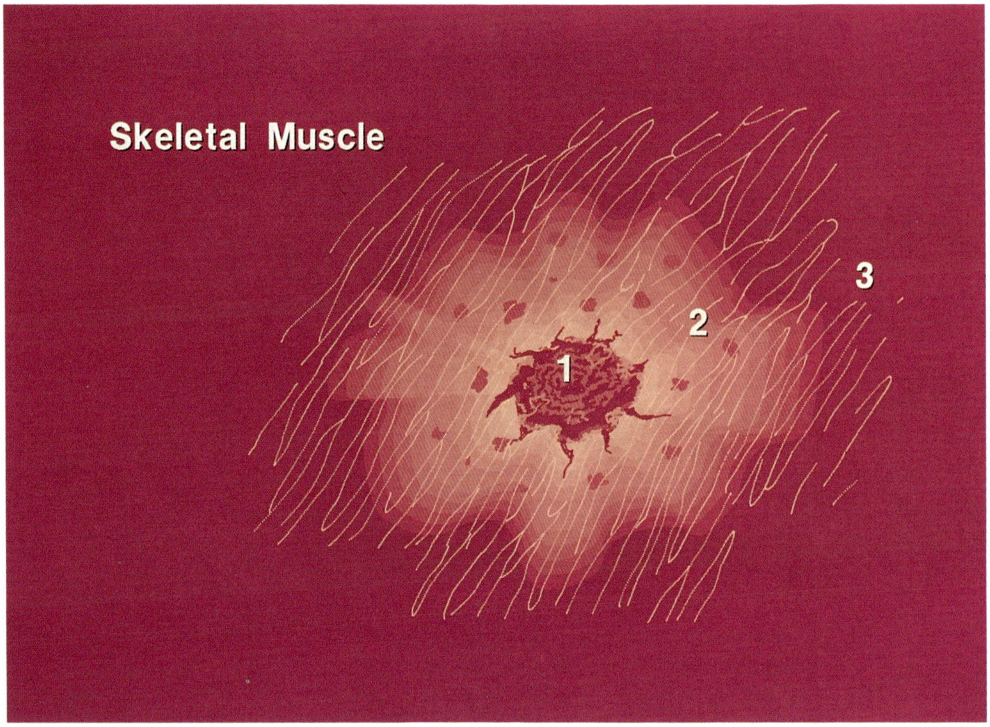

Fig. 4-28. Idealized pathomorphology of a soft-tissue wound involving skeletal muscle. The wound consists of three components: (1) the permanent cavity, (2) the zone of extravasation, and (3) the zone of concussion.

Pathomorphology of Soft-Tissue Wounds

Unfortunately, little data have been published on wound-tract morphology in humans. The Wound Data and Munitions Effectiveness Team (WDMET) database found that the median wound tract was only 60 mm long, and the largest single group of casualties had wound tracts measuring 20 mm or less. About 10% of the WDMET population had wound tracts 250 mm or longer. About 75% of casualties in whom wound-tract shape was assessed had elliptical or circular wounds. About 80% of the wound tracts were blind. Wound-tract volume was measured in about 10,000 wounds; 97% had a volume less than 99 cc. The WDMET data are consistent with the clinical observation that a 15-cm wound tract will usually either perforate an extremity or strike an internal viscus.[36]

Recent data from the Chinese conflict with Vietnam extend these observations. Of those casualties who were hit by bullets, 87% had perforating wounds, almost all of which were made by 7.62-mm bullets. The exit wounds (4.25 cm^2) were larger than the entrance wounds (1.0 cm^2). In some instances, surgeons observed very large permanent cavities (with diameters of 7.5 cm) with even larger wounds of exit. Wounds made by fragments (85%) were usually blind. The probability that a fragment would cause a perforating wound depended upon the casualty's proximity to the detonation site: Of the wounds sustained within 1 m of the explosion, 60% were perforating, while beyond 6 m, nonperforating wounds were common.[37] This finding is not unexpected; fragment velocity rapidly degrades in air (Figure 4-2).

The gross pathomorphological components of a typical wound (Figure 4-28) involving skeletal muscle are, from inside out, *(a)* the permanent cavity, which is a hole containing blood clots, detached chunks of tissue, and foreign material that may have been aspirated or carried into the wound; *(b)* the zone of extravasation, which is the grossly hemorrhagic, shredded, pulped muscle around the permanent cavity; and *(c)* the zone of concussion, which is grossly normal muscle, but with histological evidence of damage such as interstitial hemorrhage, vascular congestion, and abnormal myocytes.

The Permanent Cavity. Except in "explosive" wounds, little tissue is actually expelled from the target in forming the permanent cavity. The unopposed elastic recoil of the partly detached surrounding tissue keeps the hole open.

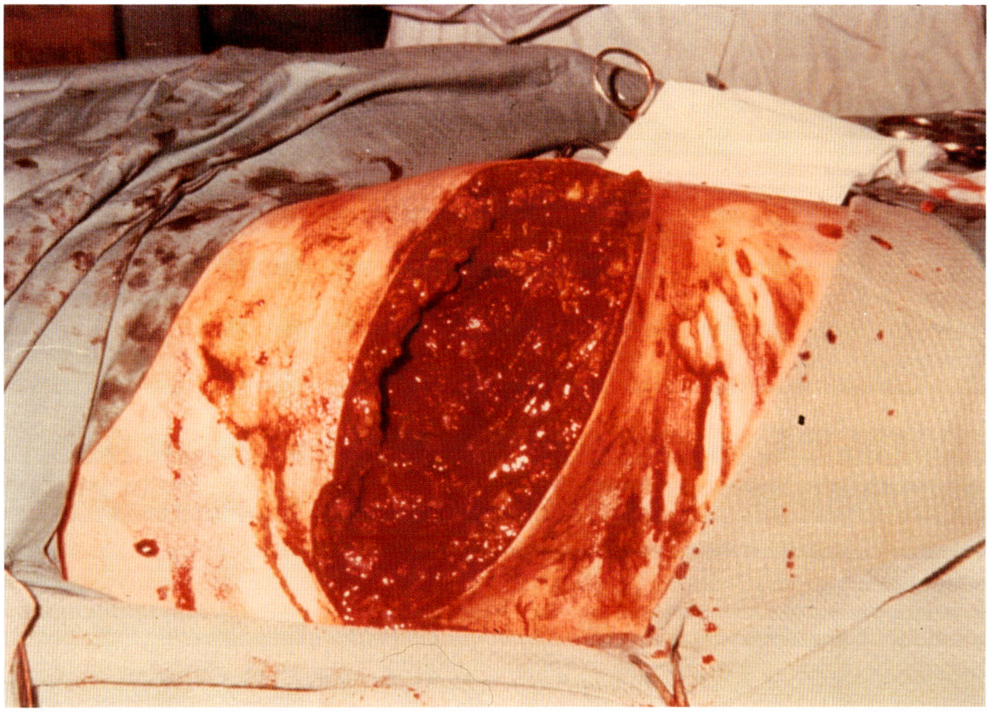

Fig. 4-29. A thigh wounded by an M43 ball at close range. The permanent cavity has been opened, exposing the hemorrhagic zone of extravasation.
Source: Wound Data and Munitions Effectiveness Team

The Zones of Extravasation and Concussion. Damage to the soft tissue surrounding the permanent cavity is probably caused by stretching during temporary cavitation, and extravasation probably results from small blood vessels being stretched until they rupture. The pulling apart of the Z bands of individual myocytes supports this contention.[38]

A representative skeletal-muscle wound made by a high-velocity bullet (Figure 4-29) shows the open permanent cavity and the typical hemorrhagic zone of extravasation. Typical animal studies show that the zone of extravasation usually extends for 5–10 mm beyond the permanent tract.[38] The zone of concussion extends another 20–30 mm beyond the zone of extravasation. The boundary between the two zones may be discrete; however, localized areas showing the typical histopathology of the zone of extravasation (that is, necrotic myocytes) are commonly found within the concussion zone. Similarly, the vascular congestion and hemorrhage within the zone of extravasation frequently extend into the zone of concussion. Bones and fascial planes control the expansion of the temporary cavity; therefore, the zones of extravasation and concussion may not be symmetrical around the permanent cavity.

The histopathology of the zones of extravasation and concussion in skeletal muscle changes with time after wounding.[38] Within 6 hours, the zone of extravasation is characterized by *(a)* necrotic myocytes with fragmentation, hyalinization, and loss of transverse bands; *(b)* dilated and ruptured capillaries and venules, with extravasation of red blood cells and plasma; and *(c)* beginning infiltration by leukocytes. In the zone of concussion, the most prominent changes after 6 hours are edema and interstitial hemorrhage in myocytes; after 12 hours, progressive dissolution of myocytes and increasing infiltration by leukocytes; after 24 hours in the zone of extravasation, the collection of large numbers of leukocytes around necrotic myocytes; and after 72 hours in both zones, inflammation, frequently with outright cellulitis, and the permanent cavity may now contain purulent exudate.

Blood flow in the tissue surrounding the permanent cavity also changes over time. In the zone of concussion, the initial generalized vasoconstriction is followed within 6 hours by vasodilation. Vasodilation persists for many hours and indicates both the ongoing inflammatory reaction and the ultimate healing of the wound. Various markers of perfusion such as radiomicrospheres, supravital dyes, and so forth, fail to label the zone of extravasation and indicate that blood flow in the tissue immediately adjacent to the permanent cavity is impaired for some time.[12, 13, 39] The resulting ischemia is probably one factor leading to cellular death in the zone of extravasation. Various studies indicate that frank necrosis usually involves less than 1 cm (and frequently less than 5 mm) of the zone of extravasation.[13] This dead tissue constitutes the slough that John Hunter had described in the eighteenth century. Ultimate healing of the wound and the death of tissue in the zone of extravasation are not incompatible. Any dead tissue not sloughed is absorbed when tissue from the zone of extravasation grows into the permanent cavity.

Tissue Damage Assessed by Debrided Muscle

Traditional soft-tissue wound surgery excises the hemorrhagic, shredded, pulped tissue of the zone of extravasation and some of its neighboring zone of concussion. This mass of debrided tissue is commonly used as an index of tissue damage, and can be correlated with measured energy transfer. Methodological considerations (specifically recognizing the tissue around the permanent cavity that needs to be surgically removed) are very important in these experiments. The criteria for making these judgements usually employ the *four Cs*: Skeletal muscle is surgically excised if its *color* is abnormal, if it fails to *contract* when pinched, if its *circulation* is impaired (that is, it does not bleed when cut), and if it has abnormal *consistency*. Skeletal muscle subject to excision should be considered damaged but not necessarily dead or devitalized.

The results of a typical experiment show the mass of debrided skeletal muscle from swine thigh plotted against energy transfer (Figure 4-30). Although it looks like a scattergram, the graph shows a definite tendency for the mass of debrided tissue to increase with greater energy transfer.[14]

Although the data can be fitted by a linear regression model, no biophysical process, especially one as complicated as a projectile's penetration through tissue, is likely to be described by a simple linear relationship. Nevertheless, Swedish ballistic researchers, on the basis of their extensive experience, estimate that each J of energy transferred damages 0.3 g of muscle.[31]

Stratifying the outcome by the behavior of the bullet might be expected to provide insight into the relationship between tissue damage and energy (Figure 4-31). Breakup or severe deformation of a bullet was usually associated with greater energy transfer, but there was a disproportionately small increase in the amount of excised muscle, indicating that some of the energy that appears to have been transferred from the bullet was actually used to alter the projectile's structure rather than to damage muscle.[14]

Total energy transfer, however, gives only part of the available information about the projectile-target interaction. Energy transfer plotted as a function of depth of penetration gives a much clearer picture. The concept is further illuminated when the magnitude of debrided tissue is seen as a function of energy transfer and both are plotted along the wound tract. Figures 4-32 and 4-33 show the results of especially elegant experiments that were designed to relate tissue damage in skeletal muscle to energy transfer along the wound tract.[2]

Figure 4-32 shows the force of retardation as a function of the depth of penetration in soap blocks for two assault-rifle rounds. (The Ak 5 is similar to the 5.56-mm M855 fired by the US M16A2, and the Ak 4 is similar to the NATO 7.62-mm round.) Note that both bullets have a marked increase in retardation (the increase in drag is proportional to a similar increase in energy transfer) beginning at about 10 cm for the Ak 5 and 12 cm for the Ak 4. Figure 4-33 shows the amount of tissue debrided from the wound tract in the thighs of anesthetized swine. The marked increase in tissue damage corresponds to the site of the bullet's maximal energy transfer in the soap blocks. The conclusion is inescapable: Tissue damage and energy transfer are closely linked. Almost all of the Ak 5 bullets disintegrated after penetrating about 10 cm. None of the Ak 4 bullets broke up or deformed, but all began to yaw and tumble after penetrating about 12 cm. These experiments are difficult to perform, but they are essential to provide comprehensive information on the biophysical aspects of ballistic tissue damage and to strengthen the field's scientific validity.

How much of this tissue damage can be attributed to the temporary cavity's stretch? Encasing a target thigh in an unyielding plaster-of-Paris cast partially suppressed the temporary cavity's formation and decreased by 40% the amount of gross skeletal-muscle damage.[40] Because the plaster cast did not completely suppress it, cavitation may have caused some of the damage observed in this experimental wound. Additional damage must have been due to direct cutting by the projectile, but the researchers suggest that stress waves may have caused most of the residual damage. This suggestion, and the estimate of damage that the cavity's forceful implosion might cause (in addition to that caused by the stretch that occurred during the cavity's initial explosive expansion), are controversial. Fragmentation and cavitation may increase tissue damage synergistically: The fragments lacerate the tissue around the trajectory and the ensuing cavitation tears the weakened tissue apart.[20]

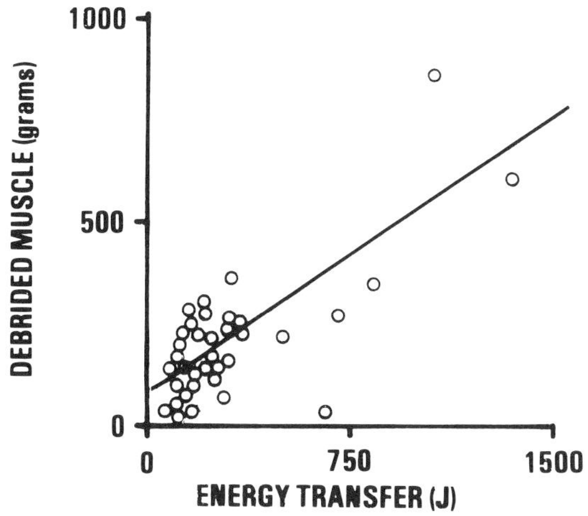

Fig. 4-30. The mass of surgically excised swine-thigh muscle is plotted against measured total energy transfer. Each symbol represents data from a single swine. A variety of different rounds were used to make the wounds: 7.62 x 51 mm; 5.56 x 45 mm; and 7.62 x 39 mm. The data are fitted by Y = 0.24x + 71.4, r = 0.74.
Source: Redrawn from Figure 4-25 in reference 14

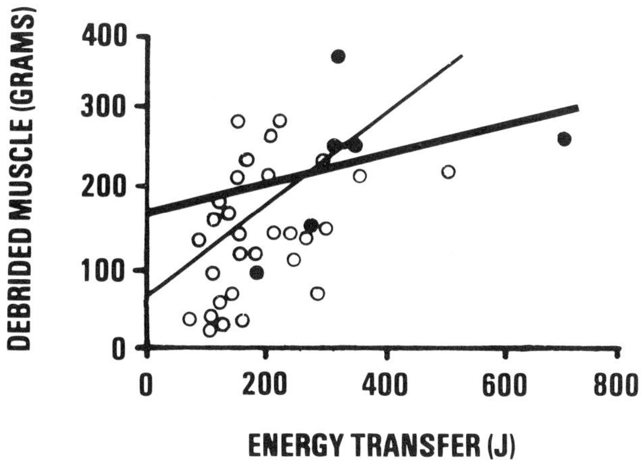

Fig. 4-31. The mass of surgically excised swine thigh muscle is plotted against measured total energy transfer. These data are from different experiments than those shown in Figure 4-30. The same rounds were used in Figure 4-30, but the data have been stratified according to whether or not the 5.56-mm bullet deformed or fragmented (solid circles). The open circles (thin line) are fitted by y = 0.44x + 65, r = 0.48. Data for damaged 5.56-mm bullets (thick line) are fitted by y = 0.18x + 168, r = 0.39. The smaller x coefficient for the latter equation compared to the former suggests that some of the energy transferred by the damaged bullets does not go into injuring muscle.
Source: Redrawn from Figure 24 in reference 14

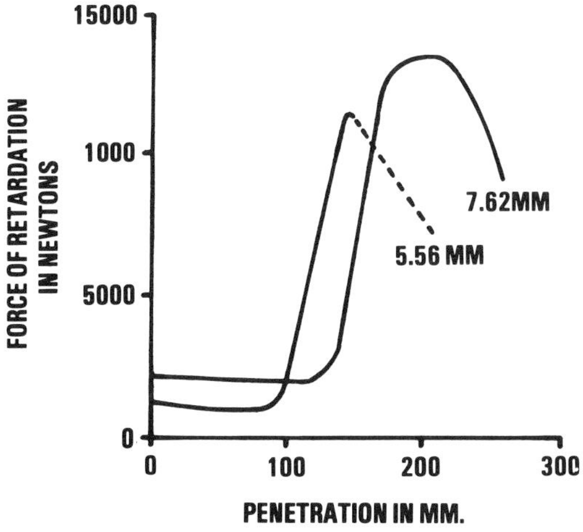

Fig. 4-32. The force of retardation measured by an X-ray methodology for 5.56-mm bullets (similar to the M855) and 7.62-mm bullets (equivalent to the NATO 7.62 x 51-mm round) as they penetrate into soap blocks. Because it is smaller, the 5.56-mm bullet experiences less retardation in the initial part of its trajectory than does the larger 7.62-mm bullet. After penetrating about 10 cm, retardation of the 5.56-mm bullet greatly increases due to yaw, tumbling, and finally fragmentation. The dashed curve is an estimate of the retardation of the fragments. The 7.62-mm bullet characteristically yaws and tumbles after penetrating 12 cm.
Source: Redrawn from Figure 4 in reference 2

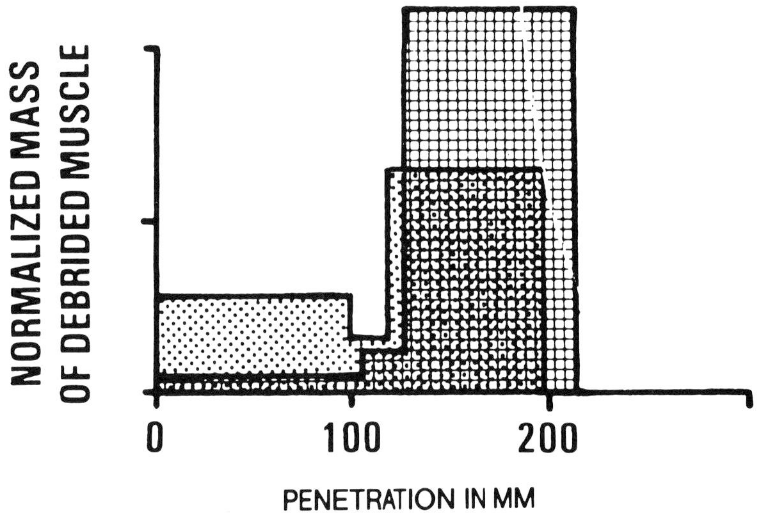

Fig. 4-33. Debrided swine skeletal muscle as a function of the depth of penetration (the abscissa, in mm) for 5.56-mm (cross-hatched) and 7.62-mm bullets (stippled). Data from one experiment with each bullet is shown. Tissue damage as assessed by debrided muscle was markedly increased at the site at which bullet instability occurred.
Source: Redrawn from Figure 4 in reference 2

ORGAN-SPECIFIC WOUNDS

Body parts other than soft tissue have unique wound-ballistics characteristics that influence the relative importance of direct (cutting) and indirect (shear and stress waves) effects as sources of injury. Controversy exists regarding the relative importance of these effects, but it is probably safe to say that in most casualties who are candidates for surgical care, injury results from the direct effects of the projectiles. That is not to say that indirect effects are inconsequential. They are important in the overall context of wound ballistics, but less so as a source of surgical treatment problems. Casualties with wounds of the head, chest, and abdomen, in whom indirect effects (especially cavitation) are prominent, are frequently not candidates for surgery: Such casualties are usually killed outright.

The Skull and Brain

Ballistic wounds of the skull and brain are often grossly destructive, and in the past have been ascribed to explosive bullets. The explosive wound of the skull shown in Figure 4-34 is typical; as Horsley and Woodruff suggested at the end of the nineteenth century, this phenomenon results when temporary cavitation occurs in a fluid-like viscus (in this instance, the brain surrounded by its subarachnoid space) enclosed in a rigid container (the bony skull).[41] Kocher and other late–nineteenth-century ballisticians observed the identical phenomenon (that is, the hydraulic or hydrodynamic effects) when they shot high-velocity projectiles into water-filled lead containers (Figure 4-35).

Harvey and his group, working at Princeton University in the 1940s, demonstrated the necessity for a fluid medium (the brain) to be present for the explosive effects associated with the temporary cavity in the skull (and other organs) to develop. They emptied cat skulls of brain and shot them with 1/8-inch steel spheres at 3,800 fps. The only damage to the empty skulls were "rather neat entrance and exit holes." But an intact cranium sustained quite different damage:

> The cavity formed by a missile in the brain of an intact cranium is of finite size, partly because brain tissue is forced through regions of less resistance (such as the frontal sinuses and the various foramina of the skull) and partly because of the stretching of the cranium itself. When the energy delivered is very great, skull bones are actually torn apart along suture lines.[28]

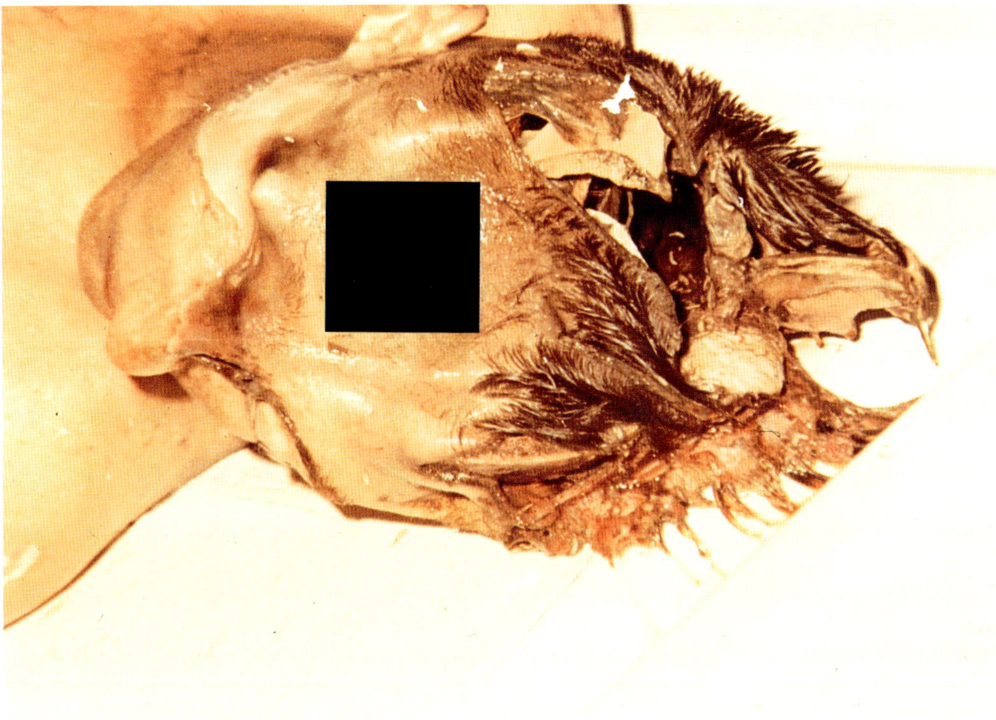

Fig. 4-34. This casualty was killed when an M43 ball fired by an AK47 blew his skull apart.
Source: Wound Data and Munitions Effectiveness Team

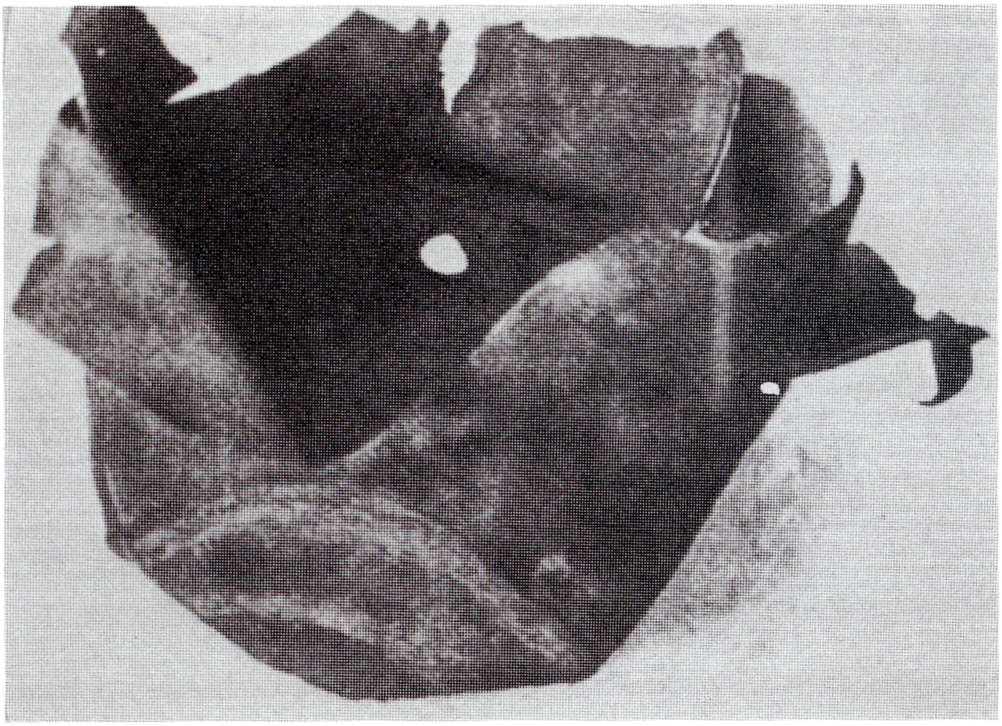

Fig. 4-35. The appearance of a water-filled lead container after it had been shot with a military rifle bullet. The bullet made the small hole at the back upon entering. The similarity between the damage shown here and that shown in Figure 4-34 should be noted.
Source: Reproduced courtesy of the Royal Army Medical College Museum

Clearly, enormous energy transfer occurred in both the skull and the lead container. Callender and French calculated that a typical rifle bullet—probably not unlike the one that caused the injury shown in Figure 4-34—undergoing maximum retardation (that is, maximum energy transfer) corresponded to 4,000–5,000 horsepower.[7]

Recently-published elegant pathophysiological studies go beyond gross observations of pathomorphology.[42] These researchers fired steel spheres with 3- or 6-mm diameters into gelatin-filled, instrumented human skulls and correlated impact velocities in the range of 376–1,015 m/s with energy transfer and intracranial pressures. In some studies, they made cine-roentgenograms as the projectile passed through the skull. Most shots traversed the skull, but some were set at an angle to hit tangentially. They found that:

- About 70 J were needed to perforate the skull
- Energy transfer on the order of 400 J caused severe breakup of the skull bones
- Shock (stress) waves with durations of less than 100 µsec and with overpressures exceeding 5,000 kiloPascals (kPa)—that is, greater than 35,000 mm Hg, perhaps equivalent to 700 psi—occasionally occurred
- *Quasi-static overpressures* (that is, the average pressure during the temporary cavity's cyclic dimensional changes) with durations of 2–3 msec and pressures of about 200 kPa commonly occurred
- A linear relationship exists between the energy of impact and the quasi-static overpressure
- Energy transfer for a tangential hit (that is, the projectile did not enter the gelatin and had no direct contact with "brain") was about one-seventh that observed for a penetrating hit

In one of the experiments, a 6-mm steel ball with an impact-velocity of only 205 m/s perforated one parietal bone and penetrated 18 mm into the gelatin. The energy transferred was about 19 J, some of which went into defeating the bone, and the quasi-static overpressure was 75 kPa. To put this in perspective, others have estimated that a penetrating projectile delivering as little as 20 J into the cerebral cortex can cause death,[43] and even less energy delivered to the brain stem will cause a fatal injury. Is there any wonder why ballistic injury to the brain is so often fatal?

Figures 4-36 and 4-37 illustrate the experimentally observed pressure transients that occurred when a 6-mm sphere with a striking velocity of 838 m/s passed tangentially across a model skull. The effect of the impact was to depress a section of skull 25-mm in diameter to a depth of 10 mm. Figure 4-36 shows the high-frequency vibrations that indicate the passage of the stress wave. The waves had a duration of about 30 µsec and an overpressure of 800–1,000 kPa (110–140 psi). The negative phases occurred when the skull reflected the wave. Within 1 msec of impact, a quasi-static overpressure of about 200 kPa developed from the initial expansion of the temporary cavity. Figure 4-37 shows the subsequent pressure perturbations that occurred over at least 50 msec, resulting from the rhythmic expansion and contractionof the temporary cavitation.

These two figures provide considerable insight into the mechanisms of ballistic injury in general, and, in particular, the importance of pressure transients. Since the time that Harvey and his group did their work, the wound-ballistics community has generally agreed that stress waves, even though associated with enormous high pressure, cause little damage. Pressure-dependent indirect injury results from shear waves. This hydrodynamic process physically displaces and injures tissue; the motion of the medium itself (in this case, the gelatin, representing brain), which the projectile is passing through, causes injury.[42]

The Chest

The two major intrathoracic viscera (the lungs and the heart and its great vessels) tolerate ballistic injury differently.

The Lungs. Lung tissue has very low density compared to other organs in the body (that is, 0.2 g/cm^3; other organs' density is about 1.0 g/cm^3, and the density of bone is about 2.0 g/cm^3). According to the drag equation, resistance offered to the passage of a projectile will be low if the target's density is low; thus, energy transfer and tissue damage may be correspondingly small. Lung is also easily stretched compared to other organs. As a result of these physical properties, lung has considerable tolerance to the stretch and shear of temporary cavitation. Figure 4-38 shows the lung of a casualty killed in the Vietnam War—not by the wound tract in the lung but by a wound to his head. The lack of ecchymosis around the probe through the wound tract may indicate that either *(a)* temporary cavitation was minimal, or *(b)* it was tolerated with little tissue damage. This does not mean that temporary cavitation cannot be a destructive process in lung, however. The post-traumatic pneumatoceles that occurred in a few combat casualties in the Vietnam War show that projectiles with high energy transfer are

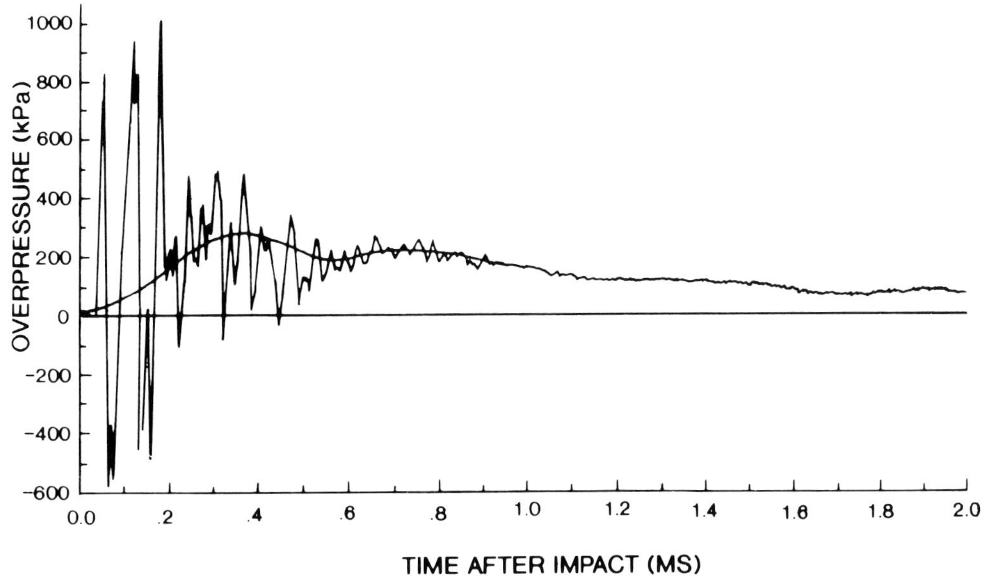

Fig. 4-36. High-frequency pressure transients observed during the first 2 msec after tangential impact of a 6-mm sphere with a striking velocity of 838 m/s on a gelatin-filled human skull. The initial vibrations are due to stress waves. The thick line indicates the development of quasi-static overpressure associated with the first expansion of the temporary cavity.
Source: Redrawn from Figure 3 in reference 42

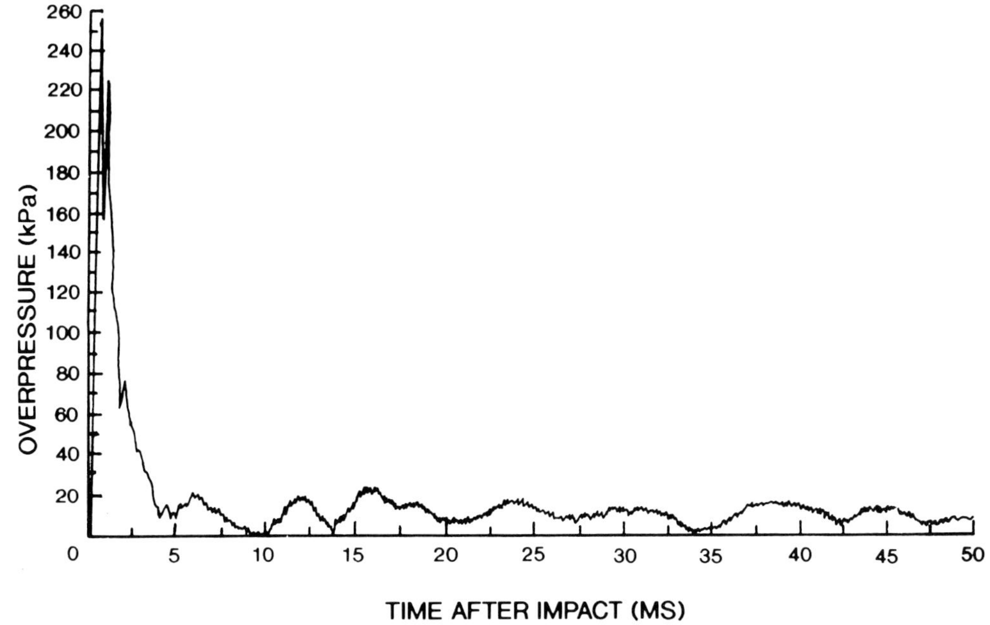

Fig. 4-37. Low-frequency pressure transients observed during the first 50 msec of the experiment discussed in Figure 4-36. The damped frequency response characteristics of the pressure transducer results in a fusion of the pressure transients associated with the stress wave and the first expansion of the temporary cavity. Subsequent expansions and contractions of the temporary cavity are apparent as the cyclic change in pressure.
Source: Redrawn from Figure 3 in reference 42

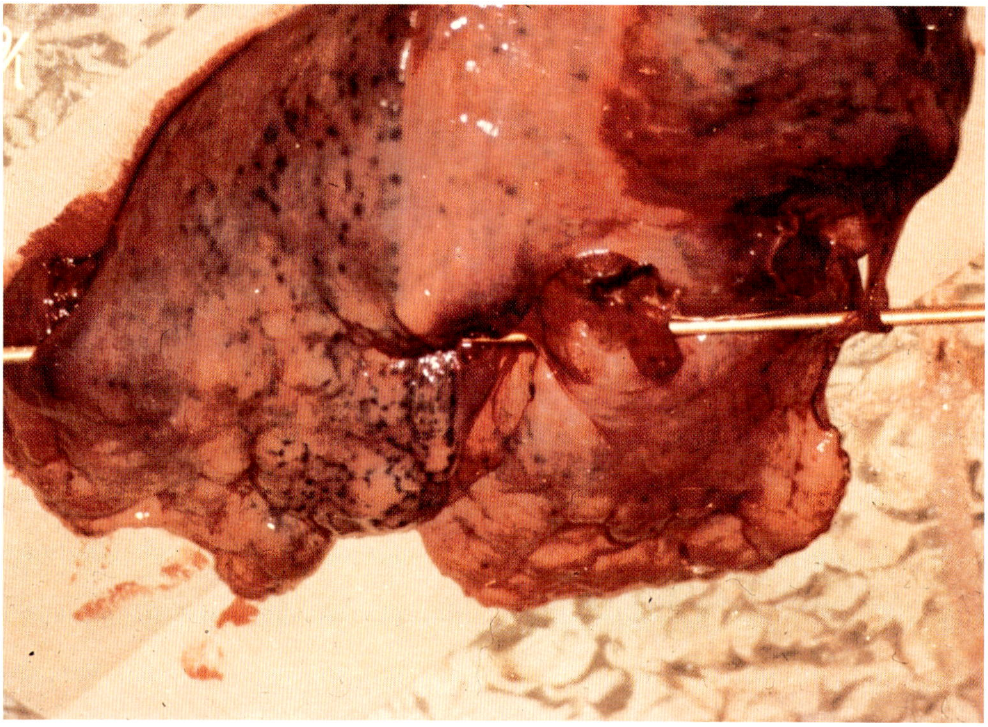

Fig. 4-38. This casualty was killed by an AK47 wound of the skull, but he also sustained the lung wound shown in this photo. There is little evidence of hemorrhage or ecchymosis around the probe, which delineates the permanent cavity.
Source: Wound Data and Munitions Effectiveness Team

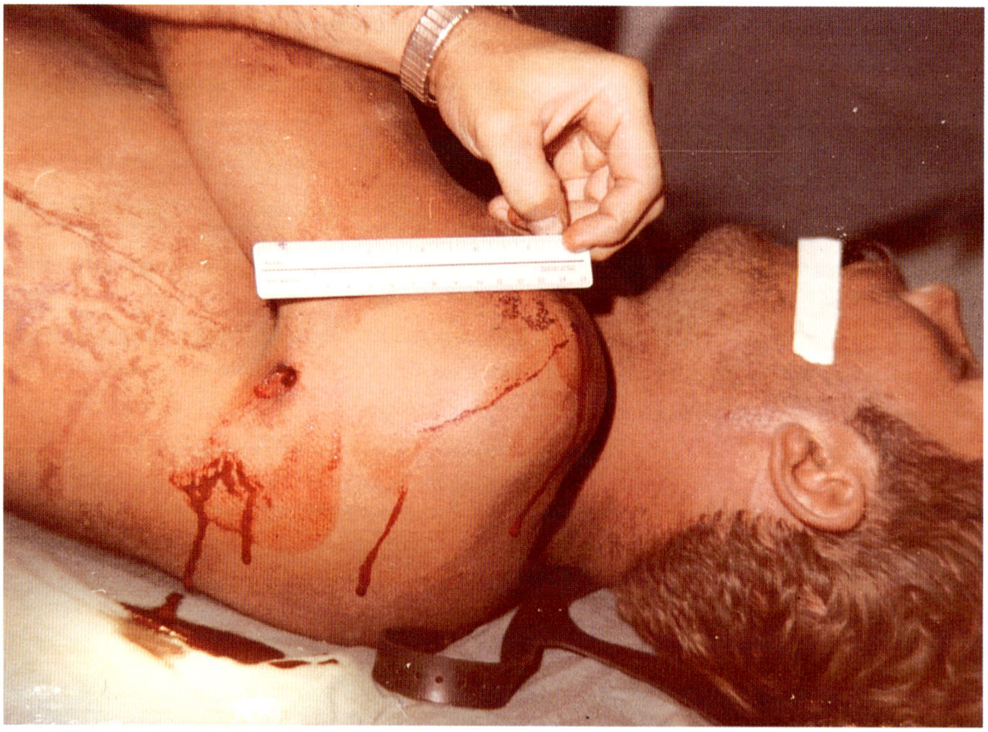

Fig. 4-39. This casualty sustained a through-and-through AK47 wound of the soft tissue of the left shoulder. The benign appearance of the wound makes it unlikely that massive temporary cavitation occurred.
Source: Wound Data and Munitions Effectiveness Team

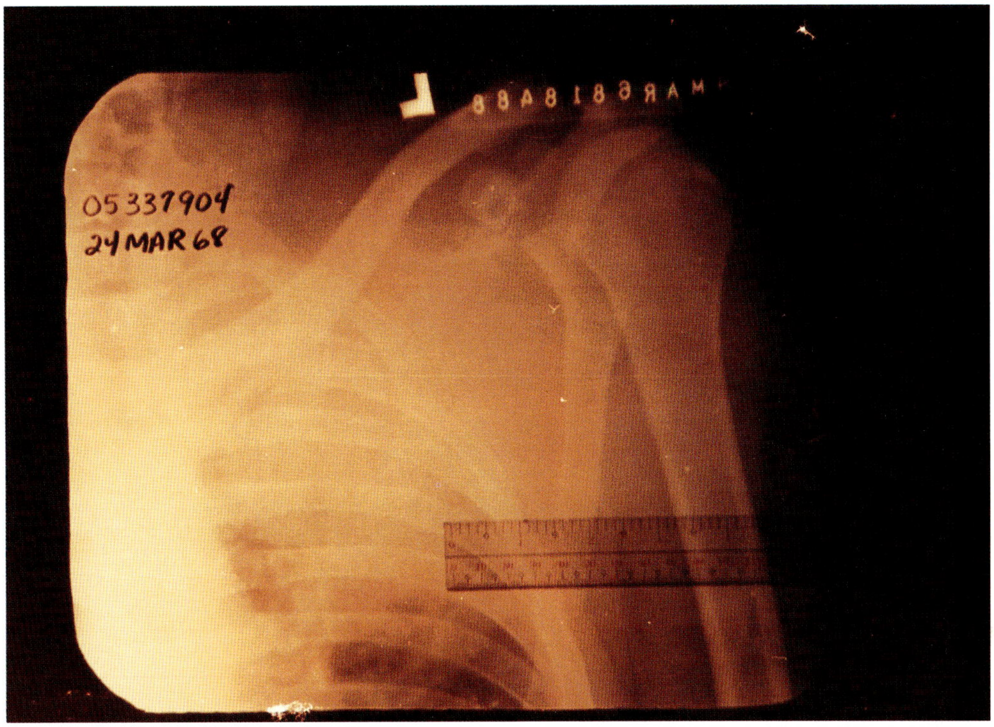

Fig. 4-40. This roentgenogram shows the chest of the casualty pictured in Figure 4-39. It was taken about 1 hour after wounding and shows a massive pulmonary contusion of the upper lobe of the left lung. The pulmonary injury may be the result of a stress (shock) wave.
Source: Wound Data and Munitions Effectiveness Team

capable of causing indirect damage to lungs.

The mechanism by which a penetrating projectile causes pulmonary injury is sometimes difficult to understand. The following example from the WDMET database may be an example of just such an injury: A soldier sustained a through-and-through wound of the shoulder made by an AK47 bullet fired from about 50 m away (Figure 4-39). A roentgenogram made about 1 hour after wounding (Figure 4-40) shows that the lung nearest the wound has an extensive pulmonary contusion. The cause of this injury is not clear. If temporary cavitation were the cause, some evidence of chest-wall damage or even a fracture of the humerus might be found. Certainly, the soft-tissue injury shows no evidence (such as ecchymosis) of the effects of massive temporary cavitation that would be necessary to have caused this distant lung injury. Could this observed injury be a manifestation of stress waves?

Lung has another distinctive biophysical property; it is perhaps the only organ in the body in which the speed of sound (50 m/s) is likely to be less than the velocity of a penetrating projectile. Thus, the potential exists for a projectile penetrating through lung to be associated with a true shock wave,[44] but whether or not this has biophysical or medical ramifications is unclear.

The Heart. Wounds of the heart, especially when made by bullets fired from military small arms, are frequently as destructive as wounds of the skull. The heart shown in Figure 4-41 was hit by an M43 ball. The bullet's trajectory, shown by the wooden rod, traverses the base of the heart (that is, the atrioventricular valves). But the most impressive feature of this injury is that the left ventricular free wall is missing; the left ventricle cavity has been blown open. This catastrophic injury is likely to have been caused by the mechanism that Woodruff described: temporary cavitation occurring in a fluid-filled viscus.[41]

The large vessels like the aorta and the pulmonary artery are susceptible to the same catastrophic damage as the heart.

The Abdomen

Intraabdominal viscera can be divided into two classes: solid organs such as the liver, and hollow organs such as the urinary bladder, which contains liquid, and the gastrointestinal tract, which can contain gas, liquids, and solids. Both types of viscera can respond similarly when penetrated by a high–energy-transfer projectile.

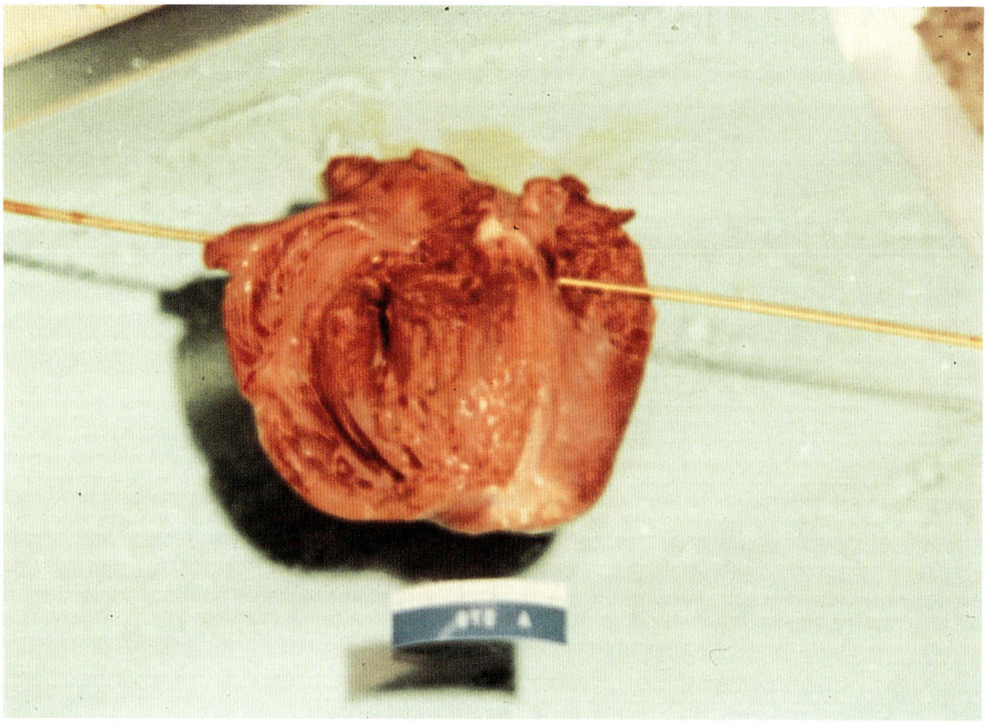

Fig. 4-41. The probe shows the line of flight of a bullet fired by an AK47 through a casualty's heart. The free wall of the left ventricle has been blown open by what must have been explosive cavitation. Since the bullet, passing as it did through the atrioventricular valves, could not have made physical contact with the left ventricular free wall, this injury must be an example of an indirect effect. The mechanism is very similar to the hydrodynamic effect that destroyed the lead container shown in Figure 4-35.
Source: Wound Data and Munitions Effectiveness Team

Liver, spleen, and kidney are highly vascular, friable organs (that is, the tissues lack elasticity; they tear when they are stretched). Temporary cavitation causes severe tissue disruption (Figure 4-42). The very large permanent cavity probably nearly matches the size of the temporary cavity. Such injuries are rapidly fatal.

The gastrointestinal tract is capable of a dichotomous response when a high–energy transfer projectile penetrates it. If the gastrointestinal tract is empty, the wound's permanent cavity will probably be the same size as the projectile. If the system is fluid-filled, however, the potential exists for severe disruption caused by the hydrodynamic forces arising from temporary cavitation that Woodruff described. Severe damage can also result from the explosive expansion of a gas pocket during the negative-pressure phase of cavitation, a mechanism that Harvey described. Figure 4-43 shows a small bowel shredded by an M43 ball fired by an AK47. The gut probably was filled with succus entericus or gas at the moment of wounding, and was ruptured in several places by temporary cavitation.

The abdomen is one body region in which damage from indirect ballistic effects may be common. The injury shown in Figure 4-42 and possibly the injury shown in Figure 4-43 are examples of indirect effects. The damage shown in these examples extends far beyond the tissue that is likely to have come into direct contact with the projectile. (Implicit in this interpretation is the concept that the temporary cavity developed within the target organ after the projectile penetrated it.)

Rigorous proof of this contention requires that there be no possibility that the projectile could have come into contact with the injured organ. If the damage was caused by an indirect effect, it cannot have been caused by the projectile's cutting. A gunshot wound of the extraperitoneal abdominal wall that caused a perforation of the underlying small bowel might be an example. There seems to be little doubt that such indirect injuries do occur,[45] but their frequency is probably quite small. The WDMET database contains only five documented examples of such rigorously defined indirect injuries out of 299 surviving casualties with intraabdominal trauma:

- A bullet passed across the first casualty's anterior abdominal wall, lacerating an inferior epigastric artery; although the

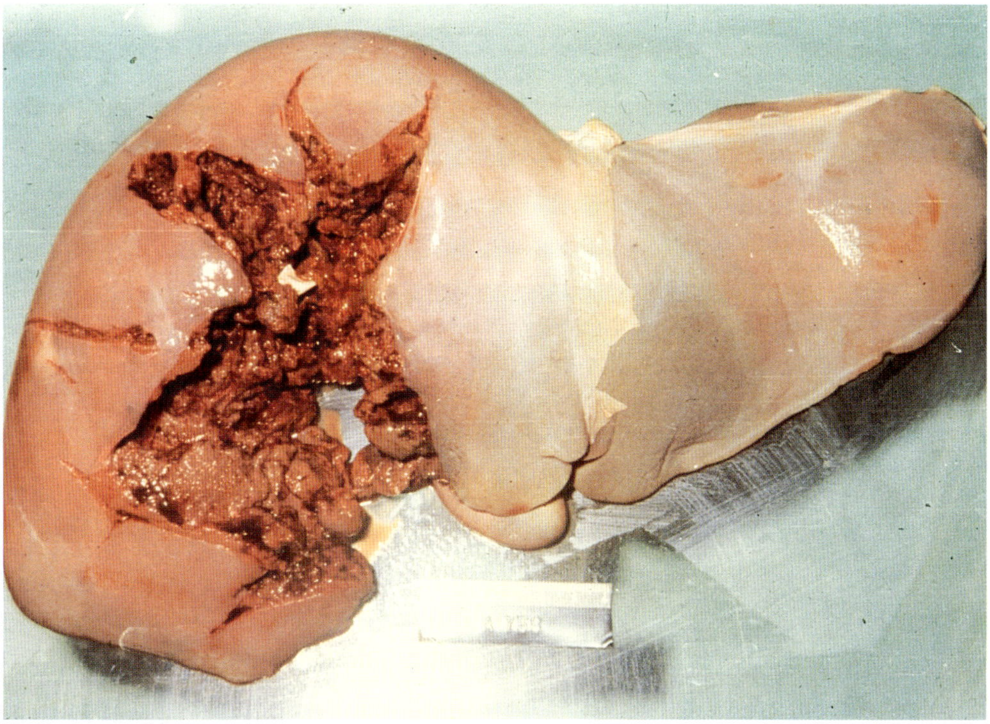

Fig. 4-42. An M43 ball fired by an AK47 caused this liver injury. The permanent cavity is probably the same size as the temporary cavity that made it.
Source: Wound Data and Munitions Effectiveness Team

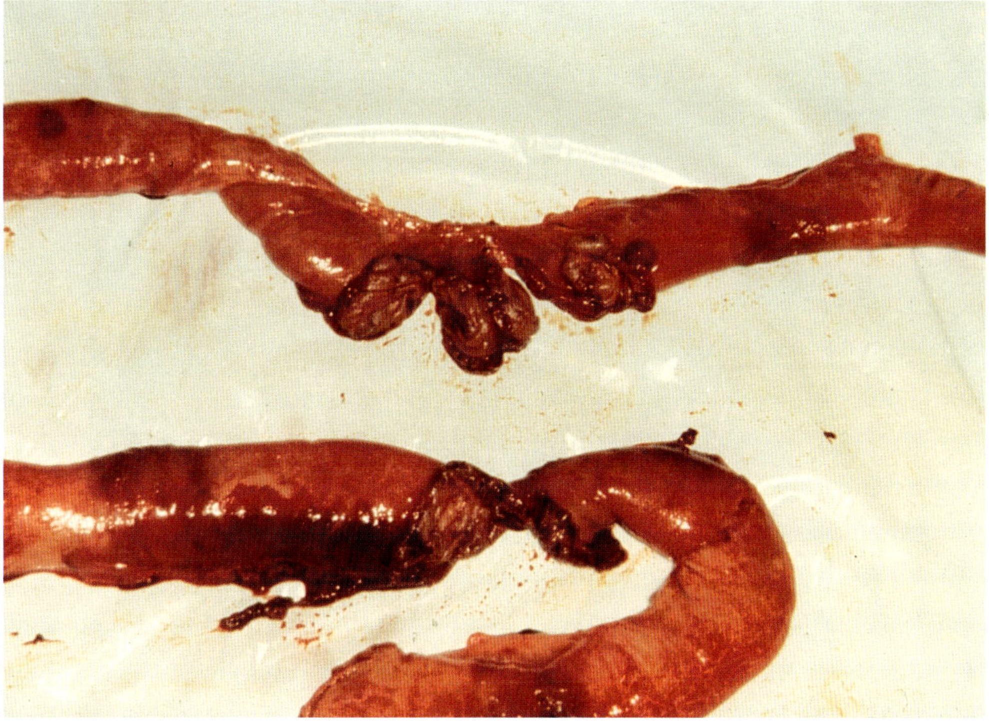

Fig. 4-43. The casualty whose injured small intestine is pictured sustained a perforating wound of the abdomen made by an AK47. The bowel looks as if it had been shredded. Although absolute proof is lacking, it is likely that at least some of this massive injury was due to cavitation in a fluid-filled bowel, rather than to direct cutting by the bullet.
Source: Wound Data and Munitions Effectiveness Team

peritoneum was intact, the cecum contained a 2-mm hole.

- A bullet entered the second casualty's right lower chest wall and exited from the right lower quadrant. The peritoneum was said to be intact (although there was an extra-peritoneal laceration of the dome of the right lobe of the liver). The small-bowel mesentery contained an extensive hematoma, and the proximal jejunum had a contusion.
- The third casualty had a gunshot wound of the buttock that fractured his sacrum. He also had a hole from "blast" in his jejunum.
- The fourth casualty had a gunshot wound in his left flank. The peritoneum was said to be intact, but the sigmoid and the descending sections of colon were "ruptured."
- The fifth casualty also had a gunshot wound in his left flank with the peritoneum intact. At laparotomy, his spleen was found to be lacerated.

A very strict definition of an indirect injury was applied to these five abdominal wounds: The projectile cannot have entered the abdominal cavity. Many more casualties probably sustain indirect intraabdominal injuries similar to the ones shown in Figures 4-42 and 4-43 (that is, the injuries occur at sites remote from the projectiles' intraabdominal trajectories).

The Extremities

After soft tissue, bone is the most frequently injured tissue of the extremities. Wounds of the neurovascular structures of the extremities are of lesser numerical (but not clinical) importance.

Bone. The spectrum of ballistic bone injury extends from tiny cortical fractures, through drillholelike perforations, through simple fractures, to grossly comminuted fractures. Tiny cortical fractures are made by slow-moving projectiles; projectiles must travel at velocities greater than 200 fps to penetrate bone. This observation, along with the facts that *(a)* penetration of skin dissipates another 150 fps, and *(b)* most wounds are inflicted at other than point-blank range, led Callender and French to criticize heavy, slow bullets:

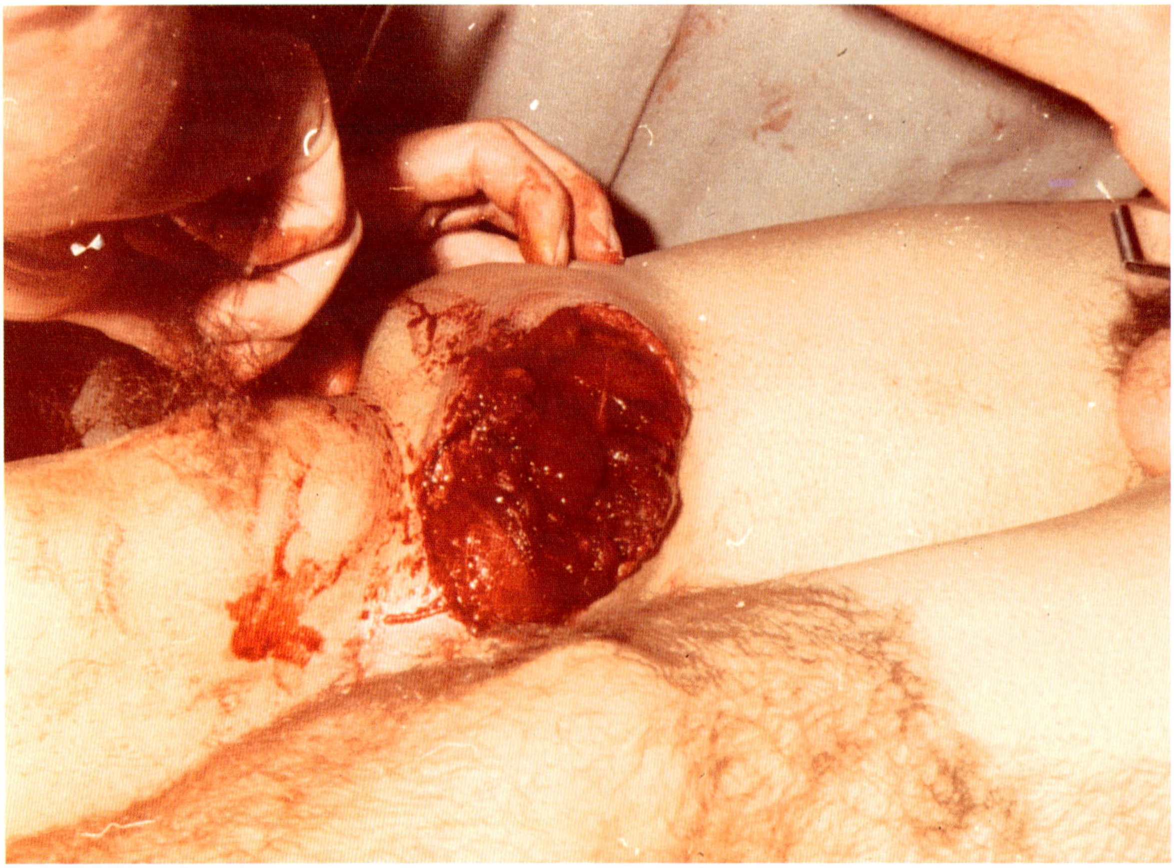

Fig. 4-44. The wound of exit in a casualty's distal thigh, made by an M193 ball fired by an M16 at close range
Source: Wound Data and Munitions Effectiveness Team

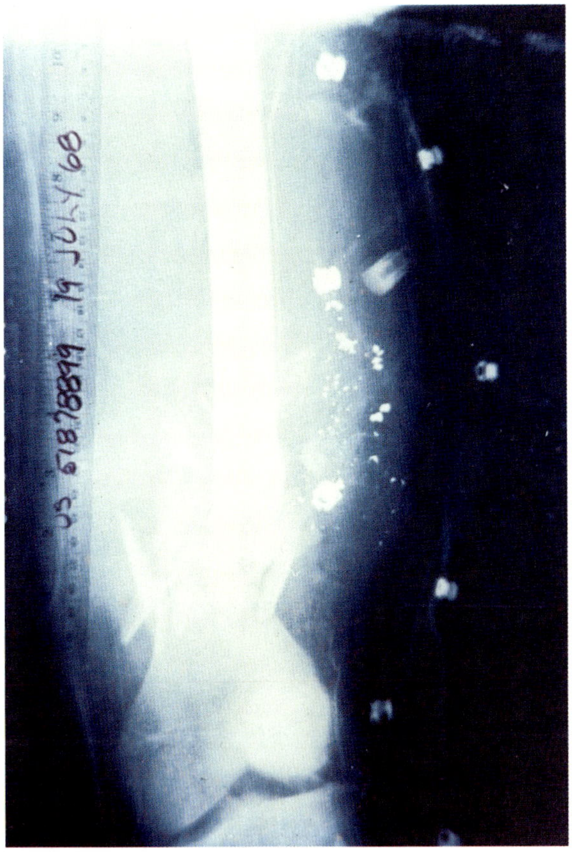

Fig. 4-45. The roentgenogram of the injury shown in Figure 4-44. Secondary missiles of bone and lead in conjunction with temporary cavitation caused the huge wound of exit. This injury is an example of an "explosive wound" such as those first described in the nineteenth century when conoidal bullets were introduced.
Source: Wound Data and Munitions Effectiveness Team

> [I]t can be readily appreciated that the .45 caliber bullet is of little value as a wound-producing agent except in the softer tissue and at near range. The bullet often fails either to penetrate or to fracture bone and practically never shatters bone in the manner common to the rifle bullet or fragment.[7]

The more serious fractures that Callender and French refer to are usually characterized by extensive soft-tissue damage that arises from secondary missiles of shattered bone. These injuries' gaping wounds of exit frequently seem to have exploded (Figures 4-44 and 4-45). A projectile that strikes bone will experience maximum drag (that is, the projectile is stopped and frequently is also deformed or broken up); thus the potential for massive energy-transfer exists. A projectile-target interaction visualized by high-speed cinematography demonstrated that the temporary cavitation may, by itself, contribute to the medical treatment problem by causing osseous sequestrations. In experiments with bones embedded in gelatin, researchers found that the tissue simulant was stripped from the embedded bone in a process that, if it were to occur in living tissue, might be expected to disrupt periosteal blood vessels.[46]

Indirect fractures (that is, those that occur in penetrating wounds in which the projectile appears not to have had physical contact with the bone) are possible in extremity wounds. These fractures, which are caused when bone is displaced by the expanding temporary cavity, have been demonstrated in laboratory experiments since Harvey's pioneering work in the 1940s.[28]

Chinese investigators have provided important data that illuminates the indirect-fracture mechanism.[47] The researchers shot the muscular portion of canine thighs with 440-mg triangular fragments at impact velocities of 460–1,500 m/s. Indirect fractures first occurred when the velocity reached 1,250 m/s (that is, impact–kinetic energy of about 340 J). When impact velocities reached 1,250–1,450 m/s,

> thigh bones 5 to 10 mm from the wound channel may suffer from indirect fracture with an occurrence rate of about 15%. When impact velocity reaches 1,450 m/s (about 460 J), the thigh bone 15 to 20 mm from the wound channel may have an indirect fracture incidence of about 29%.[47]

In a companion study, Chinese investigators measured the pressures at various distances from steel spheres as they passed through soap blocks and swine torso.[48] The pressure transients they found were similar in shape to those shown in Figure 4-36. Peak overpressures of 3,000–4,000 psi were found within 5 cm of the trajectory. The formula

$$P = k\, d^{-3.8}$$

approximates the decrement in pressure P with distance d.

They found that pressure falls very rapidly. The quasi-static overpressure was tenfold less than the peak pressure, but, within a few centimeters of the trajectory, it probably exceeded the 155 kg/cm^2 (2,200 psi) that the investigators estimated was sufficient to fracture a bone.[48]

Bearing in mind differences in bone strength and size between humans and experimental animals, these data suggest that an assault-rifle round passing within a centimeter of a long bone might very well be capable of causing an indirect fracture. Indirect fractures, in

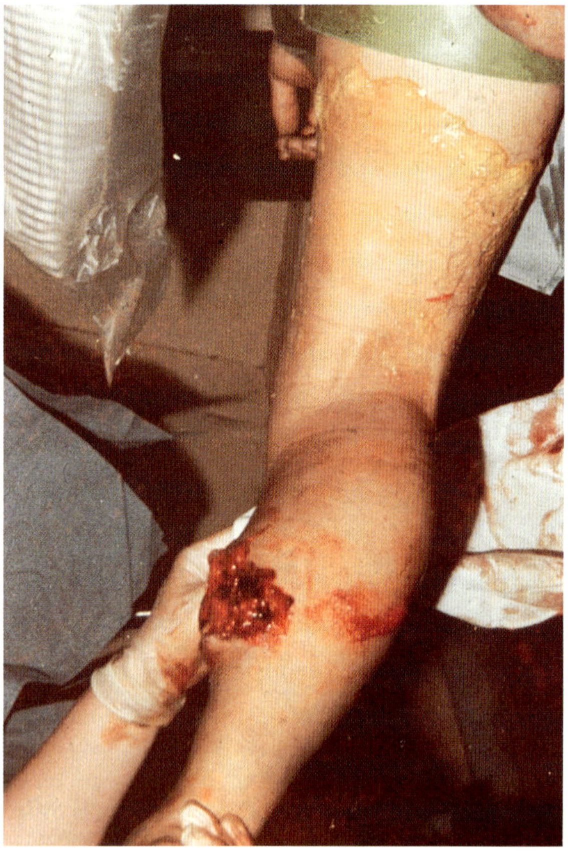

Fig. 4-46. This casualty, who was shot through his calf with an M193 ball fired by an M16, has a large wound of exit. The wound of entrance is barely visible at the medial edge of the calf.
Source: Wound Data and Munitions Effectiveness Team

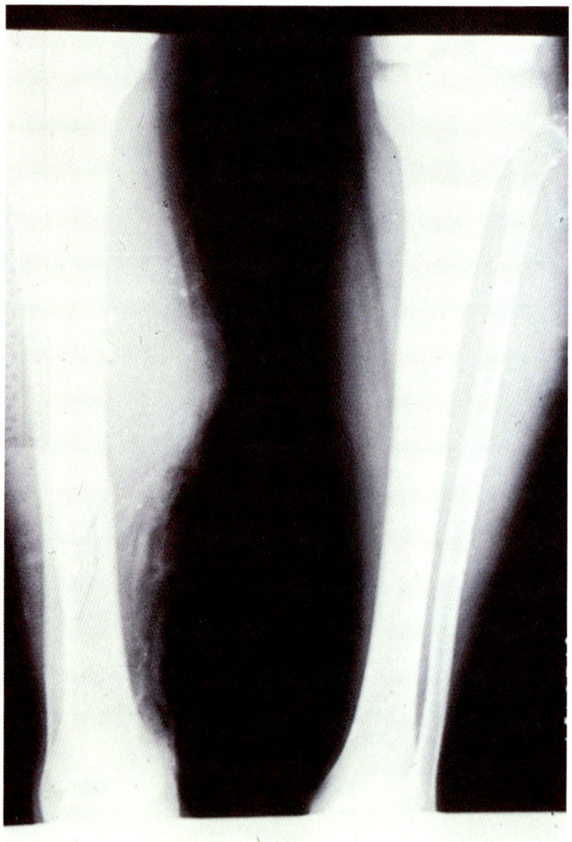

Fig. 4-47. This roentgenogram of the wound shown in Figure 4-46 shows a hairline linear fracture in the tibia about 2 inches proximal to the ankle. Pieces of lead are visible near the wound of exit. It is likely that *(a)* the bullet fragmented as it exited the calf and *(b)* the associated temporary cavitation caused an indirect fracture.
Source: Wound Data and Munitions Effectiveness Team

contrast to fractures caused by direct contact with the projectile, might be simple linear fractures. About 10% of the fractures in the WDMET database are listed as "transverse (no displacement)" and "linear".[49] These may be indirect fractures (Figures 4-46 and 4-47).

Blood Vessels. Compared to bones, large arteries and veins are much more flexible and thus better able to tolerate the stretch and shear caused by nearby cavitation. Figure 4-48 reproduces Harvey's famous roentgenogram showing the impressive distortion of a cat femoral artery caused by temporary cavitation and occurring over a few milliseconds.[28] Stretch and shear to this extent cause microscopic loss of endothelial cells, rupture of the internal elastic membrane, and focal bleeding as far as 6 cm away from the permanent cavity in experimental wounds.[50] Chinese researchers fired M193 bullets into swine thighs and found thrombi attached to the injured endothelium in about one-half of the animals 72 hours after wounding. However, the current opinion is that the only significant wounding mechanism is the cutting and crushing of direct projectile contact and "there is no evidence that resection of normal-appearing artery on either side of an injured segment is necessary."[16]

Ballisticians have speculated for years that pressure transients arising from the stress wave or from temporary cavitation (that is, the hydrodynamic effects) might propagate along major vessels and cause distant indirect injuries.[4] For example, pressure transients arising from an abdominal gunshot wound might propagate through the vena cavae and jugular venous system into the cranial cavity and cause a precipitous rise in intracranial pressure there, with attendant transient neurological dysfunction. Clinical and experimental data need to be gathered before such indirect injuries can be confirmed.

Nerves. From the standpoint of preserving their anatomical integrity, nerves resist the stretch and shear

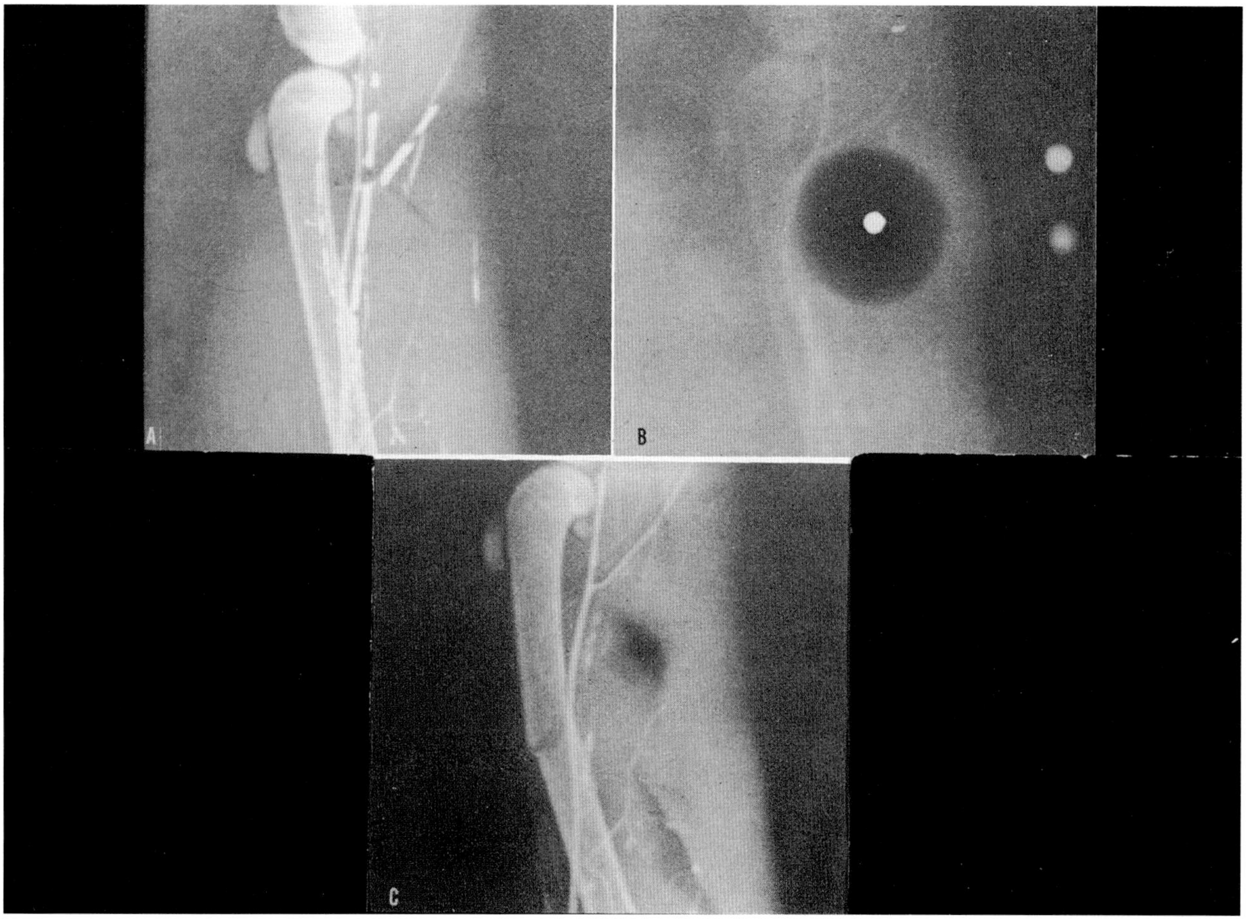

Fig. 4-48. Harvey's roentgenogram used a spark X ray to show the distortion of a feline femoral artery (containing radiopaque dye) caused by an expanding temporary cavity. The animal's thigh was shot with a 6-mm sphere fired at 980 m/s. Frame A shows the cat's thigh before it was wounded (the sciatic nerve was impregnated with barium sulfate to show its location). Frame B shows the projectile's passage and the early cavitation. Frame C was taken after cavitation had occurred, and shows an indirect fracture of the cat's femur.
Source: Reproduced from Figure 27 in reference 28

of temporary cavitation rather well. However, studies dating back to Harvey demonstrate histological abnormalities in peripheral nerves that have been subjected to stretch by a nearby temporary cavity.[28]

Experimental data, also dating back to Harvey, suggest that electromechanical effects—perhaps produced when nerves are deformed by nearby cavitation—may cause depolarization and consequent neurodysfunction.[51] The WDMET database contains at least one possible example of this phenomenon. A soldier sustained a perforating gunshot wound of the trapezius muscle in his neck. He stated that for 5 minutes after he was wounded, his body felt numb and he was unable to move any of his extremities. The subsequent physical examination revealed only soft-tissue damage to the muscle. Despite its anecdotal nature and the possibility that this was actually a combat-stress reaction, one is tempted to believe that the stress wave passing through the soft tissue of the soldier's neck indirectly caused a transient cervical-cord dysfunction.

The frequency of peripheral nerve defects caused by the stretch of a temporary cavity is unknown. However, many experienced military surgeons can recall casualties who had neurological defects in the distribution of nerves that were found to be grossly intact during surgical exploration. In fact, a training movie made during the Vietnam War shows just such an occurrence: a soldier who was wounded in the thigh by multiple grenade fragments and had a neurological defect in the distribution of the sciatic nerve. Surgeons found no gross nerve injury at surgical exploration, but the casualty's sciatic nerve lay next to a large permanent cavity.[52]

SUMMARY

The complexities of wound ballistics include not only the physical characteristics of the wounding projectile but also the biophysical characteristics of the target tissue. No single property of a projectile can explain all aspects of a wound. In the past, projectile velocity was considered to be the major determinant of a wound. Later ballisticians emphasized kinetic energy. Contemporary researchers view kinetic-energy transfer as the most important determinant of the nature of a wound. There is some truth in this contention, but even a theory of kinetic-energy transfer suffers from several limitations:

- All of the energy transferred by the projectile does not necessarily damage tissue. Projectile deformation or fragmentation requires energy, and a small portion of the energy appears as heat. The magnitude of the errors that arise from these energy-transfer mechanisms needs to be studied.
- The division of transferred energy into cutting and stretch is distinctly unequal. If Harvey's estimate is correct, one can show that very little of the energy transferred in the formation of a typical soft-tissue wound actually causes tissue damage. Even if Harvey's data substantially overestimate the amount of kinetic energy spent on temporary cavitation compared with the permanent cavity, it is apparent that total energy transfer will apparently predict tissue damage poorly.
- There may be little relationship between energy transfer, muscle damage, and the resulting medical problem. In the rather benign wounds of entrance and exit caused by an M43 ball (Figures 4-49 and 4-50), tissue damage (as quantitated by the amount of muscle in the zones of extravasation and concussion requiring debridement) was small. Yet treating this wound required substantial effort—the permanent cavity included the femoral artery (Figure 4-51).

Any meaningful theory of wound ballistics must recognize that the interaction of multiple factors determines the nature of a wound. Although a projectile's wounding potential is determined by its mass and velocity, factors such as construction, stability, and the body part that is hit determine the extent to which that potential is realized.[53]

Two combat casualties from the Vietnam War (Figures 4-52 through 4-55) may illustrate this fundamental insight. Both soldiers were struck in the forearm by bullets fired from AK47 assault rifles at ranges of about 20 m. The soldier shown in Figure 4-52 sustained a minor soft-tissue injury, while the soldier

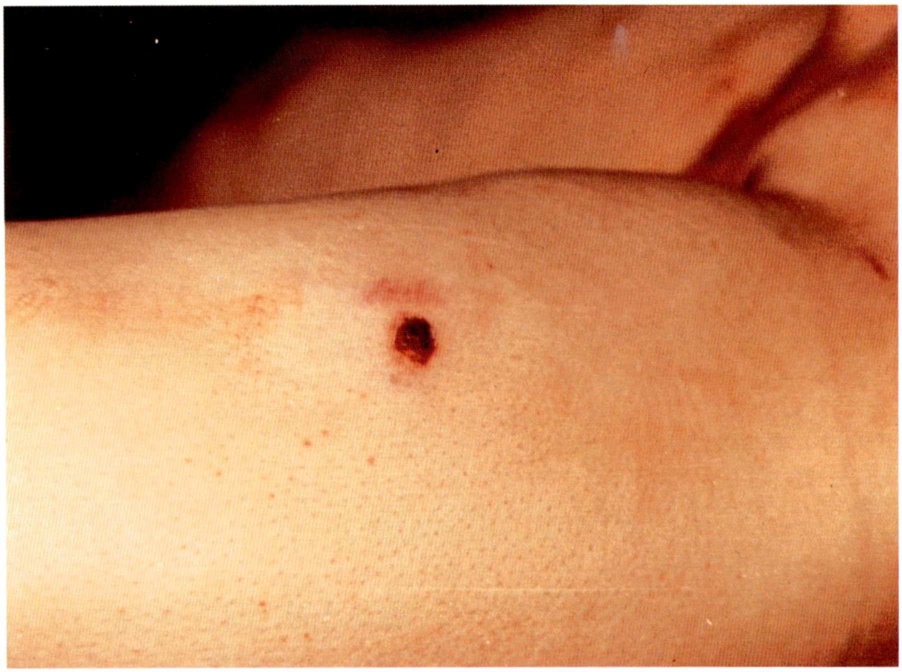

Fig. 4-49. This photograph, together with Figures 4-50 and 4-51, shows a casualty who sustained a perforating wound of the left thigh made by an M43 ball. This is the wound of entrance.
Source: Wound Data and Munitions Effectiveness Team

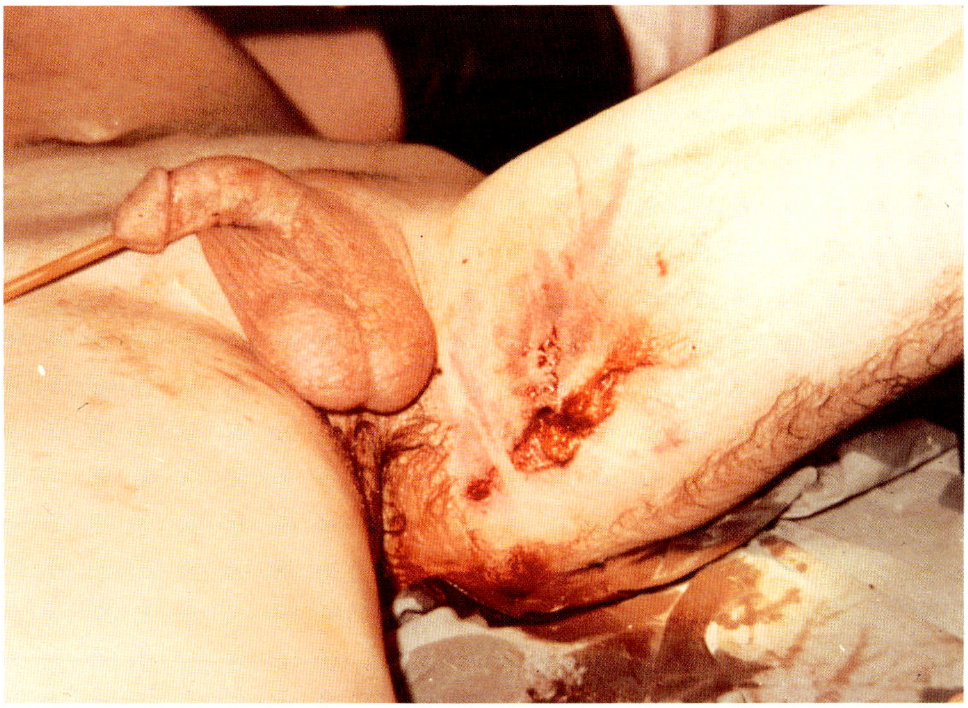

Fig. 4-50. The casualty's wound of exit. Neither this wound nor the wound of entrance shown in Figure 4-49 appears to be especially severe.
Source: Wound Data and Munitions Effectiveness Team

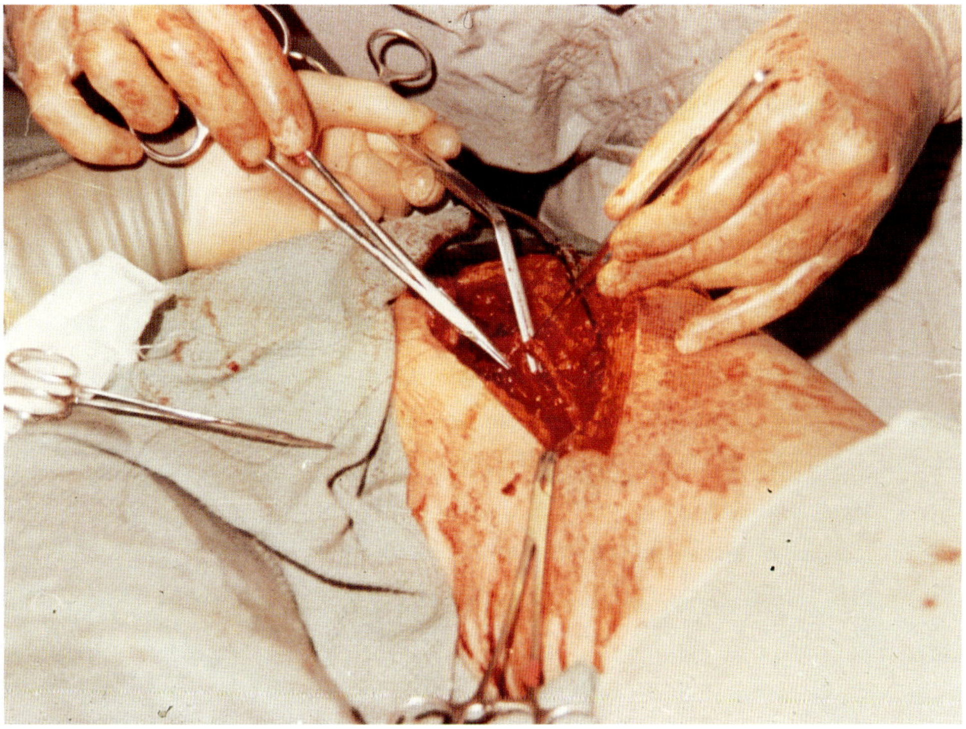

Fig. 4-51. Nevertheless, the casualty shown in Figures 4-49 and 4-50 had sustained a potentially fatal injury: The permanent cavity included the superficial femoral artery. There is little evidence of soft-tissue damage. In this case, as in many casualties, the apparent soft-tissue damage (and by implication, the energy transfer) did not correlate with the actual magnitude of the medical treatment problem.
Source: Wound Data and Munitions Effectiveness Team

shown in Figures 4-53 through 4-55 almost sustained a traumatic amputation of his arm. The bullets probably were of identical design and construction and had the same striking velocity and kinetic energy. In this instance, projectile velocity and kinetic energy clearly are not directly related to the magnitude of the wound. A meaningful theory of wound ballistics must explain such vast differences in tissue damage.

These two injuries are so different because, although the potentials for damage were identical, the full potential was realized only when the bullet hit bone. The gaping wound of exit testifies to the destruction wrought by multiple secondary projectiles arising from bone and bullet, together with "explosive" temporary cavitation. The bullet that caused the injury in Figure 4-52 transferred a tiny fraction of its kinetic energy (perhaps less than 5%, or about 50 J), and all of that went into cutting a permanent cavity similar in size to the bullet itself. In contrast, the bullet that caused the wound shown in Figures 4-53 through 4-55 transferred most if not all of its kinetic energy (about 1,600 J) and made a truly explosive wound.

The key question that medical officers attempting to understand wound-ballistics theory must ask is not: *How much* kinetic energy was transferred? but rather: *What caused* the energy-transfer to occur?

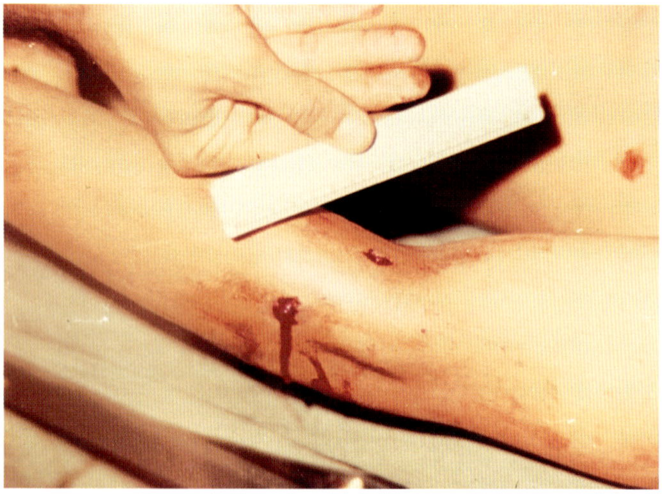

Fig. 4-52. This casualty sustained a perforating gunshot wound of the soft tissues of the forearm made by a bullet fired by an AK47 from a distance of about 20 m. The wounds of entrance and exit are small and approximately the diameter of the bullet. There is no evidence of bleeding and no ecchymosis or swelling. A similar wound could have been made by simply boring a hole through the tissue with a drill or trocar. This is an example of an en seton wound.
Source: Wound Data and Munitions Effectiveness Team

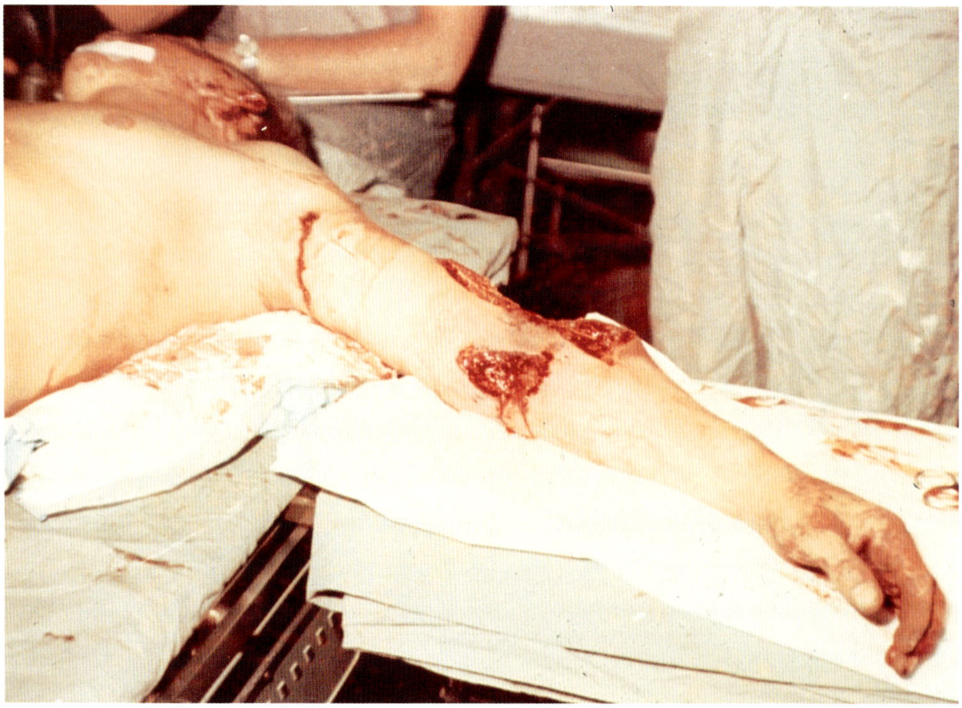

Fig. 4-53. This photograph, together with Figures 4-54 and 4-55, shows another casualty who sustained a perforating gunshot wound of the forearm made by a bullet fired by an AK47 from a distance of about 20 m. This is the wound of entrance.
Source: Wound Data and Munitions Effectiveness Team

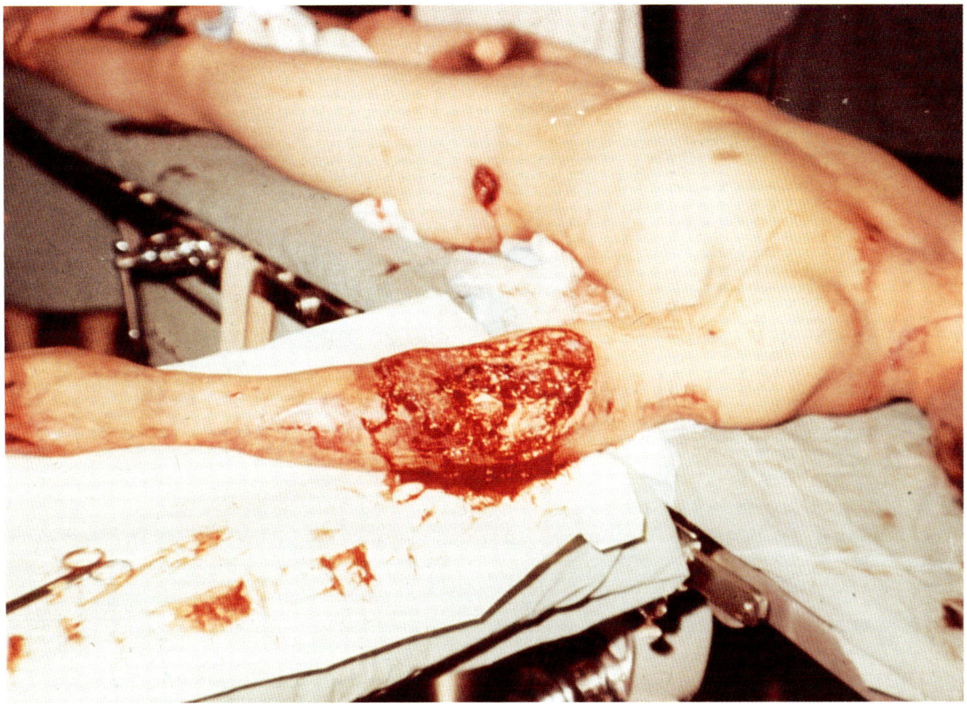

Fig. 4-54. This is the wound of exit sustained by the casualty whose wound of entrance is shown in Figure 4-53.
Source: Wound Data and Munitions Effectiveness Team

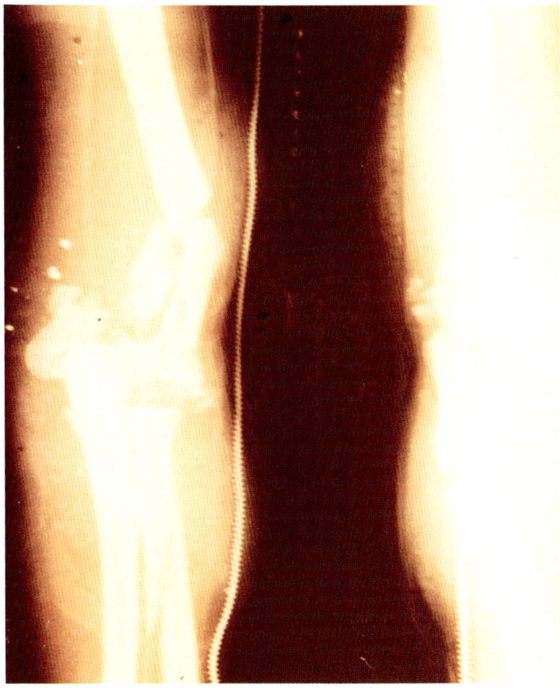

Fig. 4-55. The shattered elbow shown in this roentgenogram nearly caused a traumatic amputation of the casualty's arm, in contrast to the benign nature of the wound shown in Figure 4-52. Since the circumstances of wounding were nearly identical in the two casualties, the difference in outcome cannot be explained by theories of striking velocity and energy. In the second casualty, the bullet hit and shattered the bones of the elbow as it passed through the arm. No drill or trocar could make a wound like this. The wound looks as if it had been caused by an explosion, and it is obvious that massive energy transfer must have occurred.
Source: Wound Data and Munitions Effectiveness Team

REFERENCES

1. Hatcher, J. S. 1966. *Hatcher's notebook.* Harrisburg: Stackpole Books.

2. Berlin, R. H.; Janzon, B.; Liden, E.; Nordstrom, G.; Schantz, B.; Seeman, T.; and Westling, F. 1988. Wound ballistics of Swedish 5.56-mm assault rifle AK5. *J. Trauma* 28(2) Suppl.:S76–S83.

3. Nennstiel, R. 1990. Once again—spheres in gelatin. *J. Trauma* (China) 6(2) Suppl.:119–123.

4. Sellier, K. 1979. Effectiveness of small calibre ammunition. *Acta Chir. Scand. Suppl.* 487:13–25.

5. Ramage, C. K., ed. 1989. *Lyman pistol and revolver handbook.* Middlefield, CT: Lyman Publications.

6. Hopkinson, D. A. W., and Marshall, T. K. 1967. Firearm injuries. *Br. J. Surg.* 54(5):344–353.

7. French, R. W., and Callender, G. R. 1962. Ballistic characteristics of wounding agents. Chapt. 2 of *Wound Ballistics,* edited by J. C. Beyer, 91–141. Washington, DC: Office of the Surgeon General, Department of the Army.

8. Yu-Yuan, M.; Tain-Shun, F.; Rong-Xiang, F.; and Ming, M. 1988. An analysis of the wounding factor of four different shapes of fragments. *J. Trauma* 28(1) Suppl.:S230–S235.

9. Tikka, S.; Cederberg, A.; Levanen, L.; Lotjonen, V.; and Rokkanen, P. 1982. Local effects of three standard assault rifle projectiles in living tissue. *Acta Chir. Scand. Suppl.* 508:61–77.

10. Liu, Y. Q.; Wu, B. J.; Xie, G. P.; Chen, Z. C.; Tang, C. G.; and Wang, Z. G. 1982. Wounding effects of two types of bullets in soft tissue of dogs. *Acta Chir. Scand. Suppl.* 508:211–221.

11. Liu, X.; Chen, X.; Chen, S. L. X.; Guo, R.; Wang, X.; Fu, S.; Jiang, S.; and Xu, G. 1988. Wounding effects of small fragments of different shapes at different velocities on soft tissue in dogs. *J. Trauma* 28(1) Suppl.:S95–S98.

12. Dziemian, A. J.; Mendelson, J. A.; and Lindsey, D. 1961. Comparision of the wounding characteristics of some commonly encountered bullets. *J. Trauma* 1:341–353.

13. Mendelson, J. A., and Glover, J. L. 1967. Sphere and shell fragment wounds of soft tissues: experimental study. *J. Trauma* 7:889–914.

14. Janzon, B. 1983. *High-energy missile trauma.* Göteborg, Sweden: University of Göteborg.

15. Fackler, M. L., and Malinowski, J. A. 1985. The wound profile: A visual method for quantifying gunshot wound components. *J. Trauma* 25:522–529.

16. Bowen, T. E., and Bellamy, R. F., eds. 1988. *Emergency war surgery.* 2d U.S. rev. ed. of *The emergency war surgery NATO handbook.* Washington, DC: United States Department of Defense.

17. Fackler, M. L.; Bellamy, R. F.; and Malinowski, J. A. 1988. A reconsideration of the wounding mechanism of very high velocity projectiles—Importance of projectile shape. *J. Trauma* 28(1) Suppl.:S63–S67.

18. Fackler, M. L.; Surinchak, J. S.; Malinowski, J. A.; and Bowen, R. E. 1984. Bullet fragmentation: A major cause of tissue disruption. *J. Trauma* 24:35–30.

19. Nordstrand, I.; Janzon, B.; and Rybeck, B. 1978. Break-up behavior of some small caliber projectiles when penetrating a dense medium. *Acta Chir. Scan. Suppl.* 489:81–90.

20. Fackler, M. L. 1989. Wounding patterns of military rifle bullets. *International Defense Review* 1:59–64. Geneva: Interavia S.A.

21. Berlin, R. H.; Janzon, B.; Liden, E.; Nordstrom, G.; Schantz, B.; Seeman, T.; and Westing, F. 1988. Terminal ballistics of deforming bullets. *J. Trauma* 28(1) Suppl.:S58–S62.

22. Berlin, R.; Gerlin, L.; Janzon, B.; Lewis, D. H.; Rybeck, B.; Sandergard, J.; and Seeman, T. 1976. Local effects of assault rifle bullets in live tissues. *Acta Chir. Scand. Suppl.* 459:5–84.

23. Fackler, M. L.; Surinchak, J. S.; Malinowski, J. A.; and Bowen, R. E. 1984. Wounding potential of the Russian AK-74 assault rifle. *J. Trauma* 24:263–266.

24. Charters, A. C. III, and Charters, A. C. 1976. Wounding mechanism of very high velocity projectiles. *J. Trauma* 16:464–470.

25. Fackler, M. L.; Bellamy, R. F.; and Malinowski, J. A. 1986. Wounding mechanism of projectiles striking at more than 1.5 km/sec. *J. Trauma* 26:250–254.

26. Tikka, S.; Cederberg, A., and Rokkanen, P. 1982. Remote effects of pressure waves in missile trauma. The intra-abdominal pressure changes in anesthetized pigs wounded in one thigh. *Acta Chir. Scand. Suppl.* 508:167–173.

27. Peters, C. E. 1990. A mathematical-physical model of wound ballistics. *J. Trauma* (China) 6(2) Suppl.:303–318.

28. Harvey, E. N.; McMillen, J. H.; Butler, E. G.; and Puckett, W. O. 1962. Mechanism of wounding. Chapt. 3 of reference 7, 143–236.

29. Dziemian, A. J., and Herget, C. M. 1950. Physical aspects of the primary contamination of bullet wounds. *Milit. Surg.* 106:294–299.

30. Scepanovic, D. 1979. Steel ball—Investigation of shooting at block of soap. *Acta Chir. Scand. Suppl.* 489:71–80.

31. Janzon, B.; Schantz, B.; and Seeman, T. 1988. Scale effects in ballistic wounding. *J. Trauma* 28(1) Suppl.:S29–S32.

32. Harvey, E. N.; Korr, I. M.; Oster, G.; and McMillen, J. H. 1947. Secondary damage in wounding due to pressure changes accompanying the passage of high velocity missiles. *Surgery* 18:218–239.

33. Suneson, A.; Hansson, H.-A.; and Seeman, T. 1987. Peripheral high-energy missile hits cause pressure changes and damage to the nervous system: Experimental studies on pigs. *J. Trauma* 27:782–789.

34. Krauss, M. 1957. Studies in wound ballistics: Temporary cavity effects in soft tissue. *Milit. Med.* 121:221–231.

35. Wang, Z.; Tang, C.; Chen, X.; and Shi, T. 1988. Early pathomorphologic characteristics of the wound tract caused by fragments. *J. Trauma* 28(1) Suppl.:S89–S94.

36. Wound Data and Munitions Effectiveness Team. 1970. *Evaluation of wound data and munitions effectiveness in Vietnam* [Final Report]. In Vol. 3, Tables D.11-5; D.11-9; and D.11-11. Alexandria, VA: Defense Documentation Center.

37. Cheng, X. M.; Liu, Y. Q.; Guo, R. F.; Lian, W. K.; and Wang, D. T. 1990. Analysis of wound ballistics in 2,414 cases of battle casualties. *J. Trauma* (China) 6(2) Suppl.:169–172.

38. Wang, Z. G.; Qian, C. W.; Zhan, D. C.; Shi, T. Z.; and Tang, C. G. 1982. Pathological changes of gunshot wounds at various intervals after wounding. *Acta Chir. Scand. Suppl.* 508:197–210.

39. Hopkinson, D. A. W., and Watts, J. C. 1963. Studies in experimental missile injuries of skeletal muscle. *Proc. R. Soc. Med.* 56:461.

40. Janzon, B., and Seeman, T. 1985. Muscle devitalization in high-energy missile wounds, and its dependence on energy transfer. *J. Trauma* 25:138–144.

41. Woodruff, C. E. 1898. The causes of the explosive effects of modern small-calibre bullets. *The New York Medical Journal* (April 30):593–601.

42. Watkins, F. P.; Pearce, B. P.; and Stainer, M. C. 1988. Physical effects of the penetration of head simulants by steel spheres. *J. Trauma* 28(1) Suppl.:S40–S54.

43. M. Carey. Personal communication, 1986.

44. Cooper, C. J., and Taylor, D. E. M. 1989. Biophysics of impact injury to chest and abdomen. *J. R. Army Med. Corps* 135:58–67.

45. Ben-Menachem, Y. 1979. Intra-abdominal injuries in nonpenetrating gunshot wounds of the abdominal wall: Two unusual cases. *J. Trauma* 19(3):207–211

46. Ragsdale, B. D., and Josselson, A. 1988. Experimental gunshot fractures. *J. Trauma* 28(1) Suppl.:S109–S115.

47. Ma, Y. 1988. An analysis of the wounding factors of four different shapes of fragments. *J. Trauma* 28(1) Suppl.:230–234.

48. Ming, L.; Ma, Y.; Rong-Xiang, F.; and Tian-Shun, F. 1988. The characteristics of the pressure waves generated in the soft tissue by impact and its contribution to indirect bone fractures. *J. Trauma* 28(1) Suppl.:104–109.

49. Wound Data and Munitions Effectiveness Team. 1970. Table D.11–10, in reference 36.

50. Chen, D.; Gu, R.; Li, J.; Wang, D.; Wu, G.; and Cheng, S. 1990. The effect of high velocity missiles on adjacent blood vessels. *J. Trauma* (China) 6(2) Suppl.:76–78.

51. Wehner, H. D., and Sellier, K. 1982. Compound action potentials in the peripheral nerve induced by shock-waves. *Acta Chir. Scand. Suppl.* 508:179–184.

52. Walter Reed Army Institute of Research. 1970. *Management of Combat Wounds, Debridement, and Delayed Primary Closure of Low-Velocity Missile Wounds.* Film number 5411.

53. Fackler, M. L. Personal communication, 1985.

RECOMMENDED READING

Janzon, Bo. 1983. *High energy missile trauma: A study of the mechanisms of wounding of muscle tissue.* Göteborg, Sweden: University of Göteborg. Doctoral dissertation. This academic thesis (108 pages) is a good introduction to the field of wound ballistics and the mechanisms of gunshot trauma. While it does contain extensive experimental data, it was written to be understood by people without advanced degrees in physics or mathematics. The book may be ordered from its author, Dr. Bo Janzon, Harbrovagen 34, S-147 51 Tümba, Sweden, or from the authors of this chapter.

Chapter 5

THE MANAGEMENT OF BALLISTIC WOUNDS OF SOFT TISSUE

RONALD F. BELLAMY, M.D., FACS* AND RUSS ZAJTCHUK, M.D., FACS**

*Colonel, United States Army; Acting Chief, Department of Surgery, Walter Reed Army Medical Center, Washington, D.C. 20307-5001
**Colonel, United States Army; Deputy Commander, Walter Reed Army Medical Center, Washington, D.C. 20307-5001

INTRODUCTION

Much of a combat surgeon's time is spent in managing wounds of the *soft tissues* (that is, skin, fat, and skeletal muscle). Penetrating wounds account for more than 90% of combat casualties. These wounds not only have a soft-tissue component, but in about 50% of them, the soft-tissue wound is the major treatment problem. Since soft-tissue wounds rarely constitute immediate life-threatening problems, however, medical officers are responsible for assuring that potentially fatal injuries to viscera deep to the soft tissue are recognized and receive appropriate priority for care. A surgeon's preoccupation with soft-tissue wound management may lead to inadequate care for more seriously wounded casualties. Certainly airway, breathing, and circulatory problems must be resolved before any thought is given to soft-tissue wounds.

Deciding whether a soft-tissue wound is associated with a more serious visceral injury is not always easy. Wounds of entrance can be misleading and give no indication of the projectile's trajectory through tissue (Figures 5-1, 5-2, and 5-3). Figure 5-1 shows a wound of entrance that was made by an M43 bullet in a casualty's proximal right lateral thigh. Physical examination of the abdomen suggested an intraabdominal injury, however, which was confirmed at laparotomy; surgeons resected the casualty's severely damaged small bowel (Figure 5-2). The roentgenogram (Figure 5-3) had failed to show the bullet's expected lodgment in the casualty's right hip. Having entered the right thigh, the bullet struck and fractured the right iliac crest, was deflected across the abdomen through the small bowel, then struck and fractured the left iliac crest, and finally was deflected into the casualty's left thigh, where it came to rest.

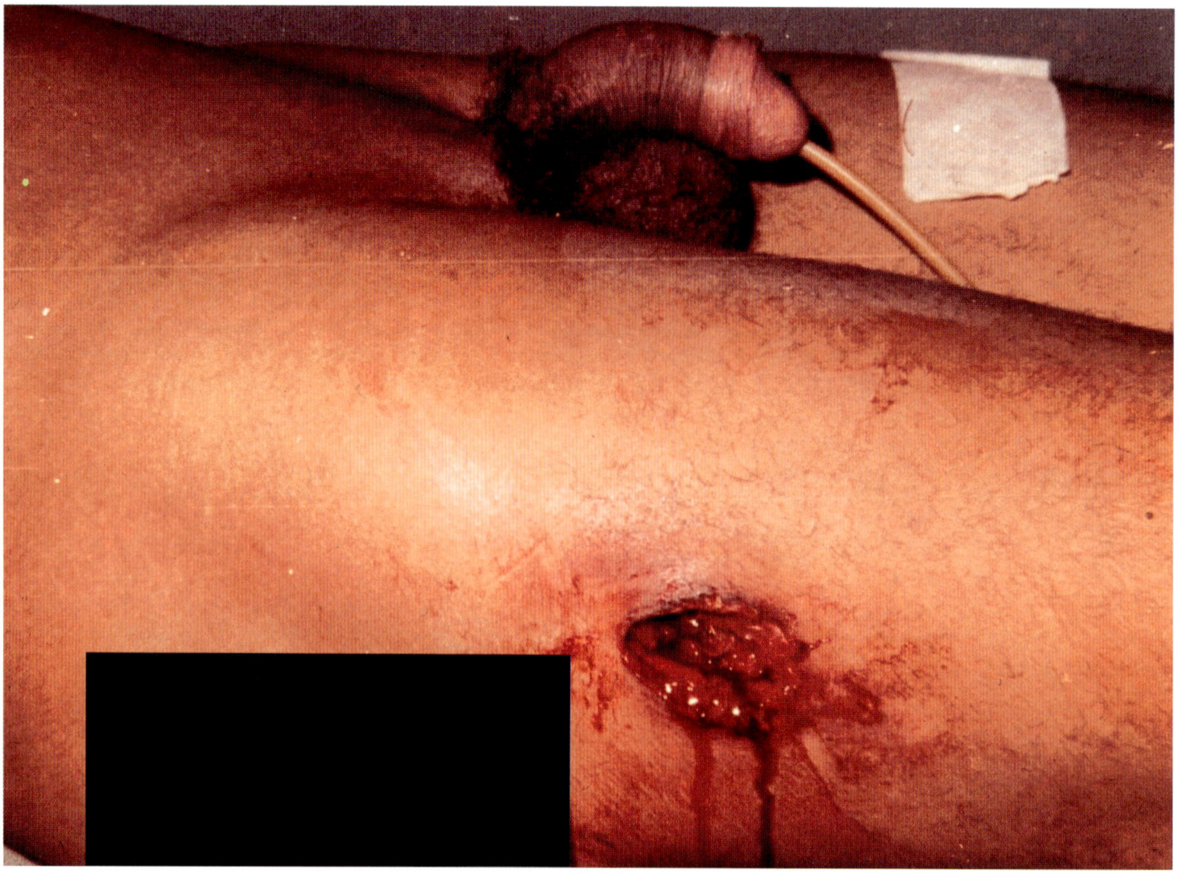

Fig. 5-1. The wound of entrance in this casualty's right hip was made by an M43 ball.
Source: Wound Data and Munitions Effectiveness Team

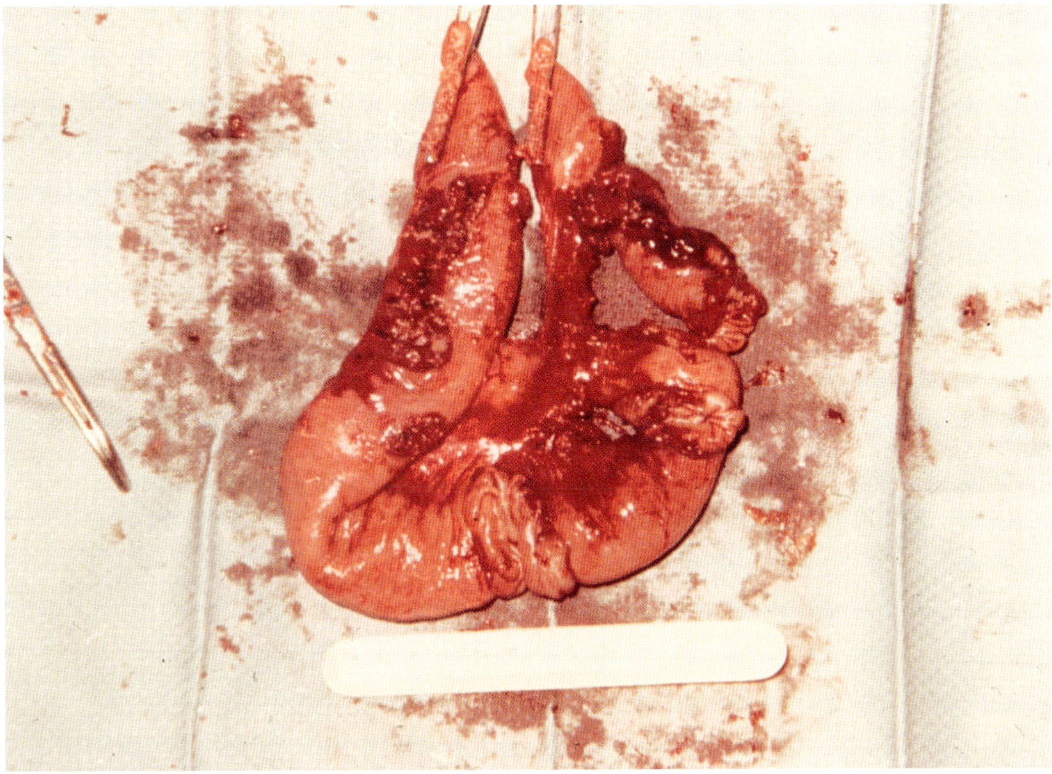

Fig. 5-2. The casualty's damaged small intestine was resected at laparotomy.
Source: Wound Data and Munitions Effectiveness Team

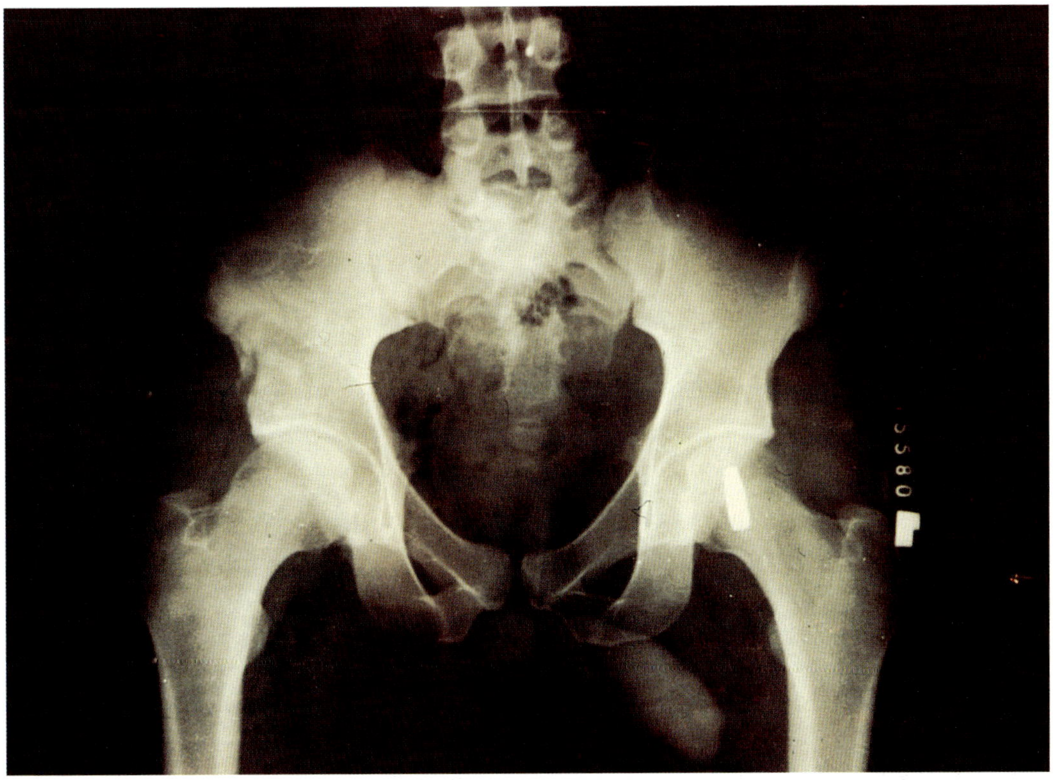

Fig. 5-3. The roentgenogram of the pelvis of the casualty shown in Figure 5-1 shows the bullet present in the soft tissue lateral to the *left* femoral head. Fractures of both iliac bones are apparent.
Source: Wound Data and Munitions Effectiveness Team

MILITARY SOFT-TISSUE WOUND CARE

The goals of soft-tissue wound care follow directly from the mission of the military medical services: to maintain the fighting power of the command. In many cases, medical officers can meet this goal by minimizing the noneffectiveness that a casualty's penetrating injuries have caused. As always in military medicine, the desired goal is achieved in the context of the greatest good for the greatest number. Infections and sepsis are the primary reasons that soft-tissue wounds fail to heal; they are also the primary reasons that a casualty with a soft-tissue wound continues to be noneffective. The military approach to managing soft-tissue wounds emphasizes simple, staged interventions that prevent infections most of the time and return most casualties to their units. Costly and time-consuming surgical interventions, even if they have perfect cosmetic and functional results, have no place during a major war.

The proper management of penetrating combat trauma, especially as applied to soft-tissue wounds, is a controversial and contentious subject. The invasiveness of military surgical management during recent wars (for example, extensive debridement) has been compared unfavorably to the the civilian approach.[1] Some have argued that traditional military management of penetrating trauma is unscientific and may even be dangerous, making the surgeon "a menace, doing more harm with his treatment than was done by the bullet."[2] Such criticisms usually focus upon the nature of the bullet, but there are other factors that need to be considered in understanding the nature of, and rationale for, the military approach to managing penetrating ballistic wounds.

Military and civilian management of penetrating soft-tissue trauma differ significantly in at least four ways:

- The potential for *tissue damage* differs because the weapons differ. High-velocity bullet wounds, and the potential for severe tissue damage, and multiple fragment wounds, which frequently coexist with blast effects, are much more frequent in the military.
- The potential for *wound contamination* differs since it depends upon the geographical site of wounding (for example, the heavily manured Flanders fields, the quite-clean South African veldt, the squalor at Stalingrad, or a downtown bank lobby). The casualty's physical condition (a cold, malnourished, exhausted combat soldier or a well-fed urban bank robber) at the time of wounding may also effect the likelihood of wound sepsis.
- The *timeliness of care* depends upon myriad tactical, logistic, administrative, and temporal (when mass casualties are involved) factors that severely constrain the capabilities of deployable medical facilities on a battlefield, but have less impact on a well-equipped urban hospital trauma center.
- Except in rare instances, military surgical management of soft-tissue wounds is staged. Not only are various stages of treatment carried out at different echelons of care, with wound debridement at the third echelon, and wound closure at the fourth, but different medical personnel treat the casualty at each stage.

In view of these distinctions, appropriate wound management for victims of penetrating trauma may be very different in military and civilian settings. For example, the wound management selected for an urban criminal who sustains a perforating soft-tissue wound of the thigh made by a 9-mm pistol bullet while he robs a bank, and who is transferred within 20 minutes to a trauma hospital capable of providing the full spectrum of needed care, may be very different from the appropriate wound management for a soldier who sustains a similar wound of the thigh while lying in a muddy field, and who stays in the muddy field for 12 hours before being evacuated to a hospital that is so busy that only 5 minutes can be allotted to caring for each casualty. Medical officers must understand that decisions regarding the optimum management of soft-tissue wounds sustained on the battlefield depend upon more than just the physical characteristics of the projectile or the biophysics of projectile-tissue interaction.

THE CONTAMINATED WOUND

The development of doctrine regarding the military surgeon's soft-tissue wound management (that is, staged intervention, debridement, delayed primary closure, and so forth) reflects the hard-won knowledge that battlefield wounds are probably *contaminated* (foreign material has been introduced into the wound), are likely to become *infected* (one or more pathogens has become established and is proliferating inside the wound), and that the major threat to the casualty's recovery is *sepsis* (pyogenic and other pathogens in the wound have invaded the surrounding tissues and are elaborating their toxic substances). The medical outcome of casualties with ballistic wounds depends upon the balance between the type and amount of bacteria that contaminate the wound, the casualty's ability to resist infection, and the extent to which that resistance has been impaired.

The Mechanics of Wound Contamination

Exactly how wounds in human casualties become contaminated can only be inferred from experimental models. Unsterile bullets and fragments are undoubtedly major sources of contamination. They contaminate the wound tract with bacteria and other foreign material that they bring in as they penetrate through the casualty's clothing and skin. The aspiration that can occur during temporary cavitation contributes less significantly to the total contamination of the wound, but has been the source of considerable speculation (Figure 5-4).

During the late 1940s, researchers at Edgewood Arsenal showed that *(a)* foreign material was aspirated into their gelatin targets during the process of temporary cavitation, and *(b)* this foreign material lined the radial fissures that extended from the permanent cavity in the gelatin. This demonstration has provided a physical model explaining the propensity of battlefield wounds to become infected.[3] Theoretically, surgically excising the lining of the permanent cavity could sterilize the wound.

But if this experimental model is valid for soft-tissue wounds, the biophysical responses of gelatin and skeletal muscle to temporary cavitation must be similar. One of these researchers' most impressive findings is foreign material 3–4 inches away from the gelatin's permanent cavity. If the equivalent depth of contamination occurs in skeletal muscle, truly radical excision would be required to decontaminate a skeletal-muscle wound.

Another researcher at the Armed Forces Institute of Pathology during the 1980s investigated the extent to which the depths of contamination around the permanent cavity in skeletal muscle are equivalent to the findings in gelatin. After attaching a packet containing a solution of fluorescein to each target at its aiming point, the researcher shot M193 balls fired by an M16A1 assault rifle into 20%-gelatin blocks and the buttocks of freshly sacrificed 80–100-kg swine from a distance of about 10 m. Then he opened each target's permanent cavity transversely and illuminated it with ultraviolet light. The morphologies of the fluorescein-contaminated permanent cavities are very different. In gelatin (Figure 5-5), numerous fluorescein-contaminated fissures, some as long as 10 cm, radiate from the permanent cavity, while the contaminating fluorescence in skeletal muscle (Figure 5-6) is not seen beyond 1 cm from the permanent cavity. Much of the partially detached muscle within the permanent cavity was contaminated, however. The therapeutic implications of this demonstration are *(a)* for all contamination to be removed, wound excision need not be carried deeper than 1 cm in muscle, but *(b)* all tissue within the permanent cavity should be removed.[4]

The Type and Magnitude of Bacterial Contamination

The relationship between bacterial counts and the likelihood of wound infection has been studied extensively in animal models. Researchers who injected *Staphylococcus aureus* or *Escherichia coli* into the subcutaneous tissue of guinea pigs failed to find clinically apparent infection when the inoculum contained fewer than 10^6 organisms, but found that infection was likely if the inoculum contained more than 10^7 bacteria.[5] Although this and similar studies conclude that clinically apparent infection will not develop unless the number of bacteria per unit volume of injured tissue exceeds a critical value, this seemingly clear-cut observation needs to be qualified. Certain organisms (such as group A beta-hemolytic streptococci) are especially virulent and can cause wound infection when present in much smaller numbers than 10^5 organisms per gram. Furthermore, criteria have not been established for typical battlefield contamination with obligate anaerobes and mixed aerobic-, anaerobic-, and polymicrobial bacterial contamination.

Experiments that correlate bacterial counts with the likelihood of infection suggest that it is the magnitude of bacterial contamination, not the elapsed time after wound contamination, that most importantly determines the likelihood of infection in an untreated wound. Thus, a wound that contains 10^5 aerobic organisms per gram of wounded tissue can be expected to heal without clinical infection, whether or not the wound is treated during or after an interval such as Paul L. Frederich's 6-hour golden period (which was discussed in Chapter Three). The host's normal resistance will eradicate the organisms. And conversely, this line of reasoning holds that a wound contaminated with 10^7 bacteria per gram of wounded tissue probably will become infected unless it is treated before the golden period has elapsed. The practical clinical problem is

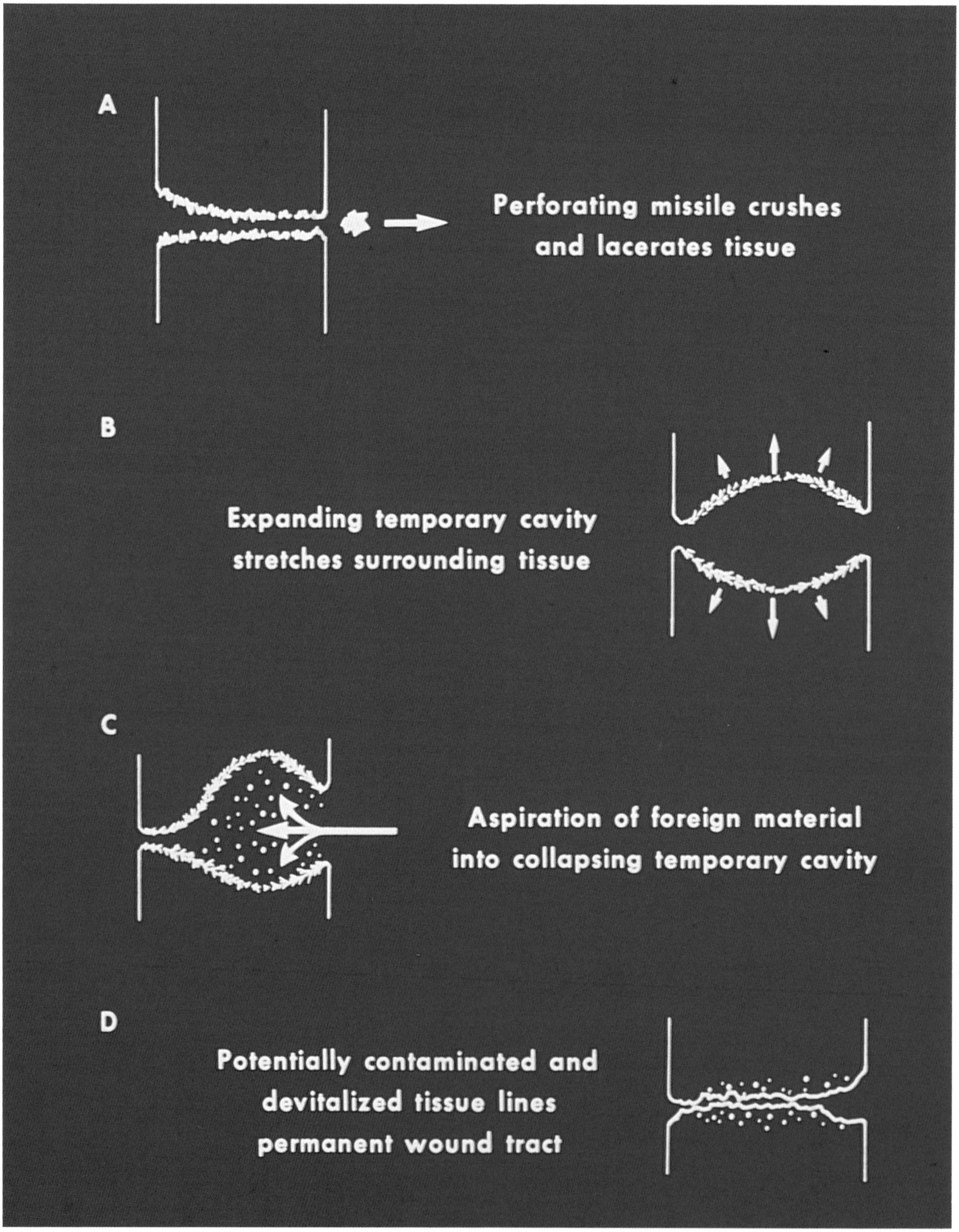

Fig. 5-4. The schematic diagram shows a mechanism by which temporary cavitation can contaminate a wound tract.

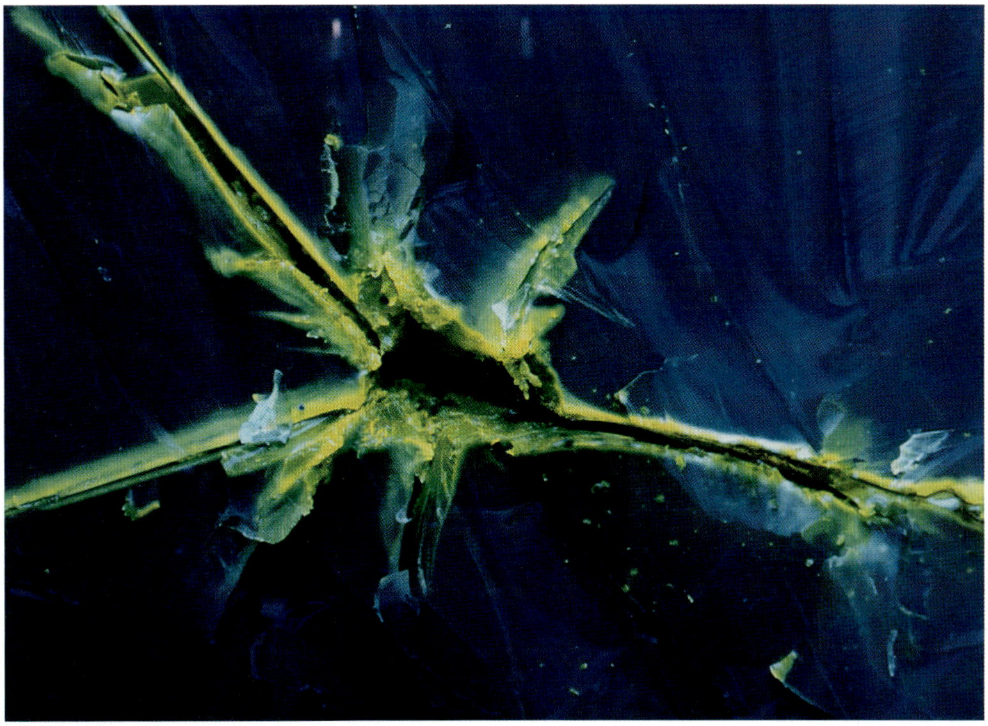

Fig. 5-5. An M193 ball has been fired through a packet of fluorescein dye into a gelatin block. The cracks in the gelatin made by temporary cavitation fluoresce, demonstrating the extent of "wound" contamination.

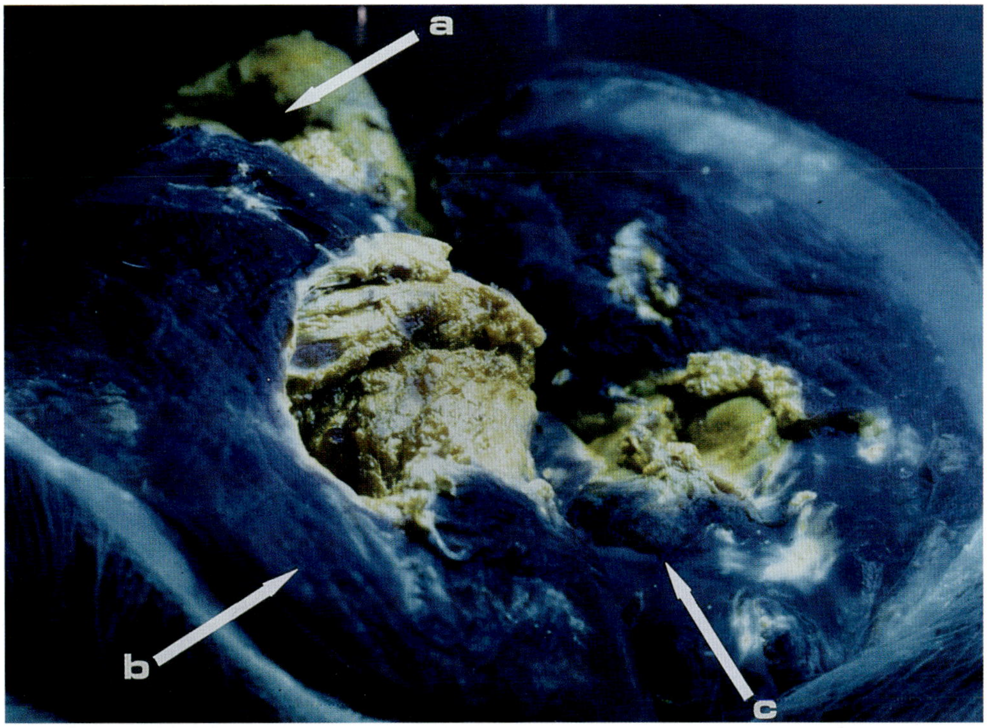

Fig. 5-6. An M193 ball has been fired through a packet of fluorescein dye into a swine's thigh. The thigh has been transected at right angles to the permanent cavity; *"a"* is a piece of detached muscle that was found in the permanent cavity; *"b"* and *"c"* are the uprange and downrange portions of the thigh. The tissue within and immediately adjacent to the permanent cavity shows intense fluorescence, but there is no evidence of the "contaminated" radial fissures that were found in gelatin.

that we have no way of knowing the actual duration of the golden period. In Frederich's experiments, it probably only indicated the time that was required for invasive sepsis to become apparent to him—the time after which local surgical measures to eliminate contamination would have had no effect on the infection's progression. The first goal of soft-tissue wound management is to reduce the bacterial count below the level that the casualty's resistance can normally eradicate.

The relationship between bacterial counts and infection in closed, contaminated wounds does not necessarily apply to either *(a)* open wounds or *(b)* contaminated wounds that are first left open and then are closed days later. Frederich knew that open wounds can resist invasive sepsis (that develops from simple bacterial contamination) better than closed wounds can.

Experimental data elegantly confirm this clinical observation: Open soft-tissue wounds that were contaminated with bacteria at the time of wounding can safely be closed after several days have elapsed (Figure 5-7).[6] In the same study, researchers found that wounds that had been left open and then were contaminated at the time of delayed closure were at greater risk of becoming septic than wounds that had been closed initially and then were contaminated several days later. The reason for this difference remains unclear, but the obvious message is to avoid fresh contamination of wounds at the time delayed primary closure is performed. Studies such as this provide experimental support for the policy of performing delayed primary closure of contaminated wounds after 4 days.

Much clinical evidence supports the importance of bacterial counts as a determinant of the time to close soft-tissue wounds. Late in World War I, some French surgeons adopted the practice of culturing bacteria from open ballistic wounds immediately after initial wound surgery. When the culture was inspected several days later, if fewer than five colonies of streptococci were present, the surgeons surgically closed the wound; otherwise, it was left open to close by secondary intent. Using this criterion, these surgeons obtained sepsis-free wound-healing in 90% of their cases, compared with 35% when they ignored the bacterial count.[7] More recently, surgeons demonstrated that only when the exudate from an open wound contained more than 10^6 organisms per milliliter was a clinically important infection likely.[8]

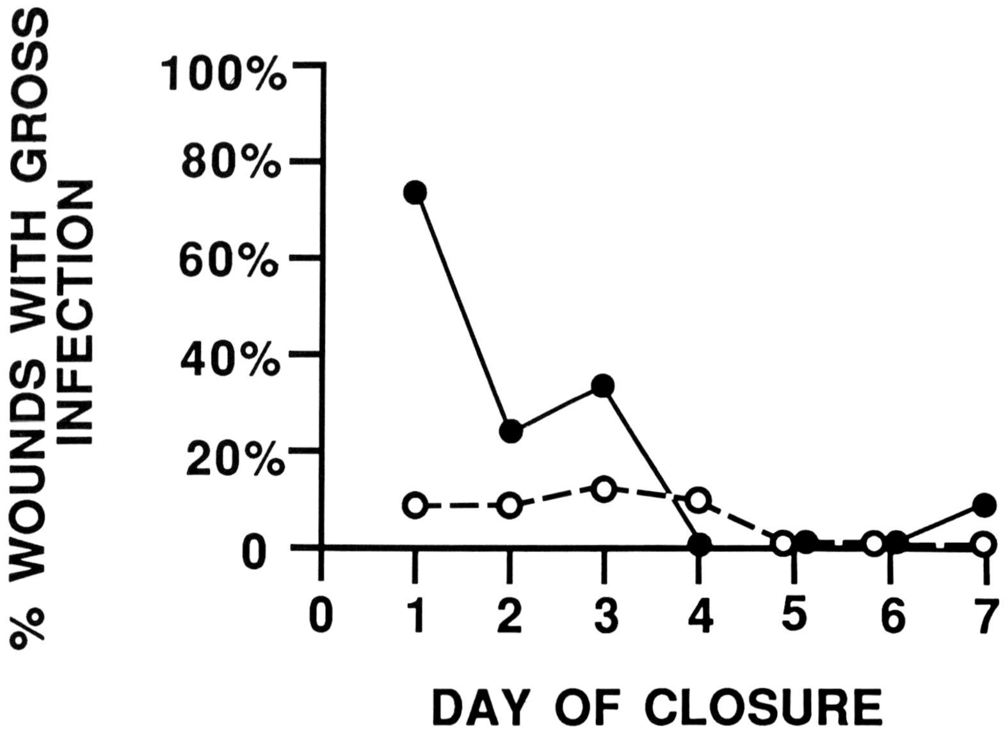

Fig. 5-7. The relationship between the time a wound was closed is plotted against the likelihood of sepsis-free healing. Wounds that were contaminated at the time of wounding (•); clean control wounds (o).
Source: Drawn from data contained in Table 1 in reference 6

FACTORS THAT CAN MODIFY A CASUALTY'S ABILITY TO RESIST INFECTION

Many factors can modify the likelihood that a soft-tissue wound will become infected. Because a penetrating wound ruptures the cutaneous barrier, conditions within the wound (that is, *local* factors), probably rival the magnitude of contamination as determinants of wound infection. The casualty's physical condition at the time of wounding (that is, *systemic* factors) have a more nebulous impact and tend to be less important, because most combat casualties, at least initially, are not compromised hosts. Some surgical techniques also introduce the possibility that a wound will become infected, and the natural process of necrosis produces an environment that favors infection.

The vast and complicated subjects of the inflammatory and specific immune responses, their dependence upon phagocytic cells, the complement system, circulating antibodies, and cellular immunity are not unique to military medicine, and therefore are best left for specialized texts such as Howard and Simmons's *Surgical Infectious Diseases*.[9]

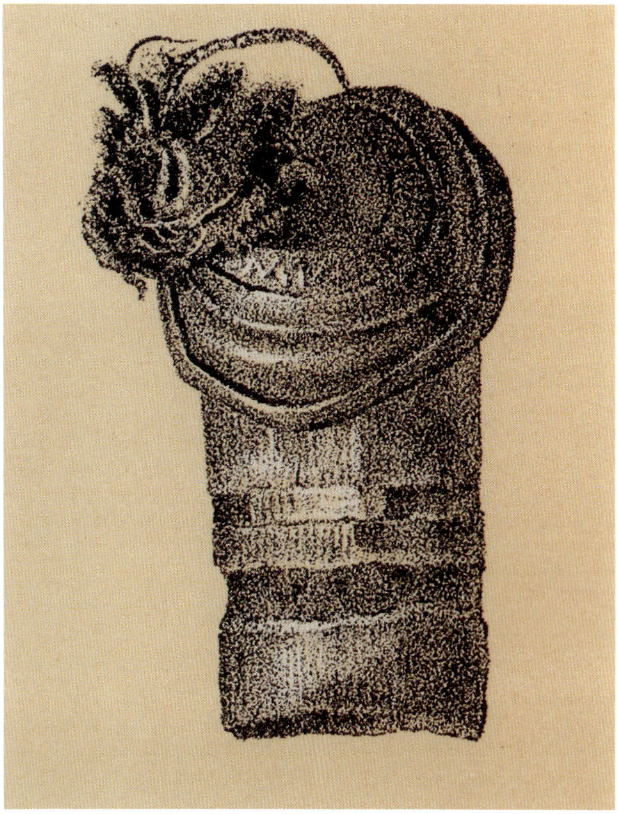

Fig. 5-8. As this bullet penetrated the body of a Civil War casualty, it carried with it a button and a piece of the soldier's uniform.
Source: Plate 39, number 4151, in reference 14

Factors Within the Wound Tract

Soil and Other Foreign Bodies. The permanent cavities of penetrating combat wounds can contain an incredible variety of foreign bodies. In addition to the obvious bullets or fragments, wounds can also contain bits of the casualty's clothing, vegetation, wood, and mud (Figure 5-8). Large objects—such as a tank tread or even parts of nearby casualties' bodies—can become imbedded in a wound.

Surgeons do not remove the penetrating projectile from the casualty's body during surgery in at least 50% of casualties. Bullets and other unsterile contaminants not only cause significant wound contamination, they also potentiate additional infection by preventing tissue-to-tissue apposition. Normal host defenses can eradicate bacteria clustered in the interspace between the foreign body and the surrounding tissue, but only with difficulty. Yet this mechanism may be a less important potentiator of infection than soil.

Although previously suspected to be implicated in reducing a host's resistance to infection, soil's role in causing infections was not shown until 1974.[10] In an experimental wound-infection model, skin on the backs of guinea pigs was incised and then contaminated with a known inoculum of *Staphylococcus aureus* and 5 mg of sterile soil, then closed and assessed for infection 4 days later. Researchers found that as few as 100 bacteria *per wound* could cause gross infection in the soil-contaminated animals. Eighty percent of the soil-contaminated animals developed infections, but none of the control animals (whose wounds were contaminated with bacteria but not with soil) did. The investigators found an active factor concentrated in the organic constituents of clay and the soils found in swamps, but which was absent in sand. They also showed that the soil-potentiating factor *(a)* interfered with normal leukocytic phagocytosis of bacteria, *(b)* impaired non-specific bactericidal activity in serum, and *(c)* possibly inactivated antibiotics.[11]

Soils differ in their ability to potentiate infection. A study performed during the Vietnam War supported this view. Researchers tested soils from ten different

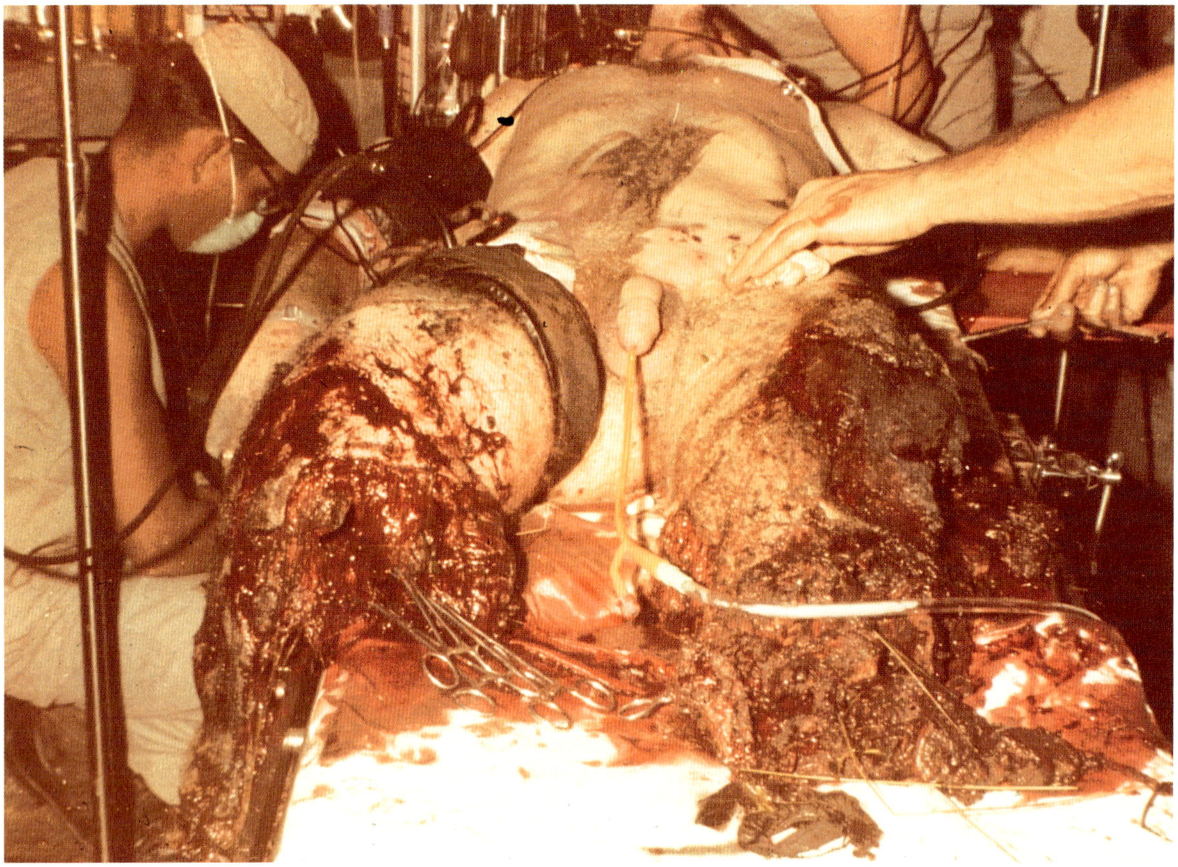

Fig. 5-9. Massive bilateral above-the-knee amputations. Note the straw and dirt that have contaminated the wounds.
Source: Wound Data and Munitions Effectiveness Team

areas of Vietnam for their ability to cause infection in an animal soft-tissue wound model. Of fifty-six animals whose wounds were contaminated with sandy soil, eighteen (32%) died of sepsis. Forty-three (90%) of forty-eight animals whose wounds were contaminated with mud or swamp soil died. Interestingly, similar bacterial flora were cultured from the wounds of both groups (for example, all samples contained pathogenic clostridia), suggesting that the size of the bacterial inoculum and the virulence of the bacteria were not the only infection-producing factors.[12] This study does not mention, but its results are consistent with, the existence of an active infection-potentiating factor in soil.

An infection-potentiating factor in some soil probably explains why battlefield wounds are so much more prone than civilian penetrating traumas are to sepsis. Soldiers wounded in the battlefields of World War I were particularly at risk:

> Many of the patients lie in trenches until the darkness of night allows of their removal: Their clothes are infiltrated with mud, while the same shell which has caused the wound often brings down the side of the trench and the injured limb may be covered with soil. Again the fragment of shell is commonly fouled with soil.[13]

A subsurface detonation of random-fragmentation shells and buried antipersonnel mines will probably massively contaminate wounds (Figure 5-9). But an improved-fragmentation munition detonating in air will cause much less wound contamination. The existence of an infection-potentiating factor in soil provides an additional rationale for surgeons to excise the tissue around a wound's permanent cavity.

The potential that civilian gunshot wounds will become contaminated has recently been emphasized.[15] Interestingly, however, the one experimental study that addressed the role of foreign bodies found that there was no apparent relationship between their presence and wound sepsis,[16] probably because the contaminating conditions are so different.

Hematomas and Extravasated Blood. Blood is an excellent substrate for bacterial growth. Expanding hematomas can impair the casualty's defenses against infection by causing extraluminal compression of blood vessels, and therefore causing tissue ischemia. Experimental animals with bacterial contaminations of their soft-tissue hematomas had a mortality rate of 75%; animals that had either a hematoma or bacterial contamination but not both had a mortality rate of 0%. Researchers do not yet understand why infections in hematomas and extravasated blood are so markedly deleterious.[17] One possibility is that oxygen-derived free radicals form. Given conditions that probably exist in damaged muscle, the reduction of molecular oxygen, which normally results in the formation of water, can potentially generate hydrogen peroxide (H_2O_2) and two species of extremely reactive free radicals: *(a)* the superoxide anion radical ($O_2^{-}\bullet$) and *(b)* the hydroxyl radical ($OH\bullet$), which is highly destructive of tissue and normally not present in the body. In the presence of ferrous iron, hydrogen peroxide and the superoxide anion radical can interact by means of the Haber-Weiss reaction to produce the hydroxyl radical:

$$O_2^{-}\bullet + H_2O_2 \xrightarrow{Fe^{++}} O_2 + OH\bullet + OH^{-}$$

The proteolysis of hemoglobin located outside blood vessels can liberate large amounts of ferrous iron. Thus, the Haber-Weiss reaction could potentially be very active in damaged tissue that contains blood clots. Furthermore, the conversion of hemoglobin and myoglobin to methemoglobin and damaged muscle will produce large amounts of $O_2^{-}\bullet$. These reactions will lead to the formation of pathological amounts of the hydroxyl radical and may decrease the casualty's ability to resist infection.[18]

Dead, Injured, and Ischemic Skeletal Muscle. One of the principal lessons of the history of the surgery of soft tissue is that dead, injured, or ischemic skeletal muscle can potentiate wound infection. In a standard guinea pig wound-infection model, wounds that contained detached pieces of skeletal muscle contained ten times more *S. aureus* than control wounds did after about 4 days.[19] Devitalized tissue impairs the bactericidal function of leukocytes, probably because the partial pressure of oxygen is low in dying tissue, and oxygen is needed for normal leukocyte function. Devitalized tissue also depresses leukocyte function *in vitro*, in the absence of bacteria, demonstrating that other factors are involved.

Muscle need not be dead to potentiate infection. Experimental studies have also shown that crushed muscle (an injury similar to that caused by the stretch of temporary cavitation) will decrease by two orders of magnitude the bacterial inoculum necessary to cause a clinically apparent infection in an animal model.[20] Studies like this provide the scientific basis for excising contused muscle from the zone of extravasation in a heavily contaminated wound.

The Casualty's Systemic Factors

Circulatory Shock. Casualties who have only soft-tissue ballistic wounds infrequently suffer shock. Some experimental and clinical studies show that circulatory shock during and immediately after wound contamination increases the likelihood that infection will develop, but the relationship is hard to demonstrate because the numbers are few. When shock does occur in casualties with soft-tissue wounds, visceral injuries—especially of the abdomen—are common. In these situations, the potential for bacterial seeding from the intraabdominal focus to distant sites of soft-tissue injury increases.

Malnutrition, Exhaustion, and Cold. Historically, the concomitants of septic combat wounds are malnutrition, exhaustion, and prolonged exposure to cold—such as might typify a winter campaign.[21] A surgeon wrote during World War I:

> The man is wounded and simultaneously inoculated with organisms [that] immediately fasten upon any dead tissue. The safety of the patient depends for the time being on his own ability to resist; and if he is collapsed from loss of much blood and is wet, cold, and starving, his leucocyte [*sic*] defense is enfeebled or absent.[22]

The casualty's resistance will clearly be impaired in such circumstances, but delayed treatment and the prevailing filthy battlefield conditions probably also contribute.

Compromised Leukocyte Response in Unconventional Warfare. Many assume that vesicant gases—such as mustard—used in chemical warfare will increase the likelihood of soft-tissue wound infections by a direct toxic effect or the systemic effect of depressing the number and action of circulating leukocytes. But the chemical warfare in World War I provides no support for this commonly held view. The nearly 900-page official World War I medical history does not mention such a synergistic interaction.[23] The very low incidence of combined injuries may partially explain the lack of such an effect; fewer than 10% of the chemical casualties had penetrating injuries as well.

While data showing a relationship between chemical agents and wound sepsis are hard to find, plentiful clinical and experimental data suggest that irradiation adversely affects soft-tissue wound healing. Most researchers believe that an otherwise nonlethal dose of systemic irradiation (that is, less than 150 centigrays) will increase the probability of dangerous wound sepsis, although the magnitude of this possible effect remains ill defined. The presence of an open wound will increase the lethality of a given dose of irradiation, an effect that is not mediated by local infection. Early wound closure (within 2 days after a combined injury was sustained) reduced lethality from 60% to 10% in experimental animals.[24] These findings have important implications for surgeons who are managing casualties with combined injuries. Current doctrine calls for delayed primary closure of open combat wounds to be performed 4–6 days after wounding, but closing the wounds during that time period did not reduce lethality in experimental animals.

Iatrogenic Factors

Certain aspects of surgical technique increase the likelihood that soft-tissue wounds will become infected.

Dead Space. A surgeon may create a dead space (that is, a void within the wound) when excising skeletal muscle during debridement. Researchers have shown that *(a)* a wound with a dead space is twice as likely to become infected than a wound that has been opened by simple incision, *(b)* the bacterial count in a dead space increases by 100-fold, and *(c)* suturing the dead space closed did not alter the likelihood of wound infection. In fact, partial closure (for example, if a suture line dehisced) was four times more likely to become infected than a wound with a simple dead space.[25] Studies like this show that if iatrogenic dead spaces have been created, immediate closure of excised penetrating battlefield wounds will be generally unsatisfactory.

Drains. When the permanent cavity is long and difficult to expose, military surgeons have occasionally treated such wounds by simply inserting a drain along the wound tract. The usual rationale for inserting a drain is to reduce the potential for infection by assuring blood drainage. But if drains promote egress of unwanted material from the wound, they also can allow undesirable material to enter. In fact, experimental studies show that drains, regardless of their composition, actually promote wound sepsis when no fluid to be drained has collected.[26] Studies such as this suggest that not only is a drain placed through a perforating wound not an adequate substitute for debridement, but also that the drain itself can introduce bacterial contamination.

Suture Material. During most past wars, military surgery has been performed using silk and gut sutures. But sutures made of such materials may actually potentiate wound sepsis. Synthetic monofilament sutures are clearly superior and should be used in lieu of the older sutures.[27]

Dead Soft Tissue Within Combat Wounds

Military surgeons frequently justify their intervention into penetrating soft-tissue wounds as the need to remove dead or devitalized tissue to prevent infection from developing. While ballistic wounds frequently do contain dead muscle, this rationale is usually overemphasized. More often than not the devitalized tissue consists of only a narrow layer that lines the permanent cavity. Two mechanisms cause muscle death: *(a)* the projectile cuts and stretches the tissue (*primary* injury), and *(b)* the vascular system is compromised either by injury to a major vessel or by compartment syndrome from a hematoma or edema (*secondary* injury). While the devitalized tissue caused by the projectile usually includes just the tissue immediately surrounding the permanent cavity, the devitalization caused by secondary injury can be extensive.

Injury to a Major Vessel. An ever-present potential exists for primary muscle injury to be exacerbated—and in fact greatly exceeded—by secondary injury if the muscle's local blood supply is disturbed either by the projectile itself or during surgery. Some muscle groups are at considerable risk of sustaining secondary injury, because the anatomy of their vascular beds features only one—or at most, several—major intramuscular vessels. Military surgeons must be aware of this potential for iatrogenic injury, and know the distribution and arrangement of the gross and intramuscular arterial supply to extremity muscles.

Compartment Syndrome. Muscles that are confined by bone and fascia in rigid anatomical compartments are at risk for secondary injury if they are subjected to a pathological increase inpressure. Intracompartmental pressure greater than 40–50 mm Hg will stop arterial flow and will cause irreversible muscle death if it persists for more than 6–8 hours.[28] The clinical syndrome that results when tension compresses muscles invested by an osteofascial envelope—the *compartment syndrome*—is more commonly seen with blunt trauma, but bleeding within a closed compartment may cause an identical problem in penetrating injuries. Although the compartment syndrome is most commonly seen following injuries to the calf, it is also seen in the gluteal muscles—the largest muscle mass in the body and a common site for gas gangrene.[29]

Some surgeons during World War I understood

that secondary mechanisms involving vascular compromise could cause muscle necrosis:

> [T]ake care to relieve all tension locally so as to allow of early re-establishment of the circulation. This may explain the advantage of "delayed primary suture" over "primary suture" in gunshot wounds.[30]

While neither the absolute amount of dead tissue that usually surrounds the permanent cavity of a soft tissue wound nor the relative importance of the two muscle-killing mechanisms is certain, useful data from both animal and human studies exist.

Animal-Tissue Experimentation. Because they *(a)* studied a large animal population and *(b)* carefully quantified the histologically dead tissue around the permanent cavities, Mendelson and Glover's landmark 1967 study is uniquely important.[16] (This is one of the most significant papers ever published on wound ballistics.) They found that the permanent cavities made by spheres and fragments were usually lined by not more than 5 mm of histologically degenerate muscle, which they measured 3–7 days after the animals were wounded. This tissue constitutes the innermost layer of the zone of extravasation. (It would be interesting to know the proportion of the zone of extravasation in relation to the total mass of damaged tissue, but since Mendelson and Glover were specifically investigating the dimensions of the permanent cavity, they did not mention the dimensions of the zone of extravasation. However, simply calculating the volumes of a hypothetical but typical wound suggests that the amount of dead tissue must be relatively small. If a 10-cm-long permanent cavity with a diameter of 1 cm and a 0.5-cm layer of dead tissue is surrounded by an additional 1-cm layer of extravasation, the volume of dead tissue is about 23 ml and the volume of the zone of extravasation is about 117 ml. Thus, only about 20% of the damaged tissue is actually dead.)

This study further suggests that, since few animals had both vascular damage and large hematomas with grossly necrotic muscle, the mechanism of death was more frequently primary injury than secondary. Furthermore, in most of these animals, clostridial infection appears to have caused the additional necrosis (beyond that attributable to the projectile). In this experimental protocol, major vascular injury was infrequent.

The researchers demonstrated that the thickness of the microscopic zone of dead tissue depended upon the projectiles' impact velocity: the higher the velocity, the larger the temporary cavity, and therefore the more extensive the primary injury. In their sample, 93% of the high-velocity (averaging 960 m/s) spheres and 77% of the high-velocity fragments caused muscle necrosis 5 mm or more thick. In contrast, only 62% of low-velocity (averaging 406 m/s) spheres and 46% of the low-velocity fragments caused muscle necrosis deeper than 5 mm.

In an earlier and less-elaborate investigation, which also spared the animals' femoral arteries, Mendelson and Glover studied skeletal-muscle death around the permanent cavities that resulted from a variety of bullet wounds and concluded: "There was no gross zone of necrosis beyond the permanent wound tract in any of the animals examined."[31] They also found that muscle death (usually associated with clostridial infection) can be massive when the arterial supply is compromised. These animal studies demonstrate conclusively that massive death of skeletal muscle is uncommon in the absence of an arterial injury.

Human-Tissue Experimentation. Although military surgeons have debrided great quantities of wounded skeletal muscle, only one published study, which was performed during the Korean War, seems to have examined the excised tissue for histological signs of death.[32] Researchers took samples from soft-tissue wounds in twelve American casualties whose wounds were caused by unspecified weapons. Surgeons had excised sixty samples of muscle that they considered to be of questionable viability from the wounds. About one-third of the samples contained muscle that was completely dead. The rest of the samples contained enough viable myocytes to have permitted the muscle to repair itself.

Whether or not battlefield surgeons can recognize dead skeletal muscle was then, and remains today, contentious. This study tested the clinical criteria for skeletal-muscle debridement—the *four Cs*:

- *Color*—dark red, red, pale, pink (normal)
- *Consistency*—mushy, stringy, soft, firm (normal)
- *Contractility*—its absence or presence (normal)
- *Circulation*—the absence or presence (normal) of bleeding

by correlating the surgeon's assessment at the time of debridement, performed 3–8 hours after the casualty was wounded, with the pathologist's microscopic determination of the degree of damage (Tables 5-1 through 5-4).

All criteria except color achieved statistical significance (using the chi-square test) as predictors of muscle necrosis. Nevertheless, using the four Cs raises problems of both sensitivity and specificity for the surgeon. For example, Table 5-1 shows that while all muscle that was likely to be dead had abnormal color, so did all the samples with histologically normal muscle. Similarly, Table 5-2 shows that three-fourths of the

TABLE 5-1

ASSESSMENT OF FOUR Cs: COLOR

5 x 4 contingency tables were constructed and statistical significance at the 5% level was determined by calculating a chi square statistic.

$p > 0.05$

Degree of Muscle Damage	Color (pink = normal)			
	dark red	red	pale	pink
Minimal	2	5	0	0
Slight	5	4	1	1
Moderate	14	5	0	1
Marked	5	4	0	1
Complete	8	4	0	0

Source: Reference 32

TABLE 5-2

ASSESSMENT OF FOUR Cs: CIRCULATION

5 x 4 contingency tables were constructed and statistical significance at the 5% level was determined by calculating a chi square statistic.

$p < 0.001$

Degree of Muscle Damage	Circulation (+2/+3 = normal)			
	+1	+2	+3	+4
Minimal	2	3	0	2
Slight	3	3	5	0
Moderate	5	9	5	1
Marked	6	3	1	0
Complete	9	3	0	0

Source: Reference 32

TABLE 5-3

ASSESSMENT OF FOUR Cs: CONSISTENCY

5 x 4 contingency tables were constructed and statistical significance at the 5% level was determined by calculating a chi square statistic.

$p < 0.001$

Degree of Muscle Damage	Consistency (firm = normal)			
	mushy	stringy	soft	firm
Minimal	1	2	0	4
Slight	0	0	7	4
Moderate	3	1	8	8
Marked	3	3	3	1
Complete	7	4	1	0

Source: Reference 32

TABLE 5-4

ASSESSMENT OF FOUR Cs: CONTRACTILITY

5 x 4 contingency tables were constructed and statistical significance at the 5% level was determined by calculating a chi square statistic.

$p < 0.01$

Degree of Muscle Damage	Contractility (+2/+3 = normal)			
	+1	+2	+3	+4
Minimal	4	1	1	1
Slight	7	1	2	1
Moderate	9	7	2	2
Marked	9	1	0	0
Complete	12	0	0	0

Source: Reference 32

samples had little if any capillary bleeding, but this defect was found with nearly equal frequency in both histologically dead and histologically normal muscle. Table 5-3 shows that muscle consistency was the most reliable predictor of tissue death. Contractility, in Table 5-4, was a less valuable predictor because, although contractility was diagnostic of viability when present, it was frequently absent—even in supposedly normal tissue. (A multiple-regression analysis might have improved the predictive value of the four Cs, but the original experimental data required to perform the test now no longer exist.)

Different and innovative approaches to assessing tissue viability—such as supravital staining with various dyes, measuring the transmembrane cellular electrical potential, and using ultraviolet light to demonstrate tissue-fluorescence—have been described, but none have been accepted, probably because they are impracticable. The four Cs, although perhaps lacking as predictors, certainly are practicable.

Human Anatomical Features That Predispose to Skeletal-Muscle Death. Many military surgeons including Raspall José Trueta have wondered whether the high prevalence of gas gangrene in wounds of the lower extremities depended upon factors other than just large muscle masses located close to the ground. In Trueta's view, ischemia of a major muscle mass was a necessary—although not a sufficient—condition for gas gangrene to develop, and the propensity for this to occur in human lower extremities depended at least partly upon the vascular anatomy of certain muscle groups.[33]

Surgeons in World War I also thought that the vascular anatomy of certain muscle groups in the lower extremities might predispose to the development of ischemic myonecrosis when vascular injury occurred. The first study to suggest this was performed near the end of World War I. During autopsies on casualties who had died of causes unrelated to injuries of the extremities, surgeons determined vascular anatomy in extremities by injecting the appropriate major artery with a barium contrast material. Muscle groups of interest were then excised and roentgenographed. On the basis of their vascular anatomy, muscle groups were divided into three categories: *(a)* those whose blood supply was derived from many sources with numerous potential anastomoses present (the deltoid, pectoralis major, and biceps brachialis muscles); *(b)* those whose blood supply was derived from one or several arteries with few potential anastomoses (the gluteus maximus, rectus femoris, and the strap muscles of the thigh); and *(c)* those whose blood supply was derived from only one artery (the gracilis and gastrocnemius muscles). The surgeons concluded that

> vascular distribution in muscle has a most important bearing on the origin and spread of gas infection in muscle. In consequence of injury to the arterial supply, the mass of muscle to which the damaged artery is distributed in classes *(b)* and *(c)* either completely dies or becomes devitalized to a marked extent. . . . When . . . the bacilli of gas gangrene invade muscle in this condition they find a nidus suitable for their growth.[30]

The arteries that these surgeons studied were not major, named arteries such as the superficial femoral or the profunda femoral, but smaller, intramuscular vessels. A study performed at the end of World War II extended this observation. Researchers determined the vascularization of muscles in rabbit extremities that were similar in shape to the strap muscles of the human thigh. They injected dye into arteries similar to classes *(b)* and *(c)* above, after interventions such as arterial ligation, partial division of the muscle belly, and experimental gunshot wounds. They found that even small lacerations of the muscle belly—such as a penetrating projectile or surgical debridement might make—caused extensive areas of persistent devascularization (Figure 5-10).

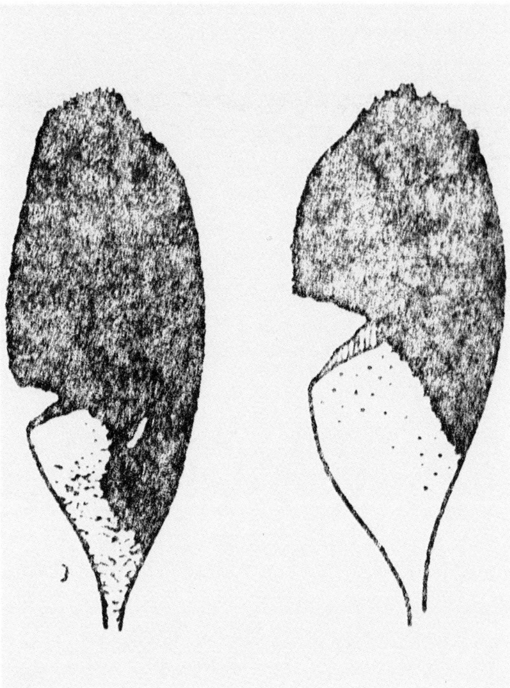

Fig. 5-10. To demonstrate tissue vascularity, a rabbit's tibialis anterior muscle was partly transected before an intraarterial dye was injected. Tissue with a normal blood flow is shown in black. The incision devitalized much of the distal portion of the muscle.
Source: Figure 3 in reference 34

Wounds made in the adductor region of the thigh (by 3/32-inch steel spheres with impact velocities ranging between 250–1,000 m/s) were usually associated with an area of unstained muscle extending 2–3 mm around the permanent cavity.

> In some cases, however, larger areas showing absence or weakness of staining were produced in the neighbourhood of the missile tract [14 mm by 8 mm]. . . . These effects are evidently due to vascular involvement, for they are too extensive to be ascribed to the direct traumatic injury of the muscular tissue by the missile. This is also shown by the fact that the areas of devascularization are usually quite asymmetrical with regard to the missile wound.[34]

Since the evidence suggested that local vasospasm contributed to producing the vascular defect, the researchers thought that direct vascular injury of intramuscular arteries was not necessary for them to become devascularized.

THE BACTERIOLOGY OF CONTAMINATED PENETRATING WOUNDS

Although many observations on the nature of the bacterial flora found in battlefield wounds have been made during the wars of this century, and our understanding of the bacteriology of penetrating wounds has been extended by animal experimentation since World War II, some important questions remain imperfectly answered:

- What is the source of bacterial contamination? Is it the host or the battlefield environment, or is it *nosocomial* (that is, hospital-acquired) or a combination of all three?
- What percentage of penetrating wounds are contaminated, and what percentage become clinically infected?
- What dynamic changes occur in the bacterial flora of contaminated and infected wounds?
- To what extent is the casualty immune to his own microflora at the site of wounding?
- What changes have antibiotics caused?

Bacteriological Observations of Battlefield Wounds

The history of military surgery is a rich source of information on the bacteriology of battlefield wounds. This textbook reviews these data in considerable detail because *(a)* much of these data are not readily available to medical officers, and *(b)* the implications of the data are more complex than we might think. Far from being a known constant, the nature of battlefield wound sepsis in each war results from a dynamic and unique interaction among various factors: the climate, the geography, the weaponry, the tactical and operational situation, the medical treatment, and perhaps even the evolving virulence of the pathogens.

World War I—Sir Alexander Fleming. Alexander Fleming, who discovered penicillin, performed some of the earliest and most comprehensive investigations of the bacterial flora in battlefield wounds. He recognized that *(a)* the flora changed over time and *(b)* the bacteria that were important immediately after wounding were absent several weeks later, having been replaced by other organisms. He performed his first study on soft-tissue and bone injuries in late autumn, 1914 (Table 5-5).[35] Several of Fleming's observations require comment:

- All the casualties had open wounds, and the chronic bacterial growth that characterizes open wounds would have been unavoidable. The reduction of the number of casualties over time appears to have been due to the healing of some wounds and the loss to follow-up in other cases.
- Mixed flora were the norm throughout the period of observation, and the organism(s) responsible for the infection is not apparent.
- The Gram-positive anaerobic bacillus *Clostridium perfringens* (known to Fleming as *Bacillus aerogenes capsulatus*) and the streptococci (Fleming did not further specify the class; the type of hemolysis is unknown, but some of the streptococci were anaerobes) were by far the most common organisms found, but they became less common as time passed. Other Gram-positive cocci predominated by the end of observation.
- Although clostridia and other anaerobic bacilli such as *B. tetani* were present in most wounds, none of these casualties developed gas gangrene.

Fleming correlated the changes that he observed in the flora with the clinical appearances of the wounds. He described three phases:

- During the first week, a foul-smelling, watery, and usually reddish-brown discharge oozed

TABLE 5-5

ALEXANDER FLEMING'S PERCENTAGE OF CASUALTIES WITH BACTERIAL SPECIES IN WORLD WAR I

Species	Time After Infection Diagnosed		
	1–7 days	8–20 days	>20 days
C. perfringens	81	34	18
Streptococcus	80	91	84
Staphylococcus	32	29	70
Coliforms	29	32	70
C. tetani	17	9	0
Other	17	17	6
Total number of casualties	127	56	27

Source: Reference 35

from the wounds, produced by the spore-bearing and intestinal coliform bacilli that grew in the old blood within the permanent cavity, but not in the surrounding soft tissue.

- During the second and third weeks, the discharge became more purulent; the earlier flora were replaced by pyogenic cocci, which caused clinical signs of invasive sepsis in and around the permanent cavity.
- During the final phase before the wounds healed, the discharge became less copious as the pyogenic cocci disappeared.

The abundance of *C. perfringens* that Fleming initially cultured from the wounds (the bacteriological correlate of the "heavily manured soil" in Flanders fields) is reflected in his simultaneous determination of the bacterial flora found on the soldiers' clothing: 83% had *C. perfringens*, 42% had streptococci, and 33% had other clostridia. No doubt a similar flora existed on the soldiers' skin. Clearly, the wound is first contaminated with the flora that the bullet or fragment collects as it passes through the soldier's clothing. To a lesser extent, contaminants are also aspirated into the wound tract if temporary cavitation occurs. But the sources of the pyogenic cocci and especially the staphylococci that dominated the latter phase remained to be determined.

World War I—Gas Gangrene. Gas gangrene—caused by the anaerobic fecal bacteria *C. perfringens*, other clostridia, and anaerobic streptococci—first achieved prominence during World War I. The exact prevalence of this most-feared of all wound infections is unclear, although at its peak early in the war, 10% of all casualties may have developed it.[36] Gas gangrene's prevalence fell to about 5% late in the war: In France in 1918, there were 221 cases among 4,377 hospitalized casualties. Although it afflicted only a small fraction of the total casualty population, gas gangrene was an important medical problem; even with optimal care, it was a major cause of death. Among 363 casualties in France who died of their wounds, gas gangrene was second only to shock and hemorrhage as the leading cause of death.[37]

A battlefield study performed in 1918 provides important data on the epidemiology of gas gangrene that remain useful today:

- Although only 51% of all wounds in this study occurred in the skeletal muscles of the shoulders, arms, hips, buttocks, thighs, and calves, 88% of all cases of gas gangrene occurred there.
- In the first 48 hours after wounding, a linear relationship exists between the probability

of developing gas gangrene and the time interval between wounding and surgery. The median time between wounding and surgery in casualties who developed gas gangrene was 40 hours.

- Fifty-four percent of all casualties in this study had wounds that cultured positive for anaerobic bacteria. (Fleming had found an 81%-positive culture rate for *C. perfringens* early in the war.)
- Two-thirds of the casualties with wounds that cultured positive for anaerobes showed no clinical evidence of gas gangrene at all.
- Only 3% of the casualties who cultured positive for anaerobes developed gas gangrene after surgery. The remainder of those who had cultured positive (about 90% of the total cases of gas gangrene) also had clinical evidence of gas gangrene at the time the cultures were made.
- *C. perfringens* was present in about 80% of casualties who developed gas gangrene. About two-thirds of the casualties also had other anaerobes.
- Streptococci, both hemolytic and nonhemolytic, were present with equal frequency in both wounds that did and wounds that did not develop gas gangrene.

And the conclusions from this research also remain valid today:

- The most important factor in preventing gas gangrene is early operation. (This is a function of rapid evacuation.)
- Most wounds are contaminated with anaerobic bacteria, but do not develop gas gangrene. (All subsequent studies agree on this point.)
- Many cases of gangrene are due to anaerobes other than *Bacillus welchii*. (This is the same bacterium that Fleming called *Bacillus aerogenes capsulatus*, which now is named *C. perfringens*.)
- In most cases of gangrene, *B. welchii* is associated with other anaerobes. (All subsequent studies agree that polymicrobial infection is the rule.)
- The streptococci (both hemolytic and nonhemolytic) are apparently of little importance in the etiology of gangrene. (We know now that anaerobic streptococci—peptostreptococci—do cause a small fraction of all cases of gas gangrene.)[37]

World War II—The Pre-Antibiotic Era. Studies carried out early in World War II extended the World War I–observations of the bacterial flora of battlefield wounds. The wounds of 105 casualties who had been evacuated from Dunkirk were cultured on admission to English hospitals. Some of the casualties had been wounded as long as 3 weeks before. Others had been wounded only a day or so before. None of the casualties had received surgical wound care, and therefore the whole population constitutes an untreated control group. The bacterial flora found in the initial wound cultures are shown in Table 5-6.[38]

Unfortunately, these results cannot be stratified by time after wounding, and thus a direct comparison with Fleming's work is impossible. Nevertheless, certain comparisons can be made between these results and those shown in Table 5-5.

- While clostridia were present in about 40% of the wounds, no cases of gas gangrene occurred in either population.
- Pyogenic cocci, and especially coagulase-positive staphylococci, predominate in both flora. (The worldwide pandemic of streptococcus infections during World War I perhaps explains the lower prevalence of hemolytic streptococci in this early–World War II sample compared to Fleming's finding.)
- *P. aeruginosa* (a latter-day scourge of intensive-care wards) first became prominent at this time, but it may have been entirely absent from Fleming's population.

Further epidemiological interpretation of these data later during World War II found that most of the species present during the first few days after wounding (including the clostridia) were contaminating saprophytes, and were killed off by host defenses or by other bacteria.[39] The pathogens that caused the most infections were the pyogenic cocci, many of which were introduced into the wound not only at the time of injury but also during the medical treatment. The researcher estimated that *(a)* almost all serious infections in battlefield wounds were caused by hemolytic streptococci or *Staphylococcus aureus* or both, and *(b)* gas gangrene had a prevalence of only a few percent.

World War II—The Early Antibiotic Era. The experience that medical officers gained in treating soft-tissue and orthopedic war wounds during late 1944 and 1945 provided evidence showing both penicillin's alteration of the bacterial flora in battlefield wounds and its potential limitations as a therapeutic agent. Perhaps the most interesting study done during this period documented the bacterial flora in thirty-six casualties who had soft-tissue and orthopedic wounds in their extremities.[40] Twenty-seven casualties had grossly infected wounds and nine had wounds that

TABLE 5-6

WOUND BACTERIA IN EARLY WORLD WAR II CASUALTIES

Bacteria	Percentage of Casualties with Given Species
Streptococci	
hemolytic	31
viridans and nonhemolytic	18
Staphylococci	
aureus	54
albus, micrococci	19
Gram-negative cocci	1
Diptheroids	8
Gram-negative bacilli:	
coliforms	25
Proteus	7
P. aeruginosa	8
Hemophilus	1
Spore-bearing:	
anaerobic	14
C. perfringens	23
C. sporogenes	10
C. septique	4
other clostridia	5
Sterile	11

Source: Based on data contained in Table 1, reference 38

appeared not to be infected. The wounds were 2–45 days old when studied. All casualties had received initial wound debridement, all had received a sulfa drug as part of their initial wound care, and all but five had received systemic penicillin both as part of their initial wound care and during their convalescence.

The bacteriological studies included both speciation and a determination of the cultured organisms' sensitivities to the antibiotics then available. Infected wounds contained five or six species of bacteria. "Clean" wounds contained two or three species. The researcher distinguished among *true pathogens* (that is, toxigenic clostridia, coagulase-positive staphylococci, and beta-hemolytic streptococci), *wound pathogens* (that is, Gram-negative organisms, nontoxigenic clostridia, and so forth) and *commensals* (that is, the diphtheroids, nonhemolytic coagulase-negative staphylococci, and so forth). Wound pathogens were distinguished from true pathogens as those bacteria unable to mount a "direct attack upon living tissue."[40] The distinction between invasive and toxigenic necrosis of living tissue (a function of true pathogens) and the septic decomposition of devitalized tissue (a function of wound pathogens) is important. It suggests that Fleming's first phase of wound infection represents only the action of wound pathogens upon blood clots and dead muscle.

The incidence of potentially invasive or toxigenic bacteria (the true pathogens) was: toxigenic clostridia, twelve; coagulase-positive staphylococcus, eleven; and beta-hemolytic streptococcus, seven. True pathogens were present in twenty-four of the twenty-seven clinically infected wounds and absent in eight of the nine "clean" wounds. Although there was only a single completely penicillin-resistant organism among the true pathogens—a staphylococcus (a harbinger of things to come)—local wound suppuration continued unabated.

The researcher's conclusions remain valid:

> Wound suppuration [is] not controlled by chemotherapy alone. . . . Invasive sepsis is controlled by the systemic use of chemotherapeutic agents. . . . Anaerobic infection is controlled by the excision of dead tissue protein and the avoidance of primary wound closure. Aerobic wound infection is controlled by preventing wound exudation through the use of splints, pressure dressing, and secondary closure of clean wounds.[40]

The researcher also offered the following practical advice regarding making decisions in the management of contaminated wounds: "The gross surgical pathologic condition of the open wound is more directly and accurately informative than any reasonable bacteriologic analysis."[40]

World War II—Anaerobic Infections. Although gas gangrene was much less prevalent during World War II than it had been during World War I, many new observations were made based on campaigns fought in the Middle East and North Africa, which established the currently accepted understanding of these infections:[41]

- About 30% of the wounds incurred in the Middle East contained anaerobic bacteria. Between 2.5%–5.0% of these contaminated wounds (that is, about 1% of the total wounded) developed clinical infections associated with anaerobic bacteria.
- In about 60% of the casualties with clinical infections, clostridia multiplied in necrotic

tissue, produced gas, spread along fascial planes, but did not invade normal muscle. This disease is *anaerobic cellulitis*.
- In about 30% of the cases with clinical infections, clostridia invaded and destroyed normal muscle. This disease is classical gas gangrene: *clostridial* or *anaerobic myositis*.
- In about 10% of the cases with clinical infections, anaerobic streptococci rather than clostridia caused muscle necrosis. This disease is *streptococcal myositis*.
- Different toxigenic clostridia were found to have different clinical characteristics. *Clostridium edematiens* had an incubation period of more than 5 days, while the more-common *C. perfringens* had an incubation period of about 1 day.
- About two-thirds of the casualties who had clinical infections also had suffered an injury to a major artery. But interestingly, in this study, the presence or absence of the vascular injury had little influence on the incubation period, the symptoms, or the end result of the infections.
- The magnitude of tissue damage predicted the casualty's outcome (Table 5-7).
- As Fleming had found during World War I, the soldiers' clothing was the source of most of the contamination: ninety-four samples taken from fifty sets of service dress cultured positive for one or more clostridial species.
- Fifty percent of the casualties with anaerobic bacterial infections died during this observation period—a rate not much different from that observed at the end of World War I. Medical officers obtained the best survival rates (70%) with surgery combined with antitoxin and sulfa drugs. Sulfa drugs by themselves were not effective.

TABLE 5-7

CLOSTRIDIAL SEPSIS: WOUND SEVERITY AND FATAL OUTCOME IN WORLD WAR II

Type of Injury	Outcome (N)	
	Fatal	Recovered
Traumatic amputation	4	1
Bony injury	4	15
Muscle laceration only	6	16
Minor injury	0	1

Source: Reference 41

These extensive observations with anaerobic bacterial infections led to several conclusions that, more importantly, helped develop the concepts that led to understanding these infections:

> Anaerobic infections are not bacteriological but clinical entities. . . . [The anaerobic bacteria's] absence from war wounds is a matter for surprise rather than satisfaction, their presence for resignation rather than alarm. . . . [T]he vast majority of these [anaerobic] organisms, including those of medical and veterinary importance, are primarily and essentially saprophytes. . . . [A]ll or nearly all [anaerobic bacteria] require special environmental conditions in their host before they can produce those effects that we speak of as a disease, before, indeed, they can even grow.[41]

The first 6 weeks of the Normandy Campaign saw one of the only studies in the history of combat-casualty care in which the experimental design allowed for a concurrent control group. The purpose was to ascertain the extent to which prophylactic penicillin would prevent clostridial wound sepsis. Out of about 4,000 British battle casualties, 436 were treated by injections of penicillin: 100,000 units as soon as possible and 50,000 units every 4 hours until their surgery. These casualties' wounds were the most likely to develop gas gangrene (that is, they included extensive lacerations of the muscles of the buttocks or thighs, compound fractures, gross contamination, long delay in providing initial care, and so forth).[42]

The results clearly indicated that penicillin markedly reduced the probability of clostridial sepsis. Only two casualties of the 436 who had received penicillin (0.46%) but twenty-eight of the nearly 3,500-member control group (0.81%) developed clostridial sepsis. Since the penicillin-treated casualties had wounds that were likely to develop gas gangrene, the difference is even more dramatic. The absence of clinical infection did not indicate that clostridia were absent from the wounds: All but one clinically benign but "dirty" wound that had been treated with penicillin grew clostridia in cultures. Penicillin did more than just prevent gas gangrene; only a small proportion of the wounds contained *Staphlococcus aureus* or *Streptococcus hemolyticus*, and about 40% of the penicillin-treated wounds that were "clean" were also sterile. The researchers cautioned that a short or inadequate course of penicillin may not totally abort clostridial wound sepsis. Profound or protracted toxemia occurred in several casualties, even though there were no local signs of clostridial sepsis. Presumably, clostridia produced their toxin even though the bacteria did not invade living muscle.

The striking difference in the prevalence of clostridial sepsis in casualties wounded while fighting over the same terrain in the two world wars is difficult to explain. Certainly, the use of antimicrobial drugs alone cannot explain the marked reduction of clostridial sepsis; the Normandy study's control group had a prevalence of only 0.8%—less than one-fifth the rate that was reported[37] at the end of World War I. Nor can differences in surgical techniques explain it; the techniques of soft-tissue wound management that were practiced near the end of World War I were surely at least as exacting as those practiced late in World War II. Could the toxigenic species of clostridia have become more benign during the period between the wars?

Korean War. The most valuable data regarding the bacteriology of battlefield wounds that has been obtained since World War II was performed by U.S. Army researchers near the end of the Korean War. One study determined the bacterial flora in skeletal muscle that was removed during the debridement of soft-tissue and bony wounds. Researchers examined 42 wounds in thirty-three casualties in the summer of 1952, and 112 wounds in sixty-nine casualties in the winter of 1952–1953 (Table 5-8). The average time between the casualty's wounding and the researchers' removing tissue for culture was about 4 hours in the summer and 8 hours in the winter. All casualties were given 300,000–600,000 units of penicillin "shortly after injury."[43]

Three of the observations that emerged from this study require comment:

- The high prevalence of hemolytic streptococci during winter no doubt reflects the expected increase in upper respiratory infections.
- No cases of gas gangrene occurred in the study group (and the overall incidence for American troops in the Korean War was less than 0.5%).
- Both the striking winter decrease in Gram-negative bacteria and the less-dramatic winter decrease in clostridia perhaps reflect a winter reduction of fecal contamination in the soldiers' environment. The fundamen-

TABLE 5-8

BACTERIAL FLORA AT THE TIME OF SURGICAL CARE IN KOREAN WAR WOUNDS

Species	Percentage of Wounds Containing Bacteria: Summer	Winter
Sterile	11	19
Staphylococcus		
hemolytic	17	46
nonhemolytic	12	33
Streptococcus		
beta-hemolytic	0	61
non-beta-hemolytic	59	76
Total Clostridia	84	36
pathogenic, including *C. perfringens*	44	21
Gram-negative bacilli	69	12
Bacillus species, including *B. subtilis*	10	62

Source: Reference 43

tally different summer and winter flora indicate that medical officers must choose carefully when considering effective antibiotic prophylaxis.

Several ancillary studies done at the same time showed:

- The larger the wound, the more likely it was to contain pathogenic clostridia. This effect was not found for aerobes.
- Soil, rather than the soldier's skin or clothing, was more likely to be contaminated with clostridia.
- Fifty-five percent of surgically removed rifle and machine gun bullets grew clostridia, and clostridia were cultured from 25% of shell fragments and 39% of grenade fragments.
- In the doses that were employed, penicillin inhibited the *in vitro* growth of only one-half to three-fourths of the isolated clostridia.

The authors of these studies emphasized that the bacterial flora "illustrate wound contamination and early proliferation of bacteria, rather than infection."[43] Unfortunately, they did not tell how many, if any, of the casualties in these studies actually developed clinical wound sepsis.

With few exceptions, studies of bacterial wound flora done before the Korean War described observations that were made at only one point in time. In the spring of 1953, researchers followed eleven casualties who had received state-of-the-art combat-casualty care and studied how their flora changed over time. They cultured skeletal-muscle biopsies that were taken at the time of initial wound surgery and again, under sterile conditions, on every second day until surgeons closed the wounds between the fifth and ninth days. The casualties had been given penicillin at the time of initial wound surgery, but not afterwards.

> All wounds contained a rich flora of Gram-positive and Gram-negative aerobes on initial culture. Without exception, these organisms persisted in the wounds during the first week of healing. . . . Nine of the 11 wounds studied contained one or more species of clostridia at the time of initial debridement. Clostridia were absent from two-thirds of the wounds when studied following initial surgery.[44]

The failure to achieve sterilization in any of the wounds might be thought to reflect inadequate wound surgery. However, the surgeon purposely excised healthy-appearing tissue (after he had performed what he judged to be an adequate debridement) on six casualties. Five of the six specimens contained bacteria of the same species that were found during debridement of the "devitalized" tissues. Two of the eleven casualties developed wound sepsis from their "clostridial and rich aerobic flora." The authors concluded that "adequate debridement was not performed" in these failures. But the clear implication from this work is not that the wounds were inadequately debrided; it is rather that surgery probably cannot sterilize a battlefield wound. Debridement reduces bacterial contamination and augments the casualty's defenses against infection by eliminating abnormal tissue.[44]

Vietnam War. Our understanding of soft-tissue wound infections advanced less than might have been expected during the Vietnam War, given the high level of medical sophistication compared to other wars. Complications of soft-tissue wounds were less frequent during the Vietnam War than they had been in prior American wars. There was less interest in the problem of wound sepsis than there had been in World War I, for example, which is not surprising. Although this favorable situation no doubt reflected the general excellence of surgical care and the liberal use of antibiotics both prophylactically and therapeutically, it is a mistake not to recognize that it was the nature of the war itself—largely low-intensity counterinsurgency operations—that made the general excellence of the medical care possible.

During the battle of Dak To in November 1967, a rare instance when a battlefield in Vietnam had the scope and intensity reminiscent of World War I and World War II, wound sepsis became a serious problem:

> The 24-hour-old wounds were uniformly purulent and the extremity wounds were often accompanied by rather marked swelling. After the first 24 hours, patients frequently became quite febrile, and while cellulitis was the rule, lymphangitis was rare. The casualties from the 173d Airborne Brigade with 2- or 3-day-old wounds demonstrated the same findings, but their fever and inflammation were more severe.[45]

The following databases clearly seem to apply to a much more benign environment than Dak To. One study followed 112 soft-tissue wounds in 110 casualties (Table 5-9). Cultures were taken at the time the casualties were admitted, but before surgery was performed. "The vast majority of patients received penicillin and streptomycin,"[46] but the researchers provided no information regarding dosages and times of administration of the antibiotics. Several striking differences seem to exist between these data and those published during previous wars:

- *Streptococcus pyogenes* was totally absent and

TABLE 5-9

BACTERIAL FLORA IN VIETNAM WAR COMBAT WOUNDS

Species	Percentage of Wounds Containing Species
No Growth	34
A. aerogenes	33
Staphylococcus aureus	30
P. aeruginosa	14
Proteus sp.	14
E. coli	11
Enterococci (group D beta-hemolytic streptococci)	7
Staphylococcus epidermidis	6
Clostridium sp.	2
Others	4

Source: Reference 46

clostridia were nearly absent, in marked contrast to the high prevalence of these organisms in wounds of previous wars. Clostridia were known to be present in all types of soils in Vietnam. Whether penicillin was responsible for the absence of clostridia in wounds is not known. The absence of *S. pyogenes* probably reflects climatic conditions: This species was also absent from Korean summer cultures (Table 5-8).

- Nearly three-fourths of the isolates were Gram-negative. Although high, these data are comparable to the Korean summer cultures.
- One-third of the cultures showed no bacterial growth. This figure is much higher than that from previous wars. It may reflect the fact that cultures were taken from wound edges, rather than from actual tissue. Or the wounds may have been sterilized by the antibiotics.

Evidence from another study supports the suggestion that the pathogens that caused such severe problems in previous wars were much less prevalent in Vietnam.[47] Clostridia and beta-hemolytic streptococci were essentially absent from cultures taken from 1,531 wounds when casualties from Vietnam arrived at fourth-echelon hospitals in Japan. All the patients had received initial wound surgery and a variety of antibiotics, so whether the absence of these pathogens reflects effective prophylaxis or decreased bacteria in the environment is unclear. However, these data do suggest that the environment and climate of the battlefield determine both the ambient bacterial flora and the consequent likelihood of wound sepsis.

One effort during the Vietnam War sought to *(a)* quantitate the bacterial counts in battlefield wounds and *(b)* determine whether applying topical antimicrobial drugs to open soft-tissue wounds could lessen the likelihood of sepsis.[8] The study population consisted of 245 wounded Vietnamese soldiers who were randomized into seven treatment groups (controls, saline irrigations, and various protocols for the topical

TABLE 5-10

BACTERIAL COUNTS DURING TREATMENT IN VIETNAMESE BATTLEFIELD WOUNDS

Species	Percentage of Wounds Containing $10^3/10^6$ Organisms per ml of Wound Exudate — Day of Culturing Bacteria			
	0	2	5	8
Staphylococcus aureus	46/17	37/29	45/30	62/40
Pseudomonas	10/5	31/26	45/39	40/30

Source: Reference 8

application of Sulfamylon, Polybactrin and Neosporin). All casualties received parenteral penicillin and streptomycin throughout the study. Cultures were taken from the wounds when the casualties were admitted, before their initial wound surgery, and on the second, fifth, and eighth days after surgery, using sterile technique (Table 5-10).

Unfortunately, this study did not report the clinical outcome of these casualties' wound-healing. Since only a few of the wounds had counts of *Staphylococcus aureus* that are known to be associated with invasive sepsis in animal models, invasive sepsis might have been uncommon in this population. Clearly, all casualties must have had surface infections, but the study did not report what happened when (or if) the wounds were surgically closed. While the details of surgical care were not specified, whatever was done surgically did not sterilize—or even decrease—the bacterial counts; *Pseudomonas* proliferated continuously. Nor did any of the antibiotics used either topically or systemically appear to decrease the bacterial counts.

TABLE 5-11

BACTERIAL SPECIES FOUND IN SOFT-TISSUE WOUND INFECTIONS DURING THE YOM KIPPUR WAR

Total Casualties = 10 Total Isolates = 41	Positive Cultures
Various Gram-negative bacilli other than Pseudomonas	15
Pseudomonas	12
Enterococci	6
Staphylococcus aureus	4
Streptococcus pyogenes	2
Clostridia	2

Source: Reference 48

Yom Kippur War. Research performed by Israeli medical officers during the 1973 Yom Kippur War yielded important information on the differences in the bacterial flora responsible for *(a)* the simple wound contamination that was found in cultures taken at the time of initial wound care and *(b)* the clinically apparent soft-tissue wound infections that were seen days to several weeks after wounding.[48] Bacterial species were cultured from the 10 of 178 casualties who had infected soft-tissue wounds, an unreported number of which were multiple (Table 5-11). The frequency of the species seen in the these infections, which also represents the flora of infected fracture wounds, is very different from the flora found during the pre-antibiotic era of the two world wars. Gone are the large numbers of wounds infected with pyogenic cocci and clostridia. They have been replaced by a large number of infections caused by Gram-negative pathogens, at least some of which are nosocomial. In a companion study, the investigators state their firm belief that the antibiotics administered in the field were primarily responsible for the changes in the flora.[49]

Insofar as the data permit comparison, the soft-tissue wound infection rate changed little, compared to late-World War II or the Korean War; only the bacterial species causing infection changed.

TABLE 5-12

BACTERIAL COUNTS OVER TIME IN MASSIVE SOFT-TISSUE WOUNDS IN GOATS

	Bacterial Counts Over Time (Hours) After Wounding				
Species	9	16	25	36	48
C. perfringens	3×10^3	4×10^4	9×10^6	3×10^7	dead
S. aureus	1×10^4	4×10^5	1×10^4	6×10^4	dead

Source: Reference 51

The Bacteriology of Penetrating Wounds in Experimental Animals

Several of the many experimental-wound studies performed at Edgewood Arsenal may help medical officers understand the bacteriology of penetrating wounds.

A study using goats with extensive soft-tissue wounds emphasized the value of distinguishing between *qualitative* assessments of bacterial flora (that is, the presence or absence of a given species) and *quantitative* measurements of the actual number of bacteria present in a wound. Researchers wounded each goat by detonating a small explosive charge near the animal's thigh. Bacterial cultures revealed little change in the flora over several days, even though the goats' deteriorating clinical status suggested invasive sepsis. A different picture emerged when bacterial counts were made: The number of bacteria per gram of tissue increased from 10^2 immediately after wounding to 5×10^3 at 6 hours, to 7×10^5 at 12 hours, and to 10^6 at 18 hours. Death occurred in most untreated animals when the quantitative measurements found more than 10^6 bacteria per gram of tissue, even though the bacterial species found in the wound when the animal died were the same as those found in the wound immediately after the animal was wounded.[50]

A companion study using a similar experimental model studied bacterial speciation and measured the growth of *C. perfringens* and *S. aureus* in a group of untreated control animals (Table 5-12).[51]

Although studies like these are difficult to perform, they are valuable because they allow investigators to quantitate the effect of a given therapeutic intervention—whether surgery or an antimicrobial agent. Subsequent research done at Edgewood that studied the bacteriology of penetrating wounds made by fragments and spheres illuminates some of the difficulties inherent in such investigations. Although *C. perfringens*, *S. aureus*, and even anaerobic streptococci, among other pathogens, were present in most wounds, there was "little consistent correlation between the organisms recovered from the wounds and the [experimental animals'] clinical course."[16] Many of the animals developed minimal, well-localized infections, and quantitative bacterial counts alone would mislead as to their extent. For example, many instances of *C. perfringens* infection contained so few organisms that the relationship between bacterial count and clinical outcome could not be determined. This study shows that the mere presence of a penetrating soft-tissue wound does not necessarily indicate bacterial contamination that will automatically progress to life-threatening sepsis. Many—in fact most—of the experimental wounds healed uneventfully.[16]

Since this pioneering work at Edgewood, many additional investigators have reported on the bacterial flora in experimental penetrating soft-tissue wounds. One of special interest combined sophisticated bacteriological studies with relevant wounds that were created under realistic controlled circumstances.[52] The investigators shot sixty-four swine (although only forty-seven were used in the study) through the soft tissues of their posterior thighs *(a)* in the field, *(b)* at ranges of 30 or 100 m, and *(c)* with a variety of military small arms including the 5.56-mm M193 ball and the 7.62-mm M43 ball. Cultures were taken *(a)* when the wounds were debrided 6 hours after wounding and *(b)* when the dressings were changed 72 hours after wounding. One-half of the animals received parenteral penicillin every 8 hours.

Important differences regarding both bacterial

counts and wound morphology appeared between the 5.56-mm and 7.62-mm bullets. When the wounds were debrided, only one of the 7.62-mm wounds contained a measurable number of bacteria (in this instance, 10^4 *E. coli*), while 50% of the 5.56-mm wounds contained various species with counts ranging between 10^2 and 10^4. None of the latter animals had received penicillin. Twelve of the swine were studied at 72 hours. All the 7.62-mm wounds were apparently sterile, but the 5.56-mm wounds were invasively infected (with bacterial flora of soil or fecal origin) and contained more than 10^5 bacteria per gram of tissue.

Wound morphology was also strikingly different in the 7.62-mm and 5.56-mm groups. The en seton wounds made by the 7.62-mm bullets appeared benign; the dimensions of the wounds of entrance and exit were the same. However, the exit wounds made by the 5.56-mm bullets (especially those made at the 30-m target distance) were more often than not "explosive," with dimensions many times larger than their corresponding wounds of entrance. The huge exposed surfaces of the large wounds of exit became the sites of invasive sepsis.

This study has several important implications for military surgeons who may treat battlefield wounds:

- Benign, perforating, (en seton) soft-tissue wounds that the 7.62-mm bullets made frequently healed without any therapeutic intervention being necessary. This study shows why: Bacterial contamination is insufficient to cause infection.
- The greater the tissue damage, the greater will be the potential for bacterial contamination. Yet the invasive sepsis that developed in the 5.56-mm wounds appears not to have been caused by the contamination that occurred at the time the animal was wounded, but by secondary contamination from the animal's environment that occurred many hours after wounding.
- Penicillin prevented the growth of the bacterial contamination that occurred at the time of wounding, but was ineffective in preventing the later colonization of the open wound.

AN OVERVIEW OF MANAGEMENT CONSIDERATIONS

The military surgeon's goal in soft-tissue wound management is to to return the combat casualty to duty at the earliest possible moment. The medical factor still most likely to delay early return, however, is the wound's failure to heal because of sepsis. Ideally, prophylactic interventions will prevent a contaminated wound from becoming infected and an infected wound from becoming septic, but if prevention fails, therapeutic interventions will have to be employed.

The potential for wounds to become infected or septic can be lowered by *(a)* decreasing the magnitude of bacterial contamination and *(b)* eliminating those factors that decrease the casualty's resistance to bacterial infections. Interventions that both decrease contamination and augment the casualty's resistance include *(a)* surgery, *(b)* mechanical irrigation, *(c)* antiseptics, and *(d)* antibiotics. Of course, civilian surgeons face many of these same situations every day, but there are aspects that are unique to soft-tissue wound management in combat casualty care.

Surgery

Surgical interventions range among *(a)* wound incision (that is, simply opening the wound tract), *(b)* simple wound excision (that is, excising all or part of the permanent cavity's wall, cutting from the inside out), and *(c)* total wound excision or excision en bloc (that is, entirely excising the tissue around the permanent cavity, cutting around the damaged tissues but never entering the permanent cavity itself). The distinction between simple wound excision and total wound excision is of academic interest only: Excision en bloc is hardly ever a practical possibility. Even the distinction between incision and excision may be more theoretical than practical, because performing wound excision is impossible without first performing wound incision. Furthermore, except when incising a grossly suppurative permanent cavity (that is, when draining an abscess), the surgeon will usually trim injured tissue from the permanent cavity's walls. Because both incision and some degree of excision are *(a)* part of the usual surgical management of penetrating soft-tissue wounds and *(b)* included in the term *debridement* (both as it has been used in the U.S. Army since World War I and compatible with its contemporary civilian use), this textbook uses debridement to describe the surgical management of penetrating soft-tissue combat wounds.[53]

Removing dead or devitalized tissue is the usual

rationale for performing debridement, but wounds usually contain little truly dead tissue. They do, however, contain significant amounts of damaged tissue: the ecchymotic, suffused, edematous tissue in the zone of extravasation. This is the tissue most likely to be contaminated by foreign material—including bacteria and soil. Therefore, debriding a layer of the zone of extravasation lying just outside the permanent cavity will both decrease the bacterial count and augment the casualty's ability to resist infection. The famous four Cs criteria—color, consistency, contractility, and circulation—while they do not absolutely identify dead tissue, do actually identify the tissue most likely to be contaminated and thus at risk to develop sepsis.

But there should be no doubt as to whether debridement can sterilize a wound: It can not. Neither can debridement sterilize an infected wound: Infection cannot be excised.

Irrigation

Large foreign bodies, blood clots, and small pieces of detached muscle and fat are easily removed from the walls of a permanent cavity by conventional irrigation (that is, lavage with large volumes of saline at low pressure). But bacteria, because of their *(a)* small size and consequent low hydraulic drag and *(b)* surprisingly great physical adherence to tissue, resist being removed by conventional irrigation, even when saline is squirted forcefully from a bulb syringe. Bacteria can be removed from tissue only if the irrigation solution floods the wound margins at a pressure of 7 psi or greater.[54] Commercial devices are available for this purpose, but a 35-ml syringe ejecting through a 19-gauge needle can obtain a similar effect.[55] Devices such as the Water Pik frequently use a high-pressure pulsatile jet. Extensive experimental work done by the U.S. Army Medical Research and Development Command has shown the value of such devices as adjuncts in the mechanical cleansing of wounds.[56] Earlier concerns that high-pressure irrigation would drive the contaminating bacteria into deep tissue recesses have been dispelled by studies showing that the benefits from physically removing the bacteria outweigh any decrement in the casualty's ability to resist infection.[57] Wounds have also been successfully decontaminated using ultrasound waves. In response to the cyclic high- and low-pressure phases of the sound waves, microscopic air bubbles expand and collapse explosively and strip particulate matter from the tissue.[58]

Modalities such as high-pressure irrigation and ultrasound, applied after the permanent cavity is opened, might seem to be attractive alternatives to excision, but their value to military surgeons is moot: Such devices are unlikely to be available in combat-zone hospitals. Battlefield medical facilities may lack even copious quantities of irrigation fluid for conventional wound lavage.

The wound must be incised before any irrigation technique can be employed, although attempts to circumvent this prerequisite occasionally occur. Some have tried to irrigate without incising by placing the nozzle of a syringe directly into the wound of entrance or exit and squirting vigorously. Obviously, the convoluted geometry of most permanent cavities precludes anything other than inadequate lavage. More recently, others have suggested that the permanent cavity could be scrubbed by pulling a sponge or gauze through it, but an unanesthetized casualty may not tolerate a surgeon's insinuating a gauze through a long permanent tract. Cleansing a wound by direct mechanical trauma may actually impair the casualty's resistance. In one experimental study, the percentage of infected wounds was increased from 0% in the controls to 40%–70% in sponged animals, depending upon the sponge's roughness.[59]

Antiseptics

Antiseptics have a long and controversial history in military surgery. Surgeons in World War I managed grossly septic open wounds by irrigating them frequently with corrosive chemicals. The best-known (but now obsolete) regimen used Carrel's technique and Dakin's 0.5% sodium hypochlorite solution. Although Dakin's solution killed bacteria and digested dead tissue, it also injured living tissue in the wound. Furthermore, the procedure required that the wound be exposed frequently, with the attendant possibility of secondary contamination with hospital bacteria.

While using antiseptics as therapeutic agents in treating grossly infected wounds seems to be reasonable, using an antiseptic prophylactically is not. Any chemical capable of killing bacteria will also kill mammalian cells. But nontoxic detergents (such as Pluronic polyol F-68), because of their ability to reduce the bacterial count in experimentally contaminated wounds, might be useful adjuncts in debridement.

Today, surgeons use antiseptics—especially those based upon iodophors (that is, complexes of elemental iodine and polymers of polyoxyethylene or polyoxypropylene)—in managing suppurating wounds. The goal remains to reduce the wound's bacterial count until secondary closure can be performed safely.

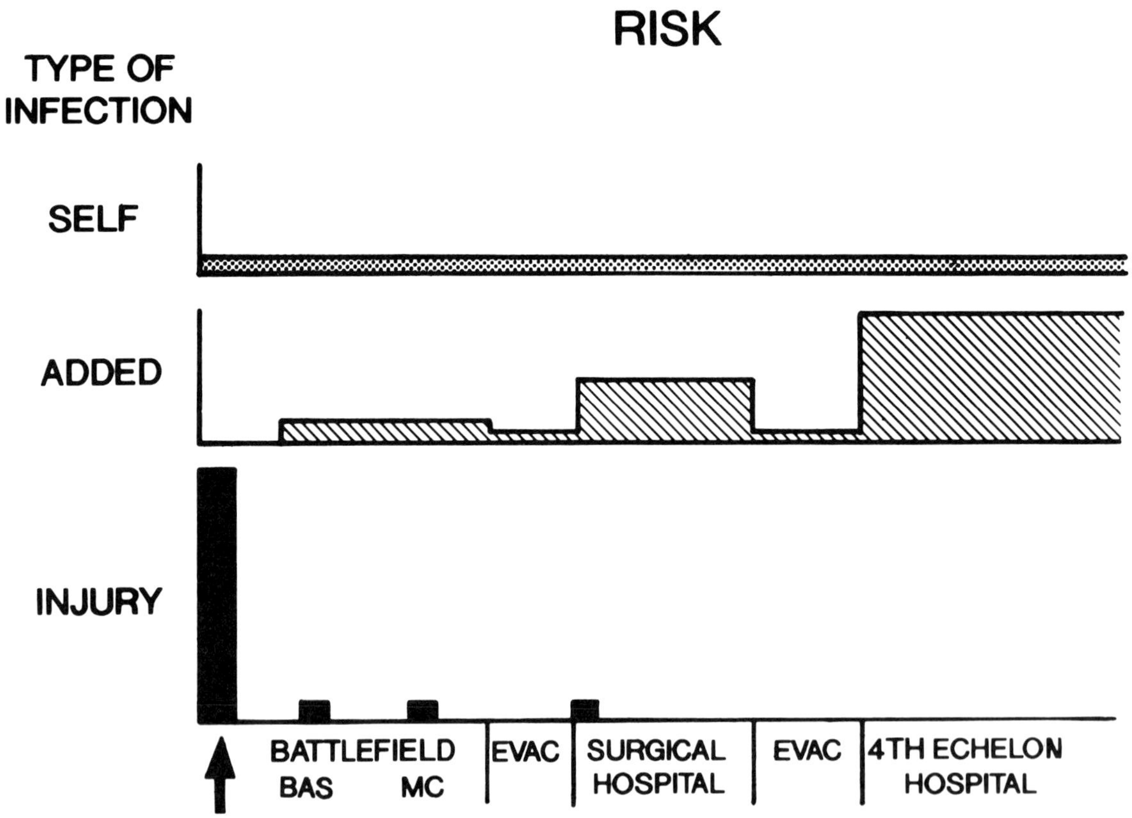

Fig. 5-11. A battlefield wound is subject to three sources of bacterial contamination: from the environment at the time of injury, from the casualty's native flora at any time, and from the medical-treatment environment during wound care. Source: Redrawn version of Figure 4 in reference 39

Antibiotics

In managing soft-tissue wound suppuration and invasive sepsis, the choice of a therapeutic agent should be predicated upon the surgeon's knowledge of the causative organisms' antibiotic sensitivities. The major conceptual problem with battlefield antibiotic prophylaxis, however, is our inability to decide (because of our lack of knowledge) which casualties really need such therapy. Therefore, doctrine states that all casualties with penetrating injuries will receive antibiotic prophylaxis, which medics and battalion surgeons will administer in the field. Many of the casualties, such as those with en seton gunshot wounds and small, blind, fragment wounds, are probably at small risk for developing wound sepsis. Others, those with huge wounds of exit or external evidence of extensive soft-tissue injury, probably will develop wound sepsis even if they receive prophylactic antibiotics, but administering them may temporarily stave off infection and compensate for delays in evacuation.[60]

Systemic Antibiotics. Although supported by animal experimentation, antibiotic prophylaxis to abort sepsis has not conclusively been proven effective in contaminated battlefield wounds. Combat casualties are exposed to numerous different pathogens, not only when they are wounded, but also when they are evacuated from the battlefield and treated at the next echelons of care (Figure 5-11). Each stage of treatment exposes the casualty to different organisms:

- During wounding—clostridia and other bacteria of fecal origin from the soil and the casualty's own clothing and skin, and *S. aureus* from the casualty's skin, are likely to be introduced.
- Continuing self-infection—as long as the wound remains open, further contamination from the casualty's own skin (especially with various staphylococcal species) remains possible.
- During treatment—at each echelon where the open wound is manipulated, contamination with a vast spectrum of nosocomial organisms can occur every time the dressing is removed. Beta-hemolytic streptococci are probably added to the flora at this time.

Obviously, the antibiotic must be effective against the organisms likely to contaminate the wound, but choosing the optimal one is difficult because *(a)* the spectrum of organisms likely to be encountered is broad, and *(b)* bacterial contamination is a dynamic process. At a minimum, toxigenic clostridia, coagulase-positive staphylococci, and beta-hemolytic streptococci must be eradicated. Penicillin is quite effective against clostridia and beta-hemolytic streptococci (the sources of the most life-threatening infections) and is also both safe and inexpensive. But penicillin, as usually administered, is active for only a short time. For that reason, military surgeons prefer a drug with more favorable pharmacokinetics, like cefazolin. (Physicians should consult the North Atlantic Treaty Organization's handbook *Emergency War Surgery*[61] for appropriate dosing information.)

Experimental studies with animals and a growing body of civilian clinical experience clearly indicate that the appropriate antibiotic, given parenterally during or immediately after wound contamination, will decrease the incidence of sepsis. Initial studies of antibiotic prophylaxis in experimental wounds demonstrated the importance of the time of administration: Penicillin administered to guinea pigs within 2 hours of a wound's contamination with *Staphylococcus aureus* prevented sepsis in 90% of wounds; its administration later than 3 hours produced an infection rate no different than that in control animals.[62] In combat-casualty care, however, a medic or corpsman might not be able to administer the antibiotic in time for the casualty to benefit from its potential effectiveness.

Recent experimental evidence shows that penicillin and possibly other antimicrobial drugs may do more than just impede bacterial growth. Measuring the mass of skeletal muscle that they debrided 12 hours after they shot experimental animals, researchers found that animals given penicillin immediately after they were wounded had only one-third the muscle damage that untreated controls had.[63] The reason for this phenomenon, and whether it might have practical significance in human medicine, remains unknown.

Topical Antimicrobials. Topical antimicrobials such as Sulfamylon have played an important role in preventing and treating sepsis in burned patients; although the concept is attractive, their similar role in managing soft-tissue wounds has not been established. Several convincing studies show that researchers can prolong animal survival by using topical Sulfamylon or penicillin on massive open wounds, where death caused by *C. perfringens* is otherwise certain.[51] But in the only trial in combat casualties of the topical antimicrobials Sulfamylon, Polybactrin, and Neosporin, researchers found no benefit, at least in their ability to control *S. aureus* or *Pseudomonas*.[8]

Unfavorable wound morphology lessens the efficacy of topical antimicrobials. The penetrating wounds that most casualties suffer have narrow wound tracts with small wounds of entrance and exit. In fact, most casualties of modern warfare have small, blind wound tracts. Few have a gaping soft-tissue wound as their major therapeutic problem. How can a surgeon deliver a topical antimicrobial to the walls of a narrow permanent cavity located deep inside an extremity without opening the wound tract?

Clinical and Experimental Therapeutic Trials in Soft-Tissue Wound Management

If randomized, double-blind trials of proposed interventions (that is, antibiotics or no treatment, wound excision en bloc or debridement with antibiotic adjuncts, and so forth) could be performed with humans, the contentious subject of the proper management of projectile wounds sustained on a battlefield could be resolved. But not only have no such trials ever been performed, none is likely ever to be done. We must make do with tantalizing reports such as this from World War II:

> The author was on the surgical staff of an evacuation hospital during two campaigns in the Southwest Pacific.... The first campaign covered a period of 2 to 2 1/2 months.... Casualties did not begin to occur in very large numbers until the campaign was about 3 to 4 weeks old. When they did occur the great majority were seen within 4 to 6 hours of injury by small surgical units very near the scene of action. These units had been directed to debride thoroughly. . . . Following surgery these patients were moved to the rear. . . . On the average they arrived about 48 hours after injury. . . . [C]omparatively few of them showed signs of toxicity.... About 10% required a more extensive or a primary debridement.... [T]here were 10 cases of gangrene [out of about 1,550 casualties]....
>
> The second campaign lasted only 3 to 4 weeks. The method of treatment of wounds of the extremities in this campaign in the forward area was only the application of sulfanilamide crystals and sterile dressings with adequate immobilization. Any further treatment required in such extremities was to be given in the rear areas. . . . Evacuation in this campaign was from the beachhead medical units . . . to our hospital. . . . The patients arrived on the average about 72 hours after injury.... [P]ractically all who had wounds of any extent showed signs of toxicity.... Of the 250 patients received during this campaign, 54% required debridement. . . . There

> were 13 cases of gangrene of which 10 were due to bacterial agents. . . . Of the 10 cases of bacterial gangrene 5 . . . had small through-and-through perforating wounds of the extremities without bony injury.
>
> A plea is made for early debridement which at least provides adequate drainage from the wound even if all devitalized tissue is not removed.[64]

Within the historical context of the pre-penicillin era, we cannot challenge the validity of the author's conclusion: Penetrating soft-tissue wounds *must* be debrided. But can his conclusion be extrapolated to the present era, with its powerful antimicrobial drugs? Since the appropriate human studies are neither practicable nor perhaps even possible, a definitive answer cannot be given. We may gain insight from animal experiments that had recovery—or at least the animals' long-term survival—as their end points; however, extrapolating the results of animal studies to the care of human casualties is always dangerous.

Penicillin Prophylaxis of Gas Gangrene. Researchers in England sought to determine the prophylactic effects of wound incision, wound excision, and penicillin in sheep that were infected with gas gangrene, with the animals' survival as their end point.[65] They shot sheep through their thigh muscles with bullets that were first passed through a piece of cloth containing a standard dose of toxigenic clostridial spores. The sheep were divided into five groups: *(a)* controls—which were untreated, *(b)* wound incision—in which the entire wound tract was opened, *(c)* wound excision—in which the wound tract was opened and all abnormal-appearing tissue was excised, *(d)* wound incision and penicillin—in which the animals received 600,000 units of penicillin 45 minutes after wounding and another 300,000 units 6 hours after wounding when they had surgery, and *(e)* nonoperative—in which the animals received 600,000 units of penicillin 1–9 hours after being shot. The researchers operated on the sheep 6 hours after wounding them. The animals were considered to have survived if they lived for 200 hours after being wounded. Average survival times (excluding anesthetic deaths and wounds in which muscle was not injured) were: *(a)* among the seven controls, 43 hours: *(b)* among the nine that received incision only, 37 hours; *(c)* among the nine that received excision, 160 hours; *(d)* among the twelve that received both incision and penicillin, 60 hours; and *(e)* among the ten that received only penicillin, 168 hours.

TABLE 5-13

EFFECT OF TOPICAL THERAPY ON GOATS' SURVIVAL FOLLOWING MASSIVE SOFT-TISSUE TRAUMA

(N = 6 in all groups at 0 hours)

Treatment	Percentage of Animals Surviving Over			
	100 hours	200 hours	400 hours	600 hours
Controls	0	0	0	0
Penicillin spray	67	0	0	0
5% Mafenide	67	17	0	0
20% Mafenide	67	50	17	17
5% Mafenide and penicillin	67	67	33	0
20% Mafenide and penicillin	100	100	100	50

Source: Reference 51

In this investigation, penicillin alone was clearly as effective as conventional wound excision in preventing death from gas gangrene.

The deleterious effect of wound incision is surprising; these researchers suggest that the incision itself created devitalized tissue that, in turn, assured that the clostridial contamination would progress to gas gangrene. This study confirms the experimental results that were obtained in 1945.[34] It also provides clear-cut evidence that systemic penicillin has an obvious role in preventing gas gangrene, and provides experimental evidence supporting the British World War II clinical finding that prophylactic penicillin reduced the incidence of gas gangrene in Normandy in 1944.[42]

Topical Antimicrobial Treatment of Large Soft-Tissue Wounds. After detonating small explosive charges on the thighs of 150 anesthetized goats to create massive open wounds, researchers sought to measure the ability of several topical antimicrobials (alone and in combination) to prolong the animals' survival.[51] They applied the topical preparations immediately after the animals were wounded and twice daily thereafter, but did not surgically manipulate the wounds at all (Table 5-13). Nor did they deliberately contaminate the wounds. They did attempt to prevent the deleterious effects of the animals' prolonged recumbency, however. *C. perfringens* sepsis developed in some of the animals' massive soft-tissue wounds, but the results clearly indicate that topical antimicrobials can prevent the deaths of animals that otherwise would have died.

Studies like this one involve a great amount of custodial care, which are both labor intensive and very costly. But this study's relevance to the management of battlefield casualties is not clear-cut, since casualties usually do not present with a massive soft-tissue injury as their only treatment problem. Furthermore, a battlefield situation in which a treatable casualty did not receive surgical care for weeks on end is hard to imagine. Its questionable relevance illustrates one of the problems medical officers encounter when results of animal experimentation are used to rationalize treatment in human casualties.

Survival Following Untreated Soft-Tissue Ballistic Wounds. Researchers sought to determine spontaneous survival in 147 goats with untreated soft-tissue wounds.[16] They shot the goats with either low-velocity (averaging 406 m/s) or high-velocity (averaging 960 m/s) spheres and fragments, and assessed the animals' survival 3 weeks later. (Animals that died within 1 hour of wounding were excluded from the study.) Of the twenty-seven goats shot with low-velocity spheres, twenty-two survived, and of the twenty-five shot with high-velocity spheres, five survived. Of the forty-seven goats shot with low-velocity fragments, thirty-one survived, and of the fifteen shot with high-velocity fragments, nine survived.

Even though the researchers performed extensive anatomical, pathological, and bacteriological studies, they usually could not determine the cause of death. By excluding those deaths that occurred within 1 hour and by performing exacting autopsies on those that died within 72 hours, they ruled out hemorrhage as the cause of death. A small number of animals appeared to have died of gas gangrene, and only about 18% of autopsied animals had evident *C. perfringens* infection. The researchers' most significant observation was that untreated projectile wounds of soft tissue can be fatal. One cannot help but wonder how effective surgical and antibiotic interventions would have altered the outcome.

This study raises more questions that it answers. The fact that 41% of the animals died, most without any obvious cause, is mystifying. Something killed these animals and the clear implication for medical officers is that soft-tissue wounds cannot be ignored.

Nonoperative Treatment of Assault-Rifle Wounds. Researchers shot ten large swine through their posterior thighs with solid brass 5.45-mm bullets (replicas of AK74 assault-rifle projectiles, specially made to prevent deformation and fragmentation from contributing to the wounding). The permanent cavities had large wounds of exit. Each animal received 2.5 million units of penicillin intramuscularly 30 minutes after wounding, and 2.5 million additional units twice daily for 5 days. This was the only treatment that five of the swine received. Researchers excised the "severely disrupted and nonviable" muscle from the other five swine. All animals survived and their wounds healed in 20–22 days. The researchers concluded that in well-drained assault-rifle wounds adequately covered with antibiotics, wound excision provides no advantage.[66]

This study has great practical significance, since it suggests that nonoperative treatment is an option even in casualties who have extensive soft-tissue wounds. But several possible limitations need to be considered before medical officers fully accept these results:

- The study gives no information about the type and magnitude of bacterial contamination of the wounds. If contamination were less than 10^6 bacteria per gram of damaged tissue, a similar outcome could be expected regardless of the research protocol. Clearly, debridement alone, antibiotics alone, or no treatment at all would yield similar results in "germ"-free animals shot in a sterile laboratory. Additionally, the real controls for this experiment, animals that received no

treatment whatsoever, are missing.
- The experimental protocol design was optimal for nonoperative care. The swine each received a large dose of penicillin soon after being wounded, and the configurations of their wounds allowed for easy drainage. This combination of characteristics is unusual—or at least not predictable—in real combat wounds.
- Although the researchers speculate about the effect that delayed primary closure would have had on this population, in fact they excluded delayed primary closure from their experimental design. The design should have included an additional control group to determine the time necessary for excised wounds to heal after delayed primary closure. Returning wounded soldiers to duty as soon as possible is accomplished both by preventing sepsis and by early closure of sepsis-prone wounds.

No laboratory experimental design can include all the salient aspects of the clinical problems being studied. Does shooting animals in a laboratory replicate the contaminating conditions associated with being shot in Flanders fields, Stalingrad, the Sinai peninsula, or Dak To? Probably not. Medical officers must remember that animal experimentation has limited relevance to combat-casualty care, and must exercise judgment when predicating changes in established policies of wound management based on the results of laboratory investigations. Animal experimentation is useful, but in the absence of clinical trials, most results cannot be extrapolated directly from laboratory animals to human battlefield casualties.

PRACTICAL ASPECTS OF MANAGING SOFT-TISSUE COMBAT WOUNDS

Battlefield surgeons may find that mass-casualty situations are more confusing and difficult than they had supposed. They must make decisions in real time with no more than a few minutes allocated to each casualty, synthesizing all that they have learned about the wounding effects of various weapons, whether and how much to debride, and which wounds are most likely to become infected. Knowledge of theoretical wound ballistics may allow the surgeon to make the necessary decisions more easily.

Management Options

The basic principles of managing soft-tissue combat wounds follow; technical aspects of implementing these surgical options are considered in greater detail at the end of the chapter. Medical officers are also advised to consult the relevant chapters of the *Emergency War Surgery* NATO handbook. The first actions to be taken must address the presence of chemical contamination and the acute life-threatening conditions considered by the Advanced Trauma Life Support (ATLS) course offered by the American College of Surgeons. The material that follows applies only *(a)* when soft-tissue wounds are the major treatment problem or *(b)* after the more seriously wounded casualties have been treated.

Infected Wounds—Incision and Drainage. The presence or absence of clinical infection when a soft-tissue wound is first seen is the most important determinant of the treatment the casualty will receive. A septic wound should be opened, its pus drained, foreign material removed, and grossly necrotic tissue excised. The surgeon must design the incision so that drainage will be optimal, and make a counterincision if good dependent drainage would otherwise be questionable. A fasciotomy is mandatory if there is any possibility that a compartment syndrome will develop.

Noninfected Wounds—Nonoperative Treatment. Two options are available to the surgeon who is managing a soft-tissue wound that has no signs of infection: *(a)* nonoperative—simply clean the wounds of entrance and exit (if there is one) and give antibiotics or *(b)* operative—give antibiotics to all casualties and proceed to debridement.

Noninfected Wounds—Minor Debridement. Open the wounds of entrance and exit (if there is one), evacuate blood clots and foreign material, and inspect the lining of the permanent cavity. Open the full extent and depth of the permanent cavity. This frequently requires that fascia must be incised; incision of the fascia is as important as incision of the skin. No further treatment is required if there is little evidence of a zone of extravasation. (In practice, however, most surgeons feel compelled to remove at least a scant amount of tissue.) By degrees, minor debridement passes into major debridement.

Noninfected Wounds—Major Debridement. An extensive zone of extravasation in the wound dictates that the surgeon perform major debridement—excision sufficient to expose normal-looking tissue (that is, the color, consistency, circulation, and contractility appear grossly normal) in the wall of the permanent cavity. Dress the wound so that drainage is not precluded and apply a splint (to minimize pain and swelling in and around the wound) whenever major debridement has been performed on either legs or arms. The wound should *never* be packed.

Wounds of the face or scalp can be closed as part of the initial management, because their sepsis rate is acceptably low. Wounds of the remainder of the body surface are closed by: *(a)* delayed primary closure, which is performed 4–6 days after the initial care or *(b)* secondary closure, which is usually performed more than 10 days after the initial care. (A more complete distinction between delayed primary and secondary closure will be made later in this chapter.) The dressing applied to the wound after the initial surgery *must not be removed* before delayed primary surgery is attempted unless there are compelling reasons such as *(a)* extensive bleeding, *(b)* pus draining through the dressing, *(c)* evidence of sepsis for which there is no apparent site other than the wound, or *(d)* severe and increasing pain.

Echelons of Care

It is not possible to consider the care of ballistic wounds of soft tissue divorced from the echelons of military medical care. The *first echelon* of care—the battalion aid station—and the *second echelon* of care—the division- or brigade-level medical company—have as their mission providing first aid, initial triage, and if necessary, preparing the casualty for evacuation to a higher echelon. Their essential function is to assure that the casualty with penetrating trauma receives an effective antibiotic upon arrival at a medical treatment facility (MTF). Since the second echelon has a holding capability, it is perfectly feasible to provide nonoperative care there to selected casualties with ballistic wounds of soft tissue. Data from the Vietnam War indicate that one-fourth or more of casualties with soft-tissue wounds need not be evacuated beyond the division-level MTF.

The *third echelon* of care—the corps-level evacuation and combat support hospitals—has as its mission providing initial wound surgery. Most soft-tissue wound debridement will be performed in third-echelon facilities. Mobile Army Surgical Hospitals (MASHs)—which are also third-echelon units, but which are usually located further forward with the division-level medical assets—have as their mission performing emergency or resuscitative surgery. Since soft-tissue wounds do not usually constitute immediate life-threatening problems, they would not usually be seen at a MASH, unless they were debrided there in conjunction with the management of severe visceral or extremity wounds. Although wound closure can be done at third-echelon facilities, their limited holding capacity and the need to maintain adequate resources for the care of incoming casualties make such surgery there undesirable.

The *fourth* and *CONUS echelons* of care—from general hospitals to medical centers—perform definitive and reconstructive surgery. Most wound closures are performed at fourth-echelon facilities. However, in mass-casualty situations and when third-echelon facilities are not fully operational, casualties with less-severe soft-tissue wounds may be evacuated from the first and second echelons to the fourth echelon (and even CONUS) for wound debridement.

Matching Injuries and Options

In the broadest sense, whether or not a penetrating wound becomes septic will be determined by the interaction of:

- the magnitude of tissue damage
- the magnitude of bacterial contamination
- the timeliness and appropriateness of care

The interaction of these three factors can be visualized in highly simplified form (Figure 5-12). These individual factors may be thought of as one-dimensional vectors, which differ from war to war (Table 5-14). The one-dimensional vectors define a vector in three dimensions; the length of this vector will, in some general sense, determine the probability that sepsis will develop in a wound. Figure 5-13 was drawn using the same coordinates that were developed in Figure 5-12 and data from Table 5-14, and demonstrates that soft-tissue wounds sustained during the Vietnam War were less likely to become septic than wounds sustained during World War I. Therefore, the minimal therapy required to prevent sepsis from developing might also have been different in the two wars, and nonoperative therapy—or no therapy at all—rather than debridement might have been feasible in some Vietnam War–casualties. Still using the same three coordinates that were used in Figures 5-12 and 5-13, Figure 5-14 generalizes this concept with two hypothetical casualty populations. The inner region indicates a population with clean wounds and slight tissue damage who receive prompt care. Nonoperative treatment suffices for this population. Beyond the inner region lies a population with dirty wounds and more massive tissue damage who receive delayed care. Nonoperative care will not be sufficient for this population; debridement offers the only hope to abort

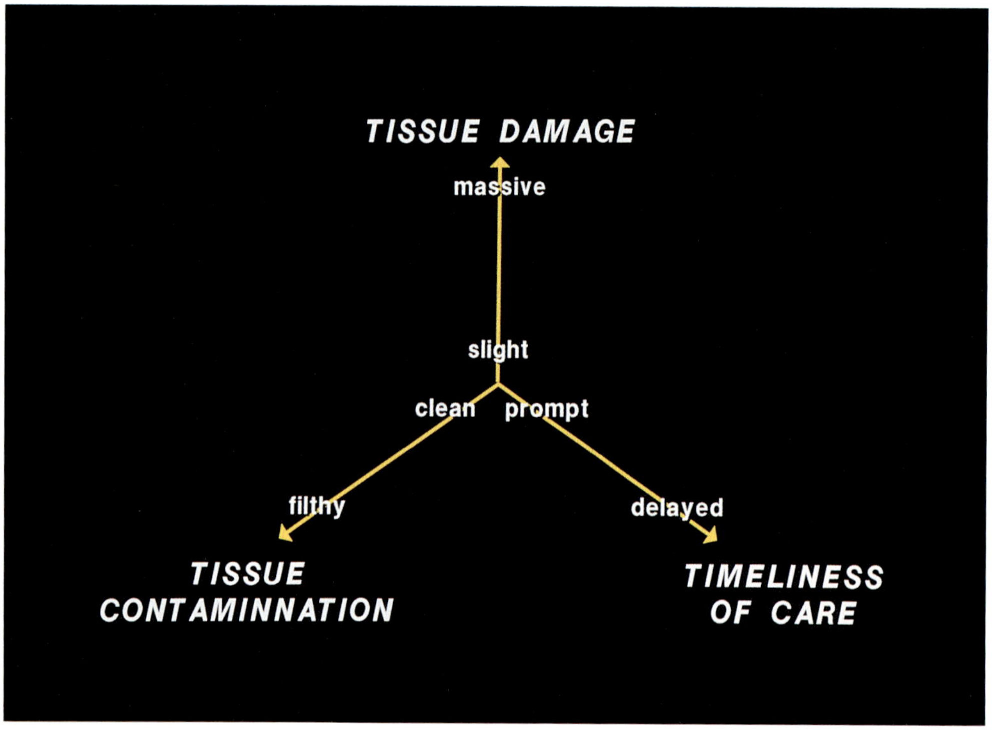

Fig. 5-12. The vertical axis shows the magnitude of tissue damage, the left horizontal axis the magnitude of tissue contamination, and the right horizontal axis the timeliness of care.

TABLE 5-14

DETERMINANTS OF WOUND SEPSIS IN VERY DIFFERENT WARS

Determinants	World War I	Vietnam War
Tissue damage (typical injury)	massive: several-gram fragments from random-fragmentation munitions	small: 200-mg fragments from improved-fragmentation munitions
Tissue contamination	dirty	clean (1/3 were sterile)
Timeliness and appropriateness of care	8–24 hours, no effective antimicrobials	1 hour, antibiotics

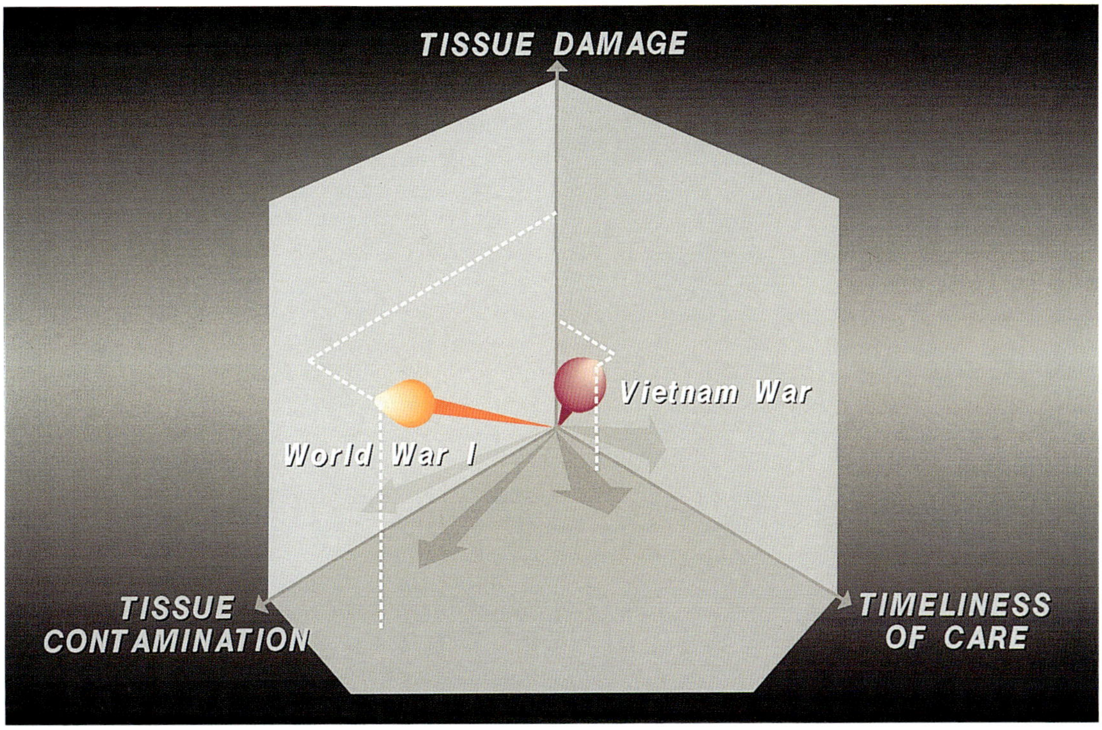

Fig. 5-13. The same coordinate system that was described in Figure 5-12 is used here. The World War I vector indicates the greater potential for wound sepsis in that war.

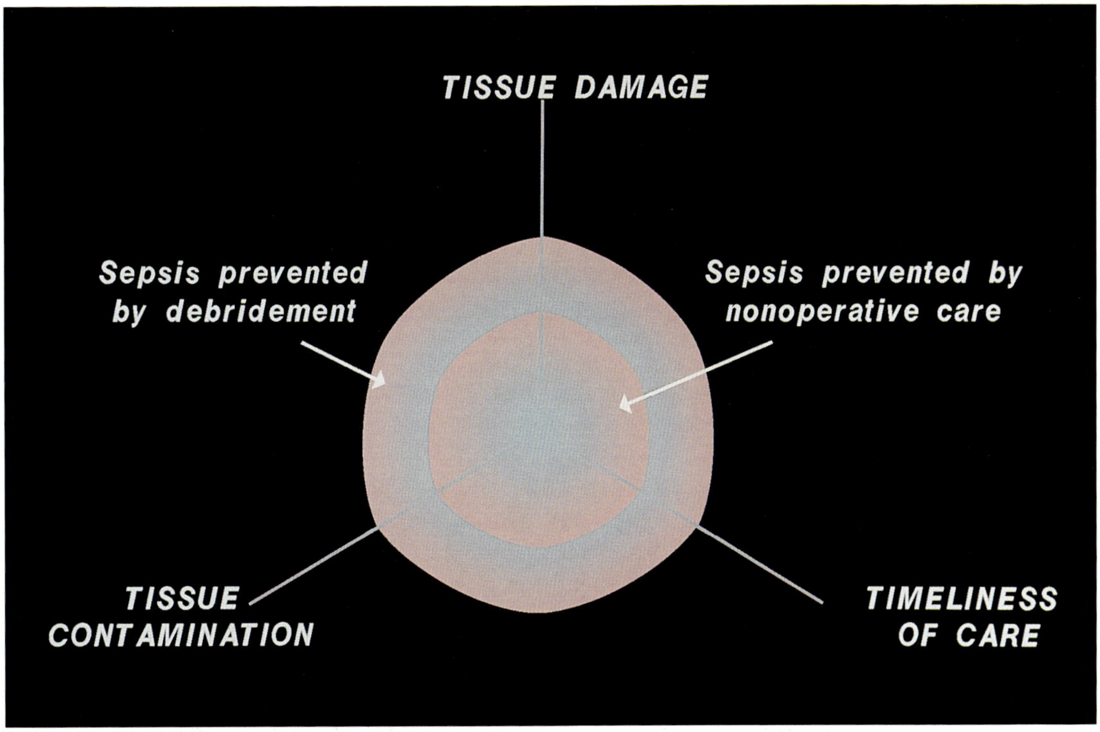

Fig. 5-14. Still using the same three coordinates that were used in Figures 5-12 and 5-13, the inner region represents a population of combat casualties with wounds that will do well with nonoperative management. Moving out from the center is a region where debridement is required to prevent sepsis. The outermost region represents a population whose severe wounds are already septic when first seen for surgical treatment.

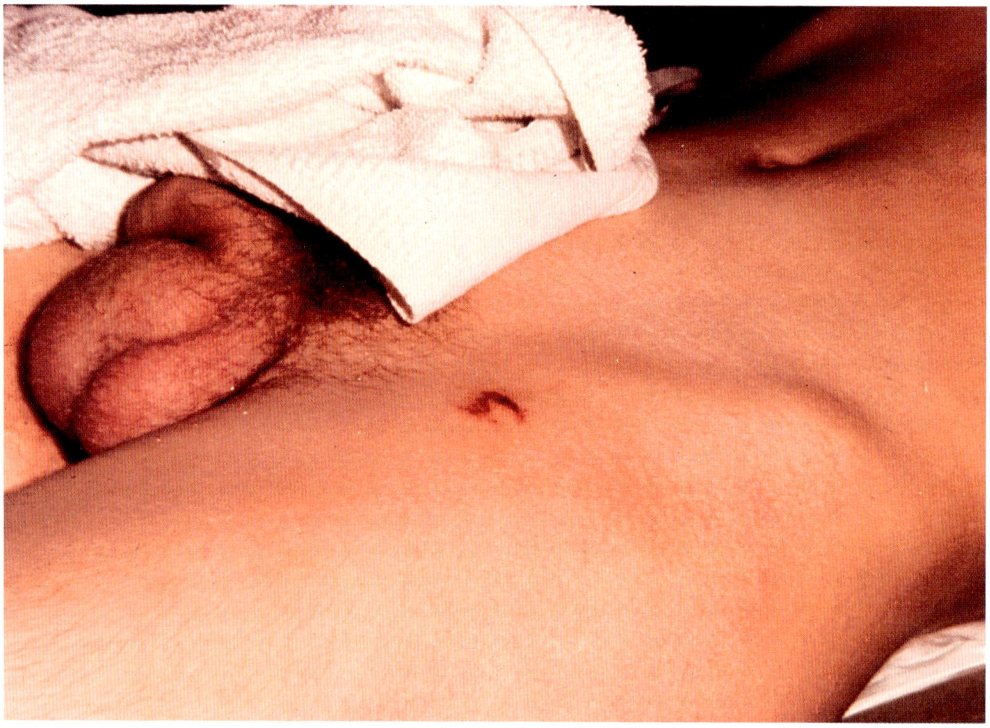

Fig. 5-15. This casualty has a small grenade-fragment wound of the left groin. Operative management is indicated, not so much because of the magnitude of either tissue damage or wound contamination, but to determine that the underlying neurovascular bundle is intact.
Source: Wound Data and Munitions Effectiveness Team

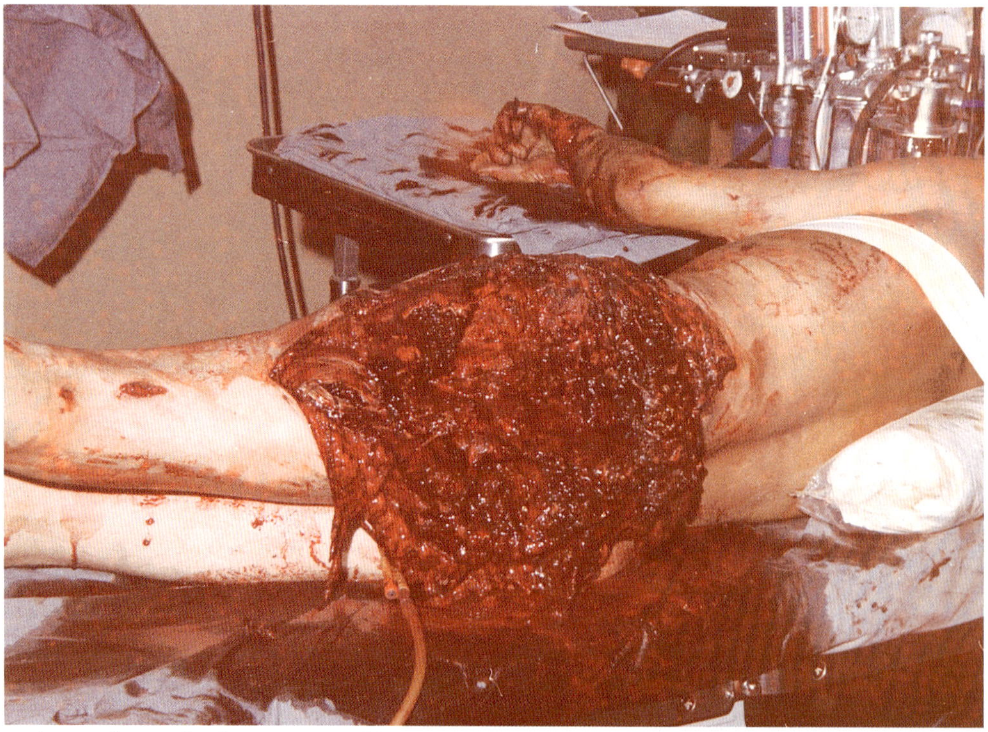

Fig. 5-16. A massive avulsion of soft tissue caused by an explosive munition. The management of this wound is beyond the scope of this chapter, but the wound must be freed of contamination and dead or injured tissue. Closure will be done in stages and will probably involve a combination of skin flaps and grafts. This wound would be an ideal one to treat initially with topical antimicrobials.
Source: Wound Data and Munitions Effectiveness Team

sepsis. All wounds lying in the outermost region are (or will become) septic due to the extent of the tissue damage, the magnitude of bacterial contamination, and delayed casualty care. What Figure 5-14 suggests should be obvious to medical officers: that possible treatment options should be matched to individual injuries. During wartime, however, mass casualties and echelon-based care may make this ideal difficult to achieve. Doctrine dictates that the treatment most likely to succeed be the treatment rendered first. In combat surgery, there is no time for a second attempt on a given casualty; thus, medical officers have a propensity to overtreat.

Soft-Tissue Trauma—An Overview of Typical Combat Wounds

The spectrum of penetrating injury to the soft tissues extends from minor wounds (Figure 5-15) to massive mutilating trauma (Figure 5-16). The necessity for surgery in managing the casualty shown in Figure 5-16 is obvious. But it may not be so obvious that surgery also has a role in managing the casualty shown in Figure 5-15. The management question that must be answered is: Where did the projectile go? This wound requires surgery, not because the surgeon expects to encounter either massive tissue damage or contamination, but because the wound is near important anatomical structures—in this case the vessels and nerves of the femoral triangle. Thus in many instances the indication for surgery is not simply one of soft-tissue wound management. (Of course, once the wound has been opened, soft-tissue wound management may be indicated.)

Some of the range of typical soft-tissue combat wounds are shown schematically in Figures 5-17 through 5-26. Consider the thigh to be the target. The permanent cavity is shown as a void, while the surrounding dotted region shows the zone of extravasation. The projectiles, not shown, enter from the left.

Figure 5-17 shows a wound that a small, low-velocity grenade fragment might make. The wound tract is blind. The small amount of tissue that may have been injured by temporary cavitation is found immediately adjacent to the wound of entrance. There is little or no swelling or tenderness deep to the wound of entrance. Many combat wounds in Vietnam were of this type, and with the advent of improved-fragmentation munitions that produce tiny projectiles, this type of wound is likely to be the one most commonly encountered in living casualties on the modern battlefield.

Figure 5-18 shows a wound that either a large, low-velocity fragment or a small, high-velocity fragment might make. There is a large wound of entrance but no wound of exit. The tissue around the wound of entrance is swollen and bruised, and the substantial injury extends inwards like an inverted cone. Many combat wounds in World War I were of this type.

Figure 5-19 shows a wound that a stable fléchette might make. This projectile easily perforates tissue, leaving a tiny permanent cavity with little if any zone of extravasation. The en seton wounds of entrance and exit are needle-like holes.

Figures 5-17 through 5-19 show solitary wounds, but medical officers will commonly encounter casualties with multiple wounds like these from fragmentation munitions and fléchettes. If the casualty is struck by projectiles in close proximity to one another, the potential exists for a synergistic interaction, producing greater tissue damage than might have been expected from the simple summation of the individual wound tracts.

Figure 5-20 shows a wound that a large-caliber, low-velocity, stable, nondeforming pistol bullet might make. The wounds of entrance and exit are small. Most of the tissue damage resulted from the bullet's cutting action. The size of the zone of extravasation is trivial. Many civilian gunshot wounds are like this.

Figure 5-21 shows a wound that a small-caliber, high-velocity, stable, nondeforming rifle bullet might make. The wounds of entrance and exit are small. The bullet's cutting of the tissue caused most of the damage. The size of the zone of extravasation is trivial. Note that the only real difference between this and the wound shown in Figure 5-20 is that the permanent cavity made by the low-velocity, but larger-caliber, bullet is larger. This is an example of an en seton bullet wound.

Figure 5-22 shows a wound that the same bullet described in Figure 5-21 might have made, except that this bullet developed significant yaw midway along its trajectory through the tissue. Consequently, both the permanent cavity and the zone of extravasation are greatly enlarged. A wound like this in an extremity produces noticeable tenderness, swelling, and skin ecchymosis. Note that the wound of exit is not different from the wound of entrance; therefore, the bullet must have displayed a small angle of yaw when it exited. Note also that the initial portion of the trajectory is identical to the one shown in Figure 5-21. Thus, because a projectile must travel a characteristic minimum distance within a target before it becomes unstable, the target's thickness is an important determinant of the nature of the wound.

Figure 5-23 shows a wound that might have been

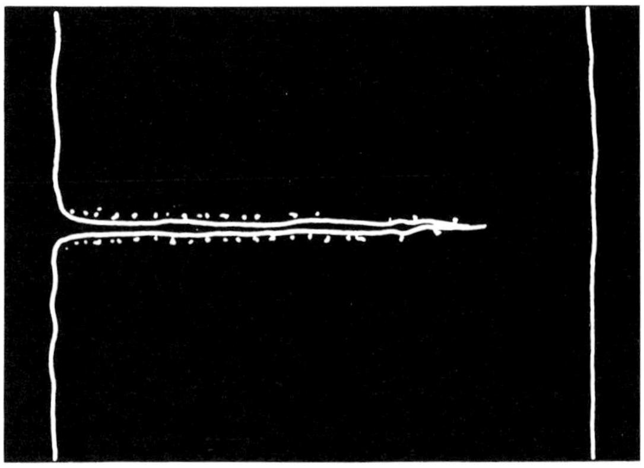

Fig. 5-17. Schematic representation of a blind wound made by a small, low-velocity fragment. The wound of entrance measures a few millimeters across. In this and all Figures 5-18 through 5-26, the permanent cavity is shown as a void and the zone of extravasation is shown as dots.

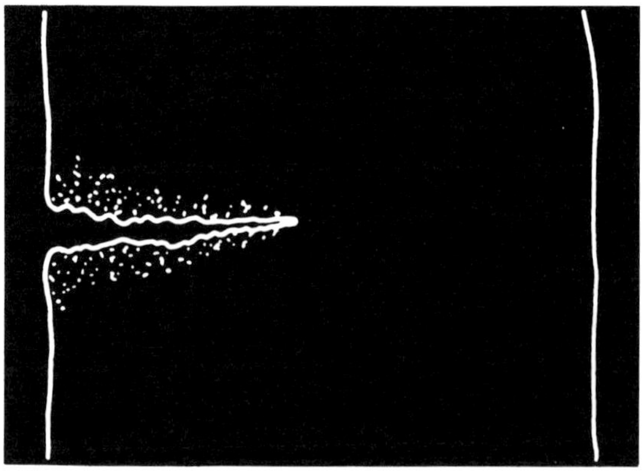

Fig. 5-18. Schematic representation of a blind wound made by a large fragment. The wound of entrance measures 1 cm across. The permanent cavity and the zone of extravasation are large.

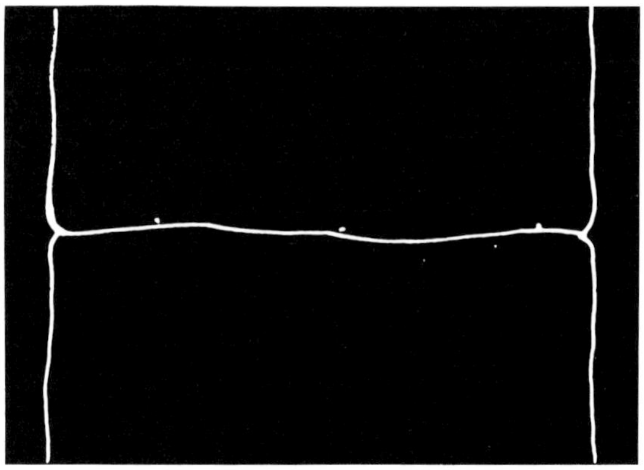

Fig. 5-19. Schematic representation of a perforating wound made by a stable fléchette. The wound of entrance is a needle-like hole and there is essentially no zone of extravasation.

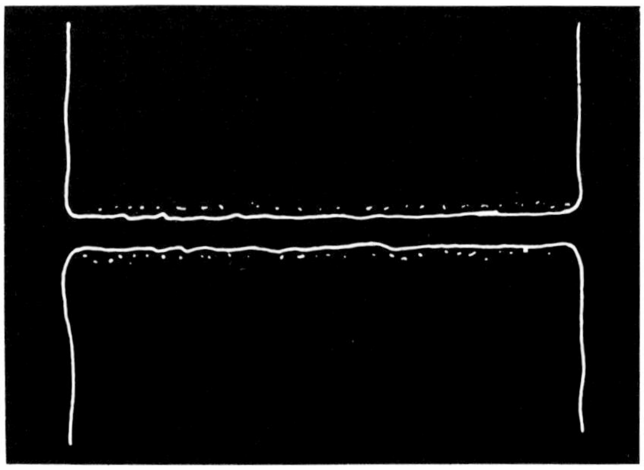

Fig. 5-20. Schematic representation of a perforating wound that a stable, nondeforming, large-caliber pistol bullet might make.

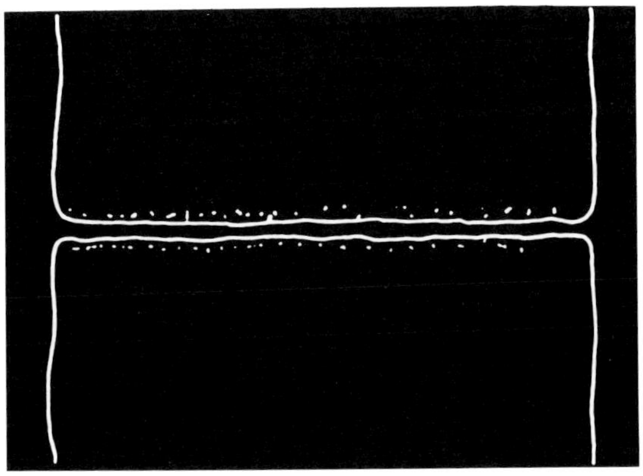

Fig. 5-21. Schematic representation of a perforating wound made by a stable, nondeforming, small-caliber rifle bullet. The zone of extravasation is small.

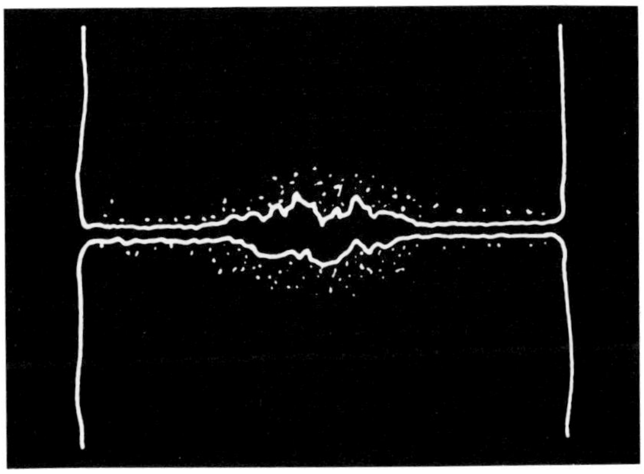

Fig. 5-22. Schematic representation of the wound that might result if the same bullet described in Figure 5-20 had developed substantial yaw midway along its trajectory through the thigh. The wound contains a large permanent cavity and zone of extravasation.

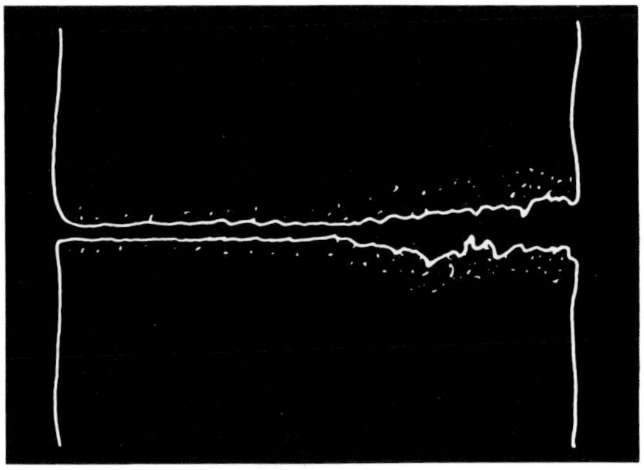

Fig. 5-23. Schematic presentation of the tissue-damage that might result if the bullet that made the wounds shown in Figures 5-21and 5-22 had yawed near the wound of exit. Note the large zone of extravasation near the large wound of exit.

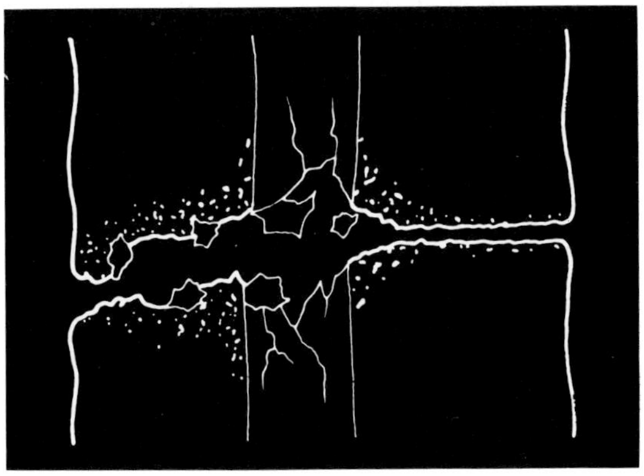

Fig. 5-24. Schematic representation showing the very large permanent cavity and zone of extravasation that might occur if the bullet represented in Figure 5-21 struck a large bone.

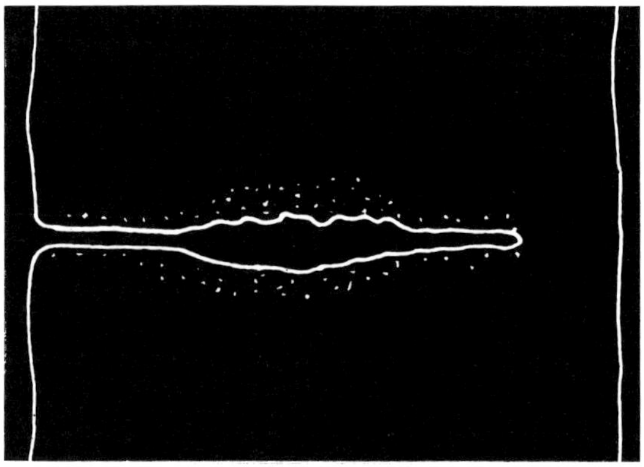

Fig. 5-25. Schematic representation of the large permanent cavity and zone of extravasation that might result from a deforming bullet.

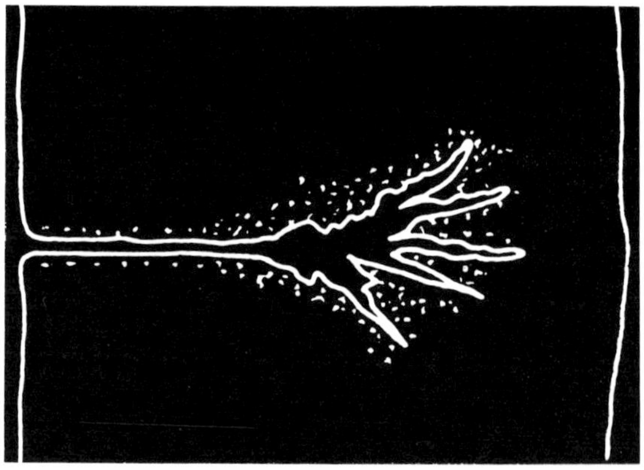

Fig. 5-26. Schematic representation of the tissue damage that might result when a bullet fragments within tissue.

made by the same bullet described in Figures 5-21 and 5-22, except that this bullet became unstable as it exited and produced an explosive wound of exit. Although this type of wound is possible, it occurs uncommonly.

Compare Figure 5-24 with Figure 5-21. A small-caliber, high-velocity, stable, nondeforming bullet perforated the target, but before it exited, it collided with the femur. Both bone and bullet shattered and formed multiple secondary missiles, creating an explosive wound of exit and an extensive zone of extravasation. This is a distinctly common type of combat wound. An extremity with this kind of wound will show obvious external evidence of significant injury such as deformity, tenderness, swelling, and skin ecchymosis.

Figure 5-25 shows a wound that a deforming soft-point or hollow-tip bullet might make. The large permanent cavity begins just distal to the wound of entrance and is surrounded by a large zone of extravasation. An extremity containing such a wound will show obvious external evidence of a significant injury such as tenderness, swelling, and skin ecchymosis.

Figure 5-26 shows a wound that a fragmenting bullet might make. The best-known current examples are the M193 or M855 bullets fired by the M16 assault rifles. After traveling 10–15 cm in tissue, the bullet destabilizes; the stresses arising from the resulting yaw cause the bullet to break up. The fragments become multiple secondary missiles that cut the tissue, which is then ripped apart by explosive temporary cavitation. A very large zone of extravasation surrounds the extensive permanent cavity. An extremity containing such a wound will show obvious external evidence of a significant injury such as tenderness, swelling, and skin ecchymosis.

Management Decisions

An algorithm can provide a theoretical framework for making management decisions in treating soft-tissue ballistic wounds, but no diagram in a textbook can reflect the actual conditions—confusion, danger, fatigue—on a battlefield (Figure 5-27). While algorithms may seem to be logical and carefully thought out, their real value will be known only when medical officers test them in the field.

The various components of the decision tree are defined by the typical schematic wounds shown in Figures 5-17 through 5-26. The drawings all show single wounds, but real combat wounds are not only frequently multiple, they may also have blast and burn components. Multiple confluent wounds in a small area (Figure 5-28) and polytraumas all speak for more

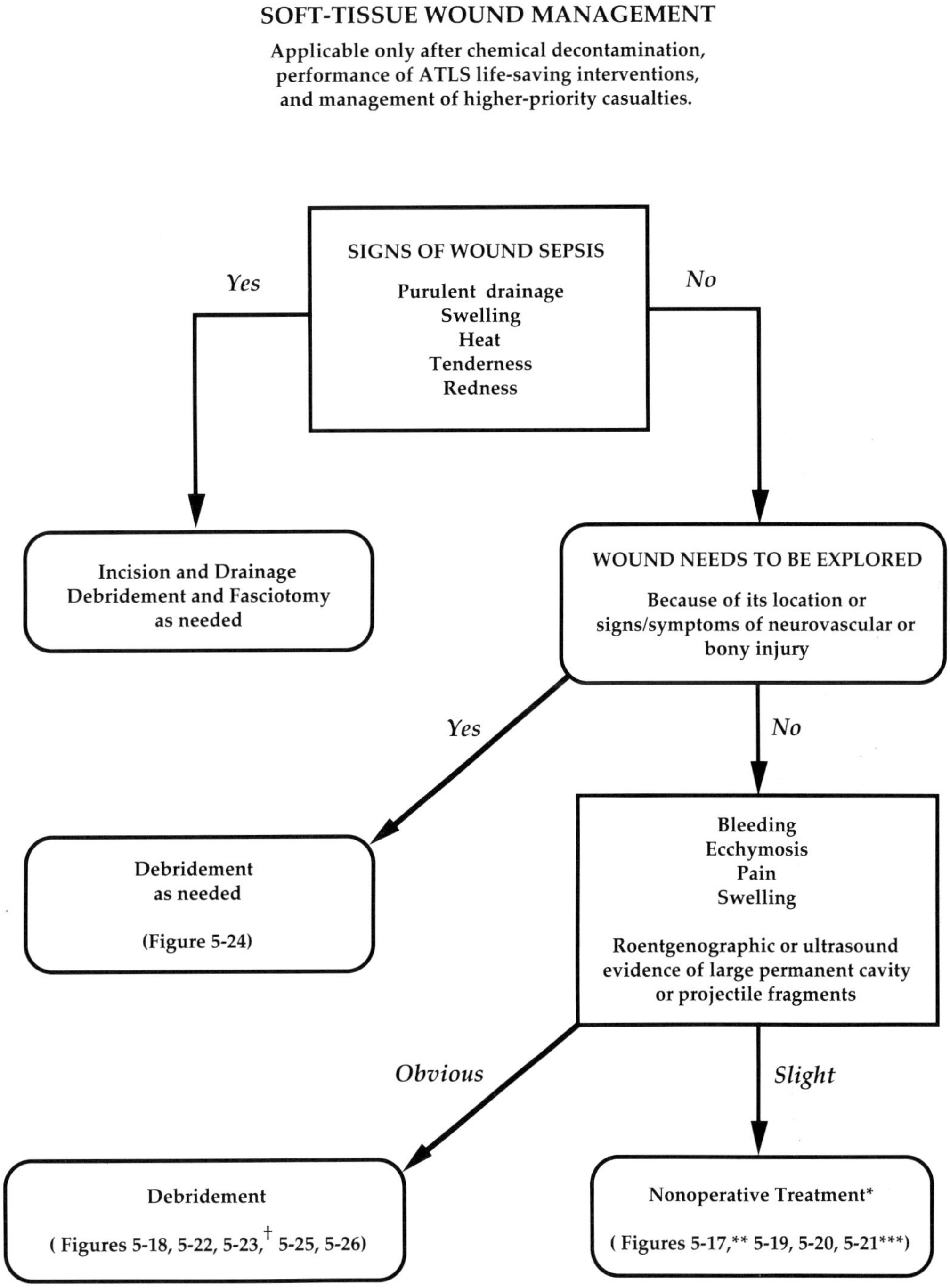

*Predicated upon the presence of effective antibiotic coverage, otherwise invalid.
**Including multiple minor superficial wounds, but multiple confluent wounds are an indication for debridement.
***At least sixty references (including English, German, and Russian sources) state that the treatment of en seton wounds need not be surgical.[67]
† Animal research has demonstrated that such wounds can be successfully treated with a nonoperative approach.[66]

Fig. 5-27. Algorithm for managing soft-tissue wounds

invasive surgical management. Furthermore, most experienced military surgeons are aware of instances, especially if the wounding projectile is a fragment, in which a seemingly benign wound of entrance conceals serious underlying soft-tissue damage.

The presence of multiple wounds in different body parts in the same casualty and the presence of multiple casualties with individual soft-tissue wounds requires that treatment be prioritized. Casualties with soft-tissue injuries only are usually assigned triage priorities of *delayed*. But those with destructive soft-tissue wounds of the buttocks or thighs may be given a higher priority for care because of their heightened propensity for anaerobic infections. Among multiple casualties with soft-tissue wounds only, those with wounds of the buttocks and thighs should be given first priority for care, followed by casualties with wounds of the calves, and finally, casualties with soft-tissue wounds of the arms.[68]

Destructive soft-tissue and orthopedic wounds resulting from buried antipersonnel mines or surface-detonations of explosive munitions of any type have the potential to massively contaminate the wound. Only radical debridement will suffice to prevent potentially fatal wound sepsis. Since the weapon that was used is an important determinant of both the degree of wound contamination and the magnitude of tissue damage, military surgeons must know the wounding characteristics of commonly encountered weapons.[69]

Surgical Interventions

For clarity of thought and expression, the description that Lieutenant Colonel Eugene H. Pool, M.D. (1874–1949) wrote of debridement, delayed primary closure, and secondary closure for the official surgical history of World War I is notable. From the broadest concepts to seemingly minor technical details, his treatise on soft-tissue wound management, excerpts of which follow, remains as valid today as it was when it was published in 1927. The original volume is largely unavailable today, except in libraries with historical collections.

During World War I, Dr. Pool served in France as Chief Surgeon of an evacuation hospital, was promoted to Consulting Surgeon to the Fifth Army Corps, and at the war's end was Consulting Surgeon to the First Army. He received the Legion d'Honneur, the Distinguished Service Medal, and a citation for "meritorious services" from General John J. Pershing.

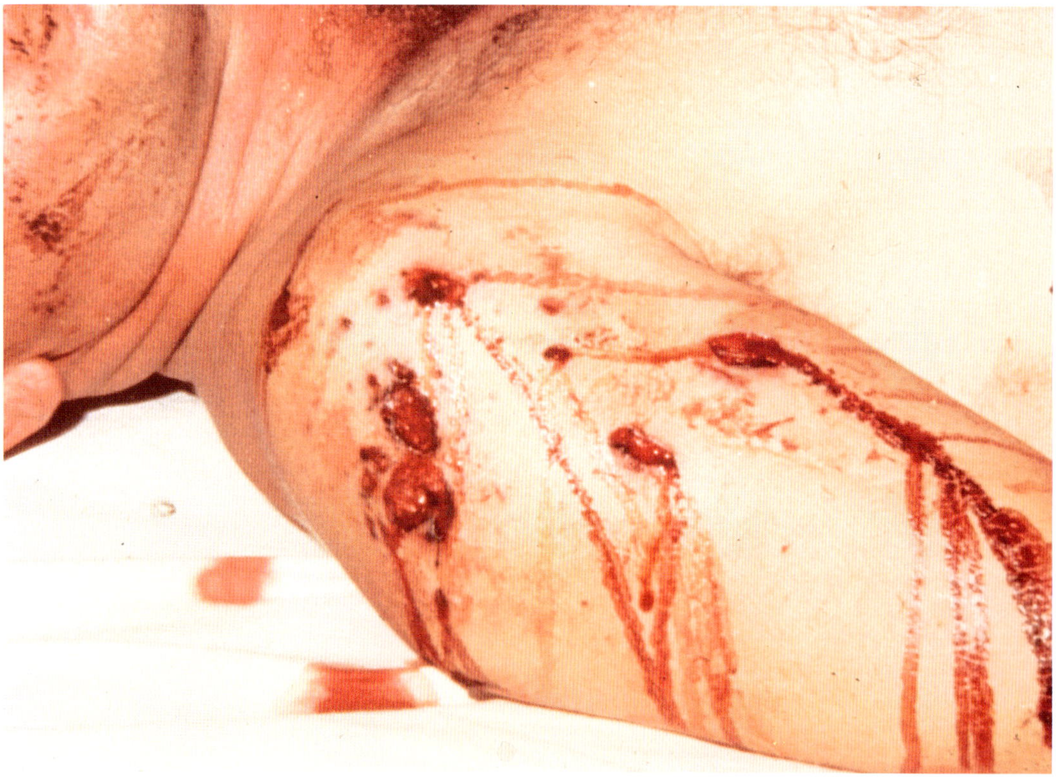

Fig. 5-28. An example of multiple, confluent, soft-tissue wounds. A nonoperative approach is contraindicated in this situation.
Source: Wound Data and Munitions Effectiveness Team

OPERATIVE TREATMENT

Operative treatment is indicated for [most casualties] as soon as possible after the receipt of the injury. Each hour increases materially the damage from infection. . . .

After the arrival of the patient at the hospital, expedition in the surgical treatment must be effected by the help of a well organized routine. The first essential is the careful sorting of cases at the admission tent. Patients presenting a considerable degree of shock should be sent to the shock ward. [Today this is called the resuscitation area. *Authors*] They must first be treated for shock, and operation deferred until reaction is evidenced by a rise in blood pressure. . . . [We know now that immediate surgery is the most effective resuscitation for an exsanguinating casualty. *Authors*] Walking wounded and slightly wounded [casualties] are referred to the dressing ward or to the service for [the] slightly wounded. Of the remainder the majority demand X-ray examination and early operation. The dressings are removed and the wounds carefully examined. Those whose condition does not contraindicate it are bathed. Cases with active bleeding, with sucking chest wounds, with penetrating abdominal wounds, with fractures of the femur, with penetrating wounds of the knee, and with multiple wounds receive the first attention. . . . Cases with uncomplicated wounds of the soft parts are, in general, cared for after the more urgent cases.

The success of operation depends largely upon the thoroughness of the roentgenologist's examination and the accuracy of his findings. . . . [Based upon our experience in subsequent wars, Pool's assessment of the value of roentgenography was overenthusiastic. *Authors*]

The patient should always be examined by the surgeon before anesthesia is begun. In wounds of the extremities, the surgeon should determine whether there is a nerve lesion and an arterial pulse. Apparently innocent wounds of the trunk may, in reality, be very serious. The possibility of intrathoracic or intraabdominal involvement should always be borne in mind. . . .

The preparation of the patient usually is done in the operating room on an extra table while the preceding operation is being completed. The wound is protected by gauze, the parts shaved thoroughly, and scrubbed with soap and water over a wide area. Application of chemicals may follow. [Pool was referring to an antiseptic such as Dakin's 0.5% sodium hypochlorite solution. Today, we would administer a systemic antibiotic. *Authors*] It is important to prepare a wide field and, in wounds of the extremities, to encircle the limb. The part is draped economically with towels and sheets.

A general anesthetic should be employed except in rare cases. . . . Local anesthesia is rarely used.

Debridement

The general plan or aim of surgical treatment is the prevention or limitation of infection, the early closure of the wound, and the preservation or reestablishment of function. The first indication is to obtain a clean wound. This is accomplished, primarily, by debridement of tissues—that is, by free incision and excision of injured and contaminated tissues, and by removal of foreign material carried by the missile into the wound.

The principle of this procedure may be visualized by considering a typical case of a wound of the soft parts with a tract from the skin to the interior of the muscles, containing a fragment of shell and pieces of clothing along its course, and having for its walls lacerated muscle. Pathogenic organisms are present throughout this tract. The devitalized, pulpified walls of the tract furnish an ideal medium for growth of bacteria. One can readily imagine that immediate wide excision of such a tract as a whole, including removal of the devitalized skin, subcutaneous tissues, aponeurosis, and muscle, together with the shell fragment, clothing, and microorganisms contained within the tract, will leave a healthy aseptic wound, provided the skin adjacent to the wound has been properly prepared and the operator has employed a technique comparable to that used in clean operations. To obtain an aseptic wound is the ideal desired, though it is doubtful whether this is actually achieved in any case. But, however skeptical one may be as to the total eradication of microorganisms under the conditions [that] prevail in these wounds, many wounds after operation undergo repair as if aseptic, and cultures and smears made from them are often sterile.

Even during times of greatest activity, debridement should be properly carried out and the best possible technique observed. The temptation to relax in these respects during periods of stress should be resisted. The time saved by careless work is not sufficient to warrant the additional risk incurred; only rarely is it justifiable to substitute incision and drainage for debridement in recent wounds.

The closure of the wound may be carried out by immediate or primary suture, delayed primary suture, or secondary suture.

Technique. [In the following passage, Pool describes the technique to use in treating a wound like that shown in Figure 5-29. Pool's original illustrations are reproduced as Figures 5-30 through 5-32. *Authors*] The skin incision, when possible, should be made parallel to the long axis of the limb. This permits wide exposure of the underlying tissues and renders subsequent suture less difficult. A transverse incision should rarely be employed. In the case of a deep

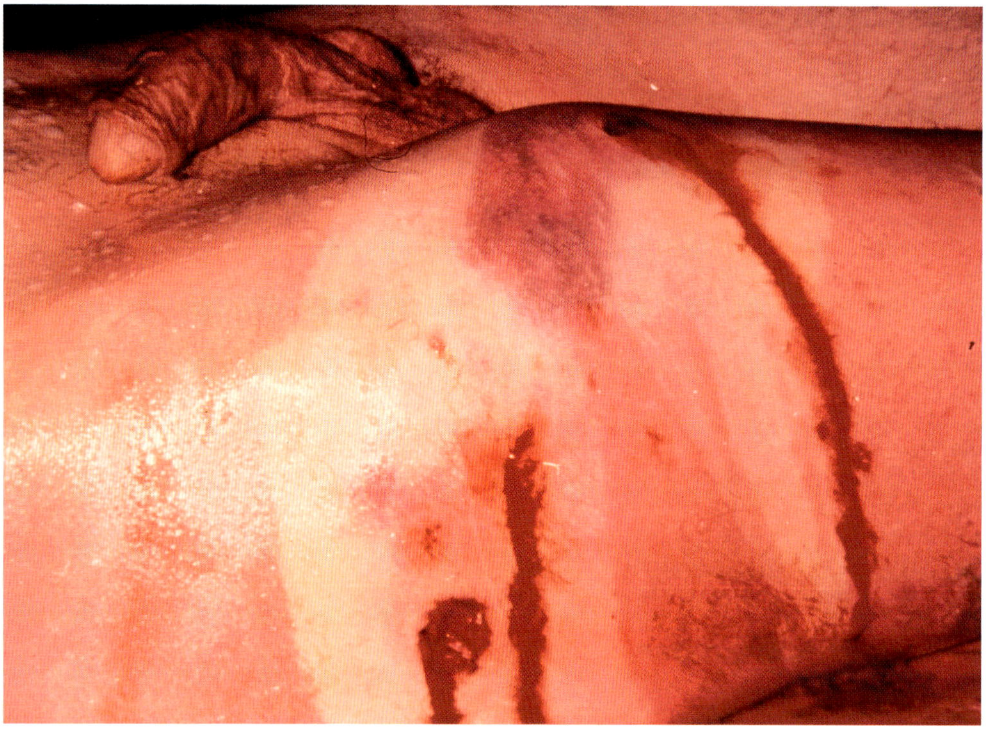

Fig. 5-29. The perforating soft-tissue wound of the thigh of a casualty who had been shot by an AK47 about 4 hours earlier. The wound of entrance is anterior. Note the extensive ecchymosis and swelling of the thigh—conditions that mandate operative intervention. The wound shown here is like the schematic one shown in Figure 5-22, and also represents the wound whose management Lieutenant Colonel Pool describes in this chapter.
Source: Wound Data and Munitions Effectiveness Team

transverse perforating wound, it is better to make two longitudinal incisions and work inward from each rather than make a transverse incision with division or excision of considerable muscle tissue. In the former case, suture is usually readily done at an early date, whereas in the latter, primary suture is often impossible because of the difficulty of uniting the severed muscle. Even when this is accomplished, the sutures frequently tear out and allow retraction of the muscle with resulting dead space and breaking down of the wound. When the transverse wound has not been closed primarily, or has reopened, secondary suture is delayed and is more difficult. The functional result is also less favorable on account of the transverse section of the muscle. [The actual management of the casualty whose thigh is shown in Figure 5-29 involved a transverse incision that divided most of the quadriceps muscle. *Authors*]

Transverse incisions should be employed in the extremities only in superficial wounds involving the subcutaneous tissues or with very superficial involvement of muscle. In the gluteal region and on the trunk the incision, in general, should be in the direction of the fibers of the underlying muscle. Occasionally, as in deep, transverse, through-and-through wounds of the calf, a long median incision may be employed advantageously; the tract is exposed in the middle of its course and debridement is carried out from this region in both directions. The skin wounds of entrance and exit are excised by small elliptical excisions and the wound edges approximated. [The midline incision, of course, is left open. *Authors*]

The operation itself consists in the free excision of all tissues with which the foreign body has come into contact and all devitalized tissues, except structures such as nerves, large vessels, and bones, whose removal would interfere with the function of the part and cause permanent disability. Free excision, however, does not mean ruthless, blind butchery of the parts but rather careful, intelligent dissection, with liberal removal of such parts as should be removed, and with equally scrupulous preservation of such parts as may be left with safety.

The wound itself, with all contused skin, is excised by removing an elongated ellipse of skin. No healthy skin should be sacrificed on the sides of the ellipse, as it is important to conserve as much skin as possible in the transverse plane of the limb to facilitate suture. This is especially important in the forearm. [During the Vietnam War, surgeons commonly excised a penny- or nickle-sized piece of skin around the wound of entrance of even tiny fragments. This served no useful purpose. *Authors*] There is no advantage in attempting debridement through a short incision. A deep debridement demands a long incision. The skin incision must always be vertical to the skin surface; the tendency

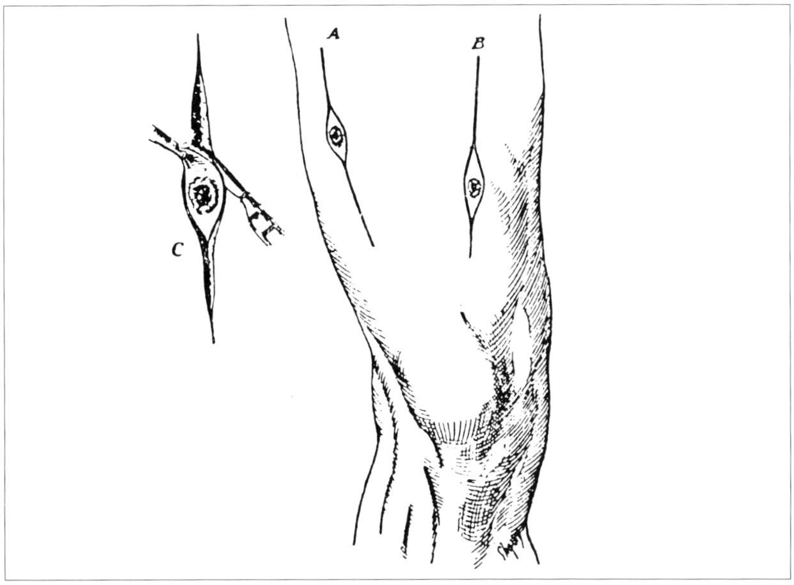

Fig. 5-30. Initial surgery for a wound like the one shown in Figure 29. Two parallel longitudinal skin incisions are made. Little skin is excised.
Source: Reference 70

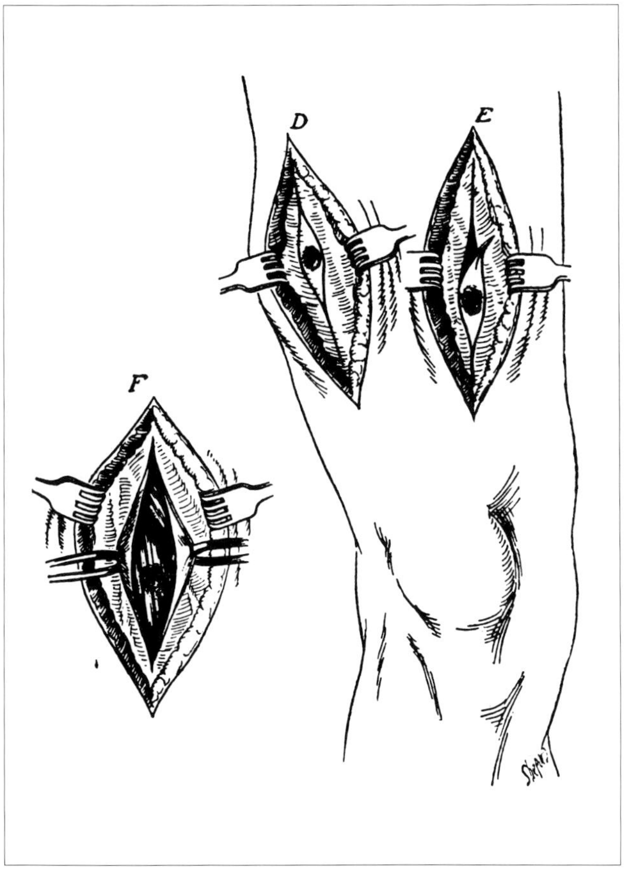

Fig. 5-31. The fascia is incised to further expose the permanent cavity.
Source: Reference 70

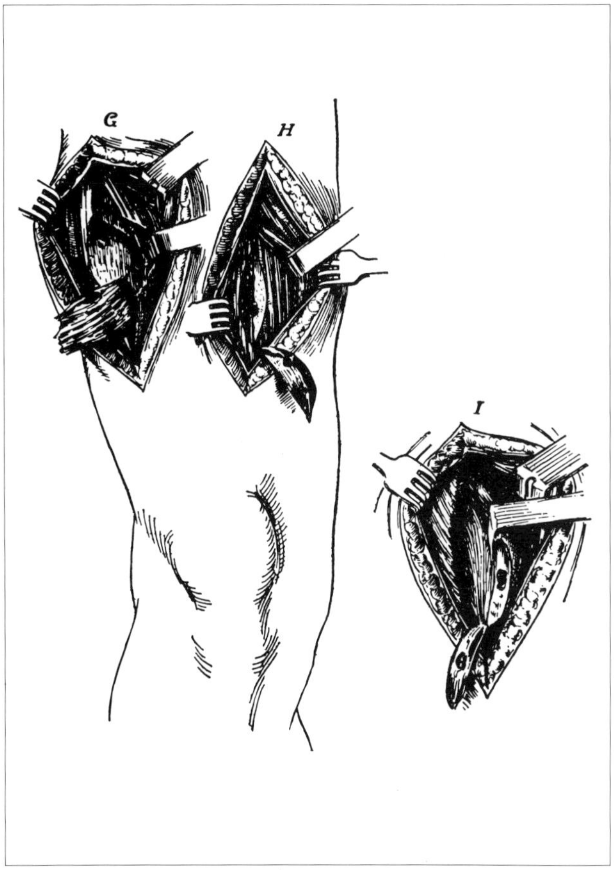

Fig. 5-32. Debridement of muscle is complete.
Source: Reference 70

to bevel the incision should always be avoided, as this interferes materially with satisfactory suture. . . .

When there are two wounds, one or two incisions may be employed as already described. Similarly, when a foreign body has taken a transverse or oblique course, penetrated a considerable distance, and lodged in the tissue, two incisions may at times be used to advantage, one over the foreign body and one to excise the wound of entrance, both being used for excision of the tract.

After excision of the skin edges, the instruments should be discarded or washed in alcohol. The skin edges are widely retracted and the subcutaneous tissues removed as far as there is evidence of laceration or contamination [Figure 5-30]. It is not necessary, however, to remove all blood-infiltrated subcutaneous tissue. In general, the fingers are kept out of the wound and dissection is made with instruments. Good exposure of every plane by retraction is essential, the edges being rolled outward and tooth retractors or some other form of clamp, such as the Allis forceps [used].

The aponeurosis is treated in the same manner as the skin—that is, by a long, straight incision with removal of the wound [that is, the permanent cavity] by a relatively narrow ellipse [Figure 5-31]. The aponeurosis is of great value in secondary sutures in the lower extremity and shoulder, and, therefore, should not be ruthlessly sacrificed. It must be emphasized that liberal excision of aponeurosis or skin is not necessary because it is not in these tissues that infection ordinarily originates or develops. The aponeurosis should be widely retracted and muscle planes exposed. It is this tissue [muscle] that favors infections. All traumatized and devitalized muscle must be removed. This demands excision for a distance of 0.5–1.0 cm on all sides of the tract. [This is the zone of extravasation. Note that the excision is not to extend for inches into the muscle; there is no need for radical excision of muscle. *Authors*] The dissection is made parallel to the fibers of the muscle; a long, relatively narrow ellipse is removed so that the sides tend to fall together after the excision. The dissection should be made by planes, muscles should be identified, and the situation of nerves and large vessels should always be borne in mind. The tract should be followed by sight, not by probing; for this purpose a reflecting headlight is indispensable. [Headlights were not issued to surgeons in Vietnam; army surgeons in the Panama campaign took their own. *Authors*] If the tract is lost between muscle planes, often slight flexion or extension of the limb will bring it into view. Careful hemostasis is necessary at all stages. Sponging of blood should be done by pressure and not by rubbing, because the latter method may carry organisms from an infected to a clean part of the wound and may cause a small tract to be lost to view. The foreign body should not be extracted until reached in the dissection, otherwise the parts fall together and the tissues immediately beyond the [foreign] body, which often contain clothing, may not be adequately excised [Figure 5-32]. When the excision is complete all exposed muscle must look healthy, contract when pinched with forceps, and ooze when snipped with scissors; otherwise its vitality has been diminished to such a degree as to favor gas bacillus infection. [Note Pool's criteria for deciding which muscle is devitalized: the four Cs; "look healthy" includes both consistency and color. *Authors*] At times the [surgeon's] finger must be introduced to search for the foreign body, but, as a rule, in cases where the tract is lost or where for other reasons difficulty arises in locating the foreign body, fluoroscopy should be employed. If this fails, the tissues should not be blindly torn up, but after a careful search one should desist, leaving the wound open and removing the foreign body subsequently, after more careful X-ray localization or under the [fluoroscope] screen. [Current practice de-emphasizes finding the foreign body. *Authors*] When the deep tissues are so markedly infiltrated with blood as to suggest the possibility of constriction of the muscle under the overlying fascia, this fascia must be incised so as to free the muscles from internal pressure.

When the fragment or tract is in proximity to a large vessel, as, for instance, the brachial vein, the vessel should be inspected. . . . [Pool goes on to describe the management of vascular injury. Not surprisingly, much World War I–doctrine pertaining to neurovascular repair is no longer valid. *Authors*] Though sudden and unexpected hemorrhage will occasionally confront the surgeon, the absence of an arterial pulse below the lesion and the widespread [bloody] infiltration of the soft tissues about the wound usually warn the operator in advance of the presence of a vascular lesion.

Care should be taken to avoid injury to nerves by careless dissection. A severed nerve should be united. . . . [Modern practice does not support nerve-repair during initial wound surgery. *Authors*]

When the excision has been completed all hemorrhage should be controlled. As little catgut as possible should be buried. [The same can be said of the synthetic absorbable sutures now available. *Authors*] The wound should be irrigated with saline. . . .

If the wound is left open, vasolined gauze is placed over the exposed skin edges and subcutaneous tissues in order to prevent the dressing from adhering and to lessen oozing and pain when the dressing is removed. . . . [Modern practice would cover the wound with fine-mesh gauze. The important point is to not pack the wound. *Authors*] Dry gauze is applied over this and the dressing kept in place with a bandage. . . .

Primary and Secondary Suture

There are two conditions under which war surgery is performed at the front: first, [during] relatively quiet periods; second, times when military activities are acute. . . .

The ultimate aim of treatment is to restore the soldier to full activity, with complete restoration of function, in as short a time as possible. Obviously, one of the conditions of such restoration is the repair of the wound. During quiet times, early closure of the wound may be undertaken successfully in a large proportion of cases. Great benefit thereby accrues both to the patient and to the service. . . .

It must be recognized, therefore, that local conditions such as the degree of battle activity alter materially the indications for suture, particularly for primary suture, in the advanced area.

[T]he general principles and [techniques] of the three varieties of suture of war wounds, namely, [*(a)*] primary suture, [*(b)*] delayed primary suture, and [*(c)*] secondary suture in wounds of the soft parts [follow:]

Primary Suture. Debridement having been completed, the choice of treatment lies between primary suture and leaving the wound open. If ideal conditions, that is, early and thorough debridement, have been approximated and the [casualties] can be watched for some days, primary suture may be made. In active periods, as in an offensive, when there are many wounded, the exigencies of a service demand haste in the primary operation, and the patient must be evacuated, passing from the operator's control soon after the operation. Under these conditions, primary suture should not be considered.

The advantages of primary suture are obvious; the disadvantages consist chiefly in the danger of closing within a wound, especially within a wound imperfectly debrided . . . anaerobes of the types [that] produce gas gangrene. A resulting gas bacillus infection, or a pyogenic infection in a few cases, will counterbalance many successful closures. . . . [Military doctrine during World War I did not absolutely prohibit primary closure. Pool discusses in detail the technical and administrative requirements for primary suture of war wounds and concludes that, as a general rule, only wounds of the face and scalp can be considered for primary closure with any frequency. *Authors*]

Technique. Thorough debridement is essential, and aseptic technique must be observed throughout the operation. Hemostasis must be complete. The wound should be washed sufficiently to remove blood clots and loose fragments of tissue. . . . The muscles and aponeuroses are approximated with interrupted catgut. As little and as fine catgut should be introduced as will approximate the tissues and obliterate dead spaces. The skin and subcutaneous tissues are closed with interrupted silkworm gut. [Modern practice employs synthetic absorbable sutures rather than catgut for the subcutaneous tissues and fine wire or nonfilamentous sutures for the skin. *Authors*] Drainage should be avoided. If employed, the drain should be removed as soon as possible, in general, within 24 hours. . . . After the dressing has been applied, the part should be immobilized.

A wound [that] has been closed by primary suture should be examined within 24 hours. . . . These precautions can not be too strongly urged. [These precautions were taken to avoid the development of gas gangrene, which Pool discusses at length. *Authors*]

Delayed Primary and Secondary Suture. The distinction between delayed primary suture and secondary suture is one of tissue repair rather than of time. Delayed primary suture is one in which the edges can be approximated and will unite without excision of tissue. Secondary suture is one in which the epidermis has grown inward and must be excised for proper union [to occur]. This is, in general, about one week. In late secondary suture, dense granulation tissue must also be excised. . . . [Pool goes on to discuss the need for bacterial cultures of the wound as a determinant of when it may be closed. His primary concern was finding hemolytic cocci; their presence precluded wound closure. Of course today the hemolytic cocci would be eradicated with an antibiotic and the wound would be closed with antibiotic coverage. *Authors*]

Delayed primary suture is usually made within 6 days after the primary operation. The advantages of this method are the practical elimination of the danger of gas bacillus infection and the marked lessening of the danger of pyogenic infection. The disadvantages are the possibility of post-operative contamination of the open wound and the subjection of the patient to a second operation. . . . [Thus the modern prohibition of changing dressings. *Authors*]

Technique. The details of [delayed primary closure] are the same as for primary suture. . . . [There are] two varieties of secondary suture:

Secondary suture of the skin. The incision surrounds the new epidermis along the wound edges. A healthy normal skin edge must be present for successful suture. The skin is freed by undermining in all directions as far as necessary in order to approximate the edges with minimum tension. The separation is made in the plane immediately superficial to the deep fascia. Only dense scar tissues or projections of granulation tissue are removed from the wound. The deep fascia are then approximated with interrupted catgut when possible; usually this may be done in the thigh and shoulder, but rarely in the leg, arm, and forearm. The skin and subcutaneous tissues are closed with silkworm gut. . . . [Modern practice would use wire. In primary and delayed primary closure (but uncommonly in secondary closure) the skin edges can sometimes be approximated with tape, which is less traumatic than suturing and therefore desirable. *Authors*] The results of suture are directly proportionate to the degree of tension. If there is extreme tension, infection may be expected. . . .

Secondary suture reconstruction. The granulation tissue and scar tissue are removed from the entire wound and all layers are reconstructed by suture.[70]

ANAEROBIC INFECTIONS OF MILITARY IMPORTANCE

Gas Gangrene

Gas gangrene is the generic name for three discrete clinical syndromes that manifest severe and frequently fatal infections. They are especially interesting to military surgeons because they are rarely seen in civilian medicine. Clostridial infections were especially common during World War I, perhaps because of the unique (that is, the heavily manured) battlefield conditions in Europe.

The three syndromes are known by a variety of names:

- *Necrotizing fasciitis,* also called *anaerobic cellulitis* and *clostridial cellulitis.* This infection involves subcutaneous and connective tissues and spreads along fascial planes without destroying either the overlying skin or the underlying muscle. The pathology is primarily due to the growth of toxigenic clostridia such as *C. perfringens* or *C. septicum,* but the usual presence of a polymicrobial flora—including streptococci and staphylococci—suggests that the fully developed syndrome requires the synergistic interaction of several bacterial species.
- *Gas gangrene,* also called *clostridial myonecrosis* and *clostridial myositis.* This clostridial infection invades and destroys living muscle. *C. perfringens* is present in most cases, but depending upon the locale, other toxigenic clostridia such as *C. novii* and *C. septicum* may also be present.
- *Anaerobic streptococcal myonecrosis,* also called *streptococcal myositis.* This infection, also characterized by necrosis of living muscle, is caused by anaerobic streptococci of the tribe Peptostreptococceae. Like the other anaerobic infections, this usually indicates a mixed bacterial flora including aerobic streptococci and staphylococci.

The effects of all the forms of gas gangrene are devastating, but because their prognoses and therapies are very different, medical officers must learn to distinguish among these syndromes (Table 5-15). While a patient with any of the three fully developed syndromes will be gravely ill, the "explosive" onset of clostridial myonecrosis is a distinguishing feature that helps make the diagnosis. The actual kind of gas that is produced is not known, but its presence can be detected on a roentgenogram. The tissue and pus contain gas bubbles that are not only visible but also can be palpated under the skin. However, gas production is not necessary to establish the diagnosis, and the presence of gas, which may have been aspirated into the permanent cavity during temporary cavitation, does not necessarily indicate an anaerobic infection. Although wounds in the buttocks and legs are most likely to become the sites of anaerobic infections, all other wounds should be considered at risk.

Prevention is more important with these anaerobic infections than with any other diseases. Traditional prophylaxis has emphasized that tissue at risk for anaerobic infections be surgically removed. In fact, preventing gas gangrene has been the raison d'etre for much of the military surgeon's soft-tissue wound management. Today, however, perhaps less emphasis should be placed on prophylaxis by radical excision. Experimental and, to a lesser extent, clinical evidence suggest that early administration of antibiotics may be as beneficial to the casualty—and far less disfiguring.

Medical officers must not forget that gas gangrene is most commonly accompanied by a major vascular injury that causes extensive muscle ischemia. No systemic antibiotic—including penicillin—is likely to be effective in this circumstance. And there should be no doubt that surgery is the therapeutic intervention of choice when confronted with established clostridial myonecrosis.

Surgical intervention is required in all cases of anaerobic infection if for no other reason than to establish the extent of the infection. However, specific aspects of the surgery and the antibiotics employed depend upon the syndrome being treated.

***Anaerobic Fasciitis*.** Make incisions that expose the underlying fascia without devitalizing the overlying skin. Since a polymicrobial flora is likely, antibiotic therapy should involve using more than just penicillin, although it remains the agent of choice when clostridia and beta-hemolytic streptococci are present. Additional drugs that have been proposed are *(a)* an aminoglycoside, *(b)* clindamycin or metronidazole, and *(c)* ampicillin. Optimal post-operative wound care usually includes continuous wound irrigation. Note that skeletal-muscle debridement is not emphasized. This is usually unnecessary, although neglected anaerobic fasciitis associated with clostridia may progress to myonecrosis.

***Clostridial Myonecrosis*.** Radically excise in-

TABLE 5-15

DIAGNOSTIC FEATURES OF ANAEROBIC SOFT-TISSUE INFECTIONS

Syndrome	Necrotizing Fasciitis	Clostridial Myonecrosis	Streptococcal Myositis
Typical Wound	dirty, old, subcutaneous contamination	large muscle group containing dead muscle	not defined
Incubation	>3 days	<1 day	3–4 days
Onset	gradual	acute	insidious
Toxicity	slight	very severe	slight, then severe
Pain	absent	very severe	variable
Swelling	slight	marked	marked
Skin	normal	pale, then tense, bronzen, bullae	tense
Discharge	slight	variable	profuse
Gas	abundant, not in muscle	rarely pronounced in muscle	little
Smell	foul	sweet to foul	slight
Muscle	no change	necrosis	early edema, then necrosis

Source: Based on Table 20 in reference 41

fected—not just necrotic—muscle. (Some surgeons use Gram stains of excised muscle as a guide to the extent of the resection.) Amputating an extremity may be necessary and can be life-saving when the patient manifests severe systemic toxicity. Give Penicillin G intravenously at the rate of 1–2 million units every 2–3 hours (a total dose of 20 million units per day). Because most infections are polymicrobial, most authorities recommend using a second antibiotic—such as chloramphenicol—as well.

Serum therapy with an antitoxin directed against the principal toxins elaborated by the clostridia was successfully used during World War II, but for unknown reasons has since fallen into disuse. The vaccine is designed to inactivate the alpha toxin, a lecithinase, and the omega toxin, a protease. However, these antitoxins are no longer available through military supply channels.

Hyperoxia inhibits the growth of clostridia and decreases their production of toxins. Civilian surgeons have used hyperbaric oxygen therapy as an adjunct to surgery and antibiotics. The U.S. Air Force is presently attempting to solve the logistic and administrative problems that impede fielding hyperbaric oxygen in third-echelon surgical facilities.

Clostridial myonecrosis, although increasingly rare (only 22 instances out of a population of 132,000 Vietnam War casualties), remains one of the bona fide horrors of war (Figure 5-33).

Streptococcal Myositis. Surgical intervention in-

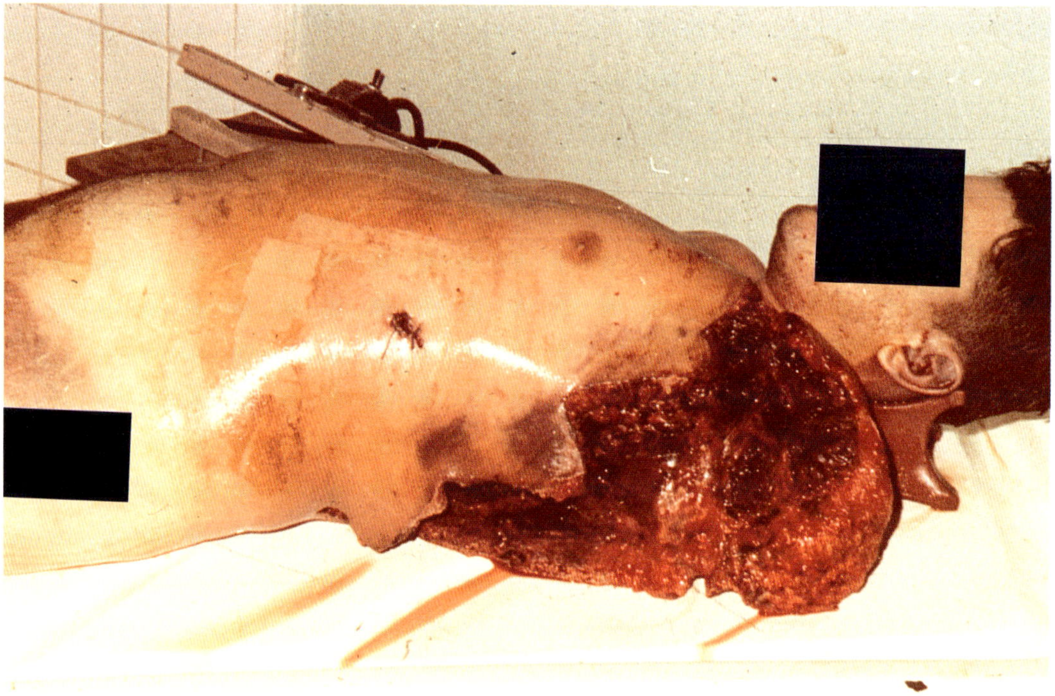

Fig. 5-33. This casualty sustained a perforating gunshot wound of his left shoulder. The bullet severed the axillary artery, which surgeons repaired during initial wound surgery. Signs and symptoms of clostridial myonecrosis were present within 8 hours after the casualty was wounded. Surgeons re-explored the wound, found that their arterial reconstruction had failed, and because gas gangrene was developing rapidly, performed a forequarter amputation. The casualty died 22 hours later. His bronzen, edematous chest wall is characteristic of this terrible disease.
Source: Wound Data and Munitions Effectiveness Team

volves excising the necrotic muscle, but because penicillin therapy will limit the spread of this disease, the extent of excision need not approach that practiced with clostridial myonecrosis. Extensive fasciotomies may be required to *(a)* alleviate vascular compromise and *(b)* allow antibiotics to reach the septic area. Administer Penicillin G intravenously at the rate of 1–2 million units every 2–3 hours until sepsis has abated.

Tetanus

Tetanus should not occur among American military combat casualties. All soldiers receive mandatory active immunization with tetanus toxoid when they are inducted, and all casualties, regardless of their injuries, receive a tetanus toxoid booster. Military medicine does not make the civilian distinction between minor, clean wounds and tetanus-prone wounds. Prophylactic administration of human tetanus immune globulin has not been necessary in past wars, no doubt because *(a)* the policy of universal active immunization is effective, and *(b)* military surgeons take excellent care of tetanus-prone wounds.

But remember that the successful tetanus prophylaxis of past wars partly depended on the fact that most soldiers were draftees who were discharged within 2 years—when their antibody levels would have been far above the minimum protective level. Members of today's professional army may serve many years after their initial immunizations; if they have not received a recent booster, they are at risk of developing tetanus if they are wounded. Data from World War I and World War II indicate that 1%–3% of nonimmunized casualties can be expected to develop tetanus.[71] In addition to the tetanus toxoid boosters that all casualties routinely receive, those at risk also require tetanus immune globulin (at least 250 units).[72]

Using antibiotics prophylactically will also decrease the occurrence of tetanus, since antibiotics such as penicillin, erythromycin, and tetracycline inhibit the reproduction of the vegetative phase of *Clostridium tetani.*

ANCILLARY ASPECTS OF WOUND BALLISTICS

Retained Projectiles

Most projectiles are nonperforating and are not removed at initial wound surgery, remaining lodged within the casualty's body. The indications for their subsequent removal include the following:

- proximity to an internal viscus, such as a bronchus or intestine, with the attendant possibility of subsequent erosion into the viscus
- ongoing infection or episodes of hemorrhage from the wound tract
- persistent pain or impairment of function
- psychological distress

These requirements are infrequently met; the overwhelming number of retained projectiles, especially those in soft tissue, cause no problems and need not be removed. Exceptions are projectiles in the central nervous system, the eyes, and the heart. Size is the main criterion for removing retained projectiles from less-sensitive areas such as the lungs and abdomen: In general, projectiles with diameters greater than 1.5 cm should be removed. No criterion has been established for removing projectiles retained in soft tissues except for the obvious indication of persistent local sepsis. But removing even large projectiles may be difficult. The foreign bodies are frequently hard to find, and the surgical exploration may cause even more tissue-damage than the projectile did. The history of military surgery contains many examples of "metal detectors," but none seem to have stood the test of time. Beyond two-view radiography, intraoperative fluoroscopy, and computed axial tomography—which are not likely to be available in combat-zone hospitals—the only additional diagnostic modality that has been suggested for use in the intraoperative localization of retained projectiles is high-frequency B-mode ultrasound.[73] Two aspects of retained projectiles require additional discussion: vascular migration and lead poisoning.

Migrating Projectiles. Rarely, a projectile may gain access to the casualty's vascular system and not cause life-threatening hemorrhage. Of course, most projectiles that penetrate into vessels that are large enough to have anatomical names cause massive exsanguination. The projectile may remain dormant at its original site for varying lengths of time, but eventually it will migrate to another part of the body where it may cause vascular obstruction. The WDMET database contains one example of this phenomenon: A casualty sustained a solitary wound in the left anterior superior chest (Figure 5-34). Surprisingly, although the roentgenogram showed a hemothorax, it showed no evidence of the projectile that caused it (Figure 5-35). Later the same day, the casualty complained of pain in his left leg, which was cool, pale, and pulseless. A roentgenogram of his left knee showed a fragment located in the area of the popliteal artery (Figure 5-36). The surgeon removed the fragment from the artery, and the patient had a benign post-operative course. The fragment must have entered a pulmonary vein and then migrated through the left atrium, the left ventricle, the aorta, the left common iliac artery, the left external iliac artery, the left femoral artery, and into the popliteal artery, where it lodged and cut off the circulation to the leg.

Among the 7,500 casualties listed in the Vietnam Vascular Registry, a team of vascular surgeons found migrating projectiles in only 22 of them.[74] Since the major clinical manifestation of projectile migration is vascular, this survey probably counted most of the cases that occurred during the Vietnam War. Assuming about 150,000 nonfatally wounded American casualties, the prevalence of migrating projectiles among combat casualties is probably less than 0.02%. About 80% of the migrating projectiles were found in the arterial circulation, which suggests that they entered through a pulmonary vein. The remaining 20% of projectiles were found in the venous systemic circulation. Although the usual pattern of migration is *antegrade* (that is, from the extremities to the lungs), retrograde venous migration has been described.[75] Fragments accounted for 90% of the migrating projectiles observed in Vietnam.

While migration can occur anytime after wounding, it most commonly occurs within 3 weeks. Removing a projectile that appears to lodged in a large central vessel before it migrates is clearly desirable, and longstanding doctrine recommends prophylactic removal of projectiles embedded in the heart.

Lead Poisoning. Most retained projectiles are fragments made of iron. But given the large number of people who have retained projectiles that are partially or completely made of lead, the number of reported cases of lead poisoning caused by retained projectiles is surprisingly low.[76] Nevertheless, lead poisoning does occur. Its clinical presentation can be quite pleomorphic and includes encephalopathy, anemia, nephropathy, and abdominal pain. Absorption of lead

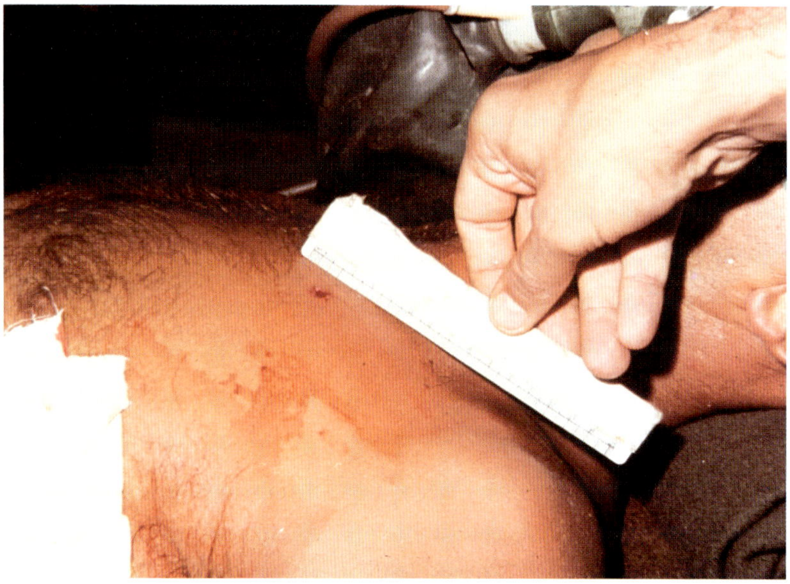

Fig. 5-34. This casualty was wounded by a fragment that entered his body through the left anterior superior chest wall. There was no wound of exit.
Source: Wound Data and Munitions Effectiveness Team

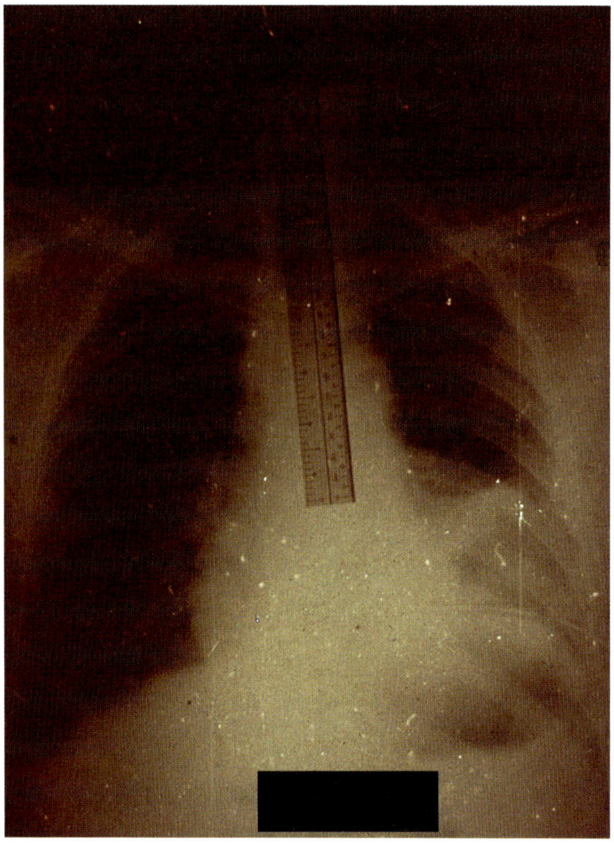

Fig. 5-35. This roentgenogram of the chest of the casualty shown in Figure 5-34 shows a hemothorax but no sign of the projectile.
Source: Wound Data and Munitions Effectiveness Team

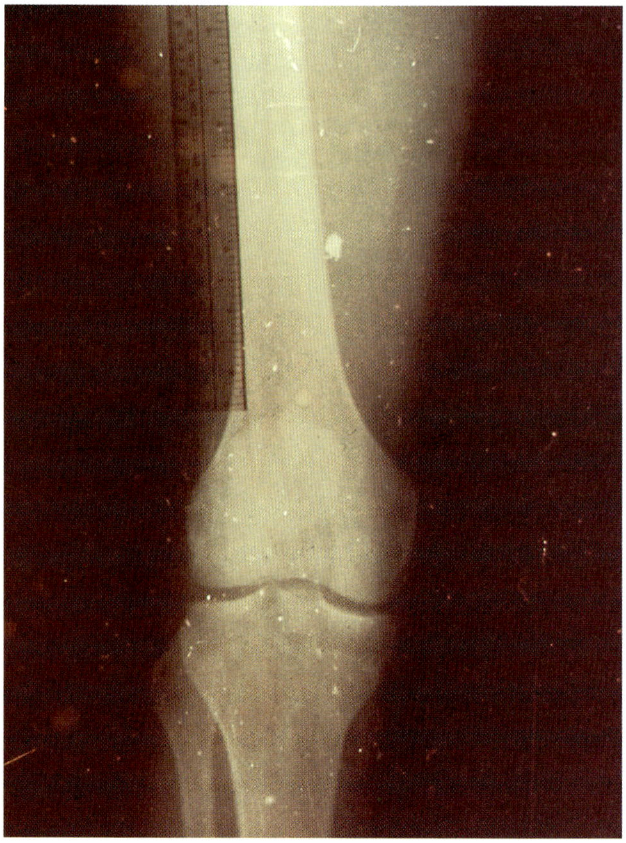

Fig. 5-36. This roentgenogram shows the missing projectile, a fragment located near the left knee of the casualty shown in Figure 5-34. The surgeon found the fragment in the popliteal artery. After it lacerated the casualty's lung, the fragment probably entered a pulmonary vein and embolized to his leg.
Source: Wound Data and Munitions Effectiveness Team

seems to be accelerated if the projectile is retained within a synovial space. Experimental studies indicate that lead concentration in the blood peaks within 4–6 months.[77]

Blunt Trauma That Results from Ballistic Projectiles

Blunt trauma may be the major injury that a ballistic projectile causes when *(a)* body armor defeats a projectile and *(b)* a projectile such as a rubber bullet is used. In both circumstances, the mechanism of injury is localized, rapid, inward deformation of the body. The more rapidly the deforming force is applied, the greater the potential for injury; the longer the duration of the impact, the greater the energy transfer. Usually a projectile's mass, not its velocity, determines the energy transfer necessary to produce blunt trauma. Both stress and shear waves may be generated at impact, although shear waves cause most of the injury. Contusion of the underlying soft tissues is the major clinical finding.

Body Armor. The nature of the injury seen when blunt trauma occurs behind body armor, especially armor worn over the trunk, depends upon the protective equipment's design. Hard, inflexible substances such as steel or ceramic plates may themselves be broken up as they defeat a projectile. The armor's breakup diffuses the projectile's impact over a wide area, and soft-tissue contusion can be extensive. When flexible armor defeats a projectile, both the impact and the underlying injury are more localized and, in that area, more intense, because the protective material protrudes into the body. Blunt trauma occurring behind body armor can be markedly decreased if its design includes a foam-rubber-like pad between the armor and the soldier's body.[78]

Rubber and Plastic Bullets. Rubber or plastic bullets, such as those used in civilian crowd control or to control rioters, are soft, broad, blunt, nonmetallic projectiles that have a muzzle velocity of about 200 fps and kinetic energy of about 370 J. When fired at the recommended range of 30 m or more, they are unlikely to penetrate the skin and usually cause only a painful bruise. When the range is 20 m or less, they can cause more serious soft-tissue injuries, fractures of small bones, and serious injuries to the eyes, brain, and lungs.[79] The original rubber bullets were notably unstable in flight, and consequently were inaccurate when aimed at a body part like the legs. Plastic bullets—designed to be more stable than rubber ones—appear to have lessened the numbers of facial and skull injuries that inadvertently occurred, with a corresponding increase in hits to the aiming point.[80]

Since soft-tissue contusion is the most common injury caused by these bullets, their introduction has not created any new management problems. In rare instances, slough of tissue has occurred, necessitating a skin graft.

SUMMARY

Infection and sepsis are the complications of soft-tissue wounds most likely to prevent a casualty's early return to his unit. Most penetrating wounds sustained on the battlefield are contaminated with a variety of bacteria, but contamination does not necessarily lead to infection. Most wounds will probably heal without infection or with only a well-localized wound abscess of little consequence. The likelihood that a wound will become infected depends upon many factors including the season, the nature of the soil, the biophysical aspects of the wound, and the casualty's physical resistance to infection.

In the past, the pyogenic cocci were the most likely sources of wound sepsis; a few casualties (certainly less than 20% and probably less than 5%) were at risk of developing life-threatening sepsis from organisms like the clostridia and (to a lesser extent) *Streptococcus pyogenes*. This group of casualties probably sustained wounds that contained more than a trivial amount of devitalized muscle.

Bacterial contamination is not constant from war to war. It depends on the battlefield environment, the local climate, the season of the year, the weapons used and the kinds of wounds they create, and probably other factors as well. Thus the medical response may need to be tailored to the conditions of the current war, not be a simple repetition of the procedures that were followed in the past.

The outcome of ballistic wounds depends upon four factors, of which the first is by far the most important:

- the body part that is hit
- the physical aspects of the projectile and the biophysical aspects of the projectile-target interaction
- the environment in which the wounding occurs
- the quality and timeliness of surgical care

Obviously, if a projectile hits one casualty in the brain stem and an identical projectile hits another casualty in a toe, their wounds will have different outcomes. With wounds of only soft tissues, the body part that is hit is less important. After all, a projectile can do only so much damage to the soft tissue at the periphery of the body before visceral or bony injuries occur.

The physical aspects of the projectile and the biophysical aspects of its interaction with the target receive disproportionate emphasis in any ballistic analysis. Certainly, high-velocity projectiles such as assault-rifle bullets have greater potential than low-velocity bullets have to cause severe soft-tissue damage, but it is unusual for this potential to be fully realized without a far more serious visceral or bony injury also occurring. Increasingly, modern munitions are being designed to cause multiple wounds. This multiplicity of wounds made by small, frequently low-velocity fragments and their possible synergy characterize many combat-related ballistic wounds.

The physical environment in which the wounding occurred is a critically important determinant of the magnitude and type of wound contamination. Identical bullet wounds sustained in a desert or a muddy farm field may represent radically different threats to the casualty. It follows that if the threats differ from one combat environment to the next, then the optimal treatments may also differ.

Treatment is the only variable over which the medical officer has any control. If there has been a dominant trend in American management of battlefield soft-tissue wounds, it has probably been in the direction of too much, rather than too little, surgical intervention. One well-respected authority[81] estimated that, among American troops in Vietnam, nonoperative treatment would have resulted in rapid and satisfactory healing in about 80% of all the casualties who had soft-tissue wounds only. Furthermore, a nonoperative approach would have returned many of those casualties to duty far sooner. The trade-off would have been the potential for serious and occasionally fatal wound sepsis in the remaining 20%. Contrast this potential outcome with the actual 5% rate of sepsis and low death rates that were obtained—with indiscriminate debridement applied to almost all casualties. The hidden costs for this achievement are *(a)* prolonged noneffectiveness (some of it iatrogenic) for many casualties and *(b)* the huge logistic burden of providing the required surgical care.

Whether or not a more selective approach, with nonoperative treatment a real option—allowing maximum return to duty and minimal septic complications—could work in a future war is difficult to say. Some would say yes; many would say no. Wound ballistics is *not* a simple subject.

REFERENCES

1. Hampton, O. P. 1961. The indications for debridement of gun shot (bullet) wounds of the extremities in civilian practice. *J. Trauma* 1:368–372.

2. Fackler, M. L. 1987. *What's wrong with the wound ballistics literature, and why* [Institute Report No. 239]. (July 1987) Presidio of San Francisco: Letterman Army Institute of Research.

3. Dziemian, A. J., and Herget, C. M. 1950. Physical aspects of the primary contamination of bullet wounds. *Milit. Surg.* 106:294–299.

4. Bellamy, R. F. 1986. Unpublished research. Washington, DC: Armed Forces Institute of Pathology.

5. Roettinger, W.; Edgerton, M. T.; Kurtz, L. D.; Prusak, M.; and Edlich, R. F. 1973. Role of inoculation site as a determinant of infection in soft tissue wounds. *Am. J. Surg.* 126:354–358.

6. Edlich, R. F.; Rogers, W.; Kasper, G.; Kaufman, D.; Tsung, M. S.; and Wangensteen, O. H. 1969. Studies in the management of the contaminated wound. I. Optimal time for closure of contaminated open wounds. II. Comparison of the resistance to infection of open and closed wounds during healing. *Am. J. Surg.* 117:323–329.

7. Hepburn, H. H. 1919. Delayed primary suture of wounds. *BMJ* 1:181–188.

8. Noyes, H. E.; Chi, N. H.; Linh, L. T.; Mo, D.,H.; Punyashthiti, K.; and Pugh, C. 1967. Delayed topical antimicrobials as adjuncts to systemic antibiotic therapy of war wounds: Bacteriologic studies. *Milit. Med.* 132:451–468.

9. Howard, R. J., and Simmons, R. L., eds. 1988. *Surgical infectious diseases.* 2d ed. Norwalk: Appleton & Lange.

10. Rodeheaver, G.; Pettry, D.; Turnbull, V.; Edgerton, V. T.; and Edlich, R. F. 1974. Identification of the wound infection-potentiating factors in soil. *Am. J. Surg.* 128:8–14.

11. Haury, B. B.; Rodeheaver, G. T.; Pettry, G. T.; Edgerton, M. T.; and Edlich, R. F. 1977. Inhibition of nonspecific defenses by soil infection-potentiating factors. *Surg. Gynecol. Obstet.* 144:19–24.

12. Matsumato, T.; Hardaway, R. M.; Dobek, A. S.; and Noyes, H. E. 1967. Different soils in simulated combat wounds. *Milit. Med.* 139:893–895.

13. Makins, G. H. 1914. A note upon the wounds of the present campaign. *Lancet* (Oct 10):905–907.

14. Otis, G. A., and Huntington, D. L. 1883. Weapons. Chapt. 11 of vol. 2, part 3, *Surgical History* in the series *Medical and Surgical History of the War of the Rebellion.* Washington, DC: Government Printing Office.

15. Smith, O'B. C. 1989. The contaminating potential of bullets fired through intermediate targets. *Milit. Med.* 154:147–150.

16. Mendelson, J. A., and Glover, J. L. 1967. Sphere and shell fragment wounds of soft tissues: Experimental study. *J. Trauma* 7:889–914.

17. Krizek, T. J., and Davis, J. H. 1965. The role of the red cell in subcutaneous infection. *J. Trauma* 5:85–95.

18. Angel, M. F.; Narayanan, K.; Swartz, W. M.; Ramasastry, S. S.; Basford, R. E.; Kuhns, D. B.; and Futrell, J. W. 1986. The etiologic role of free radicals in hematoma-induced flap necrosis. *Plast. Reconstr. Surg.* 7:795–801.

19. Haury, B.; Rodeheaver, G.; Vensko, J. A.; Edgerton, M. T.; and Edlich, R. F. 1978. Debridement: An essential component of traumatic wound care. *Am. J. Surg.* 135:238–242.

20. Cardany, C. R.; Rodeheaver, G. T.; and Thacker, G. T. 1976. The crush injury: A high risk wound. *J. Am. Coll. Emerg. Physicians* 5:965–969.

21. Amosoff, N. M. 1975. *PPG 2266.* Chicago: Henry Regnery Company.

22. Bowlby, A. A. 1915. *On wounds in war: The Bradshaw lecture.* Bristol: John Wright and Sons Ltd.

23. M. W. Ireland, ed. 1926. *The Medical Department of the United States Army in the World War.* Vol. 14, *Medical Aspects of Gas Warfare.* Washington, DC: Government Printing Office.

24. Messersschmidt, O. 1985. Results of animal experiments as a basis for recommendations on therapy of combined injuries. In *The Pathophysiology of Combined Injury and Trauma*, edited by Walker, R. I.; Gruber, D. F.; MacVittie, T. J.; and Conklin, J. J. Baltimore: University Park Press.

25 deHoll, D.; Rodeheaver, G. T.; Edgerton, M. T.; and Edlich, R. F. 1974. Potentiation of infection by suture closure of dead space. *Am. J. Surg.* 127:716–719.

26. Magee, C.; Rodeheaver, G. T.; Golden, G. T.; Fox, J.; Edgerton, M. T.; and Edlich, R. K. 1976. Potentiation of wound infection by surgical drains. *Am. J. Surg.* 131:547–549.

27. Sharp, W. V.; Belden, T. A.; King, P. H.; and Teague, P. C. 1982. Suture resistance to infection. *Surgery* 97:61–73.

28. Kitka, M. J.; Meyer, J. P.; Bishara, R. A.; Goodsen, S. F.; Schuler, J. J.; and Flanigan, D. P. 1987. Crush syndrome due to limb compression. *Arch. Surg.* 122:1078–1081.

29. Brotschi, E. A., and Canntelmo, N. L. 1990. Gluteal compartment syndrome. *Surgical Rounds* (July) 42–46.

30. Campbell, J., and Pennefather, C. M. 1919. An investigation into the blood-supply of muscles. With special reference to war surgery. *Lancet* (Feb 22):294–296.

31. Dziemian, A. J.; Mendelson, J. A.; and Lindsey, D. 1961. Comparison of the wounding characteristics of some commonly encountered bullets. *J. Trauma* 1:341–353.

32. Scully, R. E.; Artz, C.P.; and Sako, Y. 1956. An evaluation of the surgeon's criteria for determining the viability of muscle during debridement. *Arch. Surg.* 72:1031–1035.

33. Trueta, R. J. 1943. *The principles and practice of war surgery.* St. Louis: The C. V. Mosby Company.

34. Le Gros Clark, W. E., and Blomfeld, L. B. 1945. The efficiency of intramuscular anastomoses. With observations on the regeneration of devascularized muscle. *J. Anat.* 79:(1) 15–32.

35. Fleming, A. 1915. On the bacteriology of septic wounds. *Lancet* (Sept 18):638–643.

36. Owen-Smith, M. S. 1981. *High velocity missile wounds.* London: Edward Arnold.

37. Pettit, R. T. 1919. Infections of wounds of war. *JAMA* (Aug 16):494–496.

38. Miles, A. A.; Schwabacher, H.; Cunliffe, A. C.; Rose, J. P.; Spooner, E. T. C.; Pilcher R. S.; and Wright, J. 1940. Hospital infection of war wounds. *BMJ* (Dec 21):855–859.

39. Miles, A. A. 1944. Epidemiology of wound infection. *Lancet* (June 24):809–814.

40. Lyons, C. 1946. An investigation of the role of chemotherapy in wound management in the Mediterranean theater. *Ann. Surg.* 123:901–924.

41. MacLennan, J. D. 1943. Anaerobic infections of war wounds in the Middle East. *Lancet* (July 17):63–66; (July 24):94–99; and (July 31):123–126.

42. Fisher, G. H.; Florey, M. E.; Grimson, T. A.; and Williams, P. M. de C. 1945. Penicillin in clostridial infections. *Lancet* (March 31):395–399.

43. Lindberg, R. B.; Wetzler, T. F.; Marshall, J. D.; Newton, A.; Strawitz, J. G.; and Howard, J. M. 1955. The bacterial flora of battle wounds at the time of primary debridement. *Ann. Surg.* 141:369–376.

44. Strawitz, J. G.; Wetzler, T. F.; Marshall, J. D.; Lindberg, R. B.; Howard, J. M.; and Artz, C. P. 1955. The bacterial flora of healing wounds. *Surgery* 37:400–411.

45. Major, J. 1969. After Action Report, 1–30 November 1967. 71st Evacuation Hospital, APO San Francisco 96318. Typescript.

46. Kovaric, J. J.; Matsumoto, T.; Dobek, A. S.; and Hamit, H. F. 1968. Bacterial flora of one hundred and twelve combat wounds. *Milit. Med.* 132:622–624.

47. Matsumato, T.; Wyte, S. R.; Mosseley, R. V.; Hawley, R. J.; and Lackey, G. R. 1969. Combat surgery in communication zone. Part 1. War wounds and bacteriology (Preliminary report). *Milit. Med.* 137:655–655.

48. Simchen, E., and Sacks, T. 1975. Infection in war wounds. *Ann. Surg.* 182:754–761.

49. Klein, R. S.; Berger, S. A.; and Yekutiel, P. 1975. Wound infection during the Yom Kippur War. *Ann. Surg.* 182:15–20.

50. Oppenheimer, J. H.; Knecht, A. T.; Mansberger, A. R.; Gillette, R. W.; and Pon, R. S. 1958. A new preparation for the study of experimental shock from massive wounds. Part 4. *Surgery* 43:730–739.

51. Mendelson, J. A., and Lindsey, D. 1961. Sulfamylon (mafenide) and penicillin as expedient treatment of experimental massive open wounds with *C. perfringens* infection. *J. Trauma* 1:239–261.

52. Tikka, S. 1982. The contamination of missile wounds with special reference to early antimicrobial therapy. *Acta Chir. Scand. Suppl.* 508:281–287.

53. Editorial. 1944. Wound excision and wound trimming. *Lancet.* (May 20):665–666.

54. Madden, J. E.; Edlich, R. F.; and Schauerhamer, R. 1971. Application of fluid dynamics to surgical wound irrigation. *Curr. Top. Surg. Res.* 3:85–88.

55. Stevenson, T. R.; Thacker, J. C.; and Rodeheaver, G. T. 1976. Cleansing the traumatic wound by high pressure syringe irrigation. *J. Am. Coll. Emerg. Phy.* 5:17–21.

56. Gross, A.; Bhaskar, S. N.; Cutright, D. E.; Posey,W. R.; Larson, W. J.; and Mulcahy, D. M. 1972. The effect of antiseptic agents and pulsating jet lavage on contaminated wounds. *Milit. Med.* 114:145–147.

57. Wheeler, C. B.; Rodeheaver, G. T.; Thacker, J. C.; Edgerton, M. T.; and Edlich, R. F. 1976. Side-effects of high pressure irrigation. *Surg. Gynecol. Obstet.* 143:775–778.

58. Nichter, L. S., and Williams, J. 1988. Ultrasonic wound debridement. *J. Hand Surg.* 13A:142–146.

59. Rodeheaver, G. T.; Smith, S. T.; Thacker, J. C.; Edgerton, M. T.; and Edlich, R. F. 1975. Mechanical cleansing of contaminated wounds with a surfactant. *Am. J. Surg.* 129:241–245.

60. Sanford, J. P. 1985. Battlefield wound infections. In *The Pathology of Combined Injury and Trauma,* edited by Walker, R. I.; Gruber, D. F.; MacVittie, T. J.; and Conklin, J. J. Baltimore: University Park Press.

61. Bowen, T. E., and Bellamy, R. F. 1988. *Emergency war surgery.* 2d U.S. rev. of *The emergency war surgery NATO handbook.* Washington, DC: United States Department of Defense.

62. Burke, J. F. 1961. The effective period of preventive antibiotic action in experimental incisions and dermal lesions. *Surgery* 50:161–175.

63. Dahlgren, B.; Almskog, B.; Berlin, R.; Nordstrom, G.; Rybeck, B.; Schantz, B.; and Seeman, T. 1982. Local effects of antibacterial therapy (Benzyl-Penicillin) on missile wound infection rates and tissue devitalization when debridement is delayed for twelve hours. *Acta Chir. Scand. Suppl.* 508:271–279.

64. Monroe, C. W. 1944. Debridement—When and how much? *Surg. Gynecol. Obstet.* 79:478–481.

65. Thoresby, F. P., and Matheson, J. P. 1967. Gas gangrene of the high velocity missile wound. Parts 1 and 2. *J. R. Army Med. Corps* 113:32–47.

66. Fackler, M. L.; Breteau, J. P. L.; Courbil, M. D.; Taxit, R.; Glas, F.; and Fievet, J. P. 1989. Open wound drainage versus wound excision in treating the modern assault rifle wound. *Surgery* 105:576–584.

67. Fackler, M. L. Personal communication, 1985.

68. Yudenichi, V. V. 1979. Mistakes made in the surgical treatment of gunshot wounds. *Voyenno-Meditsinskiy Zhurnal* 4:39–41.

69. Garrick, J. G. 1970. Problems related to the management of combat wounds caused by specific ordnance. *J. Trauma* 10:1152–1157.

70. Pool, E. H. 1927. Wounds of soft parts. Chapt. 12 of vol. 11, *Surgery*, in *The Medical Department History of the United States Army in the World War*, a series edited under the general direction of M. W. Ireland. Washington, DC: Government Printing Office.

71. Altemeier, William A. 1952. Prophylaxis and treatment of gas gangrene and tetanus. Chapt. 27 of *Proceedings of the Symposium on Treatment of Trauma in the Armed Forces*, 10–12 March, at Army Medical Service Graduate School, Walter Reed Army Medical Center, Washington, DC.

72. Lindsey, D. 1984. Tetanus prophylaxis—do our guidelines assure protection? *J. Trauma* 24:1063–1064.

73. Yiengpruksawan, A.; Mariadason, J.; Ganepola, G. A. P.; and Freeman, H. P. 1987. Localization and retrieval of bullets under ultrasound guidance. *Arch. Surg.* 122:1082–1084.

74. Rich, N. M.; Collins, G. J.; Andersen, C. A.; McDonald, P. T.; Kozloff, L.; and Ricitta, J. J. 1978. Missile emboli. *J. Trauma* 18:236–239.

75. Schelzer, V.; Mendez-Picon, G.; and Gervin, A. S. 1989. Case report: Transthoracic retrograde venous bullet embolization. *J. Trauma* 29:525–527.

76. Linden, M. C.; Manton, W. I.; Stewart, R. M.; Thal, E. R., and Feit, H. 1982. Lead poisoning from retained bullets. *Ann. Surg.* 195:305–313.

77. Manton, W. I. and Thal, E. R. 1986. Lead poisoning from retained missiles. *Ann. Surg.* 204:594–599.

78. Liden, E.; Berlin, R.; Janzon, B.; Schantz, B.; and Seeman, T. 1988. Some observations relating to behind-body armour blunt trauma effects caused by ballistic impact. *J. Trauma Suppl.* 27:S145–S148.

79. Miller, R.; Rutherford, W. H.; Johnston, S.; and Malhotra, V. J. 1975. Injuries caused by rubber bullets: A report on 90 patients. *Br. J. Surg.* 62:480–486.

80. Rocke, L. 1983. Injuries caused by plastic bullets compared with those caused by rubber bullets. *Lancet* (April 23):919–920.

81. Mendelson, J. Personal communication, 1989.

RECOMMENDED READING

Bowen, T. E. and Bellamy, R. F. 1988. *Emergency war surgery.* 2d U.S. rev. of *The emergency war surgery NATO handbook.* Washington, DC: United States Department of Defense.

Coates, James Boyd, Jr., ed. 1962. *Wound ballistics.* A volume of the official history of the Medical Department of the U.S. Army in World War II. Washington, DC: Office of the Surgeon General, Department of the Army.

Commander in Chief, Pacific. 1970. *Fourth conference on war surgery.* Held in Tokyo, Japan, 16–19 February 1970. Surgeons (all actively engaged in the surgical care of Vietnam casualties) from the three geographic echelons of hospitals where extensively wounded casualties received care (Vietnam, PACOM off-shore and CONUS) exchanged information concerning results and complications associated with required surgical procedures. The proceedings from this meeting are the most concise statement of the management of ballistic wounds that exist in English. Typescript. Washington, DC: Department of Defense and U.S. Navy Pacific Command.

Chapter 6

PRIMARY BLAST INJURY AND BASIC RESEARCH: A BRIEF HISTORY

YANCY Y PHILLIPS III, M.D., FCCP* AND DONALD R. RICHMOND, Ph.D.**

Lieutenant Colonel, United States Army; Chief, Department of Pulmonary and Critical Care Medicine Services, Walter Reed Army Medical Center, Washington, D.C. 20307–5001, and Consultant to the Surgeon General in Pulmonary Medicine and Respiratory Therapy
***Former Director, Western Operation, EG & G, Mason Research Institute; Albuquerque, NM 87119–9024*

INTRODUCTION

Wound ballistics—the study of penetrating wounds, which have been and will likely remain the primary mechanism of battlefield casualties—is at the heart of any discussion of the medical consequences of conventional war. However, the use of large conventional munitions during this century's wars, the bombing of civilian population centers in World War II, the threat of nuclear weapons, and the advent of modern diagnostic and therapeutic capabilities have introduced the military medical officer to a newly recognized type of injury—that which occurs from the blast wave alone.

The section of this volume on blast will first discuss some civilian and military experiences with blast injury. This is followed by a brief history of the scientific advances in the blast research field. The physical basis of blast integrated with the mechanisms of blast injury will then lead into a discussion of pathology of *primary blast injury* (PBI). The final chapter of this section will then concentrate on the medical management of the blast casualty.

An explosion may kill or maim a casualty in several ways. Whether it travels through air or water, the blast wave itself may cause internal damage in air-containing organs without leaving any external sign of injury. Such PBI is the principal subject of this section. A blast may also propel fragments into a casualty, causing *secondary blast injury*, or can bodily displace an individual and cause *tertiary blast injury* upon impact.

PBI is most likely to occur during a conflict between opponents who have sophisticated weapons. Even so, the tragic worldwide increase in small-scale terrorist violence has given the medical community opportunities to supplement both wartime medical commentaries and findings from animal-model blast experimentation.

The scientific study of PBI is a twentieth-century phenomenon. The basis for most of what we know about it came out of British and German investigations during World War II. The German research, in particular, was groundbreaking in both its empirical observations and theoretical constructs. Postwar blast research has centered in Western Europe and the United States, with some work reported from the Soviet Union and the People's Republic of China. Initial investigations focused on the physical correlates of PBI and its physiological effects. Experiments in the 1980s looked at the effects of repeated exposure to blast waves and the mechanisms of PBI.

BLAST INJURY IN TERRORIST BOMBING INCIDENTS

In modern times, terrorist bombs have become commonplace elements of some political resistance movements. Although they usually do not have the potential for causing the widespread devastation that military explosive weapons can wreak, the simplicity and small size of terrorist bombs allow them to be easily hidden in areas where unsuspecting civilians are likely to congregate. They can thus capitalize on causing severe local damage, and make up in publicity what they may lack in explosive power.

By its nature, a terrorist bombing is an isolated event, and civilian casualties are usually not vulnerable to the same logistical constraints of medical care that military blast casualties might have to face. Instead, they are most likely to be treated at the site by medical professionals who are not under fire, or in nearby hospital emergency rooms that can be quickly reached by ground transportation rather than by air evacuation or by foot.

Blast-injury data from terrorist bombings are limited by the chaotic nature of an unexpected mass-casualty situation descending upon a civilian medical system. Nevertheless, retrospective reviews of many large and small bombings have yielded much useful information on the mortality and incidence of injury resulting from such attacks. Reports from Israel and Great Britain document their all-too-intimate familiarity with blast injury.

General Morbidity and Mortality Rates

Civilian bombings usually result in relatively low mortality rates unless the casualties have been exposed to *(a)* structural collapse, *(b)* a very large explosive charge, or *(c)* an explosion within a structure or vehicle. About 1%–5% of victims will die on the scene from head injuries, and most casualties who are taken to an emergency room will be slightly injured with lacerations, abrasions, and contusions. About 25%–50% of those transported will need admission for treatment or observation. A small number of victims (1%–15% of those admitted) will have significant thoracic or abdominal blast injury. Those patients are at high risk of complications and about 15% of them will die in the hospital.

The morbidity and mortality statistics from fourteen reports, involving a total of 3,357 casualties in 220 major terrorist incidents, are summarized in Figure 6-1.[1] These events ranged from the bombing of the U.S. Marine barracks in Beirut, Lebanon[2] to Irish Republican Army (IRA) bombings in Northern Ireland and Great Britain.[3–5]

The on-scene mortality ranged from less than 2% in Northern Ireland[4] to almost 70% for the Beirut barracks attack.[2] Immediate mortality was high in the Beirut bombing, as well as in the train station bombing at Bologna, Italy,[6] because a major structure collapsed in each event and many people died of crush injuries. In general, explosions that occurred indoors caused more severe primary and secondary blast injuries because the blast waves were contained within the structures and more debris was thrown about.

Although these civilian bombings generated many casualties, the overall morbidity and mortality rates were, with the exceptions noted above, relatively low; mortality was generally less than 5%. Terrorist bombs usually weigh only a few kilograms and cause mostly lacerations, abrasions, and contusions.[4] In most instances, fewer than half of the victims who were seen in an emergency room were subsequently admitted to the hospital for treatment or observation. For example, most of the victims of civilian bombings in Israel were slightly injured, according to the Injury Severity Score (ISS), a quantitative trauma rating scale.[7] Physicians at Jerusalem's Shaare Zedek Medical Center classified 87% of bombing victims who were seen in the emergency room as being slightly injured, and only 10% as severely injured.[8] Overall, 28% of patients were admitted to the hospital after initial emergency-room evaluation and stayed an average of 16 days. The in-hospital mortality rate was 2.3%.

Terrorists often hide explosives in public gather-

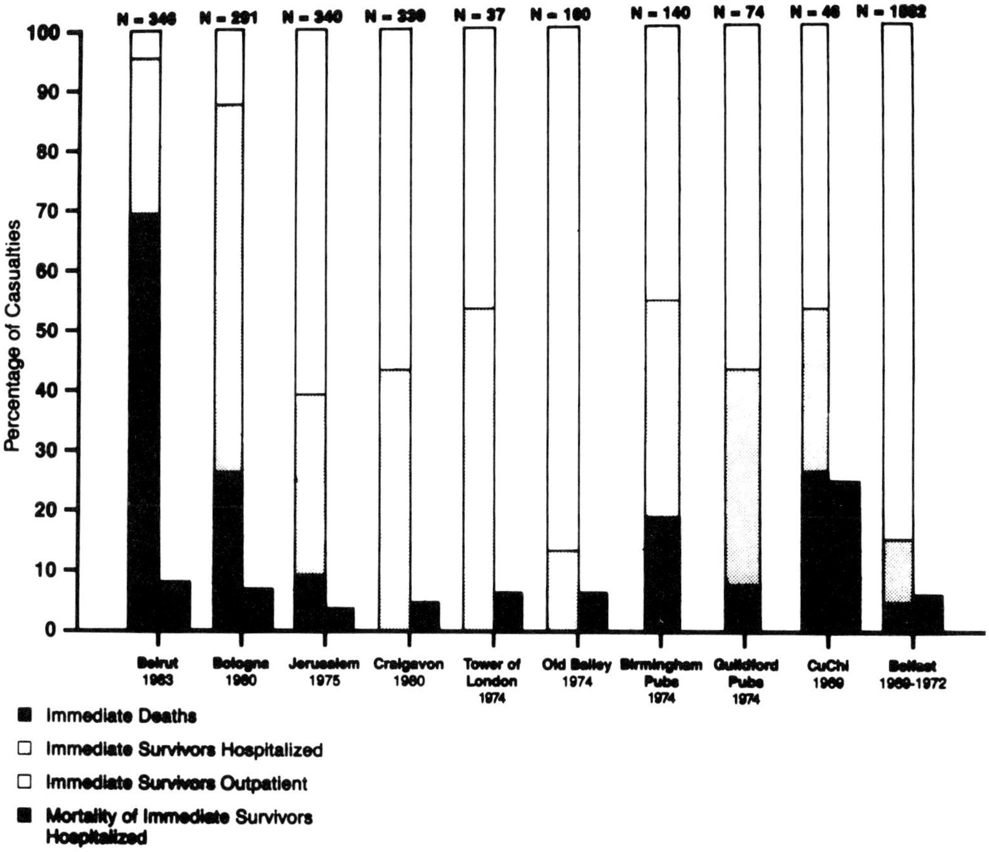

Fig. 6-1. Morbidity and mortality compiled from reports of terrorist bombings
Source: Reference 1

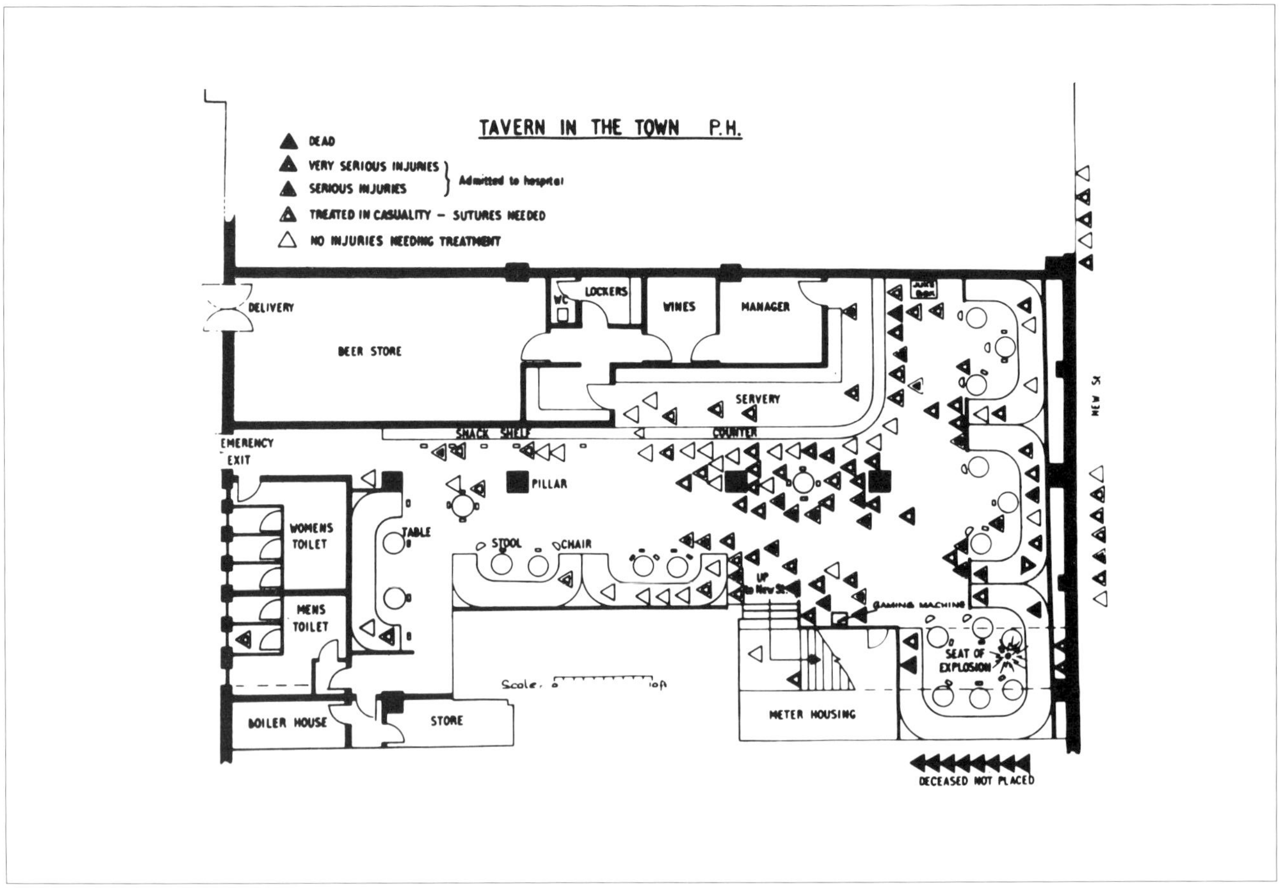

Fig. 6-2. The floor plan of the tavern in the Town Public House in Birmingham, England, depicts the locations of patrons who were killed, injured, or uninjured after a terrorist bombing.
Source: Reference 9

ing places where detonation can generate great publicity as well as many casualties. Restaurants and bars are especially dangerous because they are likely to be crowded at predictable times of the day. They also contain glassware, other light materials, and furniture that can become mutilating secondary missiles in an explosion. Figure 6-2 illustrates the asymmetrical pattern of casualty generation in the bombing of the crowded Town Public House in Birmingham, England. Although the majority of the severely injured casualties were near the explosion, some victims who were more than 35 feet away were seriously wounded or killed, and people between them and the explosion were relatively unscathed.[9]

In all fourteen terrorism reports reviewed, only one patient died after being evaluated and released from an emergency room, but the cause of death was a heart attack that was not necessarily related to the bombing.[1] Thus, there appeared to have been no overtriage of bombing victims, in which casualties who should have been admitted to the hospital would have been discharged. However, many patients with relatively minor injuries were placed in the hospital for observation (undertriage). This level of caution might have a relatively small effect on a large civilian medical facility, but in a military mass-casualty action it would severely strain the available medical resources and could result in a significant loss of fighting strength.

Mortality Associated with Specific Organ-System Injuries

The mortality and morbidity of blast injuries depend largely on which organs have been affected. Figure 6-3 illustrates *(a)* the incidence of involvement of different anatomical regions in both survivors and on-scene fatalities, *(b)* the contribution of specific injuries to mortality, and *(c)* the mortality associated with organ-system involvement in severely injured survivors who were admitted to the hospital (called *specific mortality*).[1]

The specific mortality data show that casualties who had truncal injuries were few in number but were more likely to die after being hospitalized. Blast survi-

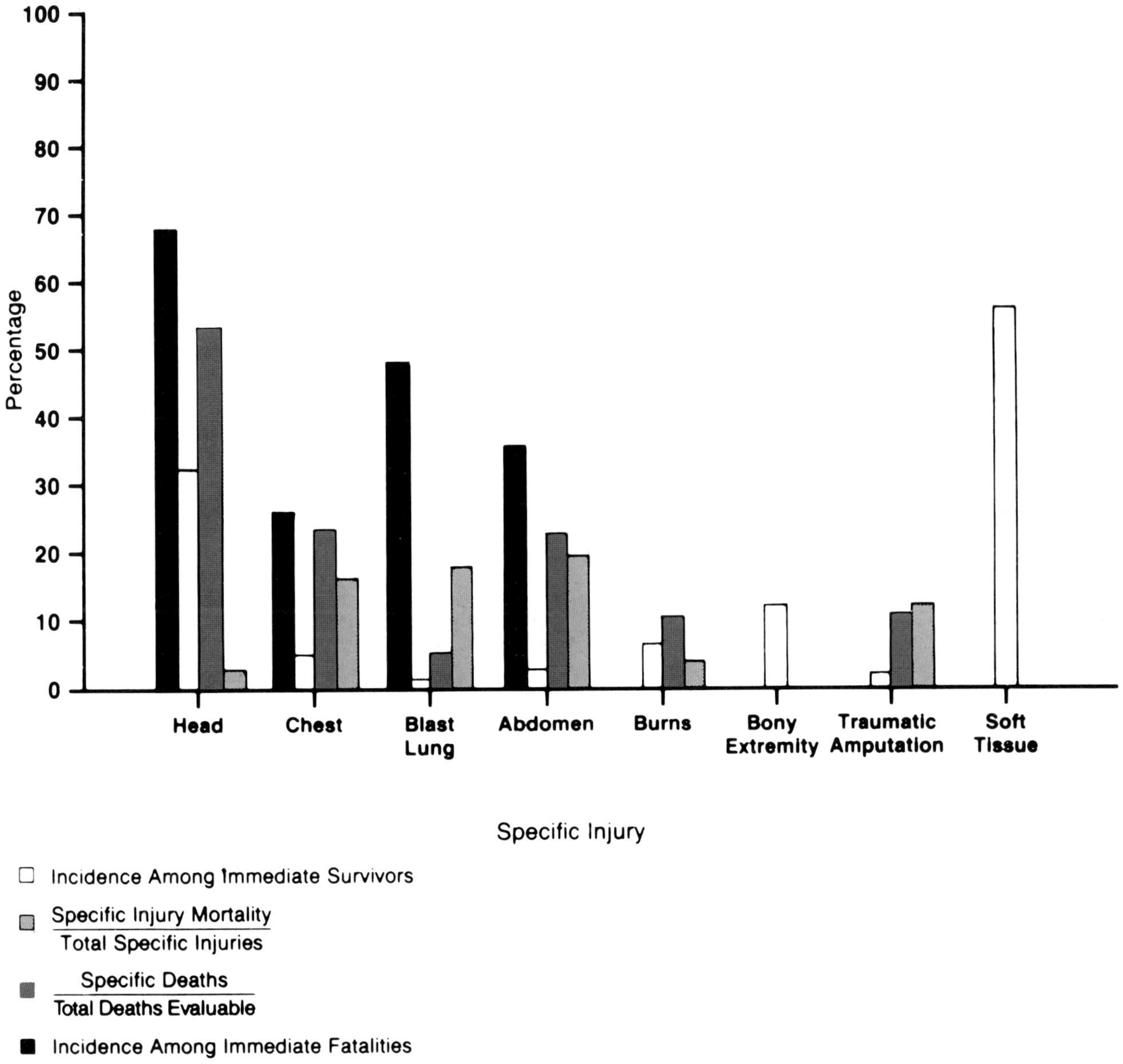

Fig. 6-3. The incidence of involvement of specific body areas in bombing victims is shown for both immediate fatalities and those surviving the attack. Unfortunately, because of incomplete reporting of autopsies, data from only a few sources are included and the figure represents less than a universal survey. The incidence of specific organ damage in immediate fatalities comes entirely from a single review of terrorist bombings in the British Isles.
Source: Reference 1

vors who were admitted to the hospital with chest injuries (2.4% of admissions) had a 15% death rate, and survivors who were admitted with abdominal injuries (3.5%) had a 19% death rate, together accounting for most of the in-hospital mortality from these incidents. Thus, the few casualties who can be expected to present to the triage officer with thoracoabdominal injuries tend to take up a disproportionate amount of medical-care resources but nevertheless represent an important focus for intervention and salvage.

Because pulmonary PBI may be an important component of a blast casualty's trauma, the use of positive-pressure ventilatory support may influence mortality and morbidity rates. Following the Bologna bombing, for example, five out of twenty victims with chest-wall or lung injuries required mechanical ventilation, and three died.[6] In three reports from Israel, a respirator was required for seventeen out of forty victims with lung injury, and four of those patients died.[10–12] Overall in these four reports, twenty-two out of sixty (37%) victims with pulmonary PBI required ventilatory support, and seven died. The specific mortality associated with blast lung was 12% overall, and 22% of those with respiratory failure died. The high mortality may have been partially due to other major injuries that were sustained, but late air embolism and barotrauma caused by mechanical ventilation were likely important (if unrecognized) factors.

The data on head and brain injuries in civilian blast incidents resemble those collected on the various anatomical sites of wounding in military conflicts. Trauma to the central nervous system is highly lethal; injuries to the head and brain were the most significant cause of death at the scene, and most fatalities from head injury occurred within a few hours of the incident.[3,13]

Wounds of the extremities were relatively common in the bombings but had low admission-mortality rates. Traumatic amputations occurred in about 1.3% of victims but carried a relatively high specific-mortality rate of 11%, probably because they occurred in victims who were very close to the detonation site and were thus vulnerable to serious PBI and other extensive tissue disruption.[4,13]

Primary Blast Injury in Terrorist Bombings

PBI is probably quite common in terrorist bombings. However, its clinical significance tends not to be emphasized because individuals so affected were usually mortally wounded by air embolism or other blast effects, particularly head trauma.[3,13] For example, according to a study of casualties who died in 5,600 separate explosions over a 12-year period, 78% of the 495 fatalities died at the scene and another 13% died within 24 hours.[13] Autopsies showed that 66% of all fatalities had brain injuries and 51% had skull fractures. PBI was found in a significant percentage of fatalities as well: 47% had the classic autopsy findings of blast lung and 45% had tympanic-membrane rupture. As a testament to the tremendous force of the explosion and the casualties' proximity to the blast, 34% had liver laceration, an injury that is more characteristic of blunt trauma.

Based upon their experience with civilian casualties, British observers have felt that survivors of a bomb attack have a low incidence of PBI.[9,13,14] For example, only 8 of the 653 IRA-bombing victims who were admitted to a hospital were thought to have had significant PBI to the lungs.[13]

However, survivors of the bombings in Paris during the early 1980s had a higher reported incidence of PBI.[15] Nine of 205 victims admitted to the hospital were diagnosed with blast lung. Of those who had traumatic respiratory insufficiency, four (44%) died.

In the bombing of the Bologna train station, 73 of the 291 casualties were killed, a higher number than might have been expected because the building collapsed.[6] Of the 107 survivors who were admitted to the hospital, nine had pulmonary contusion, pneumothorax, or pneumomediastinum. Eleven others had pulmonary injuries that were associated with rib fractures or other chest-wall trauma. Five patients developed respiratory failure and three ultimately died. Little (if any) PBI of the abdomen was observed.

Explosions within an enclosed space result in more severe PBI (Table 6-1).[11,12] In two bus bombings in Israel, sixteen patients were diagnosed with PBI to the lung, although a few also had chest-wall damage (which is not a characteristic of pure PBI). Direct blast caused some lung damage in 31% of those patients who were admitted to the hospital. Seven victims complained of significant abdominal pain; subsequent laparotomies revealed intestinal perforations in four victims, which is a relatively high rate of PBI of the abdomen for air blast. Not unexpectedly, all who were severely injured also had perforated tympanic membranes.

TABLE 6-1

MORBIDITY AND MORTALITY FROM BOMB ATTACKS ON CIVILIAN BUSES

Circumstance	(N)
Total bus passengers	104
Admitted to hospital	51
Evaluated, not admitted	46
Pulmonary blast injury	16
Killed immediately	7
Abdominal pain	7
Bowel perforations	4

Source: References 11 and 12

MILITARY EXPERIENCE WITH PRIMARY BLAST INJURY

PBI is not commonly reported in casualties of modern military operations, perhaps because the low-intensity conflicts that have occupied Western nations during the second half of this century have employed relatively light ordnance. However, the wars in the Middle East during the same period have involved massed armor and heavy conventional weapons. Israeli reports have detailed some blast injuries, although the reports are limited by a lack of definitions and autopsy data. No compilations of meaningful data from Arab nations or from the Iran-Iraq War are available, perhaps because of the limitations of their medical-care systems and the political costs of detailed casualty reporting.

The principal wounding mechanism of most military ordnance is fragmentation, a form of secondary blast injury. Perhaps because they are easier to recognize and diagnose, or perhaps because they have so many characteristics in common with ballistic wounds, secondary blast injuries have received far more attention in military circles than primary blast effects have. Nevertheless, the occurrence of PBI in certain military environments is now recognized as a factor in combat-casualty care.

PBI may be an important injury mechanism for crews of modern armored vehicles in which the threat of fragments and fire has been reduced. Blast may also have serious effects on soldiers who wear body armor, who are exposed to enhanced-blast munitions, or who are caught in underwater detonations. Hearing loss from the effects of blast or repeated loud noises also has potentially damaging effects on a combatant's ability to carry out military operations.

Data Collection

The military medical literature contains remarkably little careful documentation of PBI. Either there have been few such injuries, or whatever blast injuries occurred in a particular incident were unrecognized or unreported. American blast casualties in Vietnam, for example, were probably relatively few in number because the opposing forces there used mostly light, hand-held infantry weapons. They had few large, special-purpose explosive munitions that might be expected to cause blast injury, and little armored warfare was conducted. On the other hand, the opposing forces would have been more likely to suffer blast injuries from American weapons, but they have not reported—and probably were unable to gather—such information.

American Data Collection. The American forces went to great lengths to compile accurate casualty data in Vietnam. The most ambitious data-collection effort was conducted by the Wound Data and Munitions Effectiveness Team (WDMET), which accumulated detailed tactical and medical information on about 8,000 wounded or killed soldiers.

In all of the WDMET data, there were only two incidents in which PBI was recognized. In one case, an American patrol was inadvertently hit by a 500-pound conventional bomb dropped by an American aircraft. While fragments from the bomb's detonation caused no wounds, two soldiers presented with hemoptysis and pulmonary contusion without external evidence of injury (Figure 6-4). Both clearly had blast lung; neither required mechanical ventilation and both survived.

The second incident involved a rocket attack on an armored vehicle, in which two soldiers were killed outright. One was mutilated as he was blown through an open hatch. The other had only a scratch on his chin but was dead at the scene. Autopsy revealed that he had extensive blast injuries to his internal organs and a fatal pulmonary hemorrhage (Figure 6-5). Air embolism was the probable cause of death but was not noted, and evidence of it may not have been sought at autopsy.

Both of these wounding scenarios would have been much more common in a conflict against an enemy who used sophisticated conventional weapons.

Foreign Data Collection. Data from other countries have not always been easy to classify or interpret. According to Chinese experts, blast injuries accounted for only 0.3% of Chinese casualties during the Korean conflict;[16] however, under the prevailing hardships of that time, data collection must have been very difficult. In China's more recent border conflict with Vietnam, 20% of the injuries that were caused by artillery or mines were said to include PBI.[16] Unfortunately, other details of the injuries, including their morbidity and treatment, are not available.

The Israeli experience in the 1980s is also unclear. Israeli Defense Force physicians reported that blast was responsible for 2.3% of the casualties in Lebanon in 1982.[17] Whether this percentage refers only to PBI or also to the mutilating effects of mines and other explosives is unknown, although artillery explosions (which

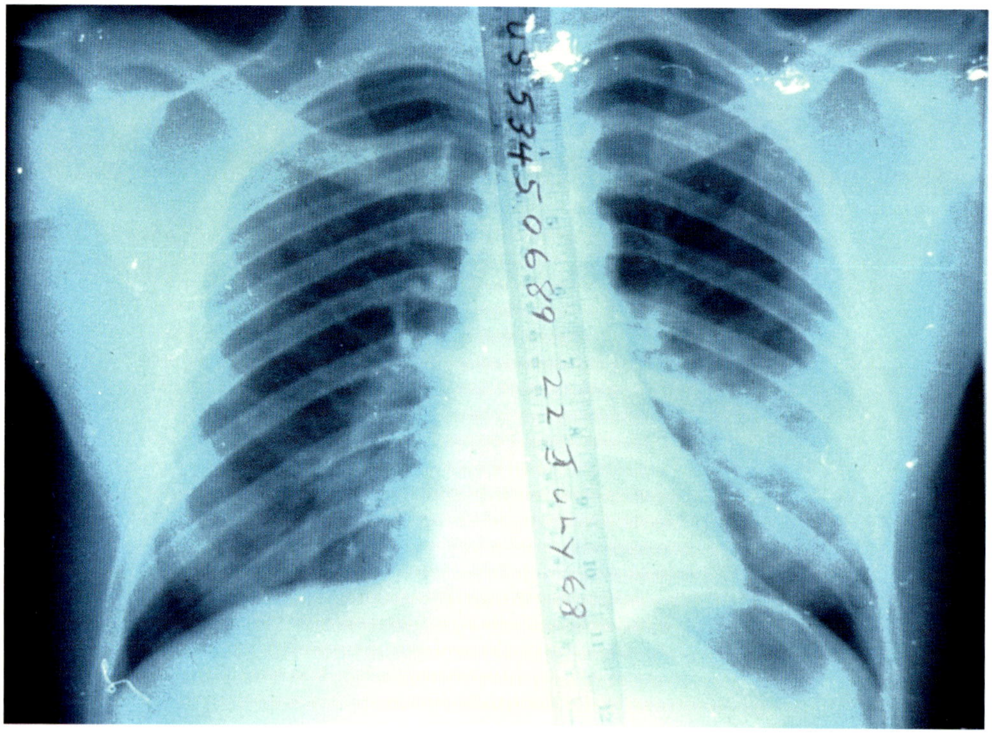

Fig. 6-4. This chest roentgenogram of a soldier who was injured by blast shows bilateral infiltrates from pulmonary contusion. The patient survived without sequelae.
Source: Wound Data and Munitions Effectiveness Team

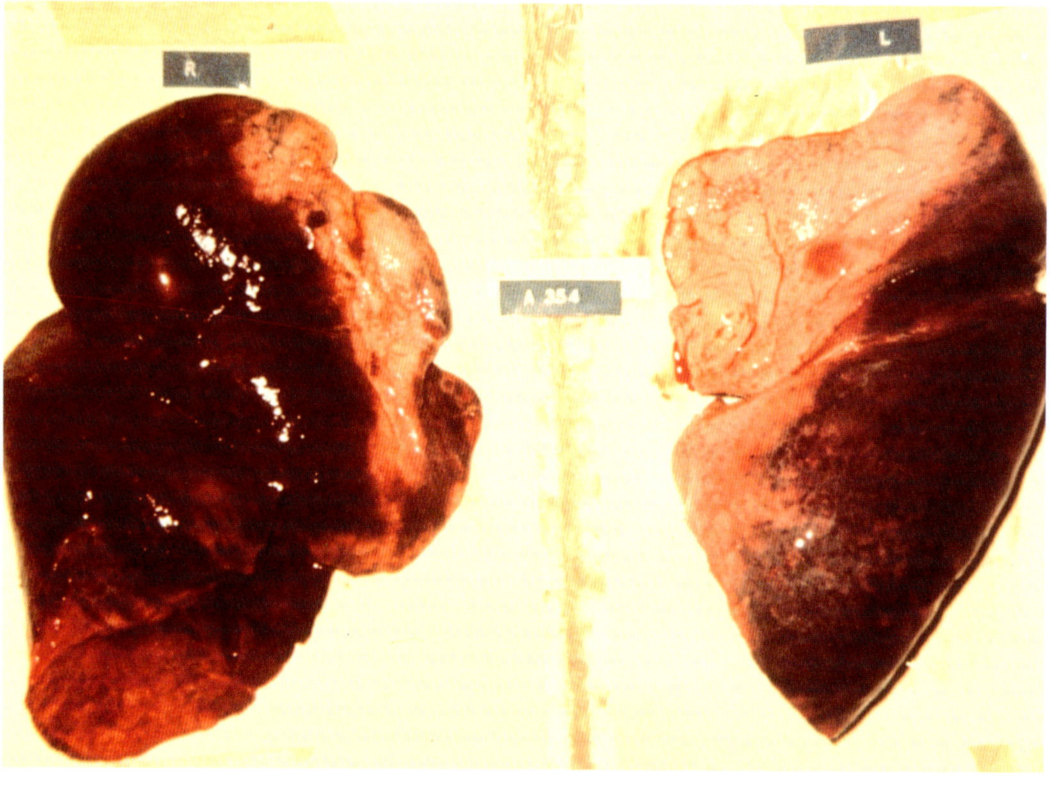

Fig. 6-5. This autopsy specimen from a soldier who was killed inside an armored vehicle by a penetrating antitank munition shows extensive pulmonary hemorrhage. The soldier exhibited no significant external injury.
Source: Wound Data and Munitions Effectiveness Team

caused 53% of battle injuries) were separated out as sources of blast injury, suggesting that the 2.3% blast casualty rate may refer to PBI only. Armored-vehicle personnel accounted for 14% of all casualties, but the data do not indicate whether PBI was a significant cause of injuries in tank crews. The collection of Israeli mortality data is complicated by religious objections to autopsy, and a definitive cause of death cannot always be determined.

A long-term British project to collect military-casualty data in Northern Ireland—called the *Hostile Action Casualty System* (HACS)—includes data from terrorist bombings as well as data from wounding by modern small arms.[18] The project reported on 828 armed-forces personnel who were injured or killed from explosions, and excluded those who were struck by bullets. Not surprisingly, the fatality statistics are similar to the civilian bombing data. There were 216 fatalities, 174 (80%) of whom were dead on the scene. Autopsies revealed a high incidence of both head injuries (33%) and pulmonary PBI (32%). Twenty-four soldiers, most of whom were wearing body armor, were killed by pulmonary PBI alone and had few external injuries. The ballistic vests they were wearing may have protected them from truncal fragment injuries but did not ameliorate the blast effects. Despite the high incidence of lethal pulmonary blast injury, only two soldiers who were admitted to the hospital required mechanical ventilatory support for blast lung as their only significant injury. Nine other soldiers died of respiratory failure in the hospital (two during surgery); blast lung was thought to play a role in most of these deaths, although sepsis and massive trauma certainly contributed to them. Abdominal blast injury was rarely noted. Tympanic-membrane rupture was seen in 86% of fatalities and in 47% of survivors. Traumatic amputations were associated with a very high lethality; only nine of fifty-two soldiers who were so afflicted survived.

Armored Vehicles

Historically, fragments and fire have caused the most injuries in armored fighting vehicles that were penetrated by antitank munitions. However, design improvements in these vehicles have significantly reduced the vulnerability of the crew to these injuries.[19] Such improvements include *(a)* spall-suppression linings, *(b)* the compartmentalization of fuel and munitions, *(c)* the extensive use of low-flammability materials, and *(d)* rapid automatic-fire suppression systems. Paradoxically, as the threat of fragment and burn injuries lessens, the threat of blast and other ancillary effects of armor penetration becomes more significant.

Many Israeli armor casualties in the 1967 War were inside armored vehicles that were penetrated by antitank guided missiles (ATGMs) equipped with shaped-charge warheads (see Chapter One). These soldiers suffered from respiratory failure and extensive (but superficial) burns, a combination of symptoms that became known as the *ATGM Syndrome*.[20] The pulmonary component was attributed to a combination of PBI and toxic-fume inhalation.

Neither British nor American casualty data from armored conflicts during World War II are particularly useful in determining the role, if any, of blast injury in that era.

In the mid-1980s, public and congressional concern focused on the supposed vulnerability of the U.S. Army's Bradley Fighting Vehicle. Some critics feared that if the vehicle's aluminum armor were penetrated, the blast inside the crew area would be tremendously increased because of the *vaporific effect*. The vaporific effect is the result of a process in which aluminum (or any material) in the armor is vaporized and fragmented, and then undergoes an explosive exothermic reaction with atmospheric oxygen in the crew area.

The U.S. Army Medical Research and Development Command (USAMRDC) conducted experiments using anesthetized sheep and pigs inside armored vehicles. These experiments demonstrated that—outside of the fragment-spall cone (see Chapter One)—significant injury to the lungs and intestine did not occur when either the Bradley or the M113 armored personnel carriers were penetrated by either small antitank munitions (such as the American-made LAW, the Soviet-made RPG6, or the Swedish-made Karl Gustav) or larger-caliber warheads (such as the American-made TOW1, the Soviet-made Sagger, or the European-made Milan).[21]

Under congressional mandate, all American military weapons systems must be tested against threat munitions under realistic operating conditions. The U.S. Army has conducted an extensive series of tests with the Bradley Fighting Vehicle, the M60A3 tank, and the M1A1 Abrams tank.[22] Casualty evaluations were made for *(a)* fragments, *(b)* fire, *(c)* acceleration/displacement, *(d)* blast, and *(e)* inhalation of toxic fumes. Although the results of these tests are classified, PBI can be expected in a few cases. The number of casualties in a modern armor conflict who will have PBI is unknowable, but it is nevertheless likely to be much lower than the number of casualties who will suffer fragment wounds. In an armored vehicle that has been defeated by a large warhead, 1%–20% of the survivors would have some degree of PBI in addition to their other wounds. Whether the blast effects would pre-

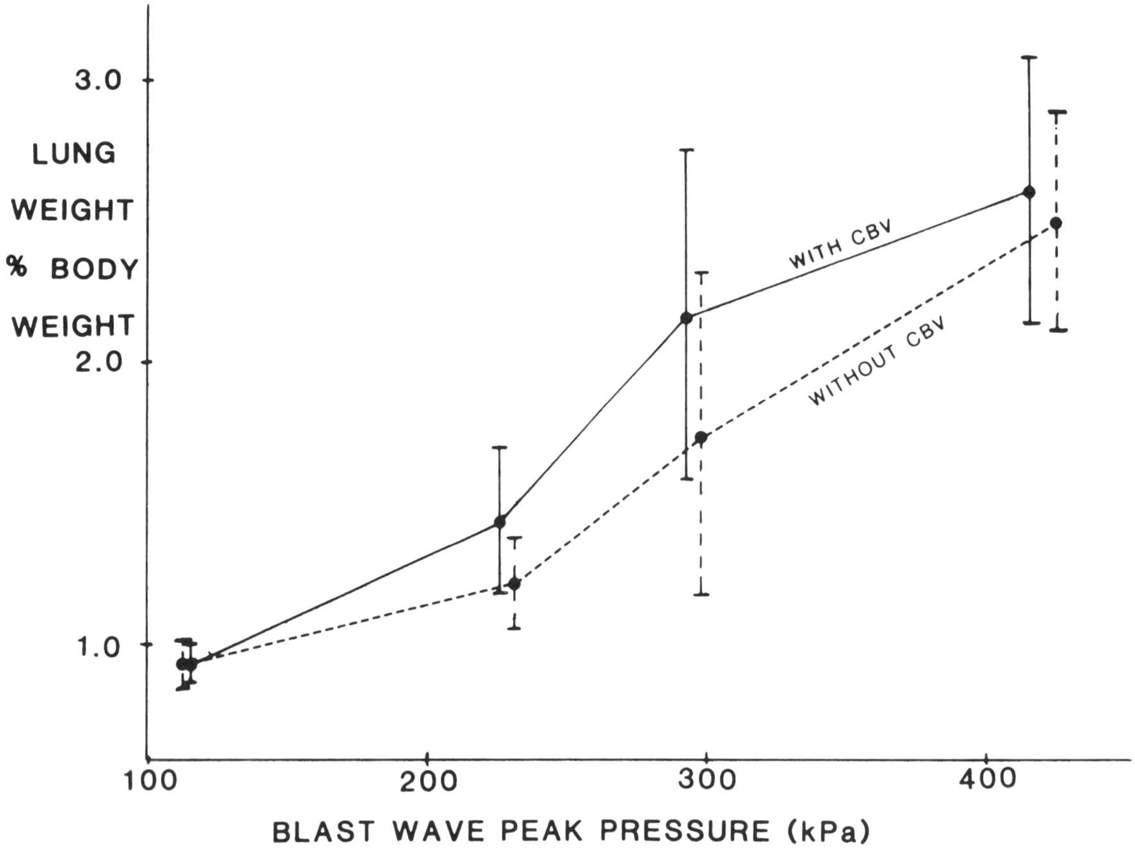

Fig. 6-6. The effect of wearing a cloth ballistic vest (CBV) on lung injury as measured by increased lung weight is shown for sheep over a range of blast-injury severity. At the highest level of blast, five out of six animals that were wearing a CBV were killed, whereas only two out of the six animals that were not wearing a CBV died of PBI.
Source: Reference 25

dominate or complicate the clinical course of these casualties is not known.

Body Armor

Just as ballistics researchers' concerns for protecting personnel from fragments led to the development of light, effective body armor, blast researchers have also sought to find a practical way to protect the individual soldier from PBI. A Swedish study demonstrated that covering a rabbit with foam rubber markedly increased a blast's lethality, whereas shielding the animal's chest with steel pipe was effective in reducing injury.[23] A study with human volunteers demonstrated that, even at the low overpressure levels that would be found in the crew areas of heavy weapons, the U.S. Army standard-issue cloth ballistic vest caused an increase in intrathoracic pressure over the intrathoracic pressure that was observed when the vest was not worn.[24] Although the minimal effects seen at such low overpressure levels were not injurious, a study using large animals and much higher levels of blast showed that the ballistic vest caused a significant increase in both lung hemorrhage and mortality.[25] Over a range of blast exposures, animals covered with the vest suffered significantly more injury than those that were uncovered (Figure 6-6). At the highest overpressure level, five of the six animals wearing the vest were killed by the blast, compared with only two of the six uncovered animals.

Although combat records do not confirm this effect, the British HACS study of IRA bombings did find lethal pulmonary blast injuries in soldiers who wore vests.[18] These soldiers had no external injuries. The vests may have saved them from potentially lethal fragment injuries, but may have done so at the cost of compounding the PBI.

Israeli soldiers commonly wear body armor, but there are no data on the incidence of PBI in soldiers who were wounded in recent Middle-East conflicts.

The mechanism for this enhancement of the primary blast effect is unknown. The vest may serve to increase the surface area that is exposed to the blast, thereby increasing the total energy delivered to the chest.[25] Theoretically, the vest may also improve the efficiency of energy transmission from the blast wave to the thorax.[25,26] A study that used small animals has suggested that effective blast protection may be afforded by putting a rigid covering over a foam material.[26] Such a protective garment might not be practical for all troops, but could be important for special clothing used by ordnance-disposal personnel.

This review of the evidence that personal body armor may enhance primary blast effects must not be construed as a recommendation for abandoning its use. Soldiers already know that body armor is hot and heavy; they do not need another excuse to shed it. The ballistic vest is a lifesaver, and the threat of injury by bullets or fragments is far greater than the threat of pure PBI on any imaginable battlefield.

Instead, these data should be used by physicians when they make triage and treatment decisions. Soldiers who were wearing vests when they were exposed to an explosion may owe their lives to the vests, but physicians should be aware that these troops may have sustained PBI to the lungs and abdomen even in the absence of significant truncal ballistic wounds.

Enhanced-Blast Munitions

Enhanced-blast munitions are designed to injure by means of their blast effects rather than by fragmentation. Most modern military powers have either fielded or evaluated enhanced-blast munitions, usually in the form of some type of fuel-air explosive (FAE). The FAE concept is described in some detail in Chapter One of this textbook.

The role of enhanced-blast munitions as antipersonnel weapons is not established. U.S. Army doctrine calls for the use of FAE weapons to clear minefields or possibly to be used against "soft" military matériel, such as vans and light structures.[27] In an example of the effectiveness of such a tactic, the Egyptians reportedly used FAE munitions to flatten and thereby disable Israeli radars during the Yom Kippur War.[28]

Although Soviet military doctrine for enhanced-blast weapons is unknown, they have been used in armored-assault training maneuvers against fortifications and dug-in troops.[29] Whether they were used for their direct casualty effects or as psychological weapons is unclear.

Large numbers of air-delivered weapons—the names of which were literally translated as "volume bombs"—were reportedly used by the Soviet forces in Afghanistan.[29] The detonation of these weapons allegedly resulted in extensive fires. Whether the munitions were primarily blast or incendiary weapons is unknown.

Unlike a fragment or a projectile, the blast effect is not limited to a linear trajectory. Not only can the blast wave go around an object, but its effect will be magnified in an enclosed area. Thus, although its potential role as an antipersonnel weapon has not been established, an enhanced-blast munition might be particularly effective against personnel in caves, rocky terrain, open foxholes, or trenches.

Underwater Blast Injury

Blast injuries were common in those World War II combatants who had been forced to abandon their ships and were in the water near a subsurface detonation of a torpedo, a depth charge, or an aerial bomb. Both American and British authors wrote of thousands of such casualties and noted that the number of dead from blast, although unknowable, was probably quite large.[30–32] Fifty casualties with abdominal blast injuries were evacuated to Pearl Harbor following the Battle of Midway in 1942.[30] One British ship's physician noted that only 90 of 125 sailors who had safely abandoned ship wearing life preservers survived a nearby depth-charge explosion.[31] Twenty-four sailors in a North Sea action were rescued after surviving an underwater explosion, but within a few days eleven of them died, seven of whom had intestinal perforations.[32]

During the 1967 War, an Egyptian missile struck the Israeli destroyer *Eilat*.[10] The crew abandoned ship and, while they were in the water, another missile detonated nearby. The number of deaths was unreported, but thirty-two survivors were rescued within a few hours. All casualties had PBI except one, who fractured his tibia while on board ship. Twenty-seven survivors had blast lung; five of them required ventilatory support. Twenty-four had abdominal signs and symptoms and underwent laparotomy; of these, twenty-two had bowel perforations. Nineteen sailors had both thoracic and gastrointestinal injuries. Four victims died, three of whom expired during or shortly after general anesthesia.

In another incident, an underwater charge was detonated near thirteen soldiers who were swimming for recreation.[33] All quickly got out of the water. However, within a minute, two sailors suffered cardiac arrest; within 10 minutes, two more died, and by 30 minutes after the blast, two more had succumbed. The remaining seven soldiers were evacuated by helicopter and, despite heroic efforts, only three ultimately survived. These casualties were almost certainly killed by air embolism to the heart and brain, which causes most of the pure-PBI deaths that occur immediately

TABLE 6-2

HEARING LOSS IN BRITISH COMBATANTS DURING THE FALKLAND ISLANDS CONFLICT

Test Group	Hearing Category	Before Blast Exposure (N)	After Blast Exposure (N)	Percentage of Combatants Whose Hearing Deteriorated
All Infantry	1+2	316	271	13.3
	3	21	52	
	4	1	15	
Infantry using small arms	1+2	105	97	7.3
	3	4	9	
	4	0	3	
Infantry using 81-mm mortars	1+2	73	55	23.7
	3	2	17	
	4	1	4	
105-mm light gun crew	1+2	78	68	11.9
	3	6	14	
	4	0	2	

*Hearing categories are by United Kingdom definitions, with 4 being the most severe.

after blast exposure.

The position of the swimmer in the water is an important factor in the severity of underwater blast injuries.[34] Sir Zachary Cope, a prominent British surgeon during World War II, observed that

> if the person were floating on the back so that neither the abdomen nor the chest were directly opposed to the blast wave, no serious injury was sustained.[31]

Because the shock wave reflects as a tension (negative) wave from the water-air interface, the effective force loading of the blast will be greater the deeper one is submerged. Thus, the abdomen will be injured out of proportion to the chest in most underwater exposures. Floating on the water's surface is the safest possible body position when exposure to underwater blast is a possibility.

Hearing Loss Data

In general, the most sensitive organ to the primary effects of a blast wave is the ear. Military personnel are at particular risk for hearing loss, not only from blast exposure but also from exposure to the loud noises that are inherent in the firing of many weapons and the operation of aircraft and tracked vehicles. Not surprisingly, hearing loss is the single largest category of medical disability for the U.S. military, resulting in the payment of more than $165 million in benefits in 1985.

Documentation of combat-related hearing loss is scanty. In a study of 338 soldiers with hearing loss sustained during the Falkland Islands conflict, patients were divided into three groups based on their type of exposure: *(a)* operators of support weapons, such as mortars, *(b)* infantrymen who used small arms, and *(c)* Welsh guardsmen who were survivors of blast injuries sustained in an attack on a transport ship.[35] Those using heavier weapons were at greater risk; the mean hearing loss from preconflict hearing levels was 5.1 dB in the right ear and 5.5 dB in the left ear. Compliance with hearing protection was so poor that no conclusions could be reached regarding its effectiveness. In a second study, 114 soldiers in the Royal Artillery were exposed to very high levels of impulse noise from the sustained firing of 105-mm artillery.[36]

Table 6-2 summarizes the British data on hearing loss during the Falkland Islands conflict.

The high incidence of tympanic-membrane rupture following blast exposure in civilian bombings and recent military conflicts attests to the frequency of aural injury to be expected in combat.[37] The complex reverberant blast environment inside a penetrated armored vehicle is likely to be very injurious to ears, should personnel escape other casualty-generating effects. In one study, large animals were placed inside armored vehicles that were penetrated by shaped-charge warheads. When a 5-inch warhead was used, tympanic-membrane rupture occurred in 71% of ears, compared to 36% when a 3-inch round was used.[21] Based on experiments with anthropomorphic mannequins, the use of conventional hearing protection (either insertional or circumaural) should greatly reduce or eliminate the risk of tympanic-membrane rupture.[38]

EXPERIMENTAL BLAST RESEARCH

Like wound ballistics, blast-injury research was spawned on the battlefield. Controlled experiments have been intertwined with military developments, not only preceding the introduction of new blast weapons or protective equipment, but also resulting from the use of innovative blast munitions by opposing combat forces or unusual blast environments that combatants may have faced in battle.

Blast Research Before World War II

Anecdotes of what can now be recognized as death from PBI were reported earlier than World War I, but this war's heavy use of high explosives exposed the potentially lethal nature of the blast wave itself.

Blast injuries to experimental animals were first studied systematically in 1914, after the Swiss researcher Franchino Rusca observed that three soldiers who had been killed by a bursting grenade during the Balkan Wars had no external injuries. To study this phenomenon, he placed rabbits inside a sand pit that had a stone cover and exposed them to blasts from 100 g of dynamite detonated within the pit. Rusca could not account for the animals' sudden deaths, which later research has proven to be the result of air embolism. However, the gross blast injuries that he described (pulmonary parenchymal hemorrhage, gastrointestinal contusions, and gastrointestinal ruptures) are now recognized as PBI.[39]

Medical personnel in World War I knew that a blast could blow a casualty to pieces, cause bodily displacement, and result in ear injury, but no systematic accounts of internal injuries or deaths from PBI were reported in the military medical literature. At that time, the blast wave was believed to affect primarily the nervous system, possibly because the many "shell-shock" casualties of World War I exhibited a variety of psychophysiological symptoms after prolonged exposure to heavy artillery barrages.

In 1918–1919, the American scientist David Hooker conducted blast-injury studies at Sandy Hook Proving Grounds in New Jersey.[40] He exposed dogs, cats, rabbits, and frogs to muzzle blasts from 10-inch naval cannons and 12-inch mortars. Hooker measured the very sudden increase in air pressure (the overpressure) that the blast produced. The blasts from the 10-inch cannons repeatedly produced shock in dogs (that is, they caused the animals' blood pressure to drop to one-half the normal level), whereas the blasts from the 12-inch mortars did not, even though they had a higher peak pressure. Hooker correctly attributed the pathophysiological abnormalities produced by the cannon's blast to the longer duration of its positive pressure phase. He took comprehensive pathological and physiological measurements, but did not find any gross or microscopic evidence of lesions in the brain or nerve tissues.

Blast Research During World War II

Some soldiers who fought during the Spanish Civil War (1936–1939) were found dead with few, if any, external injuries. However, such detonation deaths did not attract much attention until World War II, when the number of blast casualties increased considerably because of aerial bombing attacks on German and British cities.

British Studies. In Great Britain, researchers who conducted interspecies studies related the blast overpressure levels required to kill 50% of exposed animals (P_{50}) with the animals' body weight.[41] Researchers exposed mice, rabbits, guinea pigs, goats, and monkeys to blasts from 1-, 8-, and 66-pound charges, and observed a striking rise in P_{50} for increasing body size. They extrapolated these data to predict a P_{50} of 370 psi for a 60-kg human and a P_{50} of 470 psi for an 80-kg human. Based on this work with small rodents, the researchers thought that the P_{50}

would be constant for any amount of explosive. Although the explosive charges in the experiments were relatively small by human body-weight standards, they were huge by murine standards, and produced blasts that had relatively long overpressure durations for animals of such small size. Hooker's experiments over 20 years earlier had demonstrated the importance of the blast wave's duration in determining lethality.[40] It was not until after the war that British scientists acknowledged the interactive effect of duration and pressure level.

The pathological nature of the blast injuries, along with the physiological effects, were carefully described by the British researchers.[42] They also showed that the blast wave must hit the thorax directly to produce lung hemorrhage, and suggested that sponge rubber might shield the body from some direct blast effects.

German Studies. Military medical studies of blast waves were also underway in Germany throughout World War II, but the results were not made known until after the end of the war. German civil law prohibited autopsies on most bombing victims, which delayed pathological descriptions of PBI. In particular, four researchers (Hubert Schardin, Theodor Benzinger, Robert Rössle, and Hans Desaga) conducted extensive experiments on the effects of blast,[43–46] which Benzinger described as follows:

> The blast wave is a shot without a bullet, a slash without a sword. It is present everywhere within its range. Blast would be as dreaded . . . as chemical [weapons], if its range, when explosives are used, were not limited to small areas. However, it would be premature to believe that this situation will always remain the same.[44]

The Germans were the first to discover that arterial air embolism is the cause of immediate death from blast injury. They reasoned that air entered the pulmonary venous circulation from the disrupted alveoli and was then distributed to the coronary vessels, the brain, and the vascular beds in other organs of the body. By injecting very small volumes of air into the carotid artery, researchers could produce the central nervous system signs that had previously been observed in blast-injured dogs and humans. Electrocardiographic changes observed in blast-exposed animals were reproduced by injecting about 1 cc of air into the pulmonary veins of dogs. These experimental results supported autopsy findings of internal air emboli as the most probable mechanism of early death from PBI.[45]

The *duration effect* was another significant German finding.[46] The researchers found that the P_{50} for dogs decreased by a factor of three when the duration of the blast wave's positive phase was increased from 1.8 to 12.0 msec. In order to disassociate pressure and duration, the investigators used a variety of different explosive weights and placed the experimental animals at various distances from the point of detonation.

The German investigators noted that the nature of the internal pathoanatomical and pathophysiological changes caused by air and underwater blast were the same.[44] One experiment demonstrated that *(a)* the animal's head was not vulnerable to underwater or air blast, and *(b)* the blast must strike the thorax to inflict lung injury and to cause air embolism (Figure 6-7).

In another experiment, the animals' tracheas were opened widely to the air blast so that any lung injury would be intensified if the blast wave indeed entered the body through the upper respiratory passages (Figure 6-7).[44] This had been suggested by some researchers who believed that the glottis ought to protect the lungs from blast effects, because they had seen injuries to the epiglottis and hemorrhages in the laryngeal mucous membrane in exposed animals whose lungs were not injured in the blast. Five tracheotomized dogs were placed at different distances within and beyond the lethal limit for untreated blast-exposed dogs. Not only did all of the tracheotomized dogs survive, but the tracheotomies actually seemed to have some protective effect. Lung injury did not occur when the upper airway alone was open to the blast and the trunk was protected.

Unlike the British scientists, German researchers found that placing foam rubber materials around the thorax not only provided no protection from air-blast injury, but in fact intensified lung hemorrhage.[46] The injury-enhancement characteristics of this type of material have been affirmed in more recent investigations.[23,25]

Schardin took an engineering approach to the medical observations and proposed three damage mechanisms for blast injury: *(a) spallation*, *(b) implosion*, and *(c) inertia*.[43] In the spallation effect, a blast wave that passes from a more dense medium into a less dense medium reflects into the dense material as a tension wave that throws off (or spalls) material at the interface. In an experiment, a small lead azide charge was detonated in the center of a glass disk. Before the breakage cracks reached the outer edges of the glass disk, the shock front had already reflected from the periphery and spalled material from it. The same effect can also be seen when the water surface breaks up when the blast wave from an underwater explosion (for example, from a depth charge) reaches the water-air interface. Schardin speculated that a similar effect might happen at the air-tissue interface in organs that were exposed to an intense blast, but such an injuring mechanism has never been proved to exist.

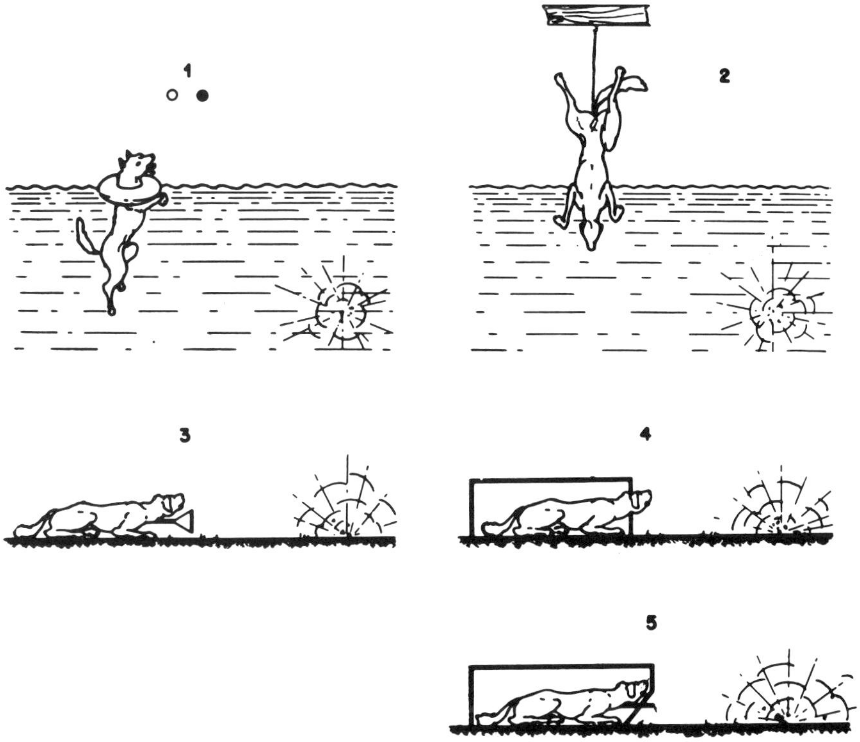

Fig. 6-7. The experiments in this pictoral summary were conducted by German scientists during World War II. The experiments resulted in several findings: The effects of immersion blast were found to be pathologically identical to those of air blast (1). The exposure of the dog's head to immersion blast or air blast resulted in no injury to internal organs (2 and 4). By using a funnel to channel air into the animal's lungs (3), researchers found that injury from air blast was not caused by air being forced down the trachea, and no injury was detected when an animal's tracheotomy was exposed to the blast while its body was protected (5).
Source: Reference 44.

In experiments designed to illustrate the implosion effect, Schardin passed a stream of air bubbles through water and sent a blast wave through them. The inwardly rushing water surrounding the bubbles accumulates considerable kinetic energy, and the bubble is compressed to a much smaller volume than would be expected from the pressure in the blast wave. As the strongly compressed bubbles expand, they become the centers of new pressure waves. Schardin speculated that a similar phenomenon might occur in the lung tissues or in the gas-containing portions of the gastrointestinal tracts of animals that are struck by a strong shock wave.[43] This hypothesis, however, has never been supported by experimental data.

In an example of the inertia effect, an intense air blast that hits a structure like a leaf blows away the delicate portions between the sturdier veins but leaves the veins themselves. Because the veins have more inertia (density) than the light tissue between them, the two materials could be expected to accelerate at different rates when struck by the blast, thereby creating great stress at their boundaries.[43] Schardin speculated that the delicate alveolar tissue between bronchi and blood vessels might be vulnerable to similar stress. Pathological studies did indeed show hemorrhage around the bronchovascular structures, which are analogous to the veins in the leaf.[45]

In keeping with a mechanistic interpretation, Schardin also suggested that, if the duration of the blast wave is less than the *natural period* of the system (that is, the frequency at which it resonates), then the *impulse* (or pressure-time integral) becomes the determining damage component of the blast wave. Thus, consideration of both peak pressure and duration are important in determining injury. If, on the other hand, the duration of the blast wave is greater than the natural period, the peak pressure alone will account for the damage observed. Such long-duration blast waves may be seen with very large bombs or nuclear detonations. Schardin's view was consistent with the British observations that blast damage in mice (which have a small mass and therefore a short natural period, and for which almost all blast waves are effectively of long duration) was dependent on peak pressure alone and independent of charge size, the main determinant of duration.

American Studies. During 1942–1945, American researchers studied the effects of air and underwater blasts using experimental animals. They concluded that PBI from a blast in air occurred only when the animals were within the radius of the blast's fireball and was not an important casualty generator.[30] These researchers studied only blasts that occurred in an open field, however, and the results may not be the same for humans who are within enclosures when they are exposed to air blasts.

During the World War II era, American researchers realized that underwater blast was an important casualty producer because of the many accounts of death and injury among sailors who had been in the water during explosions of depth charges and torpedoes.[30,47] Some experimental work was performed by the U.S. Navy on the pathology of what was then called immersion blast.

Modern Blast Experimentation

Since World War II, blast research has been driven by the increasing lethality of conventional munitions and the tremendous blast effects caused by nuclear detonations. The greatest volume of work has been done in Sweden and the United States, and much of the data is available in unclassified reports.

Swedish Studies. Research on blast injury in Sweden began about 1940 and has continued actively to the present time. Researchers have studied the relationships between the physical qualities of blast waves and changes in physiological and biochemical parameters, particularly as they apply to primary blast injury. The researchers have conducted investigations on the respiratory and circulatory changes following blast injury and on air embolism as the cause of death in blast-exposed animals.[48,49]

In studies of potential protective materials, they found that rigid materials afforded protection from blast waves, but that soft materials (such as foam plastic) did not.[23]

Swedish researchers also measured the deformation of the body wall and the overpressure at several locations inside the animal during blast exposure. They developed physical and mathematical models simulating their empirical findings.[50,51]

French-German Studies. Following World War II, German scientists continued their blast research at the Franco-German Research Institute in Saint-Louis, France. There, researchers studied the relationship between blast-wave components and mortality, and showed that animals can tolerate very high overpressures if there is no shock front—that is, if the peak pressure is reached relatively slowly. In the 1980s, they studied the effects of multiple-blast exposure in both rats and swine.[52,53]

British Studies. At the Chemical Defense Research Establishment in Porton Down, Salisbury, Wiltshire, blast research has focused on behind-armor effects, blunt body trauma, protective garments in a blast environment, and a variety of research concerns (many of which are classified) that are related to terrorist bombings and civil disturbances.[26,54]

Chinese Studies. Since the 1964 detonation of its first nuclear weapon, the People's Republic of China has conducted uninterrupted blast research.[16] Wang Zheng-Guo has led investigations to determine the blast levels required for threshold injuries, severe injuries, and mortality from nuclear and high-explosive blasts. Chinese researchers have assessed the injury potential of repeated lower-level blasts that approximate heavy-artillery muzzle blasts, and have evaluated the practicality of blast-protective garments.

Soviet Studies. Blast research has been conducted in the Soviet Union continuously since World War II, but only a few reports have appeared in the open literature. Published accounts have accurately described the pathology of PBI and have discussed the interaction of blast waves with the body.[55,56] Soviet research has drawn heavily from American and Western European reports; their medical writings often intermingle PBI with other mechanisms of blast injury and seem to stress the neuropsychiatric response to explosions.[57]

American Studies. In 1953, the Atomic Energy Commission contracted with the Lovelace Foundation to study the biological effects of nuclear blast waves, and established a blast-research facility at Kirtland Air Force Base in Albuquerque. Under a series of umbrella organizations and sponsored by many government agencies, the Kirtland facility has been the source of the most comprehensive work on blast biology in the world.

Nuclear-weapons blast research 1958–1964 aimed to develop casualty and risk criteria for both PBI and blast displacement.[58,59] Initial tests by the Lovelace group involved exposing animals to nuclear blasts while they were inside open blast shelters at the Nevada Test Site. Injury criteria were developed for personnel who were in the open field as well as inside fortifications.

For several years in the mid-1960s, researchers at Kirtland conducted tests to determine the effectiveness of FAE munitions against a variety of military targets. In 1968, an underwater test facility was constructed at Kirtland to study immersion-blast effects. In 1978, research was directed toward determining damage-risk criteria for personnel who were exposed to repeated muzzle blasts from heavy weapons that ranged from mortars to large field guns.[60] Since 1980, government researchers and contractors have been studying the physiological consequences and biomechanics of blast injury.[61,62]

SUMMARY

Although fragments cause most of the injuries that result from small terrorist bombings, PBI is often noted at autopsy and may be a contributor to early mortality in many cases. A small number of survivors will have pulmonary PBI that results in respiratory failure and high in-hospital mortality. Positive-pressure ventilation or general anesthesia will put such casualties at an even higher risk.

The determination of the incidence of PBI in military casualties may be clouded by the low-intensity nature of most American combat operations since the Vietnam War and a lack of blast-casualty data from Middle-East wars. Future military conflicts will result in casualties with PBI, usually as a component of combined injuries. PBI will continue to be an important factor in armored warfare, in underwater explosions that affect submerged or swimming soldiers, in explosions from enhanced-blast munitions, and in explosions that occur near soldiers who are wearing ballistic body armor.

Even in peacetime, hearing loss is a common injury in soldiers. The limited available data and common sense suggest that intense combat operations—even those that are as brief as the Falkland Islands conflict—will result in significant hearing loss for many combatants. Tympanic-membrane rupture and associated hearing loss will be common, especially for casualties in armored vehicles. Wearing standard hearing protection should ameliorate this form of acoustic injury.

REFERENCES

1. Frykberg, E. R., and Tepas, J. J. III. 1988. Terrorist bombing: Lessons learned from Belfast to Beirut. *Ann. Surg.* 208:569–576.

2. Frykberg, E. R.; Hutton, P. M.; and Balzer, R. H., Jr. 1987. Disaster in Beirut: An application of mass casualty principles. *Milit. Med.* 152:563–566.

3. Pyper, P. C., and Graham, W. J. H. 1982. Analysis of terrorist injuries treated at Craigavon Area Hospital, Northern Ireland. *Injury* 14:332–338.

4. Hadden, W. A.; Rutherford, W. H.; and Merrett, J. D. 1978. The injuries of terrorist bombing: A study of 1532 consecutive patients. *Br. J. Surg.* 65:525–531.

5. Roy, D. 1982. Gunshot and bomb blast injuries: A review of experience in Belfast. *J. R. Society Med.* 75: 542–545.

6. Brismar, B., and Bergenwald, L. 1982. The terrorist bomb explosion in Bologna, Italy, 1980: An analysis of the effects and injuries sustained. *J. Trauma* 22:216–220.

7. Baker, S. P., and O'Neill, B. 1976. The injury severity score: An update. *J. Trauma* 16:882–885.

8. Adler, J.; Golan, E.; Golan, J.; Yitzhaki, M.; and Ben-Hur, N. 1983. Terrorist bombing experience during 1975–79. *Isr. J. Med. Sci.* 19:189–193.

9. Cooper, G. J.; Maynard, R. L.; Cross, N. L.; and Hill, J. F. 1983. Casualties from terrorist bombings. *J. Trauma* 23: 955–967.

10. Huller, T., and Bazini, Y. 1970. Blast injuries of the chest and abdomen. *Arch. Surg.* 100:24–30.

11. Melzer, E.; Hersche, M.; Fischer, P.; and Hershko, C. 1986. Disseminated intravascular coagulation and hypopotassemia associated with blast lung injury. *Chest* 89:690–693.

12. Katz, E.; Ofek, B.; Adler, J.; Abramowitz, H. B.; and Krausz, M. M. 1989. Primary blast injury after a bomb explosion in a civilian bus. *Ann. Surg.* 209:484–488.

13. Hill, J. F. 1979. Blast injury with particular reference to recent terrorist bombing incidents. *Ann. R. Coll. Surg. Engl.* 61:4–11.

14. McCaughey, W.; Coppel, D. L.; and Dundee, J. W. 1973. Blast injuries to the lung. *Anaesthesia* 28:2–9.

15. Rignault, D. P., and Deligny, M. C. 1989. The 1986 terrorist bombing experience in Paris. *Ann. Surg.* 209:368–373.

16. Wang, Z. G. 1987. Research on blast injury in China. *Chuang Shang Tsa Chih* 6:222–228.

17. Danon, Y. L., and Nili, E. 1984. Triage, primary treatment and evacuation: The IDF experience in Lebanon. Paper presented at the Second International Congress in Israel on Disaster Management, 16–19 September, at Israel Defense Force, Jerusalem.

18. Mellor, S. G., and Cooper, G. J. 1989. Analysis of 828 servicemen killed or injured by explosion in Northern Ireland 1970–84: The Hostile Action Casualty System. *Br. J. Surg.* 76:1006–1010.

19. Kennedy, D. R. 1983. Improving combat crew survivability. *Armor* 9:16–22.

20. Owen-Smith, M. S. 1977. Armored fighting vehicle casualties. *J. R. Army Med. Corps* 123:65–76.

21. Phillips, Y. Y III; Mundie, T. G.; Hoyt, R.; and Dodd, K. T. 1989. Middle ear injury in animals exposed to complex blast waves inside an armored vehicle. *Ann. Otol. Rhinol. Laryngol.* 98:17–22.

22. Phillips, Y. Y III; Ripple, G. R.; Dodd, K. T.; and Mundie, T. G. 1989. Medical evaluation of live fire test injuries: Predicting medical effects behind defeated armor. *Army RD A Bull.* 89:16–18.

23. Jönsson, A. 1979. Experimental investigations on the mechanisms of lung injury in blast and impact exposure. Ph.D. diss. no. 80, Department of Surgery, Linköping University, Stockholm, Sweden.

24. Young, A. J.; Jaeger, J. J.; Phillips, Y. Y III; Yelverton, J. T.; and Richmond, D. R. 1985. The influence of clothing on intrathoracic pressure during airblast. *Aviat. Space Environ. Med.* 56:49–53.

25. Phillips, Y. Y III; Mundie, T. G.; Yelverton, J. T.; and Richmond, D. R. 1988. Cloth ballistic vest alters response to blast. *J. Trauma* 28:S149–S152.

26. Cooper, G. J.; Pearce, B. P.; Cater, S. R.; Kenward, C. E.; and Townend, D. 1989. Augmentation by foam materials of lung injury produced by blast waves: The role of stress waves in thoracic visceral injury at high rates of energy transfer. In *Proceedings of the International Research Council on the Biokinetics of Impacts.* Stockholm, Sweden: International Research Council on the Biokinetics of Impacts.

27. Central Intelligence Agency. Personal communication, 1987.

28. Central Intelligence Agency. Personal communication, 1987.

29. Central Intelligence Agency. Personal communication, 1986.

30. Pugh, H. L. 1943. Blast injuries. *Surg. Clin. North Am.* 23:1589–1602.

31. Cope, Z. 1953. The general effects of blast. Chapt. 18, part 1 of *Surgery,* edited by Z. Cope, 652–663. London: Her Majesty's Stationery Office.

32. Gordon-Taylor, G. 1953. Abdominal effects of immersion blast. Chapt. 18, Part 2, of reference 31, 664–672.

33. Weiler-Ravell, D.; Adatto, R.; and Borman, J. B. 1975. Blast injury of the chest: A review of the problem and its treatment. *Isr. J. Med. Sci.* 11:268–274.

34. Mellor, S. G. 1988. The pathogenesis of blast injury and its management. *Br. J. Hosp. Med.* 39:536–539.

35. Brown, J. R. 1985. Noise-induced hearing loss sustained during land operations in the Falkland Islands campaign. *J. Soc. Occup. Med.* 35:44–54.

36. Anderson, J. 1984. An audiometric survey of royal artillery gun crews following "Operation Corporate." *J. R. Army Med. Corps* 130:100–108.

37. Chait, R. H.; Casler, J.; and Zajtchuk, J. T. 1989. Blast injury of the ear: Historical perspective. *Ann. Otol. Rhinol. Laryngol.* 98:9–12.

38. Phillips, Y. Y III, and Patterson, J. H. 1988. Protection against noise and blast. *Med. Bull. U.S. Army Med. Dep.* PB 8-88-2:17–20.

39. Rusca, F. 1915. *Deutsche Ztschr. f. Chir.* 132:315.

40. Hooker, D. R. 1924. Physiological effects of air concussion. *Amer. J. Physiol.* 67:219–274.

41. Fischer, R. B.; Krohn, P. L.; and Zuckerman, S. 1941. *The relationship between body size and the lethal effects of blast* [Ministry of Home Security Report R.C. 284]. Oxford, England: Oxford University.

42. Krohn, P. L.; Whitteridge, D.; and Zuckerman, S. 1942. Physiological effects of blast. *Lancet* 1:252–275.

43. Schardin, H. 1950. The physical principles of the effects of a detonation. In *German Aviation Medicine, World War II.* Vol. 2, prepared under the auspices of the U.S. Air Force Surgeon General, 1207–1224. Washington, DC: U.S. Government Printing Office.

44. Benzinger, T. 1950. Physiological effects of blast in air and water. In reference 43, 1225–1259.

45. Rössle, R. 1950. Pathology of blast effects. In reference 43, 1260–1273.

46. Desaga, H. 1950. Blast injuries. In reference 43, 1274–1293.

47. Harmon, J. W., and Haluszka, M. 1983. Care of blast-injured casualties with gastrointestinal injuries. *Milit. Med.* 148:586–588.

48. Clemedson, C.-J. 1953. Respiration and pulmonary gas exchange in blast injury. *J. Appl. Physiol.* 6:213–220.

49. Clemedson, C.-J., and Hultman, H. 1954. Air embolism and the cause of death in blast injury. *Milit. Surg.* 114: 424–437.

50. Axelsson, H., and Richmond, D. R. 1990. The non-auditory effects of complex blast waves on personnel inside an APC attacked by shaped charge warheads. *Chuang Shang Tsa Chih* 6(2):(Supp)250–257.

51. Clemedson, C.-J., and Jönsson, A. 1976. Effects of the frequency content in complex shock waves on lung injuries in rabbits. *Aviat. Space Environ. Med.* 47(11):1143–1152.

52. Vassout, P.; Parmentier, G.; and Dancer, A. 1981. *Study of the effects of a strong shock wave on the pig: Impact of the number of exposures* [Report 89/81]. Saint-Louis, France: Institute Franco-Allemand de Recherches de Saint-Louis.

53. Vassout, P.; Frank, R.; Parmentier, G.; Evard, G.; and Dancer, A. 1986. *Mesures de pression et d'acceleration intracorporelles chez le porc exposé a des ondes de choc fortes en champ libre* [Rapport 112/86]. Saint-Louis, France: Institute Franco-Allemand de Recherches de Saint-Louis.

54. Cooper, G. J.; Maynard, R. L.; Aldous, F. A. B.; Evans, V. A.; and Kenward, C. E. 1983. *Nonpenetrating injury to the chest: An experimental study of the biomechanical principles of lung injury, the pathology of pulmonary contusions and their acute physiological effects (U)* [Technical Paper 344]. Porton Down, England: Chemical Defense Establishment.

55. Chesnokov, P. T., and Kholodnyy, A. Y. 1970. Pathomorphological shifts in the organism caused by explosive blast waves (in Russian). *Voen. Med. Zh.* 8:33–36.

56. Deneiga, V. G. 1966. Some information on the biophysics of pneumatic contusions (in Russian). *Biofizika* 11(2): 371–374.

57. Shereshevskiy, G. M. 1979. Contusions (in Russian). *Voen. Med. Zh.* 11:22–25.

58. White, C. S.; Jones, R. K.; Damon, E. R.; and Richmond, D. R. 1971. *The biodynamics of air blast* [Technical Progress Report DNA 2738-T]. Washington, DC: U.S. Department of Defense.

59. White, C. S.; Bowen, I. G.; and Richmond, D. R. 1965. *Biological tolerance to air blast and related biomedical criteria* [USAEC Civil Effects Test Operations Report CEX-65.4]. Washington, DC: U.S. Department of Commerce.

60. Phillips, Y. Y III; Dodd, K. T.; Yelverton, J. T.; and Richmond, D. R. 1985. Non-auditory risk assessment for Friedlander blast waves [Paper VII.6.1]. Paper presented at the Ninth International Symposium on Military Applications of Blast Simulators, 23–27 September, at Cambridge College, Essex, England.

61. Young, A. J.; Hoyt, R. F.; Jaeger, J. J.; Phillips, Y. Y III; Richmond, D. R. 1986. Short duration airblast does not increase pulmonary microvascular permeability. *Milit. Med.* 151:139–143.

62. Stuhmiller, J. H.; Chuong, C. J.; Dodd, K. T.; Phillips, Y. Y III. 1988. Computer modeling of thoracic response to blast. *J. Trauma* 28:S149–S152.

Chapter 7

THE PHYSICS AND MECHANISMS OF PRIMARY BLAST INJURY

JAMES H. STUHMILLER, Ph.D.,* YANCY Y PHILLIPS III, M.D., FCCP,**
AND DONALD R. RICHMOND, Ph.D.***

*Vice President, JAYCOR, Inc., San Diego, California 92121
** Lieutenant Colonel, United States Army; Chief, Pulmonary and Critical Care Medicine Service, Walter Reed Army Medical Center, Washington, D.C. 20307-5001, and Consultant to the Surgeon General in Pulmonary Medicine and Respiratory Therapy
***Former Director, Western Operation, EG&G, Mason Research Institute; Albuquerque, New Mexico 87119–9024

INTRODUCTION

An explosive is a substance that can be made to undergo a rapid chemical reaction that will transform a liquid or solid into gas, liberating a large amount of energy.[1] The products of the detonation (or *explosion*) of a conventional explosive are *(a)* a region of highly compressed gas (the *blast*) that rapidly expands to occupy a volume at least 10^5 times greater than that of the original explosive and *(b)* various solid residues from the explosive or its casing. In addition, nuclear detonations release radioactive particles when fission or fusion occur.

An explosion that occurs in the earth's atmosphere is called an *air blast*; a blast that occurs in water is called an *underwater blast*. Conventional military explosives range from a few ounces up to thousands of pounds of trinitrotoluene (TNT) equivalent. Nuclear weapons produce blast waves that are equivalent to thousands or millions of tons of conventional explosives.[2]

The rapid expansion of gas after detonation almost instantaneously compresses the surrounding air into a *shock wave* that propagates supersonically and in all directions from the explosion (Figure 7-1). The shock wave that is generated by the rapid release of gas from an explosive is called the *blast wave*. The rush of air caused by the net motion of the gas is called the *blast wind*.

Blast injury is a general term that refers to the biophysical and pathophysiological events and the clinical syndromes that occur when a living body is exposed to blast of any origin. Blast-wave physical properties, the complexity of the waveform, and the number of blast repetitions determine the potential for *primary blast injury* (PBI).

PBI occurs when the blast wave strikes and compresses the body. Energy is transferred directly from the transmitting medium (air or water) to the body surface. Damage is almost totally limited to the auditory system and the gas-containing structures of the respiratory and gastrointestinal tracts.

Secondary blast injury occurs when flying debris, collapsed buildings, or other environmental material energized by the explosion strike the body. A high incidence of casualties with secondary injuries from broken glass can be expected when blasts occur in urban areas.

Tertiary blast injury occurs when a casualty's body is thrown against the ground, equipment, structures, trees, or other stationary objects by pressure differentials or blast winds. *Mutilating blast injury* (that is, traumatic amputation) occurs as a combination of secondary and tertiary blast effects.

Blast waves that come from an explosion used to propel a soldier's own munitions are called *weapon noise*. Their principal hazard is to the soldier's hearing.

FUNDAMENTALS OF BLAST AND BLAST WAVES

The defining characteristic of a *blast wave* at any point in space is the variation in ambient pressure over time (its *pressure-time history*). The increased pressure (above normal atmospheric pressure) from a blast is termed the *blast overpressure*. The level of overpressure depends upon *(a)* the energy of the explosion, *(b)* the distance from the point of detonation, *(c)* the elapsed time since the explosion, and *(d)* the measurement technique. *Blast strength* is defined as the ratio of overpressure to ambient pressure. Some exotic explosives, such as fuel-air mixtures, can produce large overpressures with long *positive durations* (that is, the time over which the pressure is greater than the ambient undisturbed pressure). Blast waves that arise from weapon noise have small positive durations (usually less than 5 msec) and modest peak overpressures (less than 1 atm) and are accompanied by negligible blast winds. Nuclear weapons can generate blast waves that have overpressures of several atmospheres, positive durations lasting several seconds, and blast winds of hundreds of miles per hour.

The molecules of gas in the atmosphere around us are in constant thermal motion.[3] On average, at sea level, there are 30 million billion molecules in every cubic millimeter of air, moving at speeds on the order of 300 m/s and bumping into one another 100 million times each second, after traveling only 0.001 mm. This continual bombardment of gas molecules against any solid surface exerts a force on every part of that surface and is most appropriately expressed as a force per unit area, or a *pressure*.

The average energy of motion of individual molecules is measured by the temperature of the gas, while the mass of molecules in a given volume is measured by the density of the gas. Pressure, temperature, and density are measures of the *state* of the gas. Because all

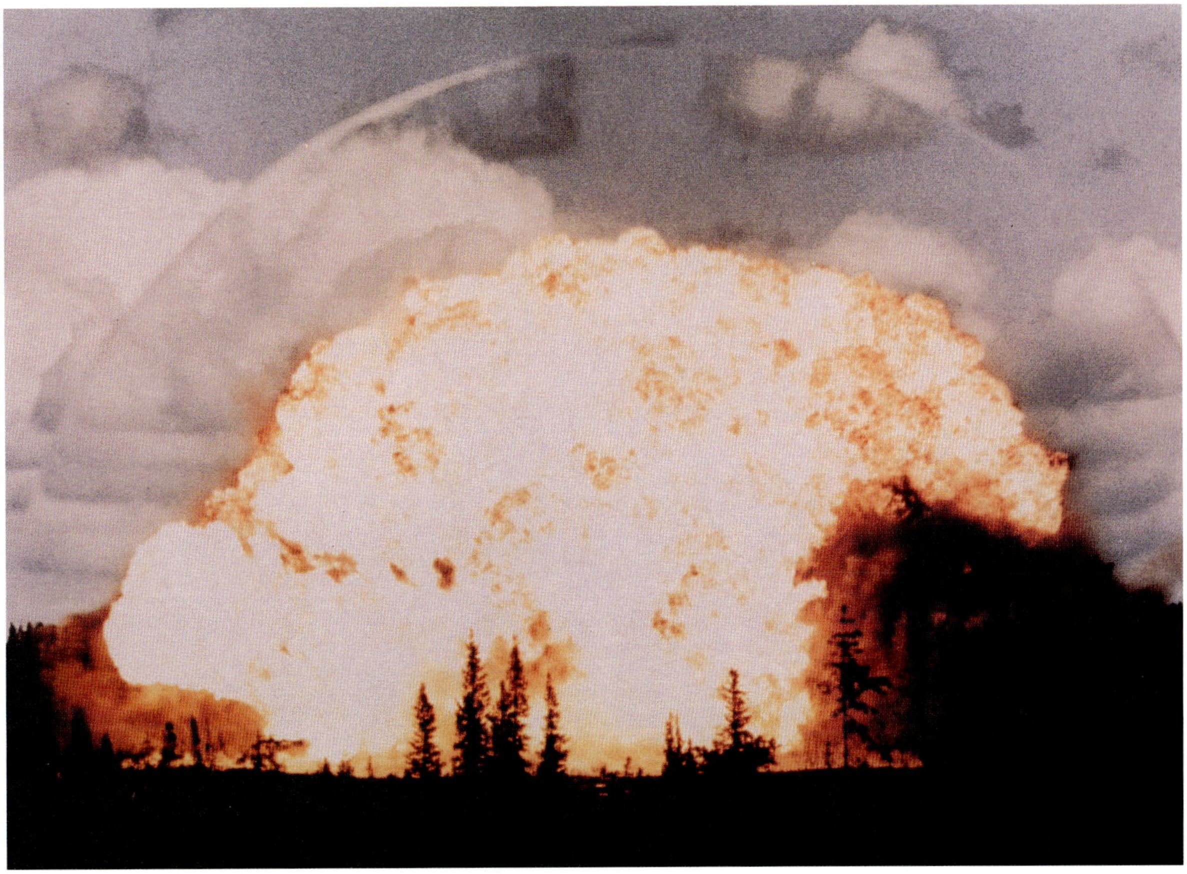

Fig. 7-1. A large conventional explosion is shown from a distance. Beyond the fireball, the blast wave appears as a sharp line, which is caused by refraction of light by the higher-density gas at the shock front.
Source: D. R. Richmond

three quantities are manifestations of the underlying motion of the molecules, they are related to one another by *equations of state*.

Physical Characteristics of Wave Propagation

When the state of a gas is disturbed, for example by opening a door into a closed room, the molecules near the door are momentarily compressed. Because the molecules move so much faster than the door, however, this local aggregation of molecules is quickly dispersed. These small compression disturbances travel at the speed of sound. The room quickly reaches a state of slightly higher but uniform pressure. Similarly, when passengers force their way onto an already crowded train, a new arrangement (in which the distance between people has evened out) takes place throughout the car without much motion of any one individual. The propagation of state changes, without the need for much motion of the individual elements, is called *wave propagation*. The speed at which such a disturbance propagates is called the *wave speed*, while the net speed at which individual elements move is called the *material speed*.

There are many examples in ordinary life of wave propagation. Sound is propagation of local concentrations of pressure through any gas, liquid, or solid. Water waves are the propagation along the surface of local variations in the water level. Electrical signals along a telephone line are the propagation of local variations in the electric and magnetic fields within the wire. In each of these examples, the material speed of the individual elements is quite small compared to the wave speed. The air that is moved in the act of speaking barely leaves the region of the vocal cords by the time the sound is heard across a room. The water molecules move at only a small fraction of the speed of the water wave. Even more dramatically, in the time the electrical signal passes from Los Angeles to New York, the electrons in the telephone wire responsible for starting the signal have moved less than 1 cm.

A different situation exists if the material speed approaches or exceeds the wave speed. When the material speed exceeds the wave speed, the individual

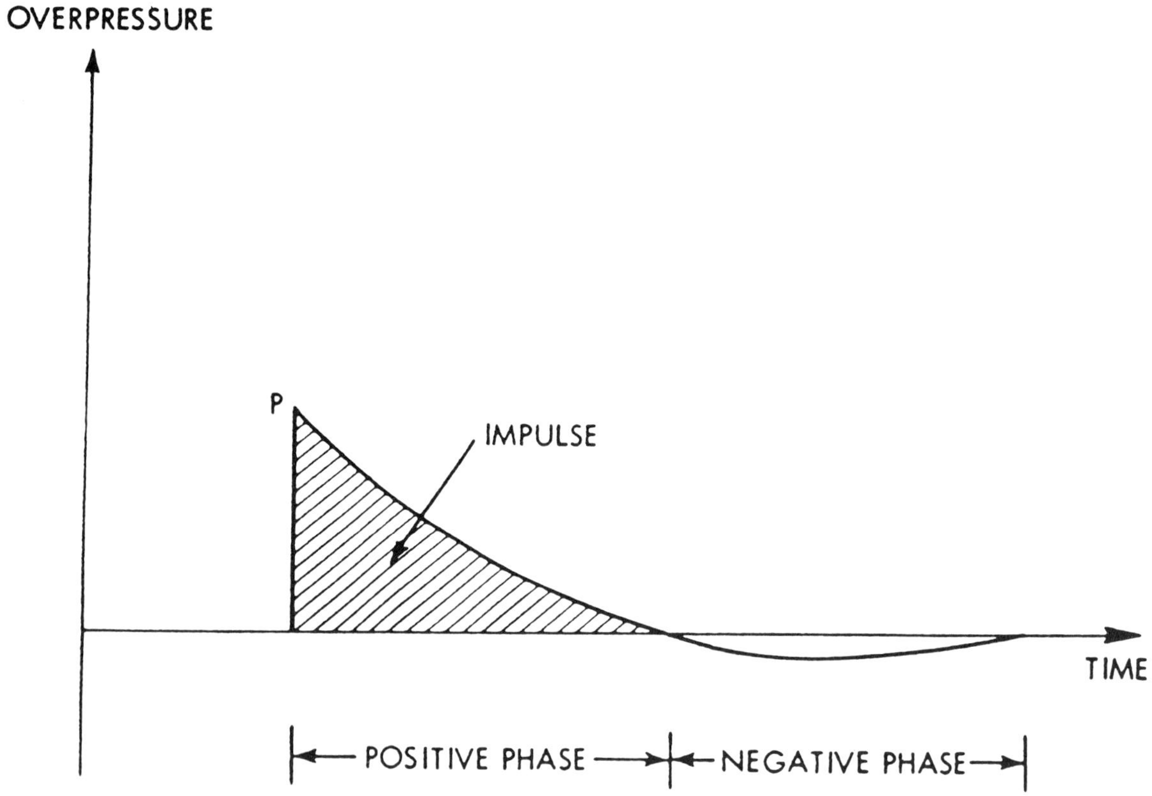

Fig. 7-2. This graph illustrates the ideal pressure-time history of an air blast in an undisturbed, free-field environment (a Friedlander waveform). The impulse is the integral of pressure over time. P is the peak overpressure.
Source: Walter Reed Army Institute of Research

elements are pushed together faster than the disturbances can be relieved by the thermal motion. Consequently, the molecules pile up and the densities, pressures, and temperatures increase rapidly. Eventually, because the wave-propagation speed also increases as these quantities increase, a state is reached in which the piling up that is caused by the material motion is just balanced by the dispersion of the thermal motion. This local high pressure, temperature, and density—the shock wave—advances faster than the speed of sound through the undisturbed medium.

The Blast Wave

The term *blast front* is often used to describe the leading edge of the blast wave as it moves into undisturbed ambient air. This front increases the density of the air through which it passes, raising its temperature and accelerating the air molecules. In the denser air at the blast front, the pressure wave travels faster than it would through ambient-pressure air.

The gases from an explosion push out circumferentially and rapidly into undisturbed air. As the blast front passes, they create both a high-pressure region (the *positive phase,* shown in Figure 7-2), and a blast wind. Because the gas is rushing away from the explosion, it not only decompresses the original high-pressure region that the explosion caused, but it also continues to expand. This creates a region of below-atmospheric pressure (the *negative phase*) that also propagates away from the explosion. Since the speed of propagation increases with pressure, the negative phase of the blast wave moves more slowly than the blast front does, and becomes separated from the front by greater and greater distances as the blast wave progresses.

In the positive phase, the air is compressed almost instantly to a peak value that decays exponentially back to and then below the ambient (baseline) pressure, into a negative phase. During the positive phase, the flow of gas, or blast wind, is away from the explosion. The direction of flow reverses in the negative phase, with a net movement of gas back towards the relative vacuum at the detonation point. The negative phase is thought not to contribute to blast injury, although definitive data do not exist.

The Pressure Waveform

A blast wave occupies a particular place at any given time, and a pressure-measuring device placed at a fixed location for a defined period of time can quantitatively describe a blast. As a result, the spatial variation of the wave is translated into a time variation, its pressure-time history or *pressure waveform.* Simple measurements of the blast wave are meaningful only when the pressure waveform has a very simple shape (Figure 7-2). Characterization of such waves, called *ideal blast waves,* includes making the following observations:

- The ambient atmospheric pressure is noted before the wave arrives
- The pressure rises almost instantaneously to the peak overpressure when the blast front arrives
- The pressure remains above ambient while the positive phase of the blast wave passes the measuring point
- The positive-phase duration is the interval between the arrival of the blast front and the first return to ambient pressure
- A lower-than-ambient pressure that slowly returns to ambient marks the passage of the negative phase

Many mathematical forms have been suggested to capture the time variation of these ideal blast waves. One equation, *the Friedlander waveform,* describes the theoretical variation of the positive pressure behind the shock front:[4]

$$P(t) = P_s (1 - t/t_o) \exp(-bt/t_o)$$

where $P(t)$ is the pressure at any given time (t), P_s is the peak overpressure (an instantaneous static pressure quantity), t_o is the positive duration (the time duration of the positive pressure), and b is a decay constant, a parameter that describes the rate at which the overpressure decreases after the peak.

Blast waves are typically measured by piezoelectric or piezo-resistive pressure transducers.[4] Less-common photographic methods include *(a)* high-speed cameras, *(b)* shadow graphs, and *(c)* Schlieren and streak films.[4,5] Figure 7-2 illustrates an ideal pressure-time pattern measured by a gauge that was oriented *side-on* (that is, the sensing surface is oriented parallel to the direction of wave propagation) to the blast in the *free field* (that is, away from any complicating surfaces that would disturb the blast wave). Major environmental features, such as buildings and vehicles, can reflect the *incident* wave (that is, the original blast wave) and lead to very complex overpressures, where measurements are suspect and the potential for injury is difficult to predict.

The pressure-time history of the ideal blast wave is characteristic of many blast waves, especially those far from the explosion. However, if the chemical reactions are slow, or if the point of observation is close to the explosion, non-ideal effects are seen. The most common deviation from the ideal waveform is a second, smaller peak that appears when the negative phase begins. This peak corresponds to a recompression of gas at the detonation site. Distortions of the ideal waveform can also occur when the combustion of slow-burning munitions continues after the blast wave has formed.

Conventional Explosives

Conventional explosives contain compounds of hydrogen, oxygen, nitrogen, and carbon. The explosive material may be a solid, slurry, liquid, or gas. *Primary explosives,* such as mercury fulminate, lead azide, and lead stefinite, are very sensitive and may be induced to explode by heat or pressure. *Secondary explosives* are less sensitive and may be either single compounds, such as TNT and pentaethyltrinitride (PETN), or mixtures. For example, Composition C4, a common plastic military explosive, contains 91% cyclotrimethylenetrinitramine (RDX), rubber, oil, and a plasticizer.[4] *Insensitive explosives* have been developed that require the impact of a high-velocity metal flyer plate to initiate a detonation. They will not detonate even when they are in contact with another explosive and are insensitive to high temperatures. Their inherent stability makes them safe to store and transport. Tables 7-1 and 7-2 give some characteristics of common single- and mixed-composition explosives.

General-purpose explosive munitions usually consist of *(a)* a detonator or a fuse containing a sensitive primary explosive, *(b)* a booster of relatively sensitive secondary explosive, and *(c)* a main charge of an insensitive explosive. The weight of the explosive charge generally increases proportionately to the total weight of the munition. The ratio of charge weight to weapon weight ranges from 0.15 for howitzer shells, 0.25–0.33 for hand grenades, 0.51 for 500-pound bombs, to 0.86 for 10,000-pound bombs. In conventional munitions such as grenades and artillery shells, an appre-

TABLE 7-1

BASIC PROPERTIES OF COMMON SINGLE-COMPOUND HIGH EXPLOSIVES

Explosive	Equivalent Weight Relative to TNT*	Density (g/cm^3)	Detonation Velocity (km/s)	Consistency
Ammonium Nitrate, AN	—	1.73	7.00	Solid
Nitroglycerin, NG	—	1.60	7.58	Liquid
Trinitrotoluene, TNT	1.00	1.65	6.90	Solid
Pentaerythritol Tetranitrate, PETN	1.27	1.70	7.98	Solid
Cyclotrimethylene trinitramine, RDX	1.19	1.80	8.75	Solid
Cyclotetramethylene tetranitramine, HMX	~1.30	1.90	9.10	Solid
Nitrocellulose, NC	—	1.2–1.7	7.30	Solid

*Based on the peak pressure produced compared to TNT

ciable fraction of the explosive energy is dissipated in bursting the casing and accelerating the case fragments. Such weapons do most of their damage as a secondary blast effect because the fragments are able to cause injuries far beyond the effective range of the blast wave.

The Scaling Laws

For any type of explosive, every combination of weight and distance from the explosion produces a particular pressure-time history. It has long been noted that if a particular peak overpressure occurs at one distance for one weight of explosive, then that same peak overpressure will occur at a smaller distance for a smaller weight and at a larger distance for a larger weight. Mathematical relationships that allow the results of one set of conditions to be determined from the results of another set are called *scaling laws.* Compilation of a wide range of experimental results produced the *cube root* or *Hopkinson's Rule:* The peak overpressure depends on the *scaled distance,* defined as the physical distance from the explosive divided by the cube root of the weight of the explosive charge. For example, 1 pound of TNT produces a peak overpressure of 0.5 atm at a distance of 10 feet. The scaled distance is $10 \div 1^{0.33} = 10$. At twice the physical distance (20 feet), 8 pounds of TNT will produce the same peak overpressure. The scaled distance is $20 \div 8^{0.33} = 10$.

Hopkinson's Rule has simplified the calculation of the peak overpressure from relying on distance and explosive weight independently to relying on a single combination of the two quantities. By measuring the peak overpressure at various distances from a single weight of explosive, the variation with the scaled distance can be determined. The peak overpressure due to any other amount of that explosive at any distance can be estimated without conducting further experiments.

Useful as Hopkinson's Rule is, it has significant limitations. New experiments would have to be conducted if another type of explosive were used or if the blast occurred at other altitudes where atmospheric conditions differed. It would be useful to have a more general scaling law.

The laws of physics governing blast waves are described by certain mathematical equations.[6] The solution of those equations provide the pressure-time history of the blast wave. To find the solution, a particular choice of explosive energy, atmospheric conditions, and distance from the charge must be made. With certain simplifications, it is possible to

TABLE 7-2

BASIC PROPERTIES OF COMMMON MIXED-COMPOUND EXPLOSIVES

Explosive*	Equivalent Weight Relative to TNT**	Density g/cm^3	Detonation Velocity km/s	Consistency
ANFO 94 AN/6 FG	0.82	~0.8	~4.7	Powder
Composition B 40 TNT/60 RDX	1.11	1.70	7.9	Solid
Octol 25 TNT/75 HMX	1.06	1.82	8.4	Solid
Pentolite 50 TNT/50 PETN	1.42	1.67	7.4	Solid
Dynamite 50 NG/0.2 NC/34 SN/15.8 C	0.90	1.40	~5.8	Solid
Bonded Mixtures				
Composition C4 91 RDX/ 2.1 rubber/ 1.6 oil/ 5.3 plasticizer	1.37	1.0–1.60	8.0	Plastic
Sheet Explosive 60–85 PETN/0–8 NC rubber and plasticizer	~1.27	~1.50	~7.0	Rubberlike sheets

*FO: Fuel oil; SN: Sodium Nitrate; C: Combustibles and chalk
**Equivalent to weights based on peak overpressure produced compared to TNT

rearrange those equations so that only dimensionless combinations of parameters appear. Solving these dimensionless equations would allow the scaling laws to be derived from basic physical principles. Unfortunately, the mathematics of the blast-dynamics equations are extremely difficult and a general solution is not known.

Blast parameters scaled to distance at sea level are given in Figure 7-3. In general, the peak pressure decreases with distance while the positive duration increases and the *positive phase impulse* (that is, the integral of the overpressure over the positive duration) falls. For a 1-pound sphere of TNT detonated in unconfined (free) air, this graph may be read directly. To use larger explosive weights, the actual distance must be scaled by dividing by the cube root of the weight of the explosive charge. The peak pressure is read directly and the scaled blast parameters are then read from the graph and converted to the actual parameters by multiplying by the cube root of the charge. To use Figure 7-3 for explosives other than TNT, the actual charge weight must be multiplied by the compound's TNT equivalency, some of which are given in Tables 7-1 and 7-2.

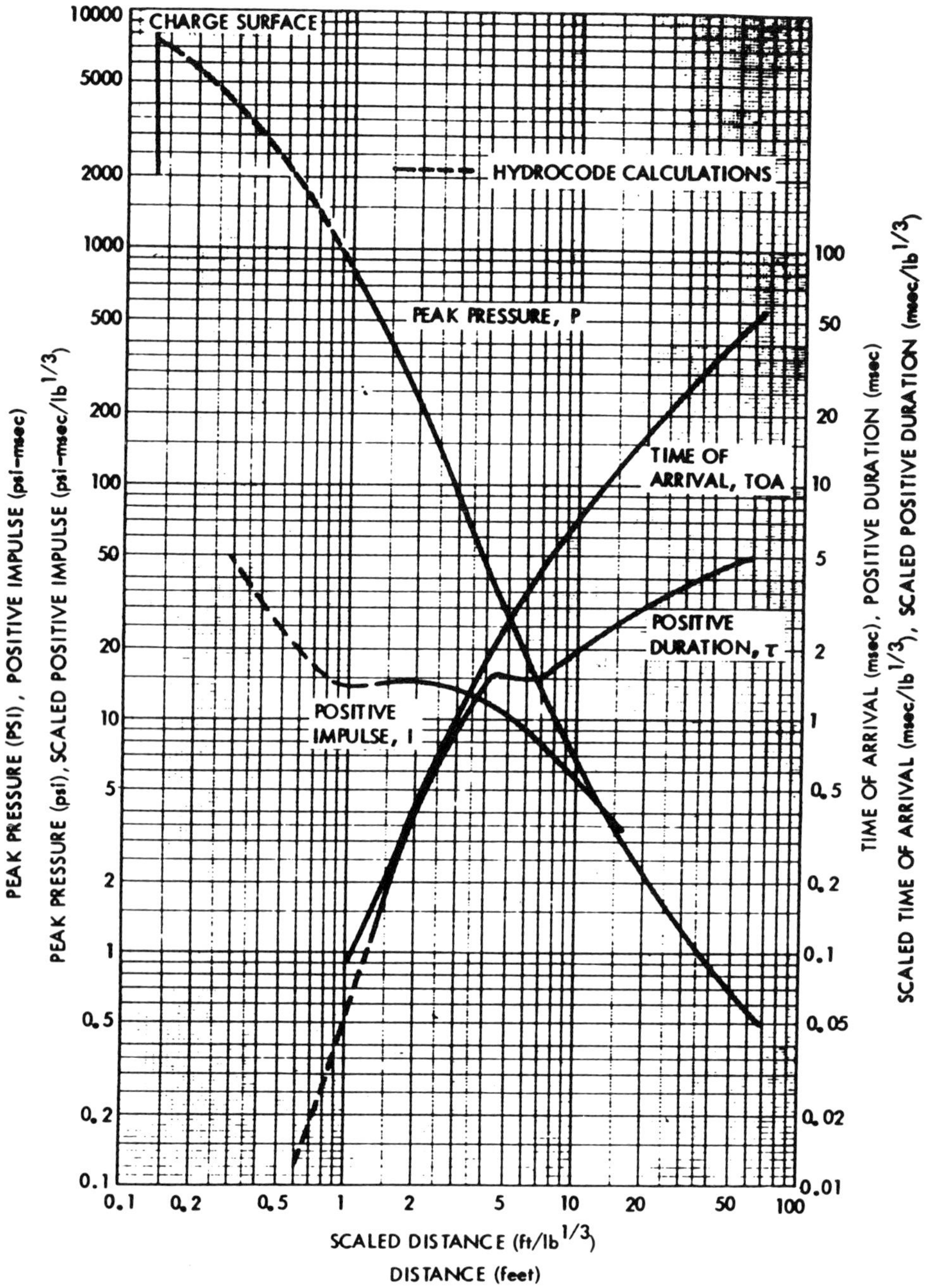

Fig. 7-3. Scaled values of positive-phase duration and impulse, peak pressure, and time of shock arrival are given for scaled distances at sea level from an explosion. For a 1-pound sphere of TNT detonated in open air, the graph may be read directly. To use larger explosive weights, the actual distance must be scaled by dividing by the cube root of charge weight. Peak pressure is then read directly. The scaled blast parameters are then read from the graph and converted to the actual parameters by multiplying by the cube root of the charge. For explosives other than TNT, the actual charge weight must be multiplied by the compound's TNT equivalency (from Tables 7-1 and 7-2). For example, to determine the blast parameters at 40 feet from a 47-pound charge of Composition C4, take its equivalent of 64 pounds of TNT (1.37 x 47) and take the cube root (4). The scaled distance is then 40/4, or 10. The peak pressure and scaled impulse at a scaled distance 10 feet are 7.5 psi and 5.5 psi-msec. The impulse is multiplied by 4 to give an actual peak pressure of 30 psi and an impulse of 22 psi-msec.
Source: Reference 7

Nuclear Blast Waves

Nuclear blast waves differ from those of conventional munitions principally in their positive-phase durations, which may last as long as several seconds, compared to milliseconds with TNT. A nuclear explosion may also produce a *precursor shock wave* under certain conditions of burst height and terrain.[2] The intense radiant thermal pulse heats the ground and adjacent air layer. The shock front near the ground travels faster in this layer of heated air and runs ahead of the main pressure wave. Because the velocity of the air flow in the precursor shock wave is greatly increased, its blast wind is several times greater than that found in an ideal wave having the same peak pressure. *Drag-sensitive equipment* (which is less massive or has a greater exposed surface) and personnel may be displaced great distances by the precursor wave, which is a tertiary blast effect.

BLAST MEASUREMENTS AND EFFECTS

Intense blasts are necessary to produce manifestations of PBI other than ear lesions. Because the intensity of the blast (the peak overpressure) decreases rapidly with distance from the detonation, personnel must be very close to an explosion to sustain PBI. At these short ranges, fragment injuries and thermal burns may mask the blast injury. In fact, fragments of conventional munitions travel in air far beyond the distance that the blast will cause injury.

The destructive aspect of a blast is due to the force it exerts. This force, called the *blast loading*, must be described as a force per unit area, or pressure, and is usually not the same on all parts of a building or a person. The blast loading on a structure depends upon its geometry and its orientation to the incident blast wave. Structural damage would be determined by the inter-relationships between material strength and local stresses produced by the external blast loading.

Blast-Pressure Measurement

Blast pressures are defined as either *static*, *dynamic*, or *reflected*. Pressure-measuring devices record the force exerted on a small sensing surface. The *static* (or side-on) *pressure* is measured by a sensing surface that is oriented parallel to the direction of propagation of the wave (gauge *e* in Figure 7-4). It is unaffected by any kinetic energy in the traveling wave front and measures the air compression that is active in all directions due to the thermal motion of the gas.

If that sensing surface is oriented so that the net motion of the wave front strikes the surface, then the *total pressure* is recorded (gauge *d* in Figure 7-4). The total pressure includes both the static pressure, due to the thermal motion, and the *dynamic pressure*, due to stopping the net air motion at the sensor surface. Dynamic pressure is the force that is associated with the blast wind (that is, the movement of air particles at the leading edge of the shock wave). It is measured as the difference in the reading between two sensors oriented at right angles, side-on and facing the blast wave (Figure 7-4).

The standard practice in blast measurement is to record the static component of the pressure and to present that measurement in terms of the peak overpressure and positive-phase duration. However, readers should not ignore the fact that the blast wind generated by nuclear and large conventional munitions may add substantially to the destructive potential of the static overpressure alone.

Structural Blast Loading and Wave Reflection

When a blast wave encounters a large, solid barrier, like the wall of a building or the ground itself, the motion of the gas molecules is impeded. If the barrier is perpendicular *(normal)* to the direction of propagation of the blast wave, the wave is said to undergo a *normal reflection*. At the barrier, the blast wave can no longer propagate forward into undisturbed gas. Consequently, the molecules are compressed even more by those following the blast front, until they are so tightly packed that they push back in the direction of the incident wave. This even greater concentration of gas molecules that builds up on the surface facing the incident wave is called the *reflected region*.

If there is a negligible amount of blast wind associated with the incident wave, then the reflected region will have an overpressure about twice that of the incident wave. As the blast winds become stronger, the overpressure in the reflected region grows proportionally and can be tenfold greater than the peak pressure in the incident wave.

The reflected region will continue to increase as long as it is supplied by the incident wave. If the

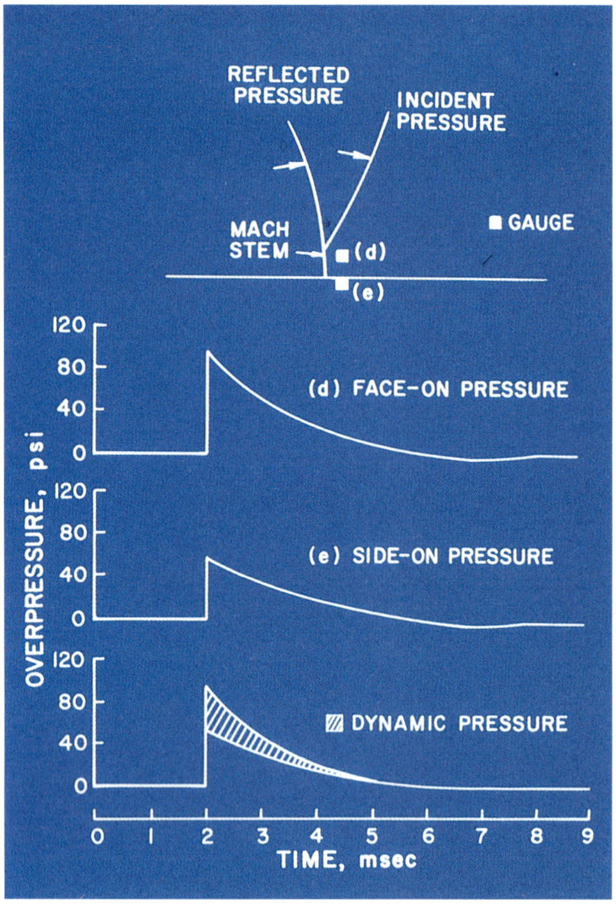

Fig. 7-4. Static and dynamic pressure measurements are depicted for an explosion occurring near the ground. The incident wave reflects from the ground. The reflected and incident waves interact near the surface to produce a strengthened wave called the Mach stem. Gauge *e* is oriented with its sensing surface parallel to the direction of propagation of the wave and measures the static (or side-on) pressure in the Mach stem. Gauge *d* is oriented face-on to the shock and measures both the static and dynamic components of the blast wave. The dynamic pressure is the difference between the two measurements.
Source: D. R. Richmond

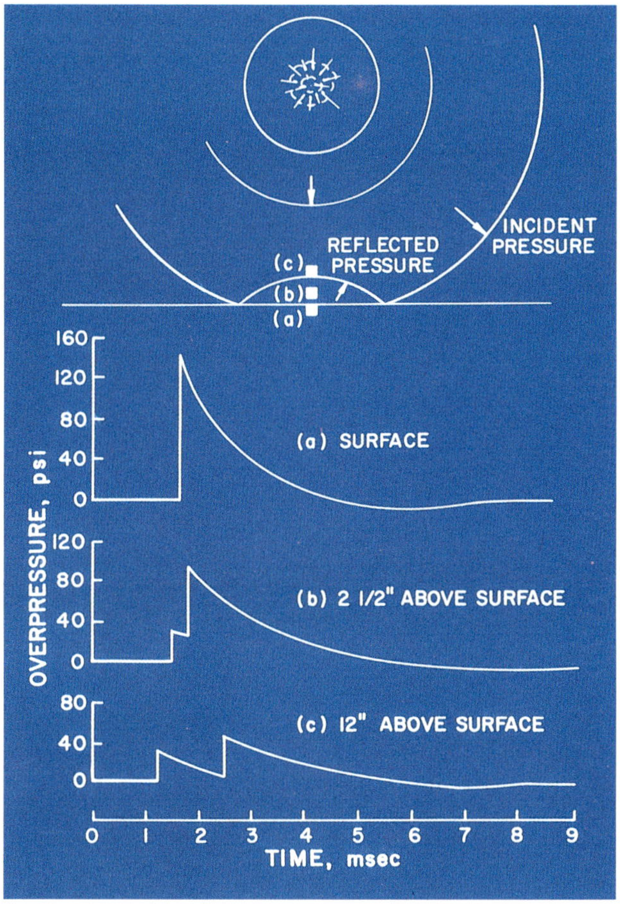

Fig. 7-5. Pressure measurements are depicted near a reflecting surface. Gauge *a* is at the surface and shows the interaction of the incident and reflected waves as a single wave with peak pressure much greater than that in the incident wave. Gauge *b* is slightly above the surface and shows the incident wave and an overlapping reflecting wave. Gauge *c* is farther from the surface and shows less interaction of incident and reflected waves.
Source: D. R. Richmond

incident wave is of finite duration, then the region of high reflected pressure will extend only a finite distance from the wall and only for an amount of time approximately equal to the duration of the incident wave (Figure 7-5). The reflection process results in a reflected wave, which moves in the opposite direction of the incident wave with a nearly identical wave form.

When the blast wave strikes a surface obliquely, the reflection process is more complex. The angle between the direction of propagation of the incident wave and the reflecting surface is called the *angle of incidence*, whereas the corresponding angle for the reflected wave is called the *angle of reflection*. If the blast is weak (that is, the overpressure is not much greater than the ambient pressure) then the angle of reflection is equal to the angle of incidence. This *regular reflection* is geometrically the same as light reflecting off a flat mirror. As the blast strength increases, the incident and reflected waves interfere with one another with the result that the angle of reflection is smaller than the angle of incidence. When the blast strength reaches a critical value, the waves combine to produce a *Mach stem*, which propagates as a single front along a reflecting surface.[7] (The Mach stem, first described by Dr. Ernst Mach in 1877, is not related to Mach numbers, although both are named for Dr. Mach.) Away from the surface, separate incident and reflected waves occur (Figure 7-4). The point at which the three waves join is called the *triple point*. In most large explosions, a person on the ground will only be affected by the Mach stem as it moves along the ground, where the peak pressure will be greater than that in the incident wave. For a surface burst, in order to account for the Mach stem, the actual charge weight in Figure 7-3 must be increased by a factor of 1.7.

When a blast wave strikes a structure, it can exert a tremendous force that can damage or demolish it. Imagine a building with one side normal to the blast. That side will be subjected to the reflected pressure for the duration of the wave, while the opposite side will be subjected to only the ambient pressure until the blast has propagated around to the back. Then the back of the building will be subjected to a pressure comparable to the static overpressure. Even modest pressure differences over the large surface area of most buildings can create enough motion to cause critical structural elements to collapse.

Quantitative values of reflected pressure, dynamic pressure, and blast-wind speed (particle velocity) at the shock front can be plotted as functions of incident static overpressure (Figure 7-6). Table 7-3 gives several examples that illustrate the nonlinear increase in both reflected and dynamic pressures with increasing static shock strengths.

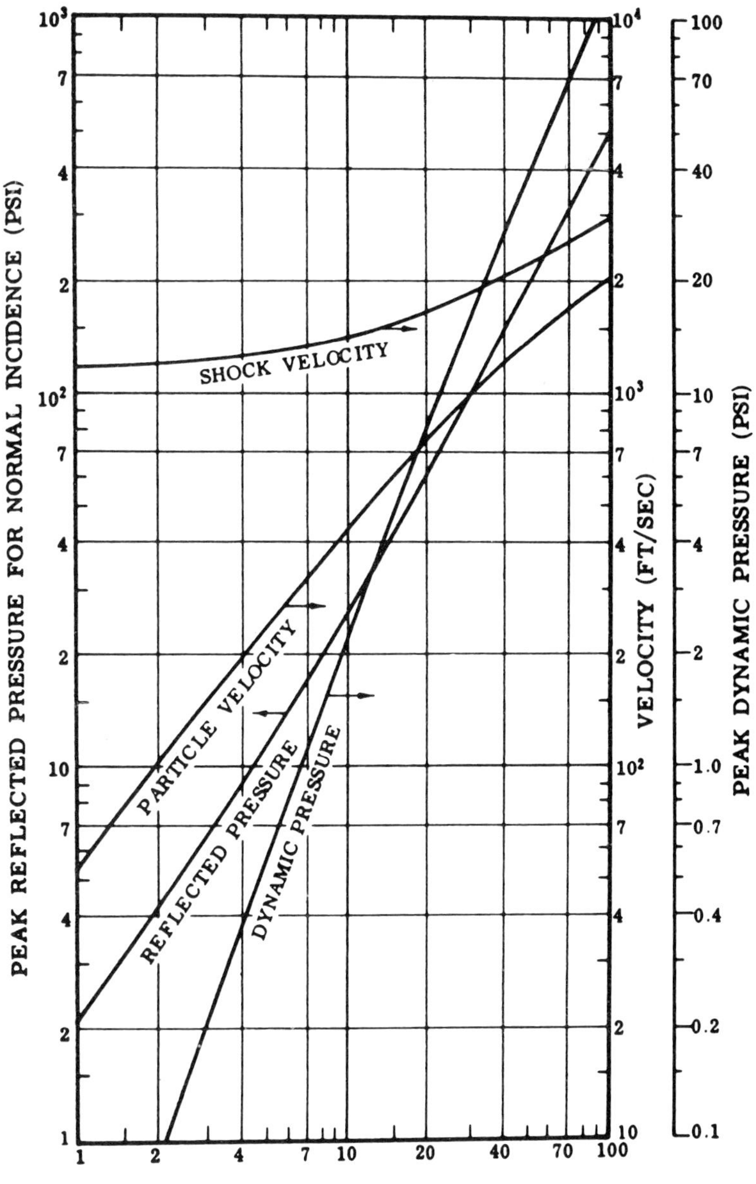

Fig. 7-6. Shock-wave parameters for dynamic pressure, reflected pressure, particle velocity (blast wind), and shock-wave velocity are plotted as a function of incident shock strength as measured by static peak overpressure. Source: Reference 2

TABLE 7-3

WIND VELOCITY RELATED TO BLAST PARAMETERS

Wind Velocity (Mph)	Maximum Pressure in Psi* Incident Static	Reflected	Dynamic
40	1	2	0.02
70	2	4	0.1
160	5	11	0.6
290	10	25	2
470	20	60	8
670	30	90	16
940	50	200	40
1500	100	500	125

*Illustrative values of peak reflected and dynamic pressures demonstrating the nonlinear increase in both with increase shock strength measured as peak static overpressure. By way of comparison, a hurricane wind of 120 mph exerts a dynamic pressure of about 0.25 psi.

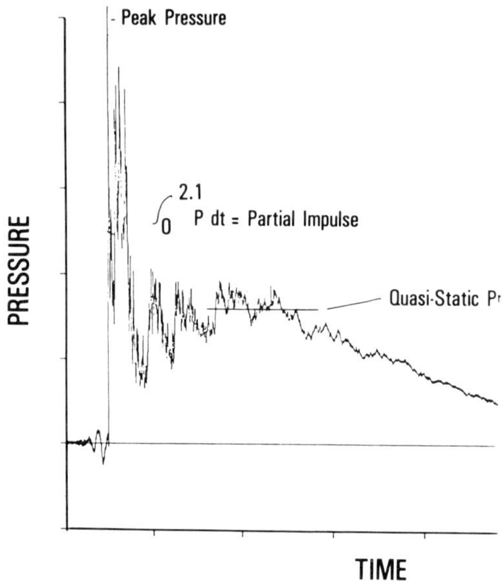

Fig. 7-7. This graph represents a complex blast wave that was recorded inside an armored vehicle that had been penetrated by a shaped-charge munition. Note the many distinct peaks of interacting reflections. After approximately 10 msecs, the ambient compartment pressure is increased by the bulk expansion of gas (quasi-static pressure).
Source: U.S. Army Ballistics Research Laboratory

Complex Blast Waves

Blast waves inside an enclosure undergo repeated reflection from the interior surfaces and create a pressure environment called a *complex blast wave*. Not only is the pressure-time history in such an environment very irregular and long lasting, but because the reflected waves will strike the sensing surface at many different angles, a measuring device does not record only the static component. As a result, even interpreting the pressure wave form is difficult.

Complex blast waveforms in an enclosure have three characteristics: *(a)* the incident blast waves, *(b)* a jumble of reflected waves, and *(c)* the static pressurization of the enclosure (Figure 7-7).

If an explosive is detonated within an enclosure, the first blast wave to arrive at a given location depends only on the explosive energy and the distance from the measuring point—the same as if the blast had occurred in a free field. After reflections begin to occur, however, the pressure-time history becomes a jumble of separate waveforms. The magnitude and timing of these waves depends on the structure of the enclosure and the orientation of the sensor. Finally, the gases liberated by the explosion heat and expand to fill the enclosure, both of which raise the ambient pressure. This static pressurization will eventually subside as the gases vent through openings in the enclosure.

On the battlefield, simple foxholes offer the potential for one of the most common occurrences of complex blast waves. Even though the blast wave propagates across the top of the foxhole and does not directly impinge upon it, the static overpressure causes a wave to propagate into the foxhole and to reverberate inside. Depending on the size and shape of the foxhole and the location of the soldier within it, the effective overpressure loading (and hence the hazard of injury) can be greater than that of the incident blast wave itself.

Blast waves can enter buildings through openings in much the same way that they enter foxholes. Structures hardened against ionizing and thermal radiation may be vulnerable to the blast effects of nuclear weapons. Radiation propagates in a straight line and can be effectively blocked by a barrier such as an earthen berm. A blast wave will propagate around or over the impediment. A useful analogy might be that light cannot be seen from behind a hill, but noise can be heard.

Complex blast waves can also be created when weapons are fired inside a structure. The exhaust gases cause weapon noise, which, in a free field, would cause only auditory injury. Inside a small enclosure, however, the reverberation of the waves and the pressurization of the enclosure lead to much greater loading and the potential for nonauditory blast damage.

Armored vehicles are also subject to complex blast effects on the battlefield. While blast waves can enter armored vehicles through openings like they do in buildings, it is more likely that blasts will be associated with enemy weapons designed to penetrate the vehicle. The penetration of the armored walls leads to both continued ignition of the original munition and secondary explosions from the fuel or other interior combustibles. Penetrating wounds from fragments remain the dominant threat, but as antispall materials are improved, blast becomes a greater potential casualty generator.

TOLERANCE TO AIR BLAST

Blast load on a person is similar to that on a building, except that the time it takes for the blast wave to engulf the body is much shorter than the time necessary for the body to respond. A person is more affected than a building by the crushing effects of the overpressure and the effects of the blast wind. Since the reflected pressure can be considerably greater than the static component, the body's orientation with respect to both the blast itself and any rigid surfaces from which the wave will reflect can affect the body's response.

Small-caliber weapons such as rifles produce blast waves of very short duration and modest overpressure that primarily threaten the auditory system. Larger-caliber weapons such as howitzers produce blast waves of many milliseconds' duration, and with overpressures of as much as 5 psi in crew locations. The principal hazard to soldiers firing these heavy weapons, however, is still to the auditory system. Shoulder-fired weapons and mortars produce high peak overpressures at the position of the soldier, precisely because the soldier is so close to the weapon at the time of firing. Fortunately, the durations are very short, and hearing loss remains the principal hazard.

Curves estimating human tolerance to free-field air blast as functions of the maximum incident overpressure and positive duration at sea level appear in Figures 7-8, 7-9, and 7-10.[8] They are based on results from studies that determined the dose-response of thirteen species subject to blast waves of various durations generated by high explosives in the open and inside shock tubes.[9] At short durations there is an

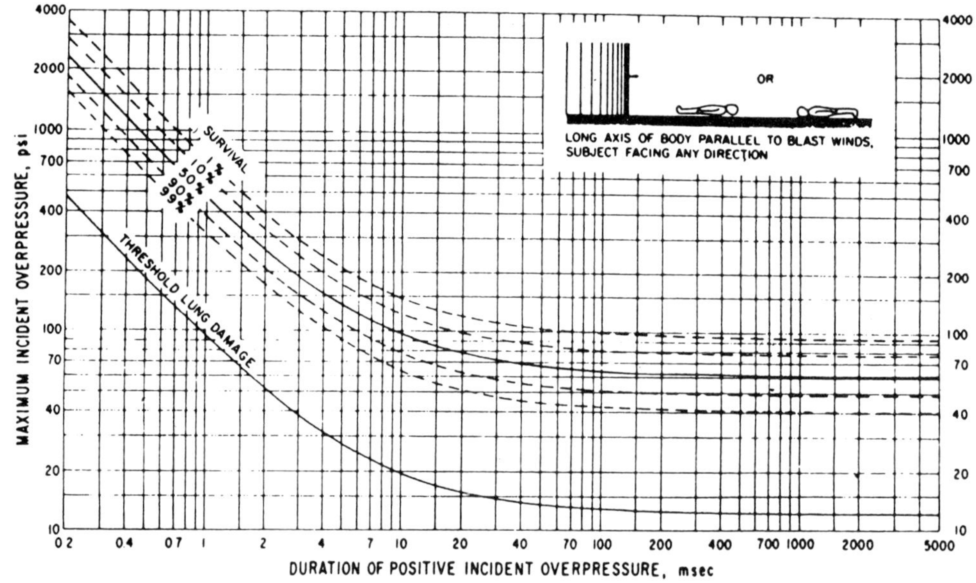

Fig. 7-8. The estimated tolerance for a single air blast at sea level is given for a 70-kg human oriented end-on to the shock wave.
Source: Reference 8

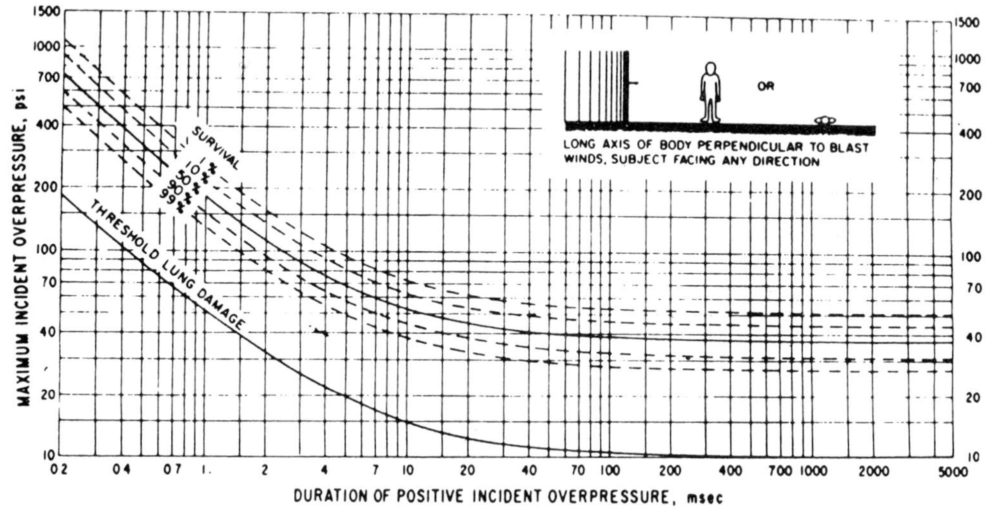

Fig. 7-9. The estimated tolerance for a single air blast at sea level is given for a 70-kg human oriented side-on to the shock wave.
Source: Reference 8

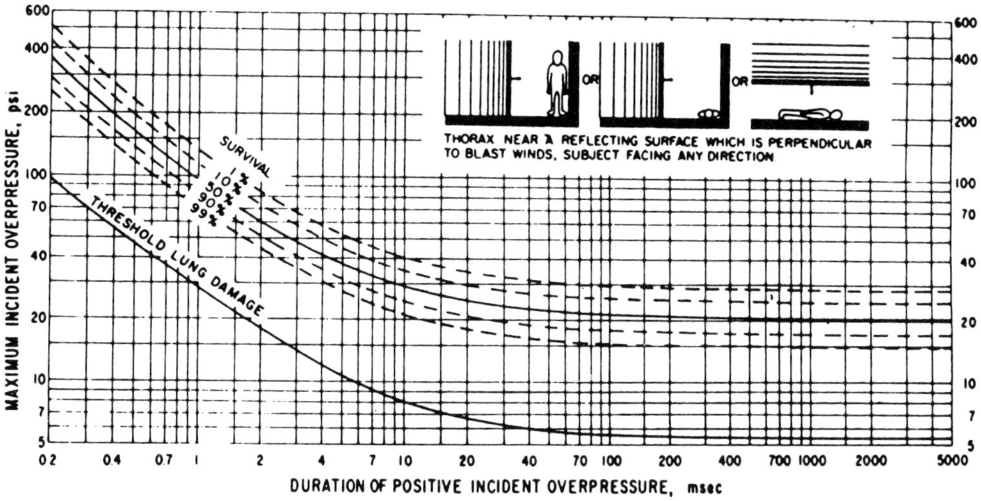

Fig. 7-10. The estimated tolerance for a single air blast at sea level is given for a 70-kg human oriented against a reflecting surface that is perpendicular to the shock wave.
Source: Reference 8

interaction between peak pressure and duration, which are the determinants of impulse. At durations longer than 20-30 msec (the range of nuclear or very large conventional explosives), the injurious effect varies directly with the overpressure level alone.

Effects of Body Positioning

Personnel oriented *end-on* to the blast wave (that is, lying down with either their head or feet pointed toward the blast) offer little resistance to the dynamic pressure component of the wave, and the incident shock (or side-on pressure) constitutes their air blast dose (Figure 7-8). The end-on orientation also gives the best protection against being displaced by the blast wind.

For persons side-on to the approaching blast wave, the dynamic pressure and incident pressure are additive (Figure 7-9). In the region of short-duration blast waves (a positive phase of 3 msec or less), there is a twofold difference in magnitude between the curves for the end-on and side-on orientations.

Individuals positioned against a large reflecting surface and normal to the incident shock would have the peak reflected pressure as their effective blast dose (Figure 7-10).

For example, the *threshold* (that is, the lowest overpressure at which trivial lesions are first detected) for lung injury is about 12 psi for blast waves of greater than 20–30 msec duration; scattered pleural petechiae are the threshold injury. Subjects end-on to the blast would require an incident shock of 12 psi static pressure to cause this lesion. If the subjects are oriented side-on, an incident shock of 10 psi (with an associated dynamic pressure of 2 psi) would cause equal damage. If the subject is against a reflector, an incident shock of just over 5 psi (reflecting to 12 psi) would cause the same injury. Although all three examples have different incident blast waves, the biologically effective blast loading is the same.

Effects of Repeated Exposure to Air Blasts

Injury from blast is a function of intensity (pressure and impulse for short-duration waves, and pressure alone for long-duration waves) and the number of shock waves.[10,11] Figures 7-11, 7-12, and 7-13 present curves relating the estimated incident static pressures and positive-phase durations producing both threshold and severe injuries in the lungs, the gastrointesti-

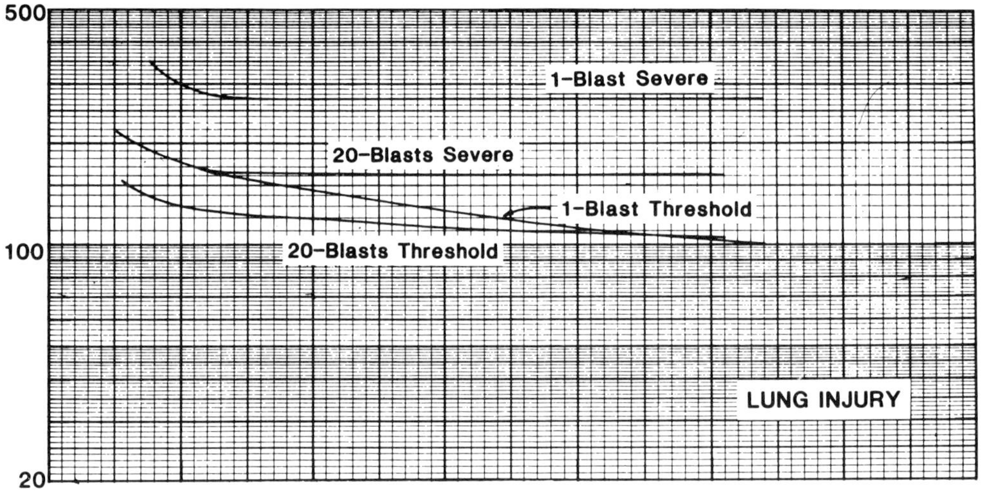

Fig. 7-11. The estimated free-field air blast conditions for one and twenty blasts are depicted for threshold and severe injury to the lungs. Threshold injury is the presence of scattered pleural petechiae, and severe injury is confluent hemorrhage covering a significant portion of the lung's surface.
Source: Walter Reed Army Institute of Research

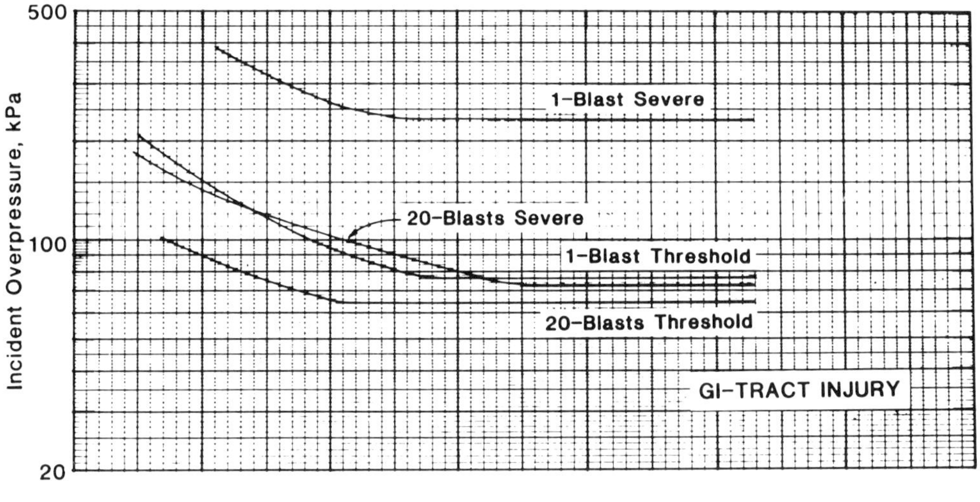

Fig. 7-12. The estimated free-field air blast conditions for one and twenty blasts are depicted for threshold and severe injury to the gastrointestinal tract. Threshold injury is the presence of scattered petechiae on the serosal or mucosal surface, and severe injury is extensive transmural hemorrhage or visceral rupture.
Source: Walter Reed Army Institute of Research

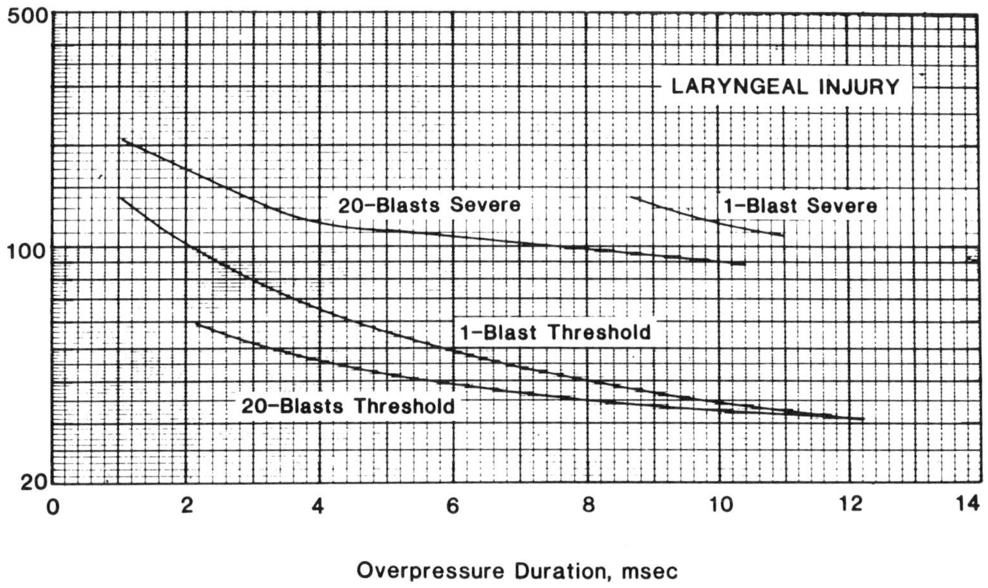

Fig. 7-13. The estimated free-field air blast conditions for one and twenty blasts are depicted for threshold and severe injury to the larynx. Threshold injury is the presence of scattered petechiae in the larynx, and severe injury is confluent hemorrhage. Source: Walter Reed Army Institute of Research

nal tract, and the upper respiratory tract of humans exposed to either one or twenty air blasts at sea level. These estimates are based on information obtained from sheep and swine that were exposed to repeated blasts from explosive charges ranging in weight from 0.5 to 64 pounds.

The larynx is the most sensitive nonauditory structure to repeated blasts, followed by the gastro-intestinal tract and the lungs. Once the threshold overpressure for injury for a single blast is exceeded, the injury worsens with repeated exposures, especially in the gastrointestinal tract and lungs. However, tolerance is high for subthreshold exposures. The effect of daily exposure to multiple blasts was tested with sheep exposed to subthreshold blasts of about 10 msec duration and 7 psi peak pressure. One group received fifty blasts at a rate of one blast per minute. Postmortem examinations at 1 hour after the fiftieth blast revealed only light contusions and ecchymoses in the lining of the upper respiratory tract. There were no lung hemorrhages or gastrointestinal tract lesions. Specimens given fifty blasts daily (one per minute) for 4 days and examined at 1 hour after the blasts ended on day 4 showed the same minor upper respiratory lesions; the lungs and gastrointestinal tract were without significant injury.[12]

In a study demonstrating the significance of repeated exposure, sheep and swine were subjected to repeated blasts at a rate of one per minute.[13] A remarkable increase in pulmonary hemorrhage and lethality was found for multiple blasts that were greater than threshold levels. A blast that resulted in 1% mortality when delivered only once produced 20% mortality when given twice, and 100% mortality when given three times. At suprathreshold levels, multiple low-dose blasts interact synergistically to enhance injury and mortality.

To evaluate the effect of varying the interval between blasts, groups of rats were subjected to long-duration overpressures of about 26 psi.[13] One exposure resulted in 5% mortality at 24 hours. Three blasts administered at 15-minute intervals produced 87% mortality. At 30 minutes between blasts, the lethality dropped to 36%; at 4-hour intervals, to 27%; and with 24 hours between exposures, to 7%. Therefore, increasing the time between individual events can ameliorate the blast-injury enhancement from multiple exposures.

Military personnel are repeatedly subjected to relatively low-intensity blasts during training and combat operations. Soldiers who fire artillery, mortars, recoilless rifles, and shoulder-launched antiarmor weapons

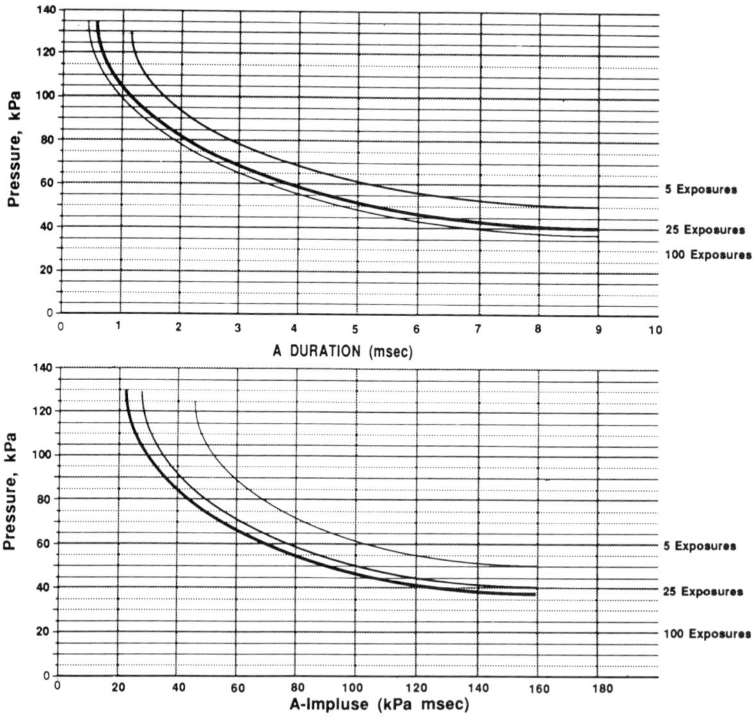

Fig. 7-14. The estimated threshold for trivial laryngeal injury in humans at sea level is given as a function of the blast wave's static peak pressure, the number of exposures, and either impulse or positive-phase duration. These data have been used to define limits for exposure to intense weapon-muzzle blast for soldiers in training.
Source: Reference 11

are in the position to receive muzzle or breech blasts from their own weapons. Although damage-risk criteria for hearing loss from repeated impulse noise have existed since the late 1960s, attempts have been made only recently to compile criteria for nonauditory blast effects at these levels.[11] Threshold injuries to the upper respiratory tract of sheep and swine produced by 5, 25, and 100 repeated blasts in relation to the incident overpressure, duration and impulse are plotted in Figure 7-14. Such estimates of threshold injury have been applied to human tolerance limits for blast from the firing of heavy weapons.

UNDERWATER BLAST

An explosive charge that is detonated underwater will produce a large volume of gaseous by-products in the form of an underwater bubble.[4] This expanding bubble sends out a compressive shock wave into the surrounding water at a speed of about 5,000 fps. As the bubble rises to the surface, it oscillates—collapses and re-expands—and sends out a series of weaker pressure waves called *bubble pulses.* As the primary shock wave reaches the surface, it is reflected as a tension wave, which spalls the surface of the water. Tiny water droplets (the spall) form a characteristic dome around the gas bubble (Figure 7-15), which soon vents, forming a spray plume (Figure 7-16).

A typical underwater blast-wave pattern for a gauge located near the surface shows the initial peak pressure and the pressure decay that is rapidly truncated by the tension wave arriving from the surface reflection (Figure 7-17).[14] In effect, the tension wave (also called the *cut-off wave*) reflecting from the surface cancels out a portion of the compressive shock wave. However, if the shock wave is reflected from a rigid underwater surface such as a rock bottom, the pressure in the primary shock wave will be increased by a reflecting compressive wave, similar to that produced in air blast. If the bottom is soft mud, there may be no reflected wave.

Studies with submerged animals have found that the positive impulse in the underwater blast (the inte-

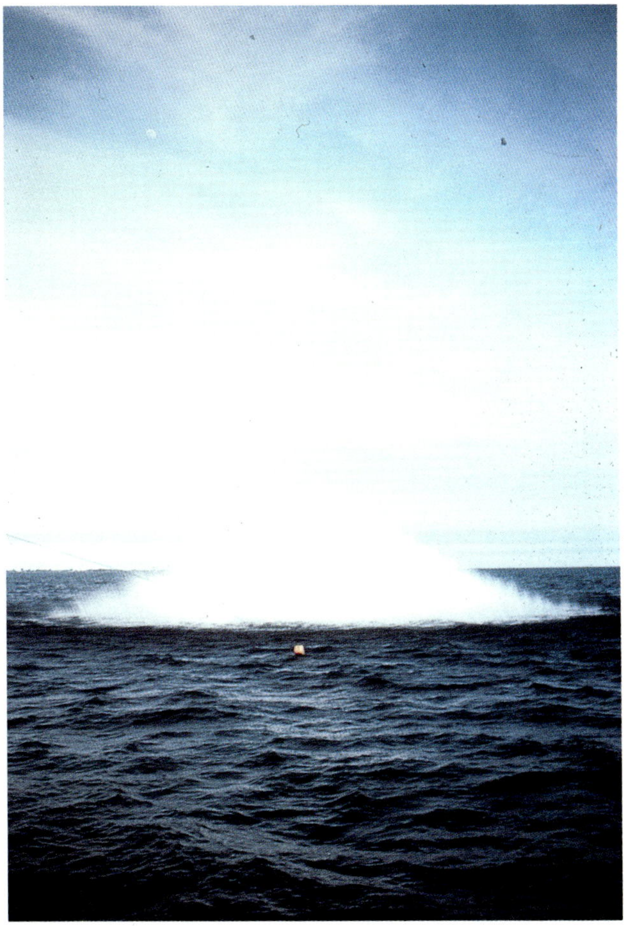

Fig. 7-15. The water surface above an underwater explosion is disrupted due to spallation as the underwater shock wave reflects off the water-air interface as a tension wave.
Source: D. R. Richmond

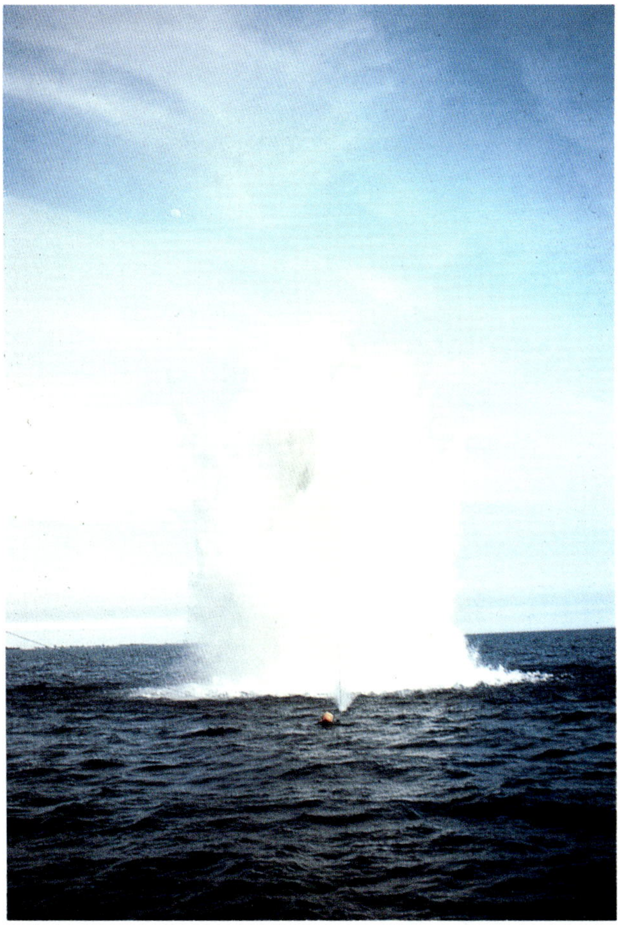

Fig. 7-16. The gas bubble created by an underwater explosion rises to the surface and expells a plume of water and gas. This follows the spallation dome shown in Figure 7-15.
Source: D.R. Richmond

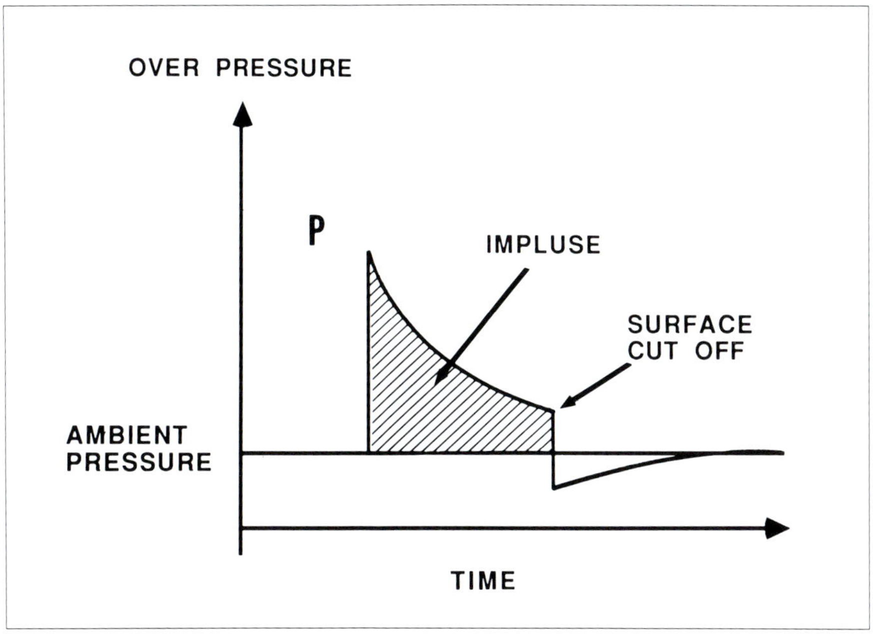

Fig. 7-17. An underwater blast wave is depicted as measured near the surface. There is a nearly instantaneous rise in pressure, with an exponential decay much like that in air blast (Figure 7-2). The incident compression wave is reflected from the surface as a tension wave, which interacts with the positive-pressure shock, effectively cancelling or cutting it off.
Source: D. R. Richmond

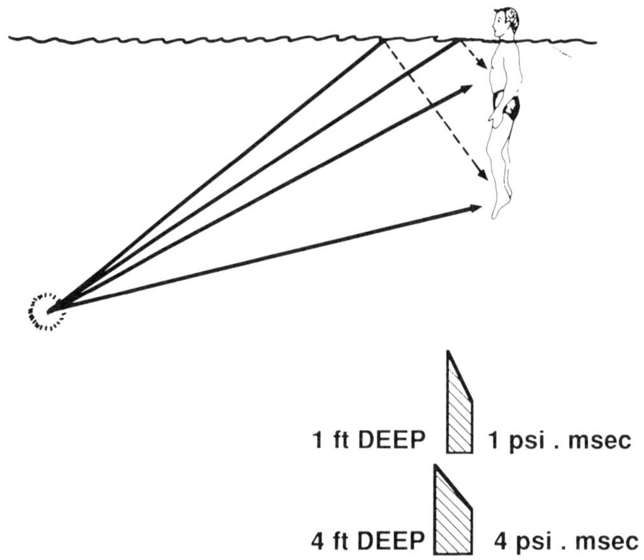

Fig. 7-18. The effective pressure-time exposure is depicted for the upper and lower body of a submerged human exposed to a nearby underwater blast. The reflected tension wave from the surface (▧) cuts off the compression wave at different times, resulting in a greater impulse loading (integral of pressure over time) for deeper structures. For this reason, the gastrointestinal tract is generally more severely injured than the lungs in underwater blast.
Source: D. R. Richmond

gral of pressure over time) is best correlated with injury and mortality (Figure 7-17).[15] For humans, it is estimated that 50% mortality is associated with an impulse of 87 psi-msec. Neither the peak pressure nor the energy (the integral of pressure squared over time) predict injury. Because of the cut-off wave from the surface, waves of high peak pressure with little impulse are common if either the charge or the target are near the surface. At depths of more than 20 feet (equivalent to a few milliseconds of wave travel) the cut-off wave is of little significance. Charges of only 0.125 pounds can kill large animals that are located about 5 feet from the detonation. With a 1-pound charge, death would occur at a distance of 23 feet. This is about three times the lethal range of free-field air blasts.

A person treading water will experience a higher impulse load on the lower portion of the body because the cut-off wave from the surface arrives later than it does at the upper body (Figure 7-18). The peak pressures will be essentially the same. Thus, the portions of the body that are deeper in the water (in most cases, the gastrointestinal tract) may be severely injured, while damage to the lungs may be much less. This observation has lead to the misconception that injuries to the gut predominate in all underwater blasts, regardless of the depth of immersion. Sheep tested at 10-foot depths, oriented with their bodies' long axes parallel to the surface (to evenly distribute the impulse load over the body), had essentially the same severity of injuries to their lungs and gastrointestinal tracts.[15] In another experiment, sheep were positioned at a 6-inch depth and horizontal to the surface. If they had been positioned vertically in the water, the blast would have been lethal, but the sheep survived with only moderate degrees of lung and gastrointestinal-tract injury.[16]

The dramatic effect of immersion depth on blast injury dictates that military personnel in danger of impending underwater blast should not tread water but should float on the surface, if possible.

THE MECHANISMS AND PREDICTIONS OF PRIMARY BLAST INJURY TO THE LUNG

Historically, researchers observed the effects of blast on physical objects, and speculated that certain phenomena (such as spallation, implosion, and inertia, which are described in Chapter Six) might be blast-injury mechanisms. These injury mechanisms have never been directly observed in a blast-exposed body; neither do they in themselves lead to a quantitative understanding of blast injury. Therefore we have to

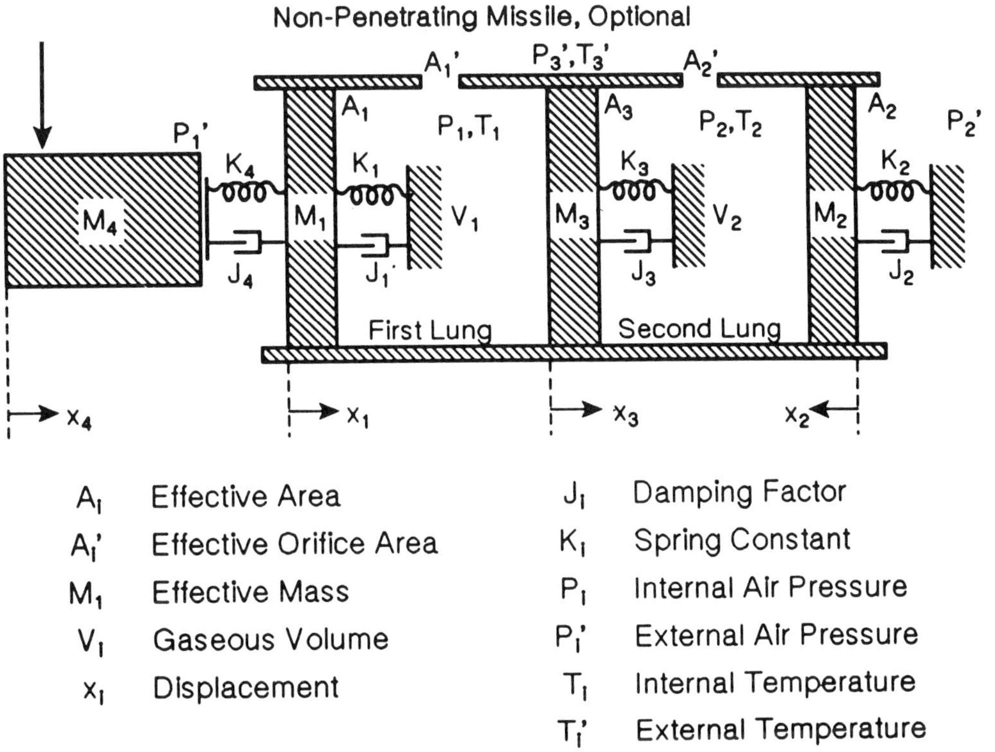

Fig. 7-19. Viscoelastic mathematical model of the thorax to simulate fluid-mechanical responses to rapid changes in environmental pressure and to nonpenetrating missile impact with the chest wall
Source: Reference 8

look elsewhere for answers.

The goal of modeling has been to assemble scientifically sound concepts of blast-injury mechanisms into a form that can be used to predict and understand the occurrence of injury. Such an approach has been successful for understanding tympanic-membrane rupture from blast.[17] PBI to the lung has received the most critical attention because its consequences are so serious. Lung damage that allows air emboli to enter the bloodstream is believed to be the primary cause of prompt death from blast effects; at lower blast levels, the loss of pulmonary function is a cause of immediate incapacitation.

The first attempt to model the body's response to blast was proposed in the 1960s, when the viscoelastic properties of the chest and abdomen were mathematically represented by the *viscoelastic thorax model.* This model visualized the thorax and abdomen as two gas-filled compartments, separated from each other and from the outside by moveable walls.[18]

Later, this mathematical model was modified to describe only the thorax, but a separate compartment represented each lung (Figure 7-19).[19] The volume of gas within each compartment would compress as the walls moved inward, and would expand as the walls moved back out. Researchers intended this model to predict lung pressures from the mechanical motion caused by the external force of the blast and then to correlate the maximum lung pressure obtained with predicted mortality.

The model used many mathematical parameters to describe the characteristics of the compartment walls and volumes of gas. Most of these had no direct relationship to physiology, however, so their values had to be selected arbitrarily. When the model was tested against blast waves of very long durations, its parameters could be chosen to give good agreement with observed pressure measurements that had been taken from the esophagi of animals. The maximum esophageal pressure appeared to correlate with the likelihood of mortality.

Direct measurements of the thoracic motion and pressure distribution within the lung were finally made in the 1980s.[20] They clearly showed that the lung did not compress uniformly, but instead contained regions of local compression that moved like waves through the parenchyma. Researchers also found that maximum esophageal pressure did not correlate with the injury found in short-duration blasts. Although the model was correctly based on the concept that the blast pushes in the thorax and compresses the lung, the mechanistic links between such gross phenomena and injury was not understood.

Modern View of the Mechanisms of Primary Blast Injury

The physical processes involved in the body's response to blast actually comprise three steps: *(a)* the body's external surface moves rapidly with the sudden increase in environmental pressure, *(b)* the air-containing organs become distorted, creating stress within the organ tissues, and *(c)* when the stress exceeds the strength of the tissue, damage occurs.

The Body's Rapid Response to Blast Loading. The amount of force exerted on the body by a blast wave is called the blast loading; the surfaces of the body that are oriented towards the blast receive the greatest load. The geometry of surrounding structures may deflect the blast wave, or it may focus the wave, particularly inside partially open enclosures where the blast loading can be significantly higher than it would have been in a free field.

The air-containing organs of the body are exquisitely sensitive to changes in air pressure. To remain functional, they rely on natural pressure-equilibrating mechanisms that keep the body's internal air pressure as stable as possible by means of *(a)* the venting of air from the middle ear through the eustachian tube, *(b)* the process of ventilation in the respiratory tract, and *(c)* the expulsion of gas from the upper and lower gastrointestinal tract.

The blast wave causes injury because of its rapid external loading. If the blast loading increases slowly enough, the internal pressures will have time to equilibrate, thus avoiding significant distortions of the tissue. A more sudden loading of the blast force, however, is not balanced by internal forces, and it quickly distorts and injures the air-containing organs.

A better understanding of the mechanics of the body's motion due to blast loading is needed to define the relationship between the blast loading and the subsequent organ distortion.

Organ Distortion and Tissue Stress. The rapid displacement of both the external and internal structures distorts the air-containing organs and stresses their tissues. For example, a pressure differential across the tympanic membrane that cannot be balanced by air flow through the eustachian tube causes a significant distortion of the membrane, with corresponding stresses on it and the stapes. A rapid displacement of the chest wall causes local compressions of the lung parenchyma that cannot be relieved through the airways, thus stressing the lung tissue. A sudden pressurization of the abdominal cavity collapses the air-containing sections of the gastrointestinal tract, which stresses the tissues of the gut wall. However, the precise relationship between organ distortion and tissue stress remains unknown.

Tissue Stress and Injury. Finally, excessive stress within a tissue leads to its mechanical failure. Some structures, such as the tympanic membrane and the organs comprising the gastrointestinal tract, can be mechanically ruptured by excessive stress. At lower levels of tissue stress, the integrity of vascular beds can be compromised, leading to local hemorrhage. The failure of alveolar walls can allow fluids into the lung (hemorrhagic edema) or air into the blood stream (air emboli). Even more subtle mechanical and biochemical damage can occur in the cochlea, resulting in both temporary and permanent hearing loss.

The failure of a material depends not only on its composition but also on its structure and the way in which the external force is applied. For example, a force applied to one end of a steel bar, whose other end is fixed, will result in greater stresses within the bar than if the force were applied uniformly along the bar.

Furthermore, the resulting stress within the material may be concentrated at certain locations called *stress points*. For example, a steel bar that is notched in the middle will fail after fewer applications of an external bending load than a similar steel bar that has no notch, because *(a)* the notch makes the bar weaker, *(b)* the bending will be concentrated there, and *(c)* the stresses will be concentrated there.

Materials have three characteristics that can be used to quantify tissue damage. First, *tensile strength* establishes the conditions at which damage will first occur. When material is pulled along its length, the resulting stress within it is called *tension*. Tensile strength is equal to the amount of stress that will cause the material to fail when it is in tension. When the tension exceeds the tensile strength, some materials will rupture, whereas materials that are more plastic will stretch without breaking. In either case, the material is damaged; that is, it is permanently changed and will not return to its original condition after the external force that created the tension is removed. Tensile strength, therefore, establishes the threshold for injury. Table 7-4 lists the tensile strength for a variety of biological and nonbiological materials, each represented by a range that reflects the variation in individual specimens.[21] The values for the biological tissues represent the composite characteristics of their component fibers and their structural arrangements.

Next, *fatigue* is a type of failure that results from repeated exposure to damaging conditions. A paper

TABLE 7-4

TENSILE STRENGTHS OF BIOLOGICAL AND NONBIOLOGICAL MATERIALS

Material	Tensile Strength (MPa)
Common building materials	
Stainless steel	1,000
Silk	400
Oak	120
Marble	6
Biological fibers	
Resilin	3
Collagen	50–100
Biological tissues	
Tracheal membrane wall	0.4–2.2
Mixed arterial tissue	1.4–1.7
Elastic arterial tissue	0.8–1.0
Venous tissue	1.7–3.0
Large intestine	0.45–0.69

clip will break if it is repeatedly bent back and forth. Each bend produces minute damage that accumulates and eventually results in failure. Experimental data for a wide variety of materials show that they have certain properties of fatigue failure in common (Figure 7-20).[21] A material's *ultimate strength* is equal to the level of stress that will produce failure from a single application of an external force. When the stress is purely tension, the ultimate strength is identical to the tensile strength. The *fatigue stress* is the stress that is required to produce failure under repeated applications of the external force, and is often proportional to the external force. For many materials, the fatigue stress decreases by about 20% for each tenfold increase in the number of applications. That is, if a material fails when 1.0 unit of external force is applied 100 times, then it will also fail when 0.8 units of external force is applied 1,000 times, or when 0.6 units of external force is applied 10,000 times, and so on. The *endurance limit* is the level of stress below which the material will not fail no matter how many times the external force is applied. Fatigue properties have not been measured for biological materials.

Finally, *irreversible work* gives a quantitative measure of the severity of the damage. Material will deform when an external force is applied to it, but if the deformation is not too great, the material will return to its original condition when the external force is removed, and any work done by that force will be recovered. For example, an aluminum beverage container that is pushed in only slightly will pop back to its original shape when the force is removed. The onset of damage occurs when the stress equals the tensile strength of the material. As the stress increases beyond the tensile strength, the work done by the excess external force will not be recovered. This is called the irreversible work, and is a direct measure of the severity of the damage done to the material. The beverage container, for example, will remain dented if it is crushed beyond a critical point.

A better knowledge of the properties of tensile strength, fatigue, and irreversible work is necessary to determine the relationship between tissue stress and injury. When the mechanisms of body motion and organ distortion are combined with the properties that describe material failure, researchers will be able to define analytically the relationship between blast and injury in contrast to the empirical relationships described to date.

New Models of Lung Injury

The three steps involved in the body's physical response to blast can be applied to models that are designed to predict blast-related lung injury. To be useful, these models need to establish three relationships: *(a)* blast to parenchymal distortion, *(b)* parenchymal distortion to tissue stress, and *(c)* tissue stress to injury.

Blast to Parenchymal Distortion. The first step in developing a predictive model of lung injury is to establish the mechanical connection between the external blast loading and distortions to the lung parenchyma. This connection is mathematically represented by *Finite Element Modeling* (FEM), which involves three stages:

First, FEM begins with a geometrically correct *mathematical representation* of the body structure under investigation.[22] Figure 7-21 shows the anatomical cross section of a sheep's thorax at the level of the seventh vertebra, selected because *(a)* it contains a representative cross section of the sheep's internal organs, *(b)* it is located where considerable rib motion occurs, and *(c)* it is a common location of lung injury in blast-exposed sheep. The cross section is then broken down into many computational elements, each representing a part of the thoracic geometry and quantifying the

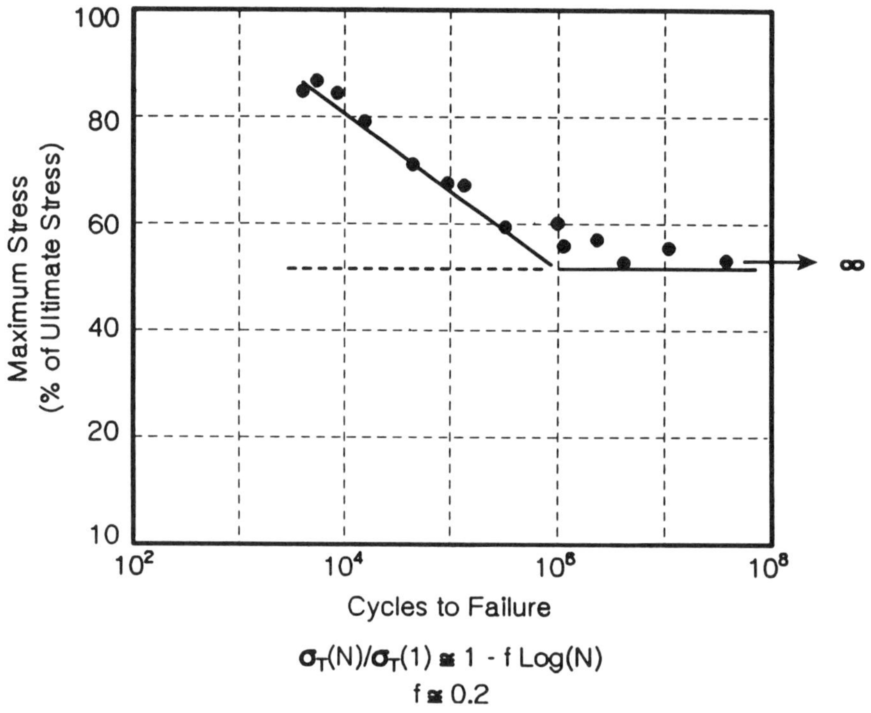

Fig. 7-20. Geometric model of the effects of repeated applications of stress on mechanical failure. The concept of fatigue is used in biomechanical modeling of blast injury to account for repeated exposures.
Source: JAYCOR

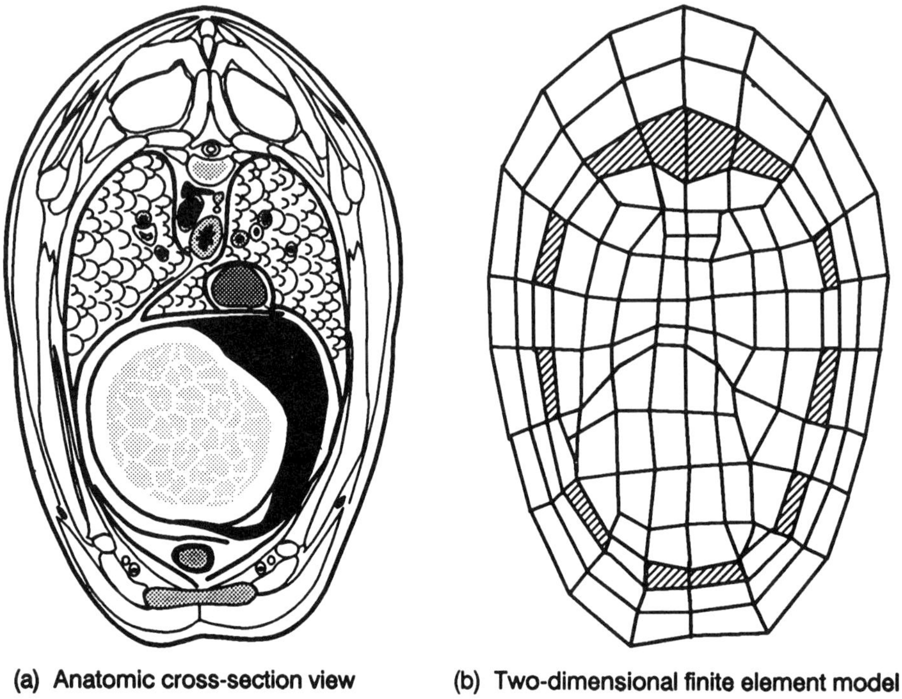

Fig. 7-21. Geometric model of a sheep thorax as represented by *(a)* a simplified anatomical cross section, and *(b)* the Finite Element Model
Source: JAYCOR

mechanical properties for that material. The chest wall contains the rib structure and musculature, which—in the two-dimensional FEM representation—provide inertia to the chest wall. The abdominal cavity, heart, and spinous process are mathematically represented by high-density, incompressible elements that do not readily deform under the rapid body motions caused by a blast. The lung parenchyma has the compressibility of air, but because it also contains tissue, it has a mass density that is one-tenth the mass density of water. These mechanical properties of the lung have been determined in laboratory measurements.[23] The model can be used to predict the dynamics of the chest wall and lung parenchyma when exposed to blast.

Next, the prediction is compared with the observed experimental data to verify its accuracy. For example, when the outer surface of a sheep's thorax is subjected to the pressure distribution of a blast wave, the chest wall is set in motion and in turn compresses the parenchyma, setting it in motion as well. The compression wave is transmitted throughout the lung and can be measured in the esophagus, where researchers often place pressure transducers during tests. The predicted intrathoracic pressure is compared with the value measured in the sheep's esophagus (Figure 7-22). FEM predictions also agree with the chest-wall accelerations and velocities that have been observed in specially instrumented test animals, supporting the accuracy of the model's chest-wall description (Figure 7-23).[20,24]

Finally, the location and magnitude of parenchymal distortions are determined. The combination of high compressibility and great inertia causes the lung parenchyma to transmit pressure waves much more slowly than either air or water do. From both theoretical considerations and direct measurements in the laboratory, the pressure-wave speed in the lung is found to be about 30 m/s.[24] Consequently, when the chest-wall velocity becomes a sizeable fraction of this value, concentrations of stress can result near the pleural surface. Other stress points occur because of the geometry of the lung and the presence of the surround-

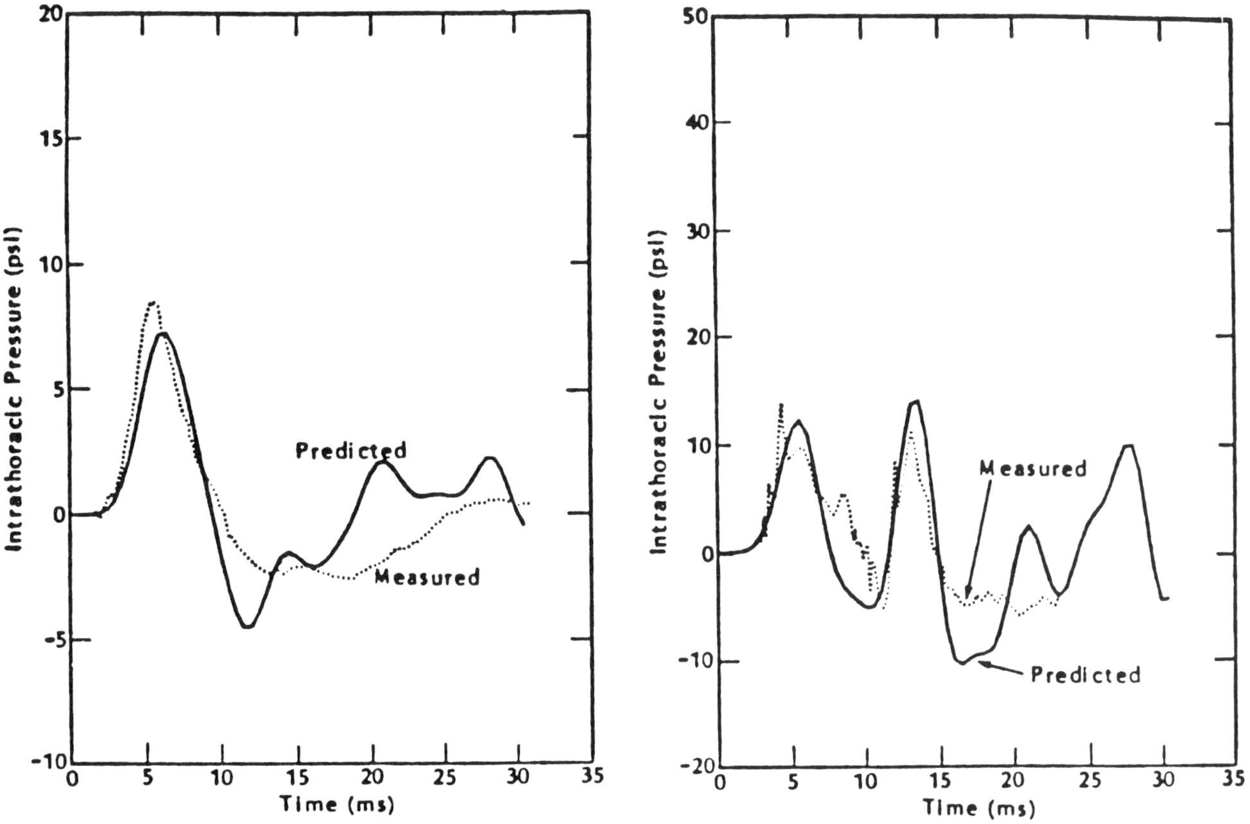

(a) Exposure to a single peak blast due to a 16 lb TNT charge

(b) Exposure to two 40 psi blast waves separated in time by 7.6 msec

Fig. 7-22. Comparison of predicted intrathoracic pressure and measured esophageal pressure in sheep
Source: Walter Reed Army Institute of Research

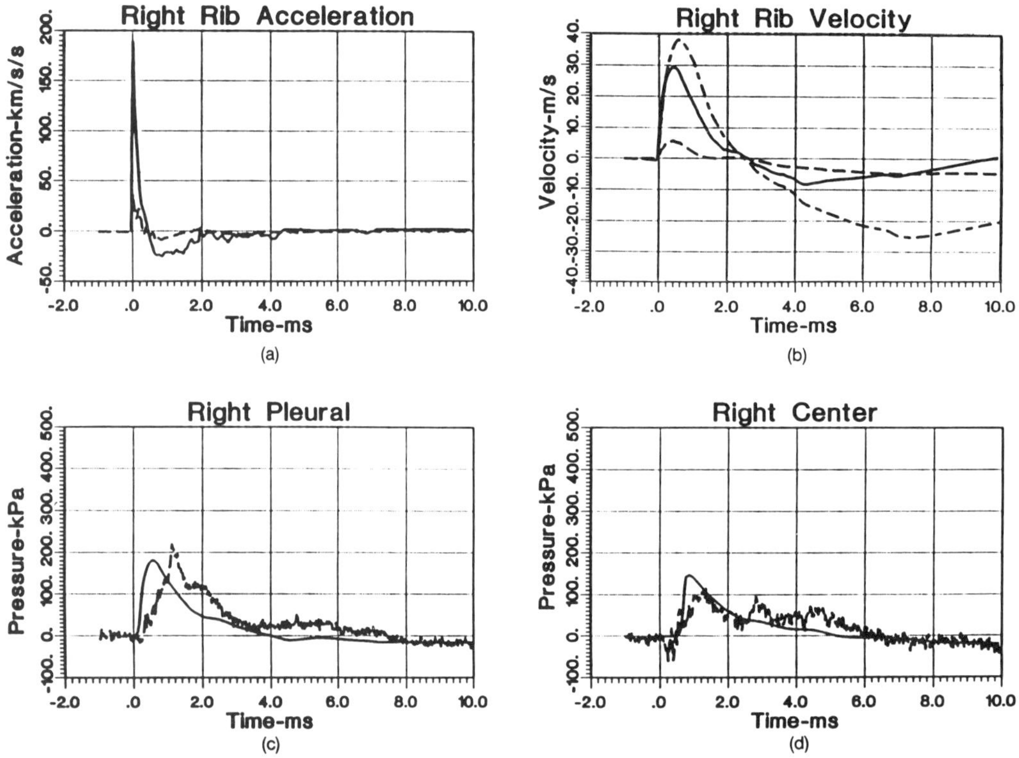

Fig. 7-23. Comparison of predicted and measured thorax dynamics: *(a)* acceleration of the right rib of a sheep subjected to a blast loading due to 1 pound of C4 explosive, *(b)* the consequent rib velocity, *(c)* the pressure in the pleural space just below the instrumented rib, and *(d)* the intrathoracic pressure as measured in an airway in the center of the right lobe
Source: Walter Reed Army Institute of Research

ing organs. For example, high stresses are predicted in the tips of the lobes, along the ribs on the side of the blast, and around the spinous process and heart (Figure 7-24). All are locations where blast injury is commonly observed.

Parenchymal Distortion to Tissue Stress. Compression does not, in itself, produce injury because it occurs in the trapped gas, not the tissue. A relationship between the compressive stress and the tissue stress must be established through a mechanical analysis of the alveolar structure when it is distorted. In principle, this relationship could be determined by FEM analysis of the parenchymal structure, but such work has not yet been done.

However, the FEM model does predict that the parenchymal pressure at the pleural surface varies over time in exact proportion to the velocity at which the chest wall is being deformed, a finding that has been confirmed by direct experimental measurement.[24] The dependence of pressure on velocity is uncharacteristic of the properties of a pure gas, and suggests that tissue distortion is involved.

Tissue Stress to Injury. The final link in the prediction of blast injury is the establishment of a relationship between the tissue stress and tissue failure.

Measurements of tissue stresses in the laboratory have attempted to determine the relationship between stress and distortion in lung tissue. The level of stress rapidly increases as the tissue is stretched to about 150% of its resting length, indicating the onset of a tensile failure. Unfortunately, the existing FEM analyses do not reveal the relationship between the stresses of wave motion within the parenchyma and the magnitude of tissue distortion. Without the establishment of this relationship, the concept of tensile strength cannot be applied.

Although tissue stress cannot quantitatively be related to injury at this time, the concept of irreversible work can be applied. Because the pleural-surface pressure depends on the chest-wall velocity, work done against it will not be recovered when the lung reexpands. Instead, the lost energy will have been dissipated within the tissue.

If the energy dissipation is due to a failure of the underlying tissue, then the irreversible work is a prime candidate for correlation with the severity of damage. There are several experimental observations that support this contention (Figure 7-25). First, the relation-

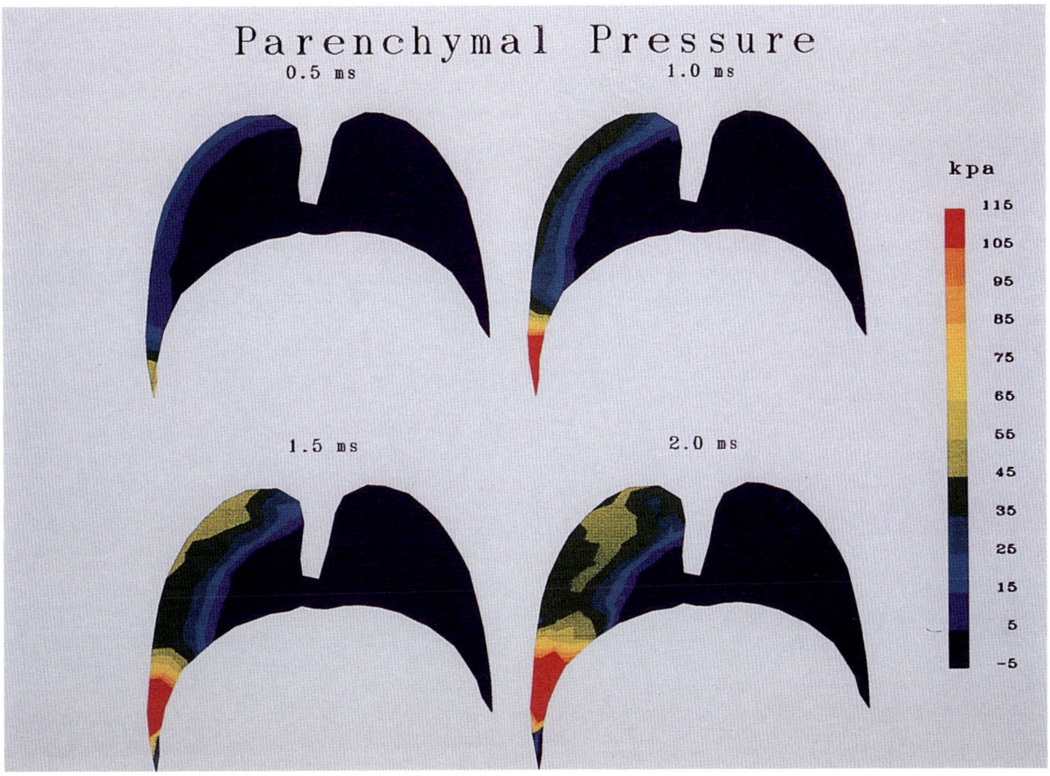

Fig. 7-24. Distribution of compressive stress within the lung parenchyma due to a blast loading on the left side of a sheep, as calculated at various points in time with the Finite Element Model
Source: JAYCOR

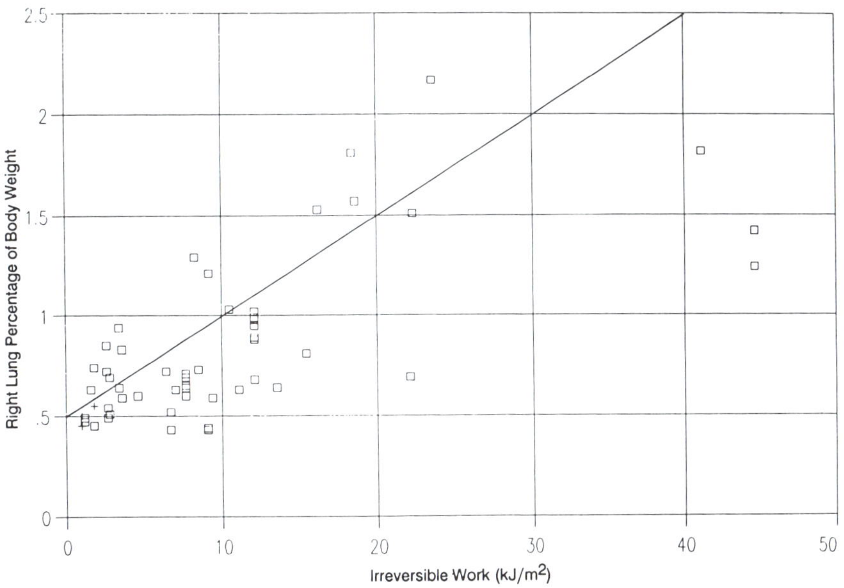

Fig. 7-25. Comparison of observed lung injury in sheep exposed to blast (as measured by the increase in lung weight over that of control animals) with the prediction of the irreversible work done to the pleural surface of the lung. Each data point corresponds to an individual animal where sufficient data were available to describe the blast environment. The exposures include single free-field explosions, multiple free-field explosions, repeated free-field explosions, and explosions inside enclosures.
Source: JAYCOR

ship is consistent with observations that lung injury correlates with chest-wall velocity.[25] Second, for ideal wave forms, irreversible work correlates with observed lethality.[26] Although the relationship between injury and lethality is not necessarily simple, it is encouraging that the observed dependence of lethality on certain blast parameters (such as peak pressure and duration) is also consistent with the concept of irreversible work. Finally, the computation of irreversible work is insensitive to the small perturbations of the external blast, such as pressure transients and baseline drift, because the inertia of the chest wall is too large to respond to such fine details.

Perhaps the correlation between lung injury and irreversible work done on lung tissue, which now unifies previous hypotheses and experimental observations, will also provide a lung-injury model that addresses both ideal and complex waves.

SUMMARY

An explosion in air or water liberates a great deal of energy as an expanding mass of gas. This creates a blast wave, which propagates in all directions throughout the medium at a speed faster than the speed of sound in the ambient medium. The blast wave consists of a sharp rise in pressure (the shock front) and a positive-overpressure phase that decreases exponentially and is followed by a longer negative phase. The effect of most explosives can be generally determined by scaling relationships, in which the physical parameters of the blast wave are proportional to the weight of the explosive divided by the cube root of the distance between the measuring point and the explosion.

At any point in space, the expanding shock front is characterized by the static overpressure—the pressure that is present in all directions and is measured by a sensing surface oriented parallel to the blast wave's path. The strength of the shock front also determines its velocity and the dynamic pressure.

When a blast wave strikes a rigid surface, it is reflected. Depending on the strength and the angle of incidence, the incident wave and the reflected wave interact to create areas of overpressure much greater than in the undisturbed incident wave. In a complicated environment, such as an explosion inside a room or a vehicle, the multiple interactions of the incident and reflected waves result in a complex blast wave.

Human tolerance to air blast has been estimated from experiments with animals. Orientation of the body with respect to the wave front and the presence of reflecting surfaces have important influences on injury potential. For blast waves of less than 20 msec in duration, consideration of both the peak pressure and positive-phase impulse are necessary to predict hazard. For the longer-duration waves that are typical of nuclear weapons, it is only necessary to know the peak overpressure to determine risk.

Repeated exposure to blast waves can greatly increase the risk of injury. The air-containing structures of the respiratory system and gastrointestinal tract are the most vulnerable to life-threatening injury. Even the relatively low-intensity blast waves that are produced by the firing of a cannon may pose a risk of injury (in addition to the well-recognized aural hazard) when repeated many times.

Underwater explosions are characterized by a much higher shock speed and a greater range of injurious effects than blasts in air. An underwater blast wave is reflected from the water-air interface as a tension wave that cuts off or cancels the shock front when it interacts with the positive-pressure compression wave. Thus, near the surface, positive waves of very high pressures and impulses with short durations are found. Such a combination would be impossible with air blasts. Injury potential is determined by positive impulse.

Efforts to model the response of the body to the physical interaction with the blast wave have been made, both as aids in predicting the relative hazard of an overpressure environment and as a means of gaining insight into the biophysical events and mechanisms of injury. Simple viscoelastic mathematical models have proven ineffective in repeated or complex-blast environments. Recent attempts to model the body as a complex geometric structure with definable physical properties have led to important predictions of physical events at the body surface (such as chest-wall accelerations and velocity) and within the lung (for example, parenchymal pressure-wave phenomena) that have been confirmed with animal experiments. A generally applicable model would deal with three important relationships: the blast-wave interaction with the body, the resultant tissue distortions and stresses caused by the motions of the body, and the failure or disruption of the tissues caused by the stresses. Although such a detailed model is presently unavailable, the finite-element model approach has suggested that irreversible work done on the body may be an important correlate of injury.

REFERENCES

1. Meyer, R. 1987. *Explosives.* New York: VCH Publishers.

2. Glasstone, S., and Dolan, P. J., eds. 1977. *The effects of nuclear weapons.* Washington, DC: U.S. Government Printing Office.

3. Rief, F. 1965. *Fundamentals of statistics and thermal physics.* New York: McGraw-Hill Book Company.

4. Baker, W. E. 1973. *Explosions in air.* Austin, TX: University of Texas Press.

5. Schardin, H. 1950. The physical principles of the effects of a detonation. In *German Aviation Medicine, World War II.* Vol. 2, prepared under the auspices of the U.S. Air Force Surgeon General, 1207–1224. Washington, DC: U.S. Government Printing Office.

6. Courant, R., and Friedrichs, K. O. 1948. *Supersonic flow and shock waves.* New York: John Wiley & Sons.

7. Swisdak, M. M., Jr. 1975. *Explosion effects and properties.* Part 18 of *Explosions in air* [Technical Report NSWC/WOL-TR-75–116]. Silver Spring, MD: Naval Surface Warfare Center.

8. White, C. S.; Jones, R. K.; Damon, E. G.; Fletcher, E. R.; and Richmond, D. R. 1971. *The biodynamics of airblast* [Technical Report DNA 2738T]. Washington, DC: Defense Nuclear Agency.

9. Richmond, D. R.; Damon, E. G.; Fletcher, E. R.; Bowen, I. G.; and White, C. S. 1966. *The relationship between selected blast-wave parameters and the response of mammals exposed to air blast* [Technical Progress Report DASA-1860]. Alexandria, VA: Defense Nuclear Agency.

10. Clifford, C. B.; Moe, J. B.; Jaeger, J. J.; and Hess, J. L. 1984. Gastrointestinal lesions in lambs due to multiple low-level blast overpressure exposure. *Milit. Med.* 149:491–495.

11. Dodd, K. T.; Yelverton, J. T.; Richmond, D. R.; Morris, J. R.; and Ripple, G. R. 1990. Nonauditory injury threshold for repeated intense freefield impulse noise. *J. Occup. Med.* 32(3): 260–266.

12. Richmond, D. R. Unpublished research performed at Inhalation Toxicology Research Institute, Kirtland Air Force Base, NM, 1982.

13. Richmond, D. R.; Yelverton, J. T.; Fletcher, E. R. 1981. *The biologic effects of repeated blast* [Topical Report DNA-5842F]. Washington, DC: Defense Nuclear Agency.

14. Swisdak, M. M., Jr. 1978. *Explosion effects and properties.* Part 2 of *Explosion effects in water* [Technical Report NSWC/WOL-TR-76–116]. Silver Spring, MD: Naval Surface Warfare Center.

15. Richmond, D. R.; Yelverton, J. T.; Gaylord, C. S.; Fletcher, E. R. 1970. *Underwater blast studies with animals* [Technical Progress Report DASA-2463]. Washington, DC: Defense Nuclear Agency.

16. Richmond, D. R.; Yelverton, J. T.; and Fletcher, E. R. 1973. *Farfield underwater blast injuries produced by small charges* [Technical Progress Report DNA-3081T]. Washington, DC: Defense Nuclear Agency.

17. Stuhmiller, J. H. 1989. Use of modeling in predicting tympanic membrane rupture. *Ann. Otol. Rhinol. Laryngol.* 98:53–60.

18. Bowen, I. G.; Holladay, A.; Fletcher, E. R.; Richmond, D. R.; and White, C. S. 1965. *A fluid-mechanical model of the thoracoabdominal system with application to blast biology* [Technical Report DASA-1675]. Albuquerque: Defense Atomic Support Agency.

19. Bowen, I. G.; Fletcher, E. R.; Richmond, D. R.; Hirsch, F. G.; and White, C. S. 1968. Biophysical mechanisms and scaling procedures applicable in assessing responses of the thorax energized by air-blast overpressures or by nonpenetrating missiles. *Ann. N. Y. Acad. Sci.* 152:122–146.

20. Stuhmiller, J. H.; Chuong, C. J.; Phillips, Y. Y III; and Dodd, K. T. 1988. Computer modeling of thoracic response to blast. *J. Trauma* 28:S132–139.

21. Yamada, H. 1970. *Strength of biological materials.* Baltimore: Williams and Wilkins Company.

22. Burton, R. 1968. *Vibration and impact.* New York: Dover Publications.

23. Fung, Y. C.; Yen, M. R.; and Zeng, Y. J. 1985. Characterization and modeling of thoracoabdominal response to blast waves. Vol. 3, *Lung dynamics and mechanical properties determination*, edited by J. H. Stuhmiller [Final Report for Contract DAMD178828C82062]. La Jolla, CA: JAYCOR, Inc.

24. Vander Vorst, M. J.; Dodd, K. T.; Stuhmiller, J. H.; and Phillips, Y. Y III. 1989. Calculation of the internal mechanical response of sheep to blast loading. In *Proceedings of the Tenth International Symposium on Military Applications of Blast Simulation,* edited by H. Reichenbach and J. H. Ackerman, 422–444. Oberjettenberg, Germany: Wehrtechnische Dienststelle für Sprengmittel und Sondertechnik.

25. Clemedson, C.-J. 1956. Blast injury. *Physiol. Rev.* 36:336–354.

26. Stuhmiller, J. H. 1988. Bio-mechanical modeling. Paper presented at Live Fire Crew Casualty Assessment Workshop, 18–19 October at Naval Underseas System Center, Groton, CT.

RECOMMENDED READING

Baker, W. E. 1973. *Explosions in air.* Austin, TX: University of Texas Press.

Jönsson, Arne. 1979. Experimental investigations on the mechanisms of lung injury in blast and impact exposure. Ph.D. diss. no. 80, Department of Surgery, Linköping University, Stockholm, Sweden.

White, C. S.; Jones, R. K.; Damon, E. G.; Fletcher, E. R.; and Richmond, D. R. 1971. *The biodynamics of airblast* [Technical Report DNA 2738T]. Washington, DC: Defense Nuclear Agency.

Chapter 8

THE PATHOLOGY OF PRIMARY BLAST INJURY

DOUGLAS D. SHARPNACK, D.V.M., M.S.,* ANTHONY J. JOHNSON, D.V.M., Ph.D.,** AND YANCY Y PHILLIPS III, M.D., FCCP***

*Major, United States Army; Chief, Department of Ultrastructural Pathology, Walter Reed Army Institute of Research, Washington, D.C. 20307-5100
**Colonel, United States Army; Director, Division of Pathology, Walter Reed Army Institute of Research, Washington, D.C. 20307-5100
***Lieutenant Colonel, United States Army; Chief, Pulmonary and Critical Care Medicine Service, Walter Reed Army Medical Center, Washington, D.C. 20307-5001, and Consultant to the Surgeon General in Pulmonary Medicine and Respiratory Therapy

INTRODUCTION

The pathological changes associated with primary blast injury (PBI) have been studied extensively for at least 75 years, since it became apparent that some soldiers who had been exposed to blasts on the battlefield were severely debilitated or killed but showed no external signs of injury. Researchers set out to study the effects of explosion-generated pressure waves on the body, and have conducted many animal experiments to document blast-related pathological and physiological changes, to determine blast-dose responses, and to develop predictive models for blast injury.

The lesions of PBI result from the complex interaction between the passing blast wave and the body tissue. When a blast wave strikes the body, it has effects that are similar to those of other kinds of blunt trauma. It displaces the body wall into the body cavities, resulting in a rapid change of organ volume and the displacement of internal tissues. Air-containing organs are the most likely to change volume as a result of blast, and thus their tissues are the most susceptible to distortion and stress. When the stress on the tissue exceeds the tissue's inherent tensile strength, the resulting failure may be manifested as detectable pathological change.

Blast may cause injury in a variety of body tissues (Table 8-1). The most common serious effects of PBI include *(a)* injuries to the respiratory system, *(b)* the introduction of air emboli into the circulatory system, and *(c)* gastrointestinal damage. Although it is usually not debilitating, the most common manifestation of PBI is rupture of the tympanic membrane, which may occur even at low blast doses. If the blast pressure is great enough, less common injuries can occur, such as solid-organ rupture.

Most blast injuries that occur on the battlefield or in terrorist bombing incidents are complicated by the more apparent secondary blast injury, which is caused by flying objects, and tertiary blast injury, which is caused by displacement of the entire body.[1] When PBI occurs in conjunction with secondary or tertiary blast injuries, or with other injuries like burns or radiation, the resulting damage is termed *combined injury.* Secondary, tertiary, and combined blast injuries are usually obvious on external examination; diagnosis and treatment of these injuries fall into the realm of ballistic injury. Because the integumentary system is very resistant to the blast wave, however, the lesions in a casualty who has pure PBI will usually not be obvious on examination of the body surfaces, and the source of the casualty's difficulties may indeed perplex the uninformed diagnostician. In spite of the fact that secondary and tertiary blast injuries are more common and more easily detected by the physician, there have been numerous reports of PBI alone and as a component of combined injuries.[2-8]

Because of the insidious nature of these potentially deadly injuries, a thorough knowledge of the clinicopathological signs of PBI will greatly enhance the medical officer's ability to provide care to these casualties. This chapter will outline, by organ system, those pathological changes that characterize PBI, based on a review of the literature and on the authors' experiences with animal blast-injury models. Several excellent reviews of the lesions of blast injury are particularly noteworthy.[9,10]

TABLE 8-1

CATEGORIES OF PRIMARY BLAST INJURIES

The Respiratory System	Pulmonary hemorrhage Alveolovenous fistula (air-embolism production) Airway epithelial damage
The Circulatory System	Cardiac contusion Myocardial ischemic change (air-embolism production)
The Digestive System	Gastrointestinal hemorrhage Gastrointestinal perforation Retroperitoneal hemorrhage Ruptured spleen or liver
The Eye and Orbit	Retinal air embolism Orbital fractures
The Auditory System	Tympanic-membrane rupture Ossicular fractures Cochlear damage

THE RESPIRATORY SYSTEM

Because the respiratory system is the only system in the body that is entirely filled with air and is therefore especially vulnerable to the effects of a blast overpressure, any discussion of PBI must begin with a discussion of respiratory-tract lesions. The respiratory system comprises *(a)* the lungs and bronchi and *(b)* the upper airways, including the trachea, the pharynx, the larynx, the nasal passages, and the sinuses.

The Lungs

Within the respiratory system, the lungs are especially vulnerable to the overpressure wave because of their unique structure and location.

The primary function of the lungs is to provide a site for the exchange of gases between inspired air and blood. To do this, the lungs contain innumerable capillaries, the walls of which are only one cell thick so that molecules of gas can pass through them. The surface area over which air comes in contact with these tiny blood vessels must be large enough to sustain a level of gas exchange that is adequate to keep the body alive, and so myriad air spaces (called *alveoli*) are embedded within the delicate capillary-containing membranes of the lungs. The resulting spongelike structure of the lungs provides the greatest possible air-blood interface within the limited anatomical space. However, it also results in the lung tissues' relatively low tensile strength and their inability—because of their contiguity with the air pockets—to withstand the effects of strong blast waves.

The location of the lungs also contributes to their vulnerability to blast. They are contained in a relatively rigid cage comprising the ribs and intercostal muscles, vertebral column, sternum, and diaphragm. In addition, they bracket the firm, muscular heart. When the thorax is struck by a blast wave, the sternum and rib cage (along with the intervening intercostal muscles) are rapidly displaced into the thoracic cavity, causing these structures to momentarily compress the lungs. The same blast wave displaces the abdominal wall, moving the diaphragm forcefully against the lungs. The lungs, in turn, are displaced into the heart and vertebral column, which act as barriers, causing further damage.

The specific lung lesions caused by the blast wave can be best understood by examining the anatomical subcomponents of the lung and the effects of the blast on each of them. Each lung consists of *(a)* the *pleura*, which covers the entire organ, *(b)* the *parenchyma*, where gas exchange occurs, and *(c)* the *bronchovascular structures*, through which blood and air flow to and from the parenchyma.

The pleura is a serous membrane that comprises a single layer of mesothelial cells and an underlying layer of connective tissue. It forms both a protective covering for the lung parenchyma and a lining for the thoracic cavity. The portion of the pleura that surrounds the lungs is called *visceral pleura;* and the portion of the pleura that lines the thoracic cavity is the *parietal pleura*. The visceral pleura contains numerous blood and lymphatic vessels, and it is thin enough to be relatively transparent, so that damage to underlying tissue can often be seen through it.

The parenchyma is the functional portion of the lung. After being transported by the conducting airways, the air arrives at the sites of gas exchange, which are tiny respiratory units called *acini*. Acini comprise the respiratory bronchioles, alveolar ducts, and alveoli, but because the surface area of the alveoli is much greater than that of the other structures, most of the gas exchange occurs there.

The wall between adjacent alveoli (called the *alveolar septum*) is a thin, delicate membrane that is 10–15 microns thick (Figure 8-1). Lining the air space on either side of the membrane is a continuous layer of epithelial cells with underlying basal lamina. Sandwiched between these two epithelial layers is the septal interstitium, which contains a meshwork of capillaries, fibroblasts, and connective-tissue fibers, along with occasional macrophages, mast cells, and lymphocytes.

The wall between the capillary lumen and the alveolus consists of *(a)* capillary endothelium and its basal lamina, *(b)* a scant interstitial space, and *(c)* a single layer of alveolar epithelial cells over its basal lamina. As the site of gas exchange, this blood-air barrier may be as thin as 0.2 microns, and averages only 0.5 microns.[11]

The bronchovascular structures (which include the branches of the pulmonary vessels and the intrapulmonary conducting airways) are embedded in the parenchyma. They are considered together because they are located anatomically in the same arborizing pattern throughout the parenchyma, and because they are of relatively similar density when compared with the surrounding low-density alveolar tissue.

Hemorrhage. The most obvious and consistent

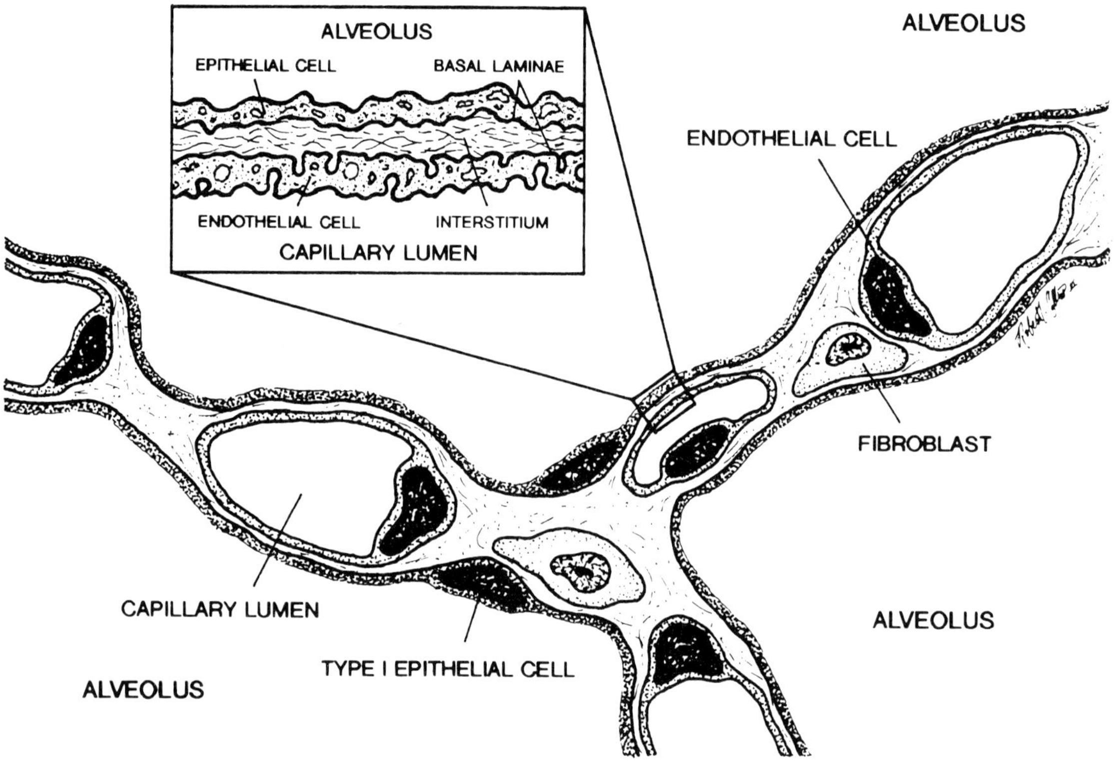

Fig. 8-1. This drawing shows the position of the alveolar capillaries within the alveolar septa. The weakest point of the wall is at the *diffusion membrane* (inset). The interstitium in this delicate membrane may vary from the relatively thick width suggested in the drawing to a much thinner width; in some cases, the interstitium of the diffusion membrane may be absent and the basal laminae of the endothelial and epithelial cells may be fused.
Source: Walter Reed Army Institute of Research

lesion of pulmonary PBI is hemorrhage, the amount and distribution of which depends on the level of blast exposure. The only external sign of lung hemorrhage is froth or blood that can be seen within the oral cavity or surrounding the nose and lips. At autopsy, hemorrhage is visible through the thin pleural membrane, and blood can be found oozing from the face of a cut section of the lung.

Although they frequently occur in combination, pulmonary hemorrhages can be divided anatomically into three distinct types: *(a)* pleural and subpleural hemorrhage, *(b)* hemorrhage that is multifocal or diffuse within the parenchyma, and *(c)* hemorrhage that surrounds the airway and vascular structures that are embedded within the parenchyma.

The first type of pulmonary hemorrhage is visible through the lung's thin pleural surface. With the exception of a small amount of extravasated erythrocytes that are found in the loose connective tissue of the visceral pleura, this hemorrhage is actually located in the subpleural alveolar tissues (Figure 8-2). It is visible at autopsy on the surface of the lungs in a bilateral and generally symmetrical pattern, although it will be more extensive on the side facing the blast source.

Pleural or subpleural hemorrhage may be visible as *(a)* a few petechiae as a consequence of a low blast dose, *(b)* ecchymoses from a medium blast dose (Figure 8-3), or *(c)* coalescing ecchymoses or diffuse subpleural hemorrhage (or both) from a high blast dose (Figure 8-4). Pleural rupture and hemopneumothorax (in which both blood and air escape into the thoracic cavity) may occur in the latter case. Lungs of casualties who have died from severe PBI exhibit such a distinctive appearance at autopsy that pathologists have come to recognize this damage as blast lung. A diffuse hemorrhage makes the entire organ, which is normally pink, look dark red or black. This corresponds to the same term used in the clinical setting, where blast lung refers to the signs and symptoms indicative of PBI.

Petechiae and ecchymoses appear in a multifocal pattern on the pleural surface and have a predilection

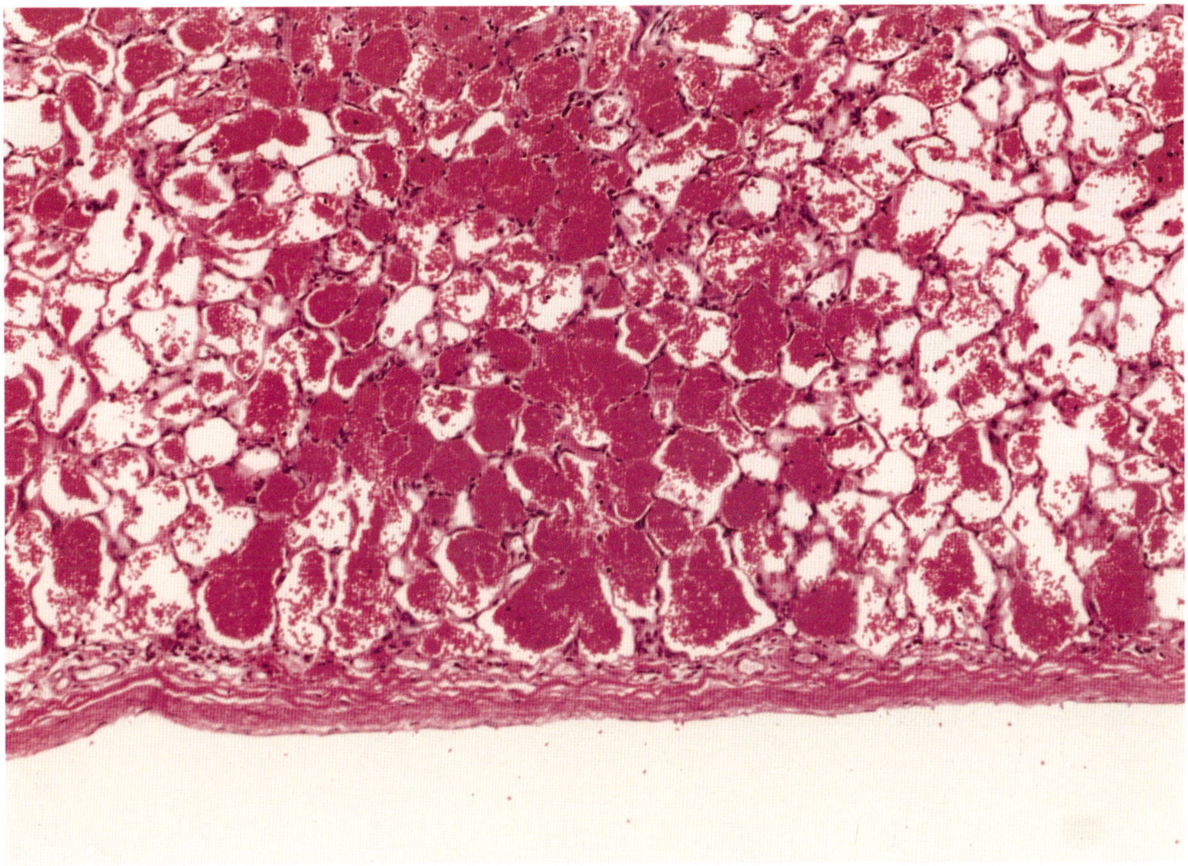

Fig. 8-2. Most of the hemorrhage that is visible at the pleural surface of this blast-exposed sheep's lung is actually contained within subpleural alveoli.
Source: Walter Reed Army Institute of Research

for certain sites, such as adjacent to the diaphragm, on the lung surfaces next to the heart, and on the posterior surfaces where the left and right lungs are in contact.

In addition, hemorrhages on the lateral lung surfaces often exhibit distinctive *rib markings* (Figure 8-4). The source of the rib markings has been the subject of thorough experimentation. At one time, the hemorrhagic rib markings were thought to correspond with the overlying ribs and to result from the ribs' displacement into the lung tissue. However, when a small amount of dye was injected into rabbits' intercostal spaces and the animals were exposed to blast, the rib markings corresponded in every case to the ink punctures from the intercostal spaces rather than to the ribs themselves.[12] When segments of the rats' ribs were removed in a later study, creating an artificially large intercostal space, this space was marked by a similar hemorrhage after the animals were exposed to blast.[13] Finally, thoracic-wall measurements of rabbits showed that intercostal tissue responded to the blast wave by moving inward faster and farther than the ribs did.[14] Thus, *intercostal markings*—rather than rib markings—would probably be a more appropriate name for these hemorrhages.

A second site of pulmonary hemorrhage is found in the parenchyma beneath the subpleural region. It probably occurs as the result of the stress that is concentrated at various sites in the parenchyma when the lungs are distorted by the blast wave. This stress may cause the delicate alveolar septa to rupture. The alveolar spaces and associated bronchioles rapidly fill with blood from severed alveolar capillaries, producing hemorrhagic foci that are visible when cross-sections of the lungs are examined at autopsy (Figure 8-5). Because alveolar-septal tears are difficult to see histologically, these hemorrhages appear as blood-engorged alveoli, with the acinar structures remaining essentially intact (Figures 8-1 and 8-6).

A similar tear may occur between the alveoli and the wall of an intralobular venule.[9] This is known as an *alveolovenous fistula*, and the resulting direct communication between the air space and the circulatory system plays an important role in the production of air emboli. (Air emboli are the primary cause of imme-

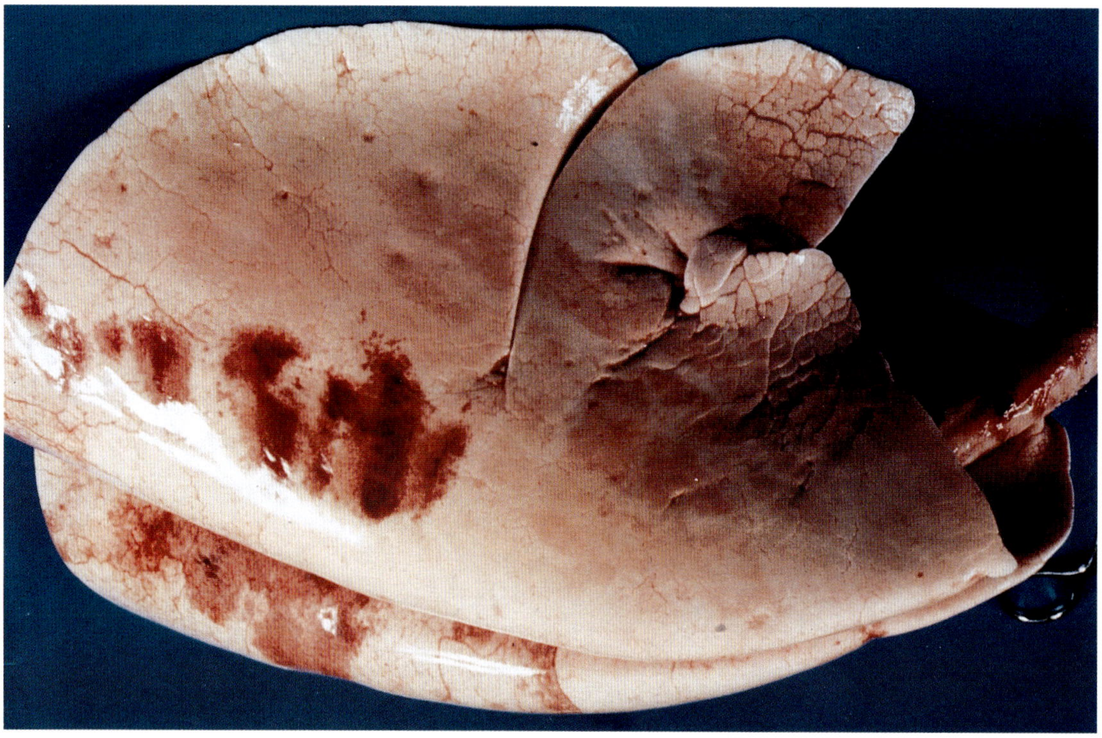

Fig. 8-3. Subpleural ecchymoses and petechiae over the diaphragmatic lobe of the lung of a sheep that was subjected to a single blast of moderate pressure
Source: Walter Reed Army Institute of Research

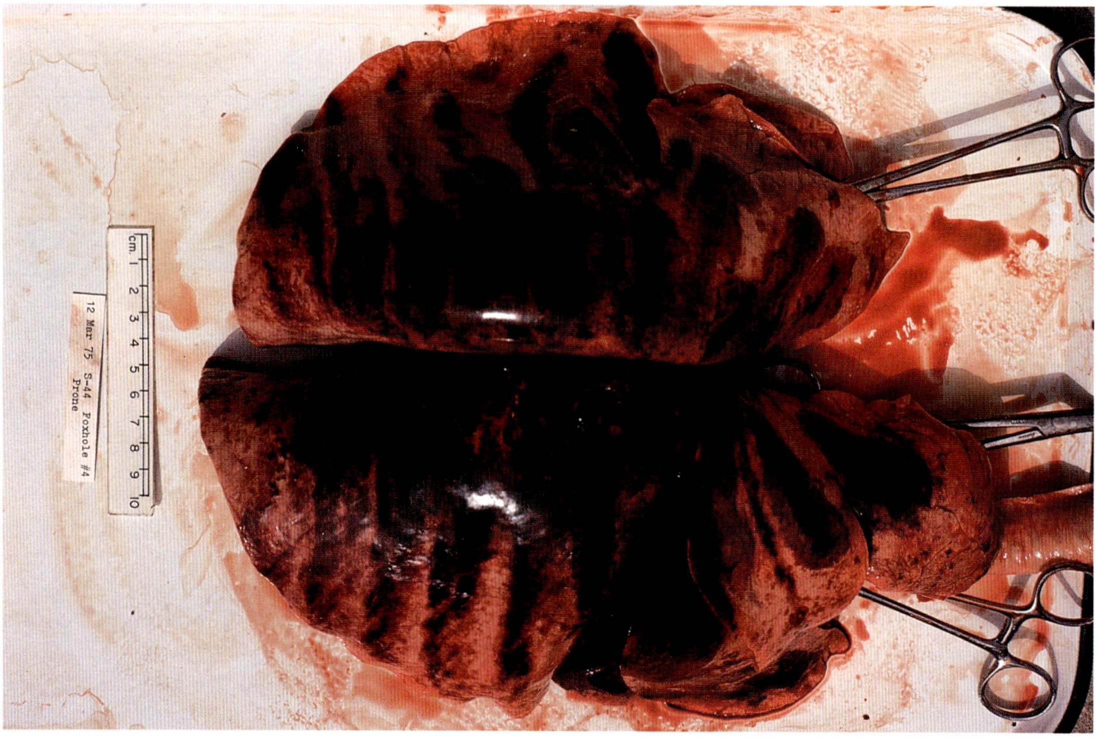

Fig. 8-4. This subpleural hemorrhage involves the entire posterior (dorsal) surface of the lung of a sheep that was subjected to a high-pressure blast. The darker portions of the hemorrhage that appear over the lateral surface of the diaphragmatic lobe actually mark the intercostal spaces, even though they are commonly called rib markings.
Source: D. R. Richmond

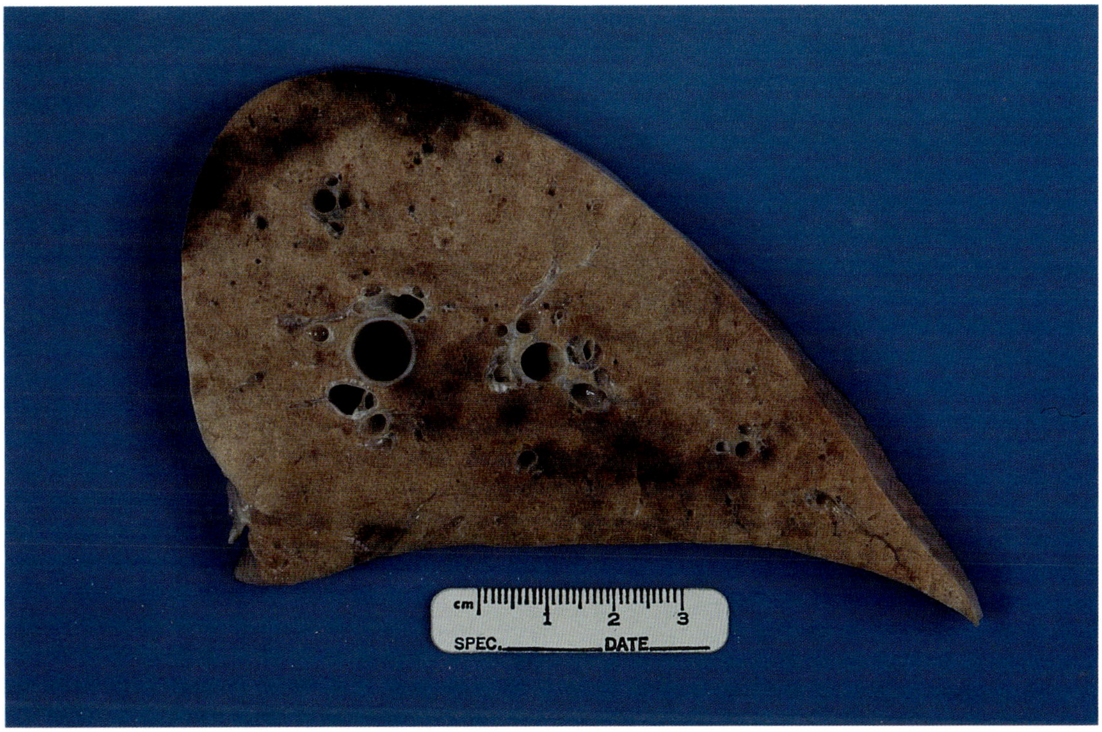

Fig. 8-5. In this cross-sectional wedge from the right diaphragmatic lung lobe from a sheep that was exposed to a single blast, note the dark-brown areas of subpleural and peribronchial hemorrhage.
Source: Walter Reed Army Institute of Research

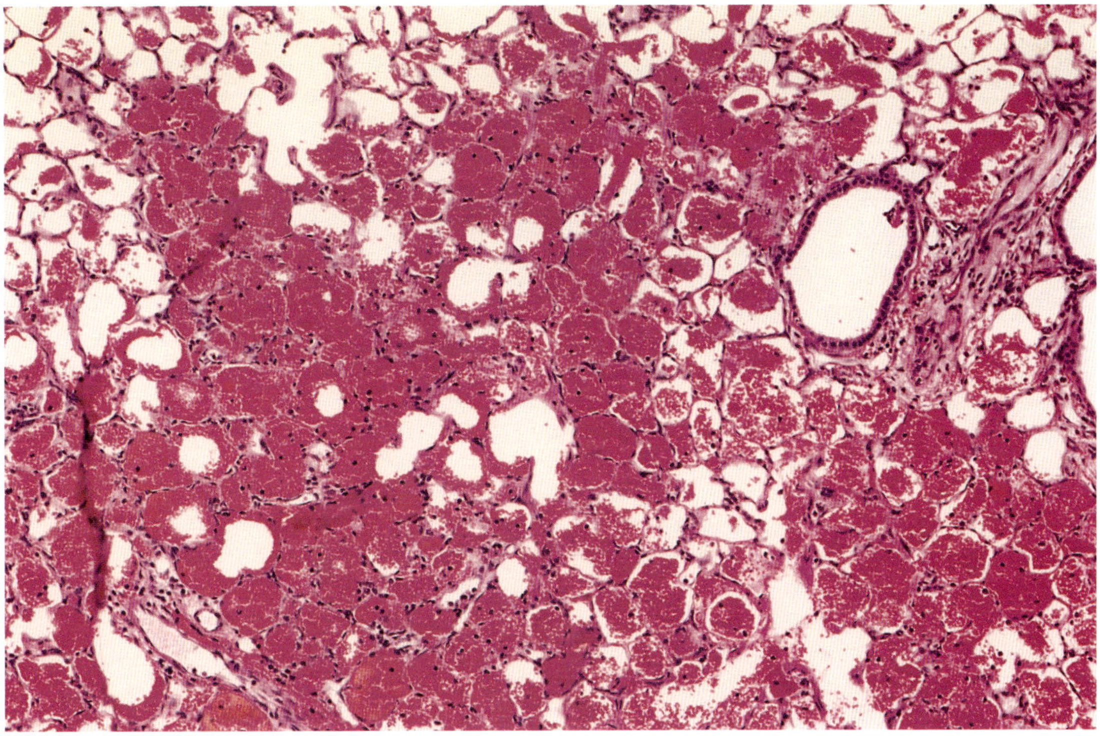

Fig. 8-6. In this histological section of lung parenchyma from a sheep exposed to a single blast, the alveoli are slightly dilated and filled with erythrocytes.
Source: Walter Reed Army Institute of Research

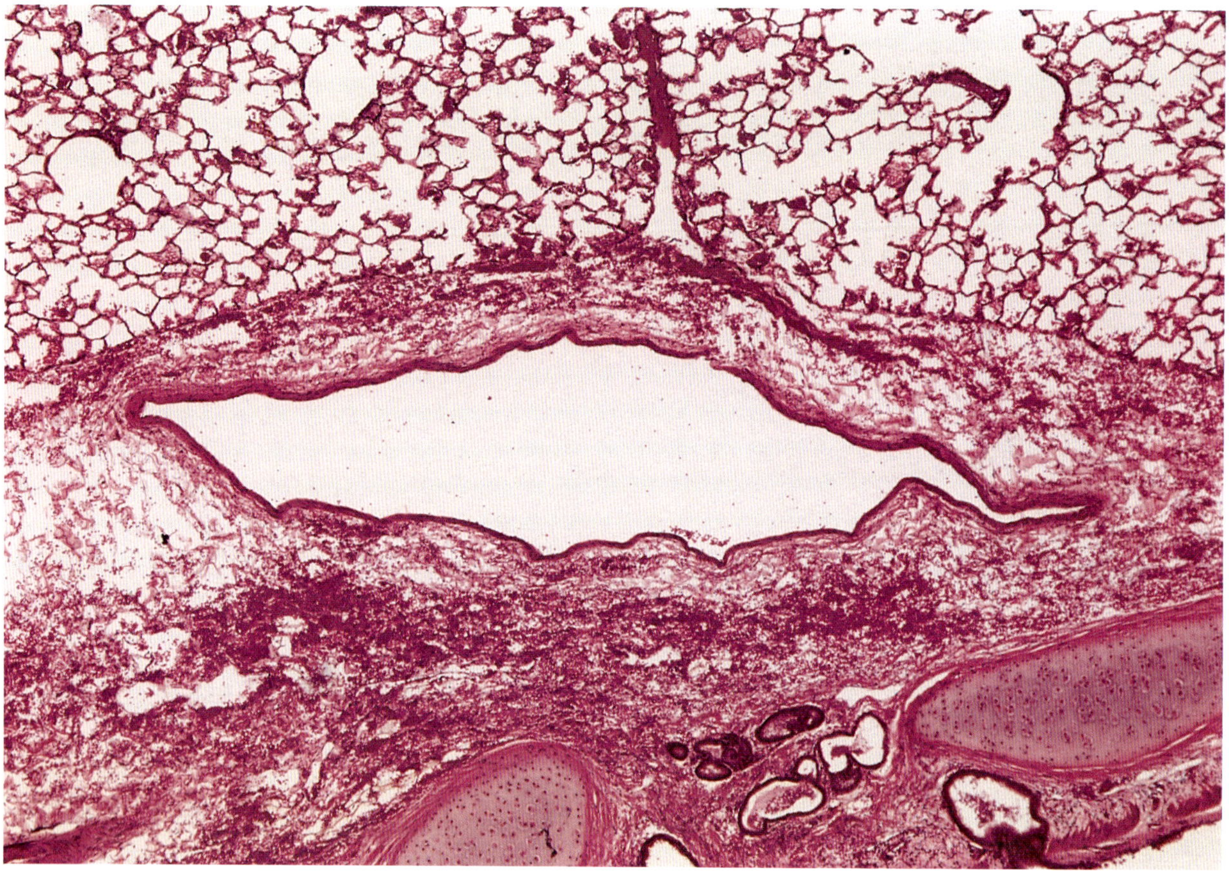

Fig. 8-7. In this histological section of lung parenchyma from a sheep exposed to a single blast, note the hemorrhage within the connective tissue that surrounds this blood vessel. This phenomenon is called ring hemorrhage.
Source: Walter Reed Army Institute of Research

diate death in blast victims, and their generation and pathophysiological effects are discussed in the next section of this chapter.)

A third site of pulmonary hemorrhage is in the thin interstitial band that surrounds vascular and airway structures. When damaged by blast, the interstitium may be filled with erythrocytes and plasma, forming hemorrhagic bands of erythrocytes surrounding airways and blood vessels. These are often called *ring hemorrhages.* They may occur far from the foci of alveolar hemorrhage, and thus they appear to develop independently. This site is particularly vulnerable to hemorrhage because of the difference in density between *(a)* the relatively rigid airways and blood vessels and *(b)* the fine meshwork of surrounding connective tissue and alveolar septa. When the bronchovascular structures (which have more inertia) resist displacement, the surrounding connective tissues are stretched and some of the capillaries are broken, with resultant hemorrhage (Figure 8-7).

Although blast researchers would like to be able to correlate the amount of hemorrhage with other blast-induced changes (such as alterations of the lung's physiological parameters, the presence of air emboli, or even mortality), the amount of hemorrhage within the lungs is difficult to quantitate. The most common way to indicate the extent of blast-related lung hemorrhage is by measuring the increase in lung weight after blast exposure. In experimental animals, the increase in gross lung weights is proportionate to the intensity of the blast, and is caused primarily by hemorrhage.

To standardize lung weights for various species and sizes of experimental subjects, the lung weight is commonly expressed as a percentage of the whole-body weight. Most uninjured lungs can be expected to fall within the normal range, usually 0.6%–1.2% of the whole-body weight. After blast exposure, lung-weight percentages that are higher than those in the normal range indicate the presence primarily of hemorrhage, with edema fluid and congestion (the pooling of blood within pulmonary blood vessels) being much less significant. In the larger proximal airways, only a small amount of blood-tinged froth (indicating hemorrhage) will typically be present; most of the hemorrhage will be in the lung parenchyma, especially in the dependent distal lobules, suggesting a gravitational

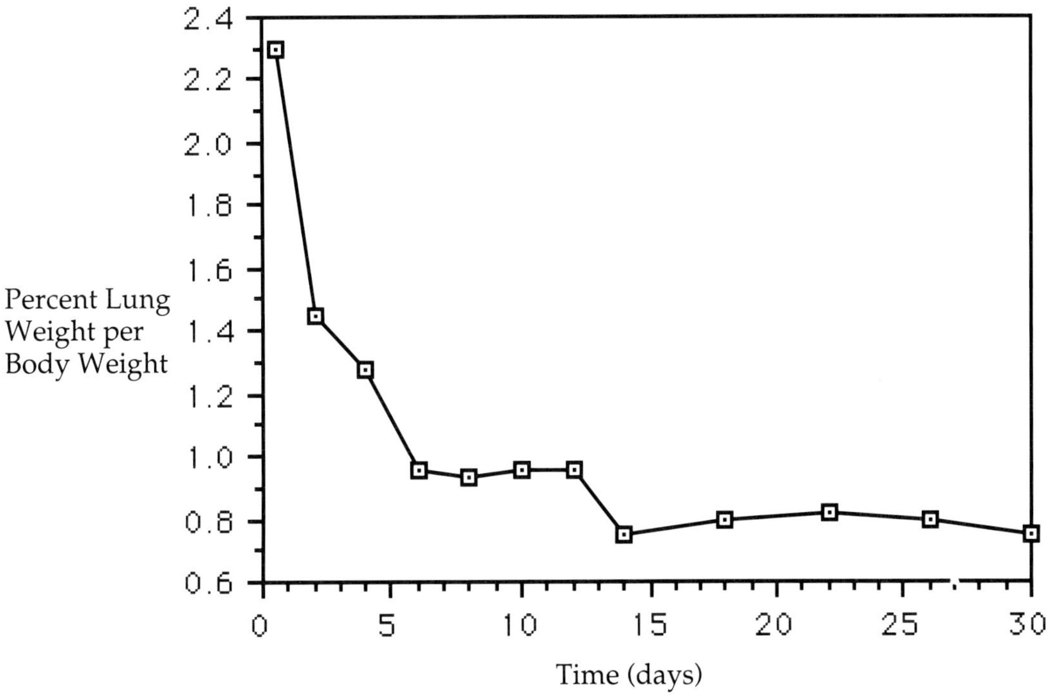

Fig. 8-8. Lung weight (expressed as a percentage of body weight) plotted against the time after a blast
Source: Redrawn from reference 9

pooling of blood.

The lung weight reaches its peak almost immediately after the blast (Figure 8-8) and returns to a near-normal level several days later. Similarly, most histological evidence of hemorrhage will be gone by the sixth day after the blast. However, many hemosiderin-laden alveolar macrophages will remain and may not be cleared for several weeks. Months after a blast exposure, experimental animals have exhibited multifocal fibroplasia around alveolar ducts.[9] These residual scars are the only evidence that the animal was ever exposed to a blast.

The extent of parenchymal hemorrhage is an important determinant of mortality (Figure 8-9). The hemorrhage within the acini may lead to increased mortality from suffocation in some subjects because it reduces the surface area that is available for gas exchange. However, the connection between parenchymal hemorrhage and increased mortality may more likely be explained by the fact that a blast that produces more severed alveolar septa is likely also to produce more alveolovenous fistulae, and subsequently more air emboli. Most PBI-related deaths are caused by air embolism, rather than by hemorrhage.

Emphysema. When the alveolar septa tear, the alveoli themselves coalesce, producing giant air spaces and causing pulmonary emphysema. Subpleural cysts are formed if the air accumulates near the surface of the lung and the pleura remains intact. If the pleura ruptures, a pneumothorax may occur.

Pulmonary Edema. Some blast researchers believe that diffuse edema is a significant component of PBI.[15,16] In theory, the same blast forces that sever alveolar septa and cause hemorrhage in the regions that are subject to the greatest distortion may also compromise the functional integrity of the endothelial-epithelial fluid barrier of the alveolar walls throughout the lungs. Then, although the barrier would remain intact enough to prevent erythrocytes from leaking, plasma would escape, producing alveolar edema and resulting in a condition that would, if the edema were diffuse, be identical to *adult respiratory distress syndrome* (ARDS). ARDS refers to the clinical syndrome that is evident when noncardiogenic pulmonary edema results from diffuse damage to the alveolar wall. It does not connote a specific etiology,

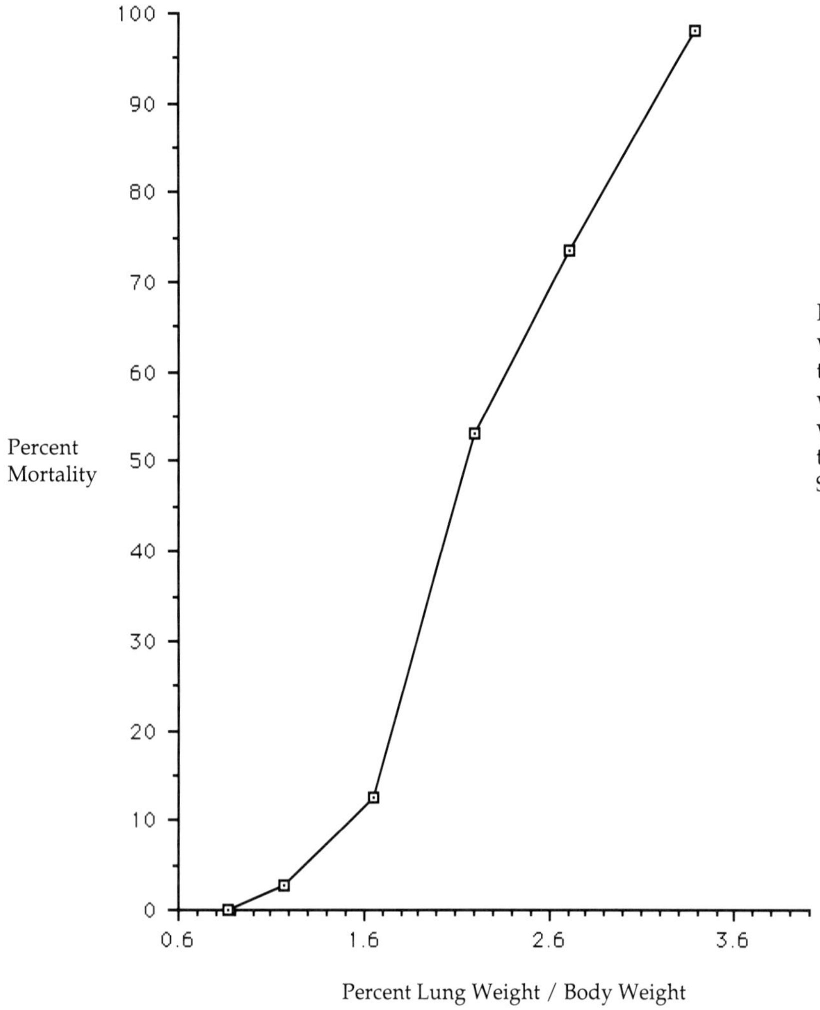

Fig. 8-9. In a study of 556 guinea pigs that were exposed to fast-rising overpressures that lasted 6–8 seconds, the animals' lung weights (expressed as percentages of their whole-body weights) were proportionate to their mortality.
Source: Redrawn from reference 9

but rather has been associated with a variety of causes, such as *(a)* oxygen toxicity, *(b)* pneumotoxicity from substances like paraquat, and *(c)* septic or traumatic shock.

However, most blast studies do not indicate that this kind of widespread pulmonary edema exists.[9,10] One study, for example, estimated the amount of pulmonary edema by measuring the amount of fluid delivered to a cannula placed in the caudal mediastinal lymph node of a sheep.[17] Blast doses that produced pleural petechiae did not increase the amount of fluid in the cannula, indicating that the permeability of the pulmonary capillaries was not significantly increased. In other studies, animals that were exposed to higher blast doses did not show significant alveolar edema, and histological sections of sites away from the foci of hemorrhage were devoid of fluid accumulation.[9,18]

Some blast effects (such as hemorrhage) are obviously localized, but other effects (such as edema), which some investigators may have assumed to be diffuse, may be localized as well. The same mechanistic aspects of blast injury that are responsible for the multifocal nature of lung hemorrhage may also cause edema that is usually localized in the same regions as the hemorrhage. In animal studies, for example, edema has been seen in the hemorrhagic regions of the lung parenchyma at autopsy (Figure 8-10).

Blast casualties in whom death is delayed may show diffuse alveolar edema at autopsy, which could be explained by *(a)* the presence of multifactorial cardiopulmonary distress or *(b)* therapeutic interventions, such as fluid resuscitation or mechanical ventilation.

Stripped-Epithelium Lesions. The tissues that line the larger conducting airways within the lungs are not immune from the consequences of the passing blast wave.

The most commonly reported lesion in airways is a *stripped-epithelium lesion,* which results when bronchial or bronchiolar epithelium is stripped from the underlying basal lamina (Figure 8-11). When these lesions are severe, they may manifest as ulcerations

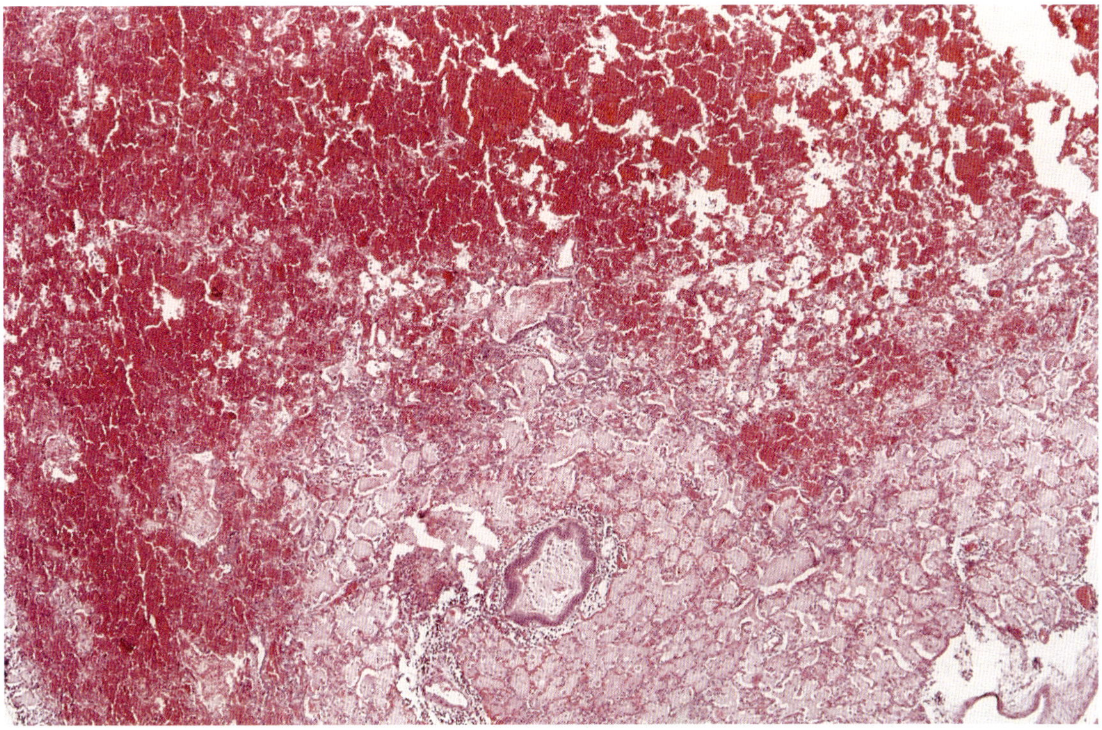

Fig. 8-10. In this histological section of lung parenchyma from a sheep exposed to a single blast, note the large area of alveolar edema (lower right) adjacent to the area of alveolar hemorrhage (upper left).
Source: Walter Reed Army Institute of Research

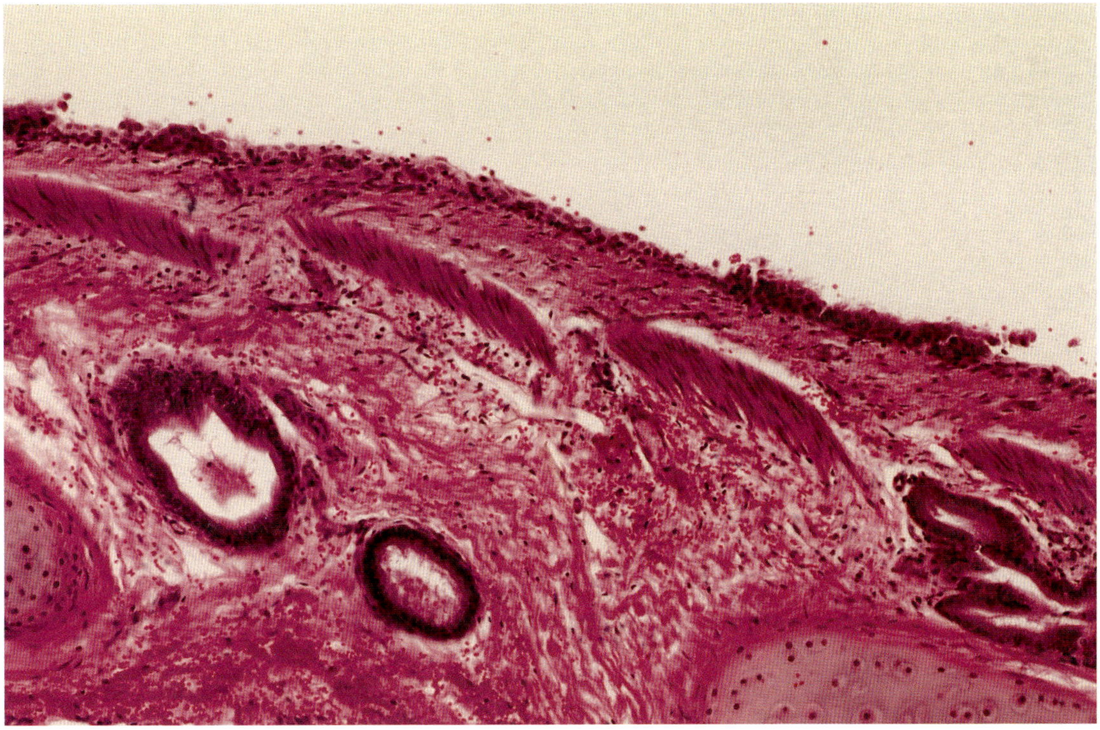

Fig. 8-11. In this histological section of lung parenchyma from a sheep exposed to a single blast, note the loss of pseudostratified ciliated epithelium from the bronchiolar surface and the hemorrhage in the underlying submucosa.
Source: Walter Reed Army Institute of Research

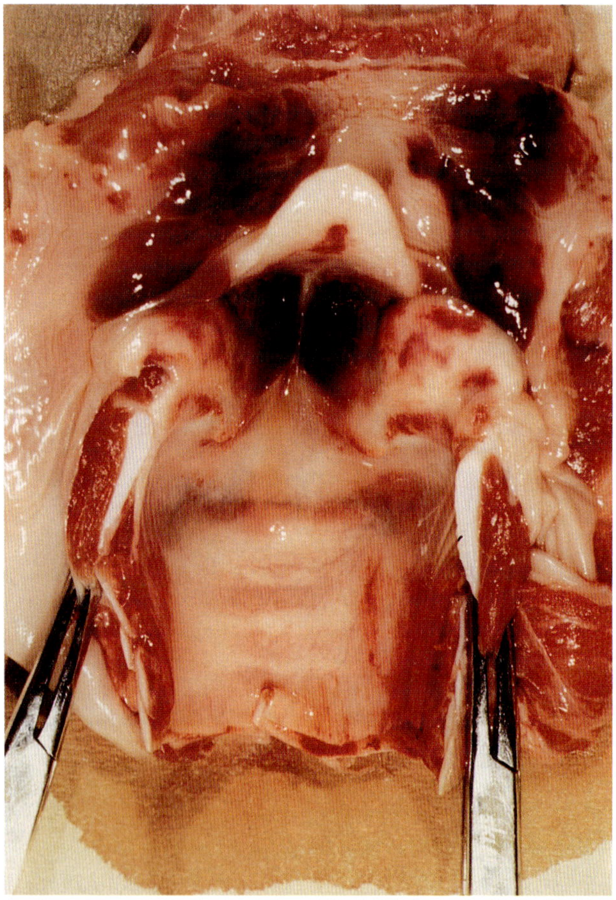

Fig. 8-12. In this autopsy specimen of the larynx of a sheep that was exposed to blast overpressure, the trachea was bisected dorsally and pulled apart to expose the larynx and proximal trachea. Note the hemorrhage within the mucosa of the posterior pharynx, laryngeal vestibule, and aryepiglottic fold.
Source: D. R. Richmond

through the basal lamina and into the underlying submucosa.[9] The hemorrhage that results contributes to the blood and fluid that collects in the distal airways and parenchyma.

Although the injuring mechanism is difficult to determine, one hypothesis suggests that spalling might be responsible for epithelial lesions in these airways. In nonliving materials, spalling occurs when a pressure wave passes through material of one density into material of a different density, throwing off fragments at the interface of the two materials.[19] If this hypothesis is applied to living tissue, a pressure wave that hits the tissues of the conducting airway is transmitted through the denser supporting cartilage or smooth-muscle layer before it reaches the less-dense attached mucosa. At the interface of the two, according to this hypothesis, spalling causes fragmentation of the mucosa. Although the applicability of this hypothesis to living tissue has never been validated, blast researchers have seen multifocal stripping of epithelium from the basal lamina. A more current explanation of injuring mechanisms in the respiratory system is discussed in some detail in Chapter Seven.

Regardless of the precise nature of the injuring mechanism, these lesions are caused by the blast's distortion of the airway, which stretches the mucosal layer and results in both the stripping of the epithelium and the rupture of small submucosal blood vessels.

Stripped-epithelium lesions can occur even when blast dose levels are below those associated with parenchymal hemorrhage, particularly if exposures are repeated.[18] In fact, these lesions may represent the most significant type of respiratory-tract injury following low-intensity blast doses. The denudation of airways and the loss of portions of the mucociliary apparatus may significantly inhibit the ability of the lung to clear particulate material, thereby creating an environment that is conducive to secondary infections after blast injury.

The Upper Airways

The upper-respiratory passages are vulnerable to the same damaging phenomena that the large airways of the lower-respiratory tract are, resulting in similar hemorrhages and stripped-epithelium lesions. These proximal airway injuries may be sentinel injuries, signalling that more blast damage has occurred distally.

Autopsy studies reveal multifocal submucosal and mucosal petechiae and ecchymoses in the trachea, larynx, pharynx, and both paranasal and nasal sinuses. These hemorrhages have been shown to occur at blast doses lower than those that cause lung hemorrhage.[20] Within the trachea, the hemorrhages appear at random or in a transverse pattern over cartilaginous rings.[9] Within the larynx, the hemorrhages often occur over the vestibule and on the posterior face of the epiglottis (Figure 8-12). There are no reported cases or studies in which upper-airway competence has been compromised by these lesions.

The loss, or stripping, of surface epithelium that occurs in the bronchi also commonly occurs in the trachea and larynx. In one study, researchers used an electron microscope to examine lesions from rats that were exposed to 20 repetitions of blast.[21] The lesions ranged from *(a)* a flattening of epithelial cells without cell loss to *(b)* the focal loss of epithelial cells with disruption of the basal lamina. When ulceration occurred, the defects were covered by fibrinocellular

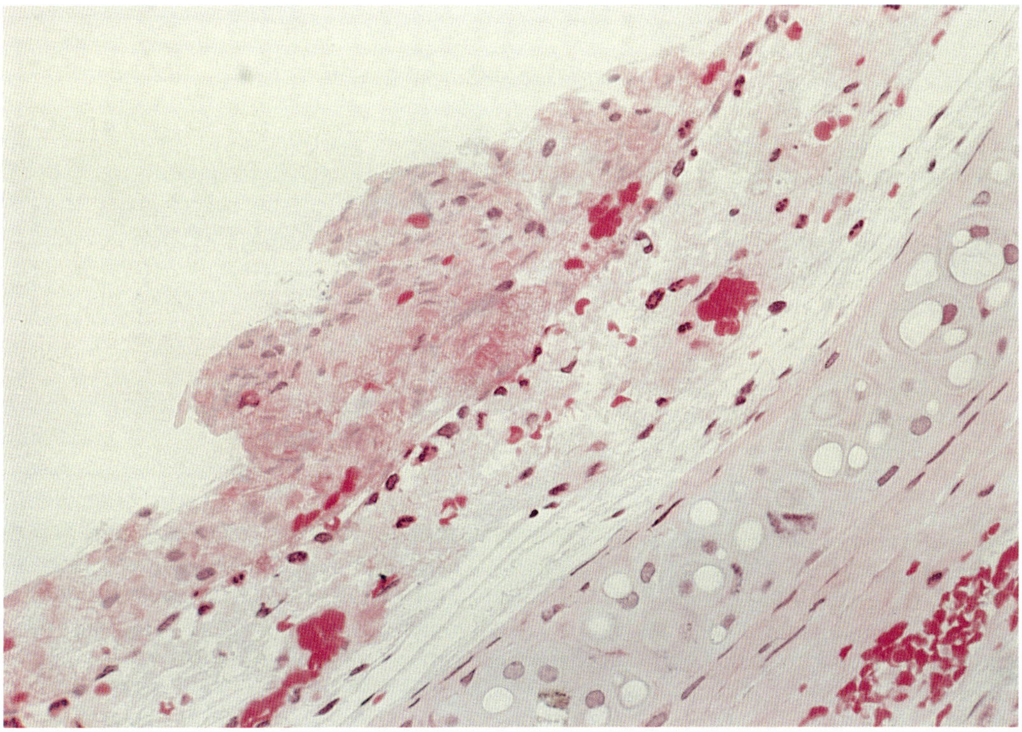

Fig. 8-13. In this histological section of the trachea from a rat that was exposed to twenty repetitions of blast at 27.5 psi on 2 consecutive days, the epithelium is focally flattened and partially denuded, with a fibrinocellular clot overlying the area of injury.

clots with admixed leukocytes (Figures 8-13 and 8-14). These lesions first appeared at or below the threshold blast dose for hemorrhage within the rats' lungs. Similarly, sheep that were exposed to fifty repetitions of blast overpressure developed tracheal lesions at peak pressures of 5 psi, although they did not develop significant lung hemorrhages until peak pressures exceeded 15 psi.[18]

The protective mucociliary apparatus extends from the larynx to the terminal bronchioles. It is made up of the cilia of the epithelial cells, which continuously carry mucus from the lungs to the pharynx. The stripped-epithelium lesions of the trachea are similar to those in the conducting airways within the lung (that is, the bronchi and bronchioles), and whether the blast wave's disruption of either of these portions of the protective mucociliary apparatus is significant has yet to be determined.

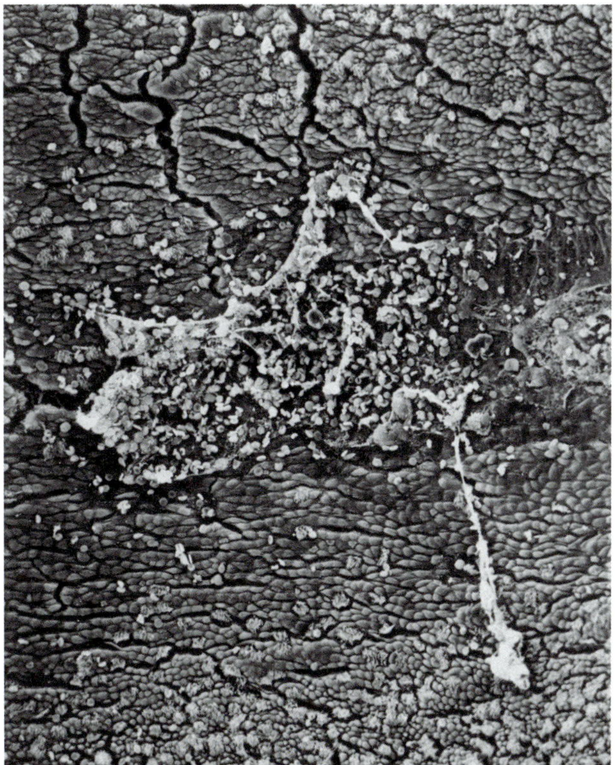

Fig. 8-14. In this scanning electron micrograph of the tracheal epithelium from a rat that was exposed to twenty repetitions of blast at 22.5 psi, the focal denudation of the epithelial lining is covered by a fibrinocellular clot.
Source: Walter Reed Army Institute of Research

THE CIRCULATORY SYSTEM

The circulatory system, which comprises the heart and blood vessels, may be directly injured by the blunt effects of the blast wave itself. However, the indirect effects of the blast on the circulatory system can be much more significant: Air emboli, which originate in the lung as a sequela of pulmonary PBI, can occlude coronary blood vessels and cause cardiac arrest.

Air Emboli

Since the early days of blast experimentation, investigators and pathologists have believed that the amount of hemorrhage seen in those animals that died after blast exposure was insufficient to explain their rapid deaths.[9] Neither the amount of lost blood nor the decreased pulmonary surface area that was available for gas exchange appeared to account for such high mortality.

In one key experiment, animals were exposed to underwater blast while their thoraces were submerged and their heads were above water. In spite of the fact that their heads were not subjected to the blast wave, they suffered deficits in neurological control as well as alterations in consciousness.[22] Previously, researchers had believed that these effects were caused by PBI to the brain, but careful pathological studies ultimately revealed the presence of air emboli in cerebral and coronary arteries following blast exposure.[9,10,22] Investigators then demonstrated that an injection of small quantities of air into the carotid artery could reproduce these abnormalities in the central nervous system.

Air emboli originate in the lungs, and are thought to enter the circulation through traumatic alveolovenous fistulae. Mortality is proportionate to the extent of both lung hemorrhage and air emboli at autopsy (Figure 8-15). Thus, the more severe the lung hemorrhage, the greater the likelihood of significant

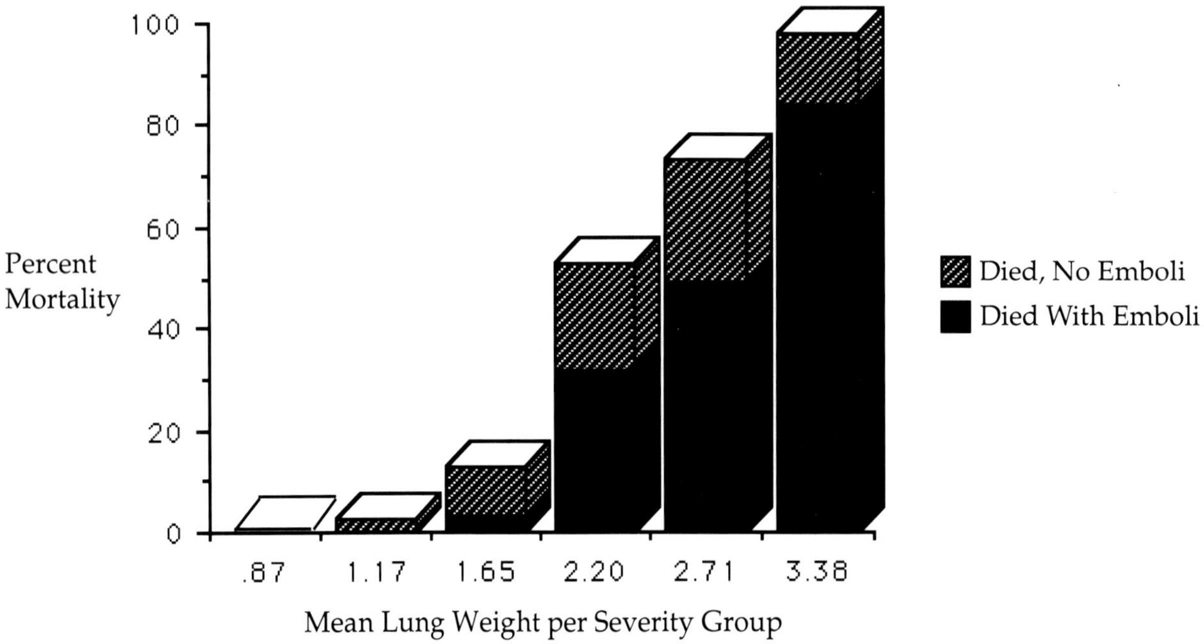

Fig. 8-15. In this graph, each of the six bars represents a group of animals categorized by severity of lung hemorrhage. The mean lung weight below each bar represents the mean lung weight for that particular severity group. Lung weight is proportionate to mortality. In addition, the proportion of dead animals that showed air emboli at autopsy increased in proportion to the amount of hemorrhage.
Source: Redrawn from reference 9

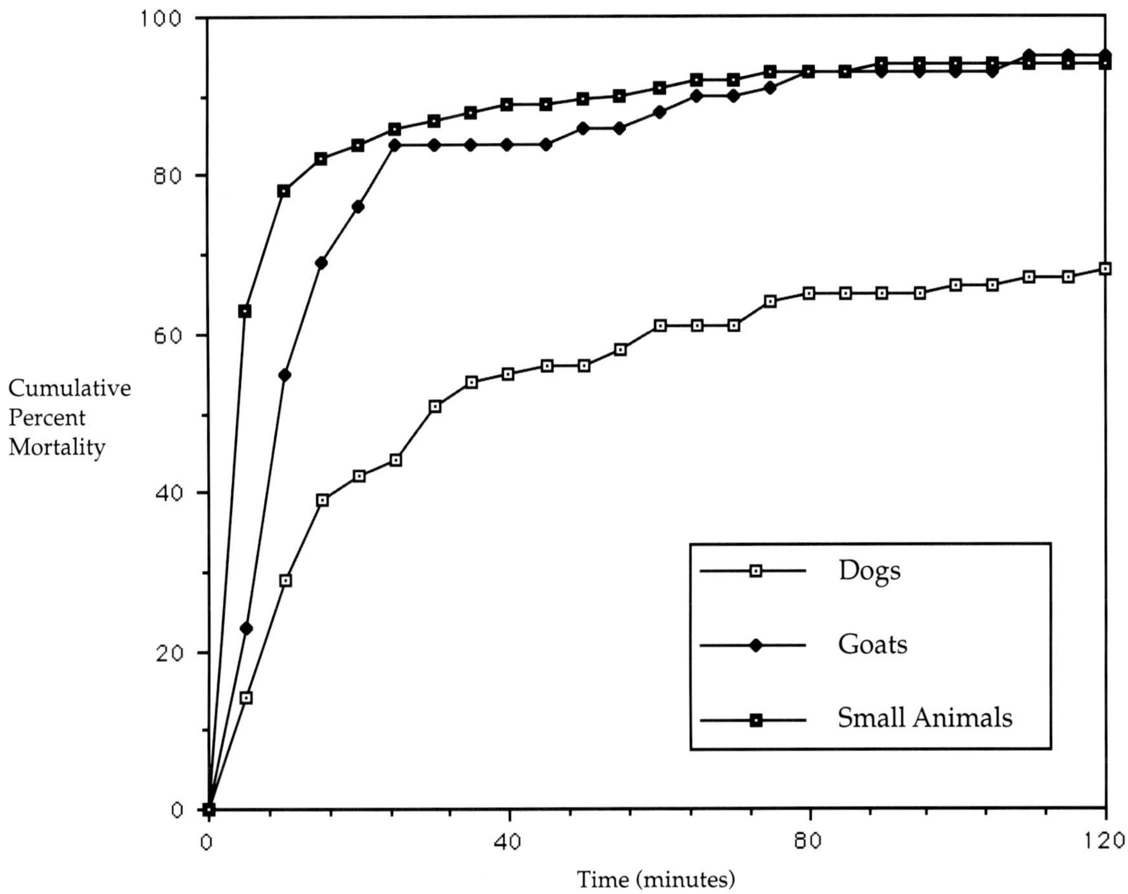

Fig. 8-16. This graph illustrates the cumulative mortality rates for various species of animals exposed to blast overpressures. The initial mortality rates appeared to be lower for the larger species.
Source: Redrawn from reference 9

embolism, which may be the principal cause of deaths that occur within the first hour after blast. In most studies, more than 50% of the deaths from PBI occurred within the first 30 minutes—and 75% during the first 2 hours—after the blast (Figure 8-16).[23] Autopsies on experimental animals that die soon after blast often reveal many air emboli.

No one knows how long air emboli may continue to be produced after a casualty is exposed to blast, nor how common emboli that are not clinically detected might be. In a study of only one animal, researchers used Doppler ultrasound to detect showers of air emboli in the carotid artery for up to 30 minutes after blast exposure.[24] However, most investigators believe that the clinically significant air emboli occur within the first 10 minutes.[9,10,22]

Emboli may be difficult to see at autopsy because the air bubbles may be absorbed after death.[10] Conversely, the prosector may accidentally introduce air into a blood vessel, leading to a false diagnosis of air embolism. In animal studies, the prosector is likely to see air bubbles within coronary arteries (Figure 8-17) or in arteries at the base of the brain (Figure 8-18). Air emboli have also been found in renal arteries after blast exposure.

The Heart

The heart may be damaged by blunt trauma from the blast wave, which may result in hemorrhage, or by the effects of air embolism.

Hemorrhage. As is the case in other organs, hemorrhage is the most common blast-related lesion found within the heart. Cardiac hemorrhage is rarely seen without accompanying pulmonary hemorrhage, although the production of cardiac lesions may require higher blast doses than the production of pulmonary lesions does.

Epicardial hemorrhage usually occurs along the posterior surface where the heart directly apposes the diaphragm (Figure 8-19). Thus, the mechanism of

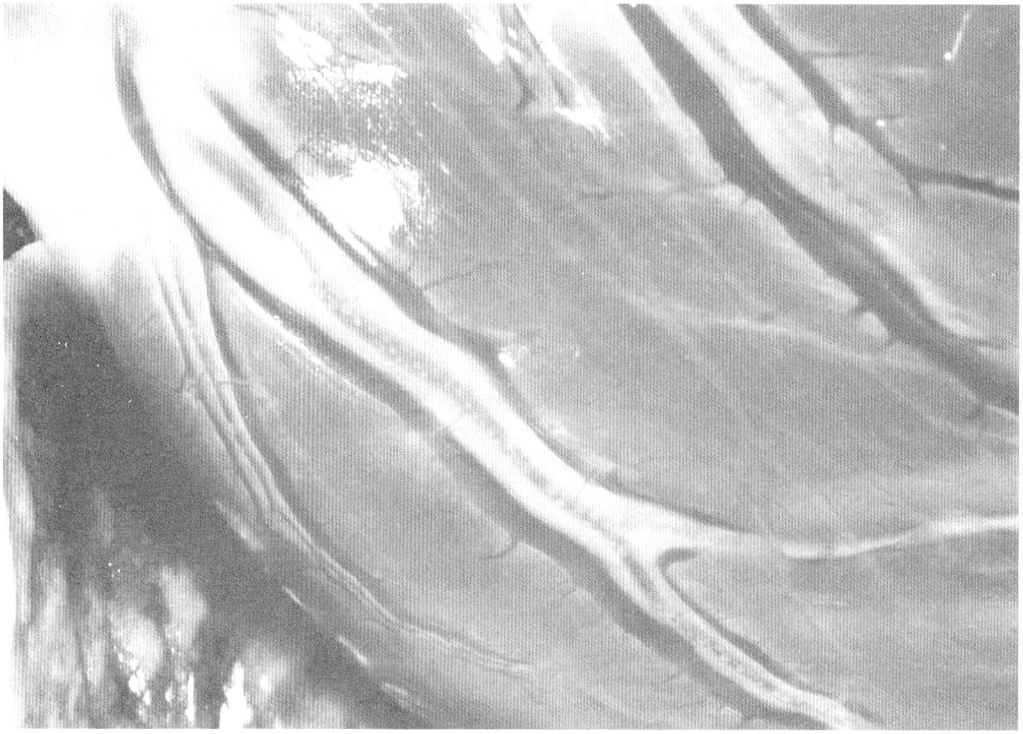

Fig. 8-17. This autopsy specimen from a dog exposed to a lethal blast dose shows air emboli within branches of the left coronary artery.
Source: D. R. Richmond

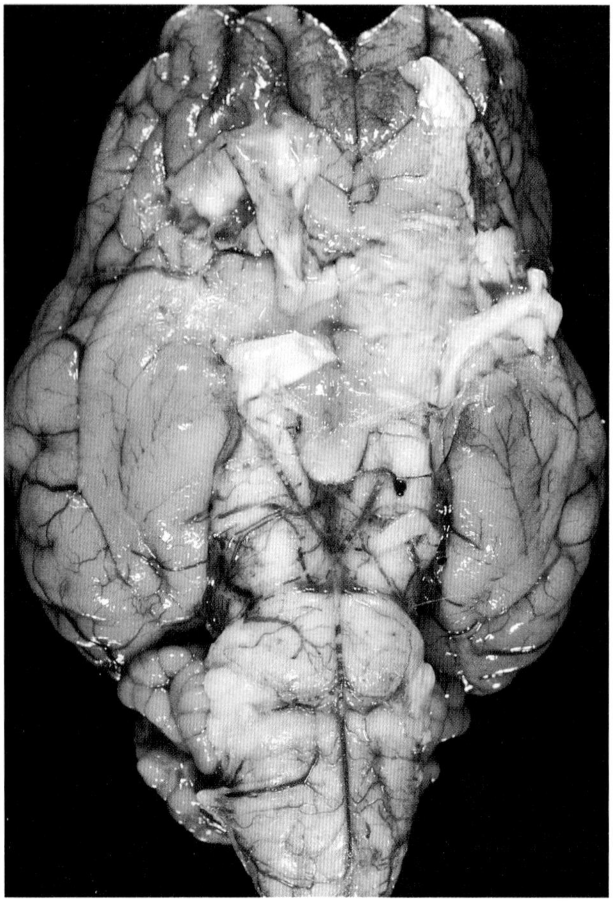

injury is probably direct contusion, which results from the diaphragm's rapid upward displacement. Myocardial hemorrhage is less frequent,[10] and an occasional cardiac tear or laceration has been documented.[9]

Endocardial hemorrhage can commonly be seen at the base of the papillary muscles, in the surrounding ventricular endocardium, and occasionally on the valve leaflets (Figure 8-20). Histologically, erythrocytes infiltrate the endocardial connective tissue and may be seen surrounding the Purkinje fibers.

Cardiac Effects of Air Embolism. Changes within the myocardium from the presence of air emboli in coronary vessels are thought to be a major cause of death in blast casualties. The emboli may produce ischemia, which leads to subsequent degeneration and necrosis of myocytes (infarction). In the living subject, electrocardiography is a useful method for detecting these changes. Myocyte degeneration has rarely been described histologically in postmortem examinations of blast subjects.[25,26]

Fig. 8-18. This autopsy specimen from a sheep exposed to blast overpressure shows air emboli within the basilar artery and the posterior portion of the arterial circle of the brain.
Source: D. R. Richmond

The Blood Vessels

The blast wave affects the blood vessels in vulnerable organs, inasmuch as every hemorrhage involves some blood-vessel damage. Although this damage may be widespread, it does not result from an injuring event that affects the circulatory system as a whole; rather, it is localized and is intrinsically related to the unique structures of the organs in which the vessels are found.

Autopsies of animals that had PBI have shown fibrin thrombi in the small blood vessels of the kidneys, adrenal glands, and heart.[23] These microthrombi have appeared as early as 5 minutes after the blast, and may be related to ischemic changes caused by the presence of air emboli. They may also be a manifestation of *disseminated intravascular coagulation* (DIC), rather than the result of direct ischemic injury to a blood vessel. For example, of five casualties of a civilian bus bombing who had lung injuries and severe respiratory failure, three also had DIC.[27]

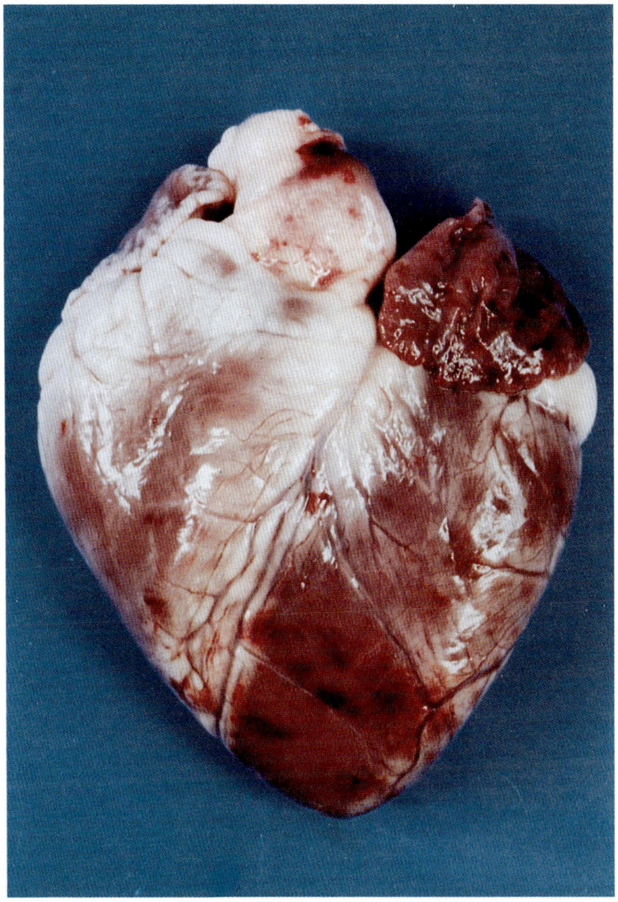

Fig. 8-19. This autopsy specimen from a sheep exposed to blast overpressure shows focally extensive epicardial and subepicardial hemorrhage. The hemorrhage is most severe on the left ventricular wall at the apex. In addition, ecchymoses can be seen on the right ventricle.
Source: Walter Reed Army Institute of Research

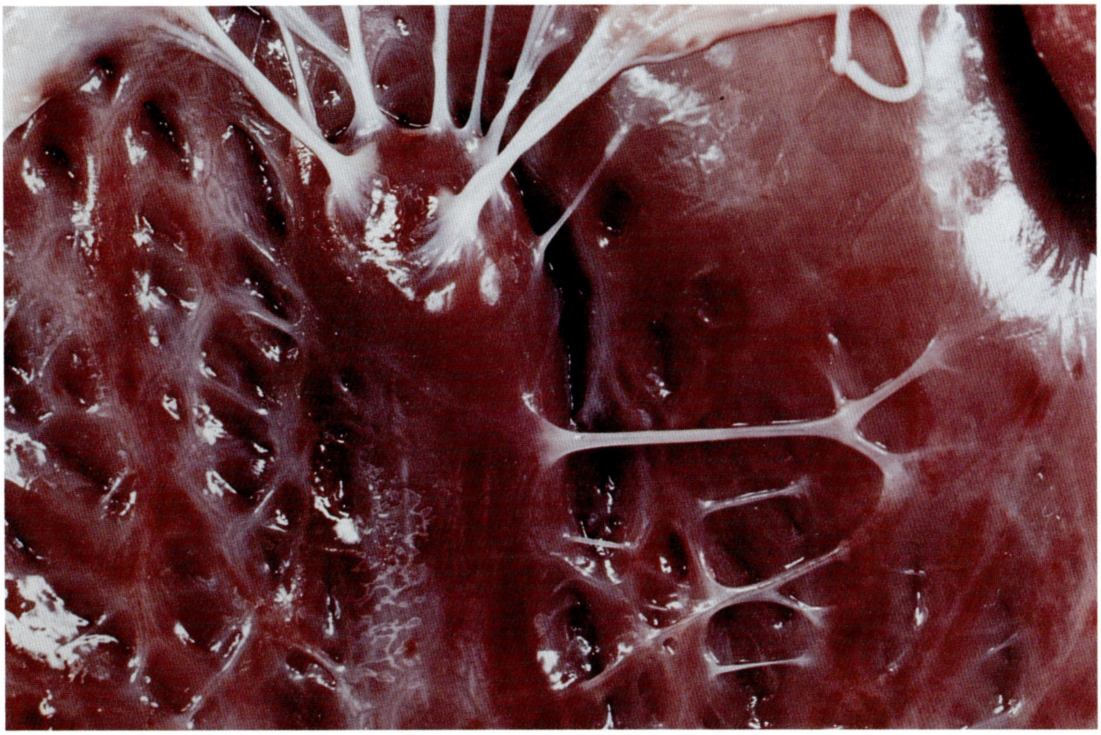

Fig. 8-20. This autopsy specimen from a sheep exposed to blast overpressure shows endocardial hemorrhage within a papillary muscle and the surrounding septal wall of the left ventricle.
Source: Walter Reed Army Institute of Research

THE DIGESTIVE SYSTEM

Like the organs of the chest cavity, the organs within the abdominal cavity that contain gas pockets—such as the gastrointestinal tract—are the most susceptible to blast injury. Solid abdominal organs may also be damaged at higher blast doses.

The Gastrointestinal Tract

Next to the damage they do to the respiratory system, pressure waves from air blasts most often injure the gastrointestinal tract, causing hemorrhages and tearing some organs within the abdominal cavity, particularly at high blast doses. For example, of twenty-nine casualties of a civilian bus bombing, four had injuries to the intestinal tract and eleven suffered lung injury.[28] Most studies of single air-blast exposure, however, indicate a much lower incidence of gastrointestinal injury.[2]

Studies performed on sheep have shown that gastrointestinal injuries from air-propagated blast waves may be more significant if the animals have been exposed to repeated blasts.[18,20] Sheep exposed to fifty blasts showed gastrointestinal lesions at overpressure levels that were actually lower than those that produced lung lesions. This information may be most important for those casualties who receive occupational-blast exposures, such as artillery personnel. Blast waves that are propagated in water, however, are much more likely to cause gastrointestinal lesions than those that are propagated in air.

Although they have been less thoroughly studied, the characteristics of blast injury in the abdominal cavity resemble those of blast injury in the thoracic cavity: *(a)* the blast wave strikes and displaces the body wall, causing distortion of the tissues within that results in their stress and failure; *(b)* no external injury is visible on the body wall; *(c)* tissues that contain gas are more vulnerable to injury; and *(d)* the most common lesions are hemorrhage and tearing of tissue.

Hemorrhages. Hemorrhages may appear along the entire gastrointestinal tract, but are most often found in the lower small intestine and the cecum, where gas commonly accumulates. They also seem to have a predilection for the antimesenteric surface.[29]

Hemorrhages that involve the intestinal tract range from small petechiae to large hematomas that may be found within the intestinal or gastric walls. Higher doses of blast pressure may cause a hemorrhagic ring, or annular band, which involves the entire circumference of a segment of gut wall (Figure 8-21). This damage may be the result of vascular compromise and is a likely site for perforation several days after the blast has occurred.

Within the gut wall, most of the extravasated erythrocytes are found within the submucosal or subserosal spaces.[9,10,18,30] The mildest hemorrhages are almost always located in the submucosa, although they have rarely been seen in the mucosa.[29] If the hemorrhages are the result of very high blast pressures, they may extend beyond the submucosal or serosal layers, and, as transmural hemorrhages, may involve the entire intestinal wall. Blood clots are commonly found within the lumen of the intestinal tract at the site of severe mural hemorrhage.

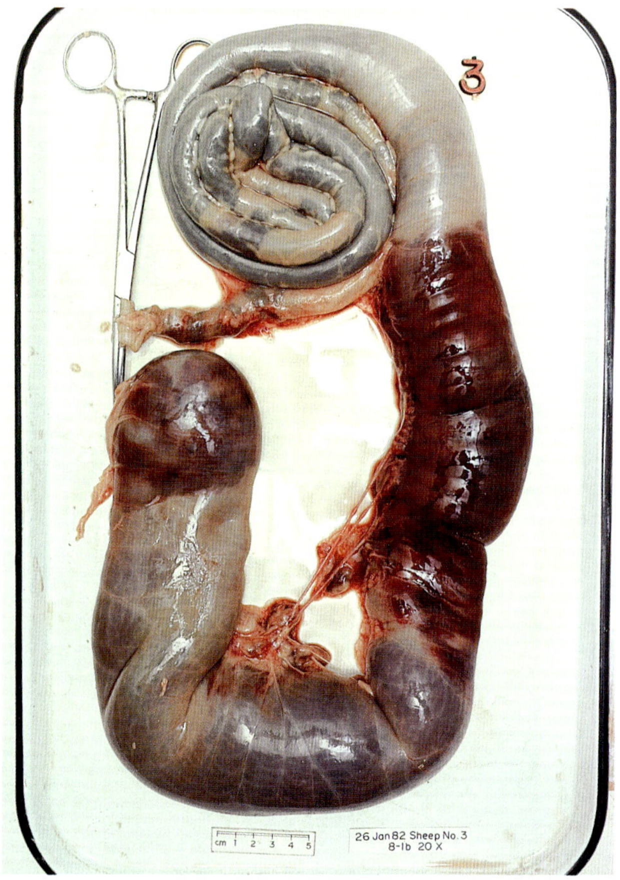

Fig. 8-21. This autopsy specimen from a sheep that had been exposed to blast overpressure shows segmental hemorrhage of the intestinal wall.
Source: D. R. Richmond

Perforations. In the most severe blast exposures, the intestinal wall may actually rupture, resulting in blood and ingesta spilling into the peritoneal cavity.[9,18] The rupture may occur either immediately or up to many days after injury.

Like hemorrhage, gastrointestinal perforation tends to occur in the tissues surrounding gas pockets. In humans, for example, the ileocecal junction is a common site of intestinal perforation.[28,29,30] In sheep, the large gas-filled rumen is the most frequent site of both hemorrhage and perforation.[18]

Other Abdominal Organs

Other regions within the abdominal cavity also suffer the effects of the blast wave. *Paint-brush ecchymoses,* which are produced by approximately the same blast dose that causes intestinal hemorrhage, will commonly be seen multifocally throughout the mesentery, and occasionally will be associated with mesenteric tears.

Hemorrhage may also occur within the retroperitoneal space. In one pathological study of twelve casualties who had been exposed to immersion blast, ten of them had retroperitoneal hemorrhage into the loose areolar tissue behind the right colic flexure.[30]

The spleen and liver may be damaged by the violent displacement of the abdominal organs after the blast wave strikes. Relatively small, multifocal, subcapsular hemorrhages may occur in the parenchyma of these two organs. The capsules surrounding them may be ruptured, or the organs themselves may be fractured. The rupture of either organ will cause hemoperitoneum.

Subcapsular hemorrhage occurs in other organs (such as the pancreas, adrenal glands, and kidneys) but seems to be of minor clinical significance.[9,29] In one case, a laceration was found in the head of the pancreas.[10] A common lesion in male immersion-blast casualties is hemorrhage into the tunica albuginea of the testicle.[29] The urinary bladder and gall bladder are rarely affected by blast.[10]

THE EYE AND ORBIT

Because the globe of the eye has relatively equal density throughout, it is quite resistant to blast overpressure waves. Blast casualties may rarely experience transient blindness after exposure, as well as hyphema and conjunctival hemorrhage. Fundoscopic studies have revealed air emboli within retinal vessels, which may be the cause of transient blindness.[6]

One unusual blast effect in the orbital region, called *orbital blowout,* involves portions of the frontal, sphenoid, and lacrimal bones on the medial surface of the orbital wall. In studies using dogs, these bones fractured from the force of the blast, and projected medially into the nasal fossa.[9] However, such orbital bone fractures have not been reported in humans, and may be unique to the shape of these dogs' skulls. In addition, the fractures occurred at such high overpressure levels that only a supralethal blast dose, such as might be caused by a nuclear bomb, would be likely to cause them. Such fractures cannot be easily detected, and may be missed on clinical or postmortem examination unless a retrobulbar hemorrhage has resulted in proptosis.

THE AUDITORY SYSTEM

The ear is the organ that is most frequently damaged by blast waves, and, at low blast doses (those below the level at which minimal respiratory lesions appear), may be the only anatomical site of detectable PBI. As is the case in other body systems that are vulnerable to PBI, the ear is damaged when the blast wave strikes and causes tissue distortion, tissue stress, and ultimately tissue failure. The ear is unique, however, in that its primary function is to transmit pressure waves from the environment to the inner ear, where they are converted into nerve impulses that are sent to the brain. Its structure amplifies any pressure waves—including damaging blast waves—along this existing conductive pathway, increasing the ear's sensitivity to levels of blast overpressure that might not be sufficient to cause PBI in other organs.

The auricle collects the sound waves, which are then focused within the external ear (auditory) canal. These waves cause the tympanic membrane at the end of the canal to vibrate. The air waves are transduced to mechanical vibrations and are transmitted through the ossicles to the perilymph of the inner ear (through the apposition of the stapes with the membranous oval window of the inner ear). These mechanical vibrations are transmitted through the fluid-filled chambers of the membranous labyrinth to the organ of Corti in the

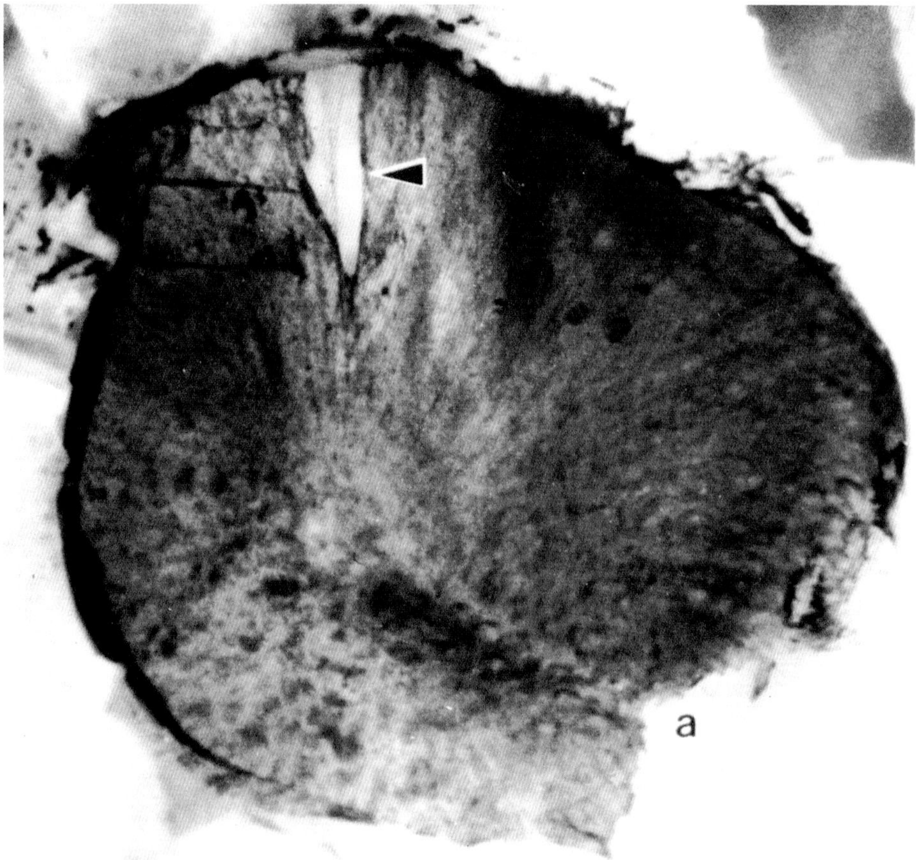

Fig. 8-22. This osmium-stained example of a triangular rupture (arrow) in the tympanic membrane of a chinchilla is viewed from the external ear canal. The *a* in the lower right corner refers to artifact.
Source: R. P. Hamernik

cochlea, where transduction again occurs and mechanical vibrations become nerve impulses.

Waves with sufficient peak pressures may overload the auditory system and cause damage to any of its component parts, including *(a)* ruptures of the tympanic membrane, *(b)* dislocations or fractures of the ossicular chain, and *(c)* damage to the organ of Corti within the cochlea.

In addition to the damaging effect of the transmission of the blast wave along the auditory conduction pathway, the rapid overpressure that develops within the air-filled tympanic cavity of the middle ear as the tympanic membrane is pushed inward by the blast wave may play a role in auditory blast damage. Normally, pressure equilibration within the tympanic cavity occurs via the auditory (or eustachian) tube, which connects the middle ear with the pharynx. This conduit is usually closed, but will open to equilibrate pressure during chewing, swallowing, or yawning. A blast wave, however, increases the air pressure within the tympanic cavity so suddenly that the overpressure cannot be relieved quickly enough through the auditory tube. The resulting distortion of the surrounding tissues damages them, especially the delicate tympanic membrane that separates the cavity from the external ear canal.

The ear facing the blast will usually be more severely damaged, although injury is frequently bilateral, especially when the casualty is within an enclosed structure and vulnerable to complex blast waves that can damage the contralateral ear.

The Tympanic Membrane

Most of the tympanic membrane comprises the *pars tensa,* a thin, bilayered, collagenous sheet that is sandwiched between an external layer of skin and an inner layer of simple squamous epithelium. A small portion of the membrane in the anterosuperior quadrant is devoid of collagen fibers, and is called the *pars flaccida.*

Tympanic-membrane rupture frequently occurs with blast exposure (Figure 8-22). In humans, the pars

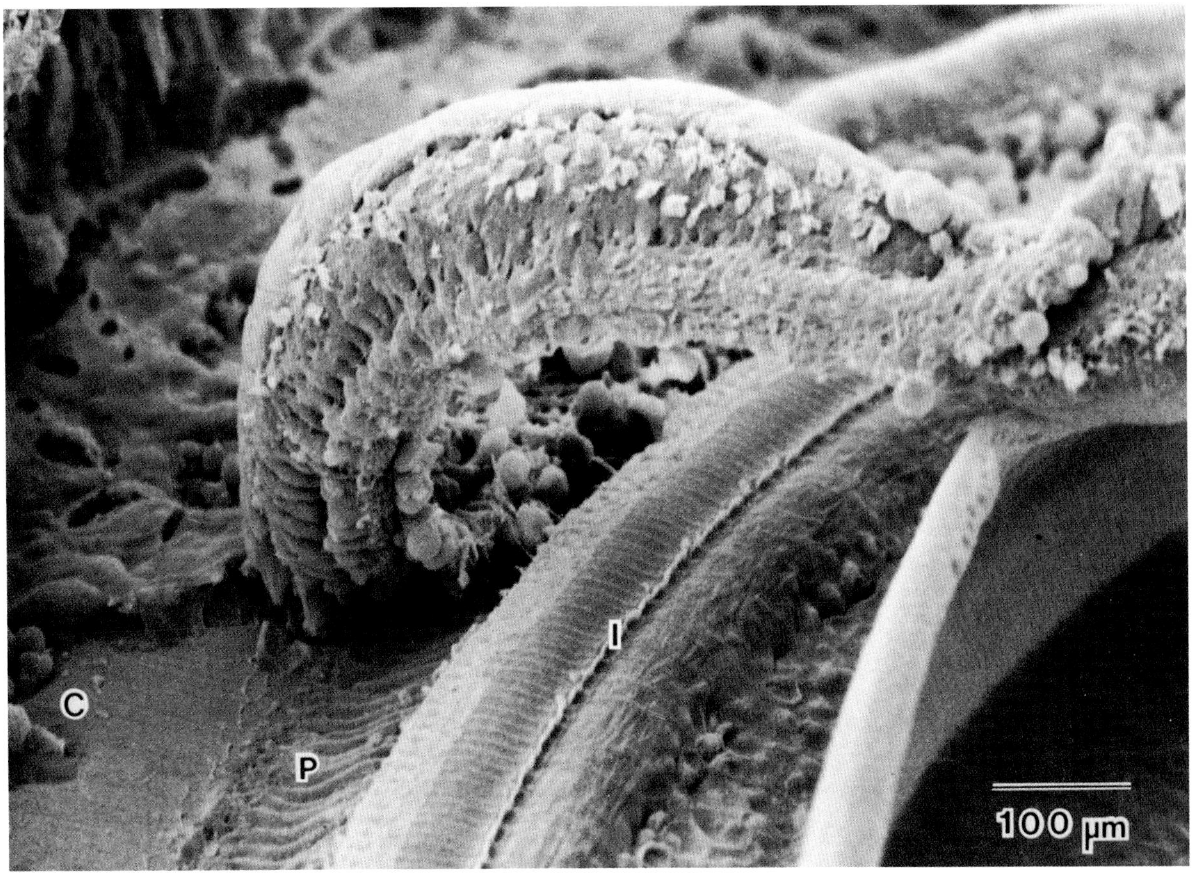

Fig. 8-23. This scanning electron micrograph shows a noise-induced dislocation of the organ of Corti. Note the relatively intact line of inner hair cells (I) and outer pillar-cell processes (P). Some Claudius cells (C) also have been dislodged.
Source: R. P. Hamernik

tensa is the portion of the tympanic membrane that is perforated by blast waves.[31] Perforations of the pars flaccida have been documented in experimental animals that were exposed to blast, but even these ruptures were less frequent than and always occurred in conjunction with ruptures of the pars tensa.[32] At doses below those that cause perforation, abnormal tympanograms indicate the probable rupture of radial collagen fibers, producing a flaccid but not perforated membrane.[33] In humans and animals, perforations usually involve less than one-third of the surface area of the tympanic membrane.

Experimental animals with blast-induced auditory trauma may suffer hemorrhage within the lamina propria of the tympanic membrane, which may progress to form a hematoma. This hemorrhage is often found around the periphery of the pars tensa or immediately below the anterior and posterior malleal folds.[32]

Although most perforations of the tympanic membrane heal spontaneously, cholesteatoma formation may be a sequela in rare cases.[31] Cholesteatoma is formed when the epidermis from the external tympanic membrane grows through the site of perforation into the middle ear, and forms a cystic structure into which layers of keratin admixed with cholesterol crystals are secreted. These cysts can grow, eventually impairing hearing and eroding surrounding structures.[34]

The Ossicular Chain

The tiny ossicular bones lie within the middle ear. The *malleus* is attached to the tympanic membrane laterally, the *stapes* is attached to the inner ear at the oval window, and the *incus* is suspended between the two. These bones normally transmit and amplify mechanical vibrations from the tympanic membrane to the inner ear.

During blast exposure, the ossicular chain may be damaged by direct displacement of the bones, or—more likely—by a severe distortion of the tympanic membrane at the attachment of the malleus. Ossicular damage is rare, however, even if the tympanic membrane has been injured. In fact, even blast doses that are strong enough to cause inner-ear injury may not damage the ossicular chain.[35]

When blast-induced ossicular damage does occur, pathological changes may include *(a)* medial displacement of the malleus handle with disruption of the incudomalleal joint, or *(b)* less commonly, incudostapedial joint separation with and without stapes fracture.[36] In studies with experimental animals, researchers noted that 29% of animals that had rupture of the tympanic membrane also had fractures of the malleus handle.[32]

The Cochlea

The transduction of mechanical vibrations into neural impulses occurs within the cochlea at the organ of Corti, a highly specialized epithelial layer that lies upon the basilar membrane and is comprised of sensory hair cells, sustentacular cells, and a tectorial membrane. The apical surface of this epithelial layer is bathed in the endolymph of the cochlear duct and is called the *reticular lamina*. Here, vibrations in the basilar membrane cause distortions of the hairs and a subsequent neural impulse within the auditory branch of the eighth cranial nerve.

In blast injury to the cochlea, abnormally intense mechanical vibrations reach the oval window of the inner ear through the ossicles, where they are transferred to the perilymph of the labyrinth and loaded onto the basilar membrane. The delicate organ of Corti cannot withstand the resulting stress.

Researchers who study the effects of blast waves on experimental animals have noted severe damage to the organ of Corti.[32] Scanning electron microscopy most commonly revealed fracture of the reticular lamina and dislocation of portions of the organ of Corti from the basilar membrane (Figure 8-23). Less severe changes include loss or fracture of inner and outer hair cells.

SUMMARY

Casualties who have been exposed to blast waves suffer a variety of lesions, the extent and severity of which depend upon the dose. Despite the multisystemic nature of these lesions, it is important to remember that it is the lung injuries—the occurrence of alveolar hemorrhage and the production of air emboli—that are usually involved in the casualty's death.

Much of the knowledge of blast pathology presented in this chapter has been attained through animal experimentation that has been conducted over the past half-century. These lesions qualitatively correspond well with those that have been described in reports of autopsies of human blast casualties. Difficulty arises, however, in predicting the extent of injury for a given dose of blast exposure. Researchers have expended extensive time and resources to model and predict injuries in humans based upon experimental-animal data. This chapter has emphasized the qualitative aspects of PBI; evaluation of the dose-response data is beyond its scope.

Current studies of the pathology of PBI are being conducted on several fronts. Using some of these data, researchers are developing computer programs that can predict injury and lethality thresholds in humans based on blast dose. Further studies are also needed to understand the factors that may complicate the progression and resolution of PBI, such as exercise and infectious disease. Research is being initiated to study the role of inflammatory mediators and cytokines in the progression of PBI, as well as the development of more specific diagnostic tests and therapeutic regimens.

Medical officers who may have to treat blast casualties need a thorough understanding of this trauma, which is often hidden from visual inspection. Familiarity with the pathology of PBI can help medical and triage officers to recognize its signs and initiate proper clinical intervention.

REFERENCES

1. de Candole, C. A. 1967. Blast injury. *Can. Med. Assoc. J.* 96:207–214.

2. Cooper, G. J.; Maynard, R. L.; Cross, N. L.; and Hill, J. F. 1983. Casualties from terrorist bombing. *J. Trauma* 23: 955–967.

3. Coppel, D. L. 1976. Blast injuries of the lungs. *Br. J. Surg.* 63:735–737.

4. Hadden, W. A.; Rutherford, W. H.; and Merrett, J. D. 1978. The injuries of terrorist bombing: A study of 1,532 consecutive patients. *Br. J. Surg.* 65:525–531.

5. Huller, T., and Bazini, Y. 1970. Blast injuries of the chest and abdomen. *Arch. Surg.* 100:24–30.

6. Phillips, Y. Y III. 1986. Primary blast injuries. *Ann. Emerg. Med.* 15:1446–1450.

7. Roy, D. 1982. Gunshot and bomb blast injuries: A review of experience in Belfast. *J. R. Soc. Med.* 75:542–545.

8. Waterworth, T. A., and Carr, M. J. T. 1975. An analysis of the post-mortem findings in the 21 victims of the Birmingham pub bombings. *Injury* 7:89–95.

9. Chiffelle, T. L. 1966. *Pathology of direct air-blast injury* [Technical Progress Report on DA-49–146-XZ-055]. Albuquerque, NM: Lovelace Foundation for Medical Education and Research.

10. Rössle, R. 1950. Pathology of blast effects. In *German Aviation Medicine, World War II.* Vol. 2, prepared under the auspices of the U.S. Air Force Surgeon General, 1260–1273. Washington, DC: U.S. Government Printing Office.

11. Fawcett, D. W. 1986. *Bloom and Fawcett: A Textbook of Histology*. Philadelphia: W.B. Saunders Company.

12. Clemedson, C.-J. 1949. An experimental study on air blast injuries. *Acta Physiol. Scand.* 18(Suppl. 61): 1–200.

13. Zhao, M.; Wang, Z. G.; Tang, C. G.; and Zhang, Q. H. 1988. The rib markings are actually intercostal markings. Paper presented at the Sixth International Symposium on Wound Ballistics, 1–4 November, at the Third Military Medical College, Chongquing, People's Republic of China.

14. Clemedson, C.-J., and Jönsson, A. 1964. Differences in displacement of ribs and costal interspaces in rabbits exposed to air shock waves. *Am. J. Physiol.* 207:931–934.

15. Fishman, A. P., and Pietra, G. G. 1980. Stretched pores, blast injury, and neurohemodynamic pulmonary edema. *Physiologist* 23:53–56.

16. Wang, Z. G. 1989. An experimental study of blast injury. *Chung Hua I Hsueh Tsa Chih* 69:7–11.

17. Young, A. J.; Hoyt, R. F.; Jaeger, J. J.; and Phillips, Y. Y III. 1986. Short duration airblast does not increase pulmonary microvascular permeability. *Milit. Med.* 151:139–143.

18. Clifford, C. B.; Moe, J. B.; Jaeger, J. J.; and Hess, J. L. 1984. Gastrointestinal lesions in lambs due to multiple low-level blast overpressure exposure. *Milit. Med.* 149:491–495.

19. Schardin, H. 1950. The physical principles of the effects of a detonation. In reference 10, 1207–1224.

20. Dodd, K. T.; Yelverton, J. T.; Richmond, D. R.; Morris, J. R.; and Ripple, G. R. 1990. Nonauditory injury threshold for repeated intense freefield impulse noise. *J. Occup. Med.* 32(3): 260–266.

21. Moe, J. B.; Clifford, C. B.; and Sharpnack, D. D. 1987. Effects of blast waves on non-auditory epithelial tissue. In *Basic and Applied Aspects of Noise-Induced Hearing Loss,* edited by R. J. Salvi, D. Henderson, R. P. Hamernik, and Y. Colletti, 473–485. New York: Plenum Press.

22. Benzinger, T. 1950. Physiological effects of blast in air and water. In reference 10, 1225–1259.

23. White, C. S.; Jones, R. K.; Damon, E. G.; Fletcher, E. R.; and Richmond, D. R. 1971. *The biodynamics of airblast* [Technical Report DNA 2728T]. Washington, DC: Defense Nuclear Agency.

24. Mason, W. V.; Damon, E. G.; Dickinson, A. R.; and Nevison, T. O. 1971. Arterial gas emboli after blast injury. *Proc. Soc. Exp. Biol. Med.* 136:1253–1255.

25. Roberts, J. E.; White, C. S.; and Chiffelle, T. L. 1953. Effects of overpressures in group shelters on animals and dummies [USAEC Civil Effects Test Group Report WT-798]. Washington, DC: Office of Technical Services, Department of Commerce.

26. Wilson, J. V., and Tunbridge, R. E. 1943. Pathological findings in a series of blast injuries. *Lancet* 1:257–261.

27. Melzer, E.; Hersch, M.; Fischer, D.; and Hershko, C. 1986. Disseminated intravascular coagulation and hypopotassemia associated with blast lung injury. *Chest* 89:690–693.

28. Katz, E.; Ofek, B.; Adler, J.; Abramowitz, H. B.; and Krausz, M. M. 1989. Blast injury after a bomb explosion in a civilian bus. *Ann. Surg.* 209:484–488.

29. Gordon-Taylor, G. 1953. Abdominal effects of immersion blast. Chapt. 18, part 2, of *Surgery*, edited by Z. Cope, 664–672. London: Her Majesty's Stationery Office.

30. Goligher, J. C.; King, D. P.; and Simmons, H. T. 1943. Injuries produced by blast in water. *Lancet* 245:119–123.

31. Chait, R. H.; Casler, J.; and Zajtchuk, J. T. 1989. Blast injury of the ear: Historical perspective. *Ann. Otol. Rhinol. Laryngol.* 98 (Supp.):9–12.

32. Roberto, M.; Hamernik, R. P.; and Turrentine, G. A. 1989. Damage of the auditory system associated with acute blast trauma. *Ann. Otol. Rhinol. Laryngol.* 98 (Supp.):23–34.

33. Eames, B.L.; Hamernik, R.P.; Henderson, D.; and Feldman, A. S. 1975. The role of the middle ear in acoustic trauma from impulses. *Laryngoscope* 85:1582–1592.

34. Cotran, R. S.; Kumar, V.; and Robbins, S. L. 1989. Diseases of the head and neck. In *Robbins Pathologic Basis of Disease*, 811–826. 4th ed. Philadelphia: W. B. Saunders Company.

35. Kerr, A. G., and Byrne, J. E. T. 1975. Concussive effects of bomb blast on the ear. *J. Laryngol. Otol.* 89:131–143.

36. Sudderth, M. E. 1974. Tympanoplasty in blast-induced perforation. *Arch. Otolaryngol.* 99:157–159.

Chapter 9

THE MANAGEMENT OF PRIMARY BLAST INJURY

YANCY Y PHILLIPS III, M.D., FCCP* AND JOAN T. ZAJTCHUK, M.D., FACS**

*Lieutenant Colonel, United States Army; Chief, Pulmonary and Critical Care Medicine Service, Walter Reed Army Medical Center, Washington, D.C. 20307-5001, and Consultant to the Surgeon General in Pulmonary Medicine and Respiratory Therapy

**Colonel, United States Army; Chairman, Division of Otolaryngology, Uniformed Services University of the Health Sciences, Bethesda, Maryland 20307-4799

INTRODUCTION

Explosions are ubiquitous in modern warfare. Although fragmentation and thermal effects cause by far the most combat injuries, the detonation of explosive munitions can create pressure waves that are powerful enough to injure the internal organs of casualties who are directly exposed to them. This injury—called primary blast injury (PBI)—may debilitate or kill the casualty by causing severe damage to the gas-containing organs of the body while leaving no external trace of injury. The damage caused by PBI is a kind of *barotrauma,* an injury caused by a local pressure differential. It results from the interaction between the passing blast wave and the body tissues, which creates an imbalance between the ambient pressure and the pressure within the affected cavity of the body. The symptoms and treatment of PBI will depend upon which organ has been affected.

Victims of an open-air blast will usually also have penetrating or nonpenetrating secondary blast injuries from fragments or objects that have been hurled through the air from the force of the blast. These wounds do not differ from classic ballistic wounds that are caused by bullets or fragments from conventional explosive munitions.

Tertiary blast injury refers to the blunt trauma that can occur when the victim is bodily lifted and thrown against a nearby structure by the force of either the blast wave itself or the venting of the blast wind or combustion gases through a constricted opening. Tertiary blast injuries may complicate primary and secondary blast injuries, especially when nuclear and larger conventional weapons are used.

The true incidence of significant PBI is unknown, perhaps in part because it is difficult to diagnose a problem that one is not prepared to recognize. Medical officers who wait for a patient who exhibits classic,

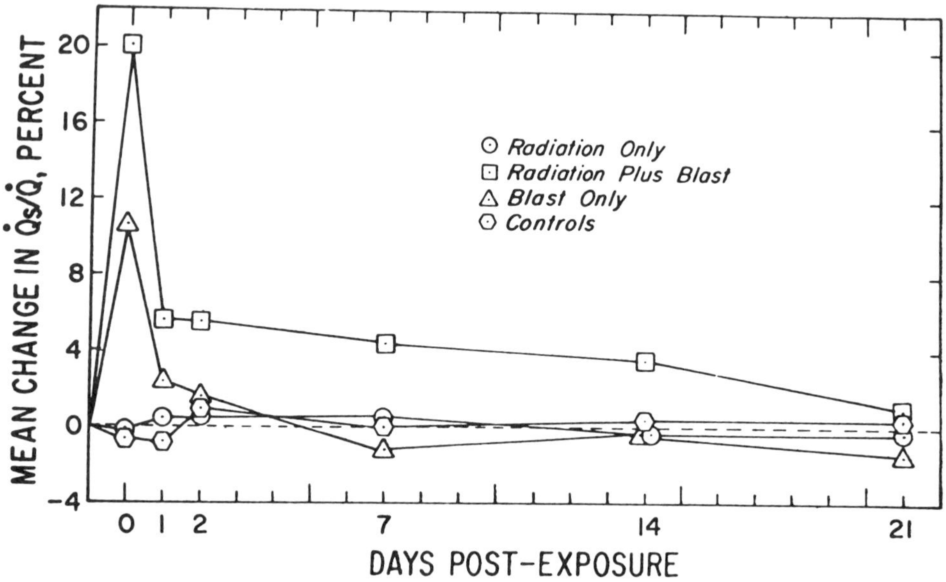

Fig. 9-1. Researchers studied the effect on the ability of sheep lungs to transfer oxygen over time following radiation only (ooo), blast only (ΔΔΔ), or radiation plus blast (□□□). Controls are indicated on the graph by hexagons. The animals that were subjected to both insults showed both the greatest decrement in oxygenation and the longest-lasting effects, even though the radiation alone had no detectable effect on pulmonary gas exchange. The development and resolution of lung injury is measured by venous admixture (shunt fraction or Qs/Qt) following injury.
Source: Reference 1

pure PBI—that is, who has neurological deficits and respiratory failure without so much as a scratch—will miss most of the PBI cases that they can expect to encounter in a trauma-care environment. An explosion might result in a mix of traumatic amputations of limbs and penetrating fragment injuries, as well as PBI to the casualties' abdomens, lungs, or ears. The thermal pulse from a detonation may burn exposed skin, or secondary fires may be started by the detonation and more serious burns may be suffered. Smoke and fumes from fires contain toxic chemicals and may cause inhalation injury. Victims may also be crushed in the collapse of a building.

Given such dramatic combined injuries, the primary blast component may be hidden but nevertheless significant, and the physician must be aware of the possibility of such occult injury lest it further complicate the patient's care. In addition, the effects of combined injuries may be synergistic rather than additive. For example, radiation injury will combine with blast or burn injury to cause much more severe and long-lasting damage than would be expected from each of the injuries individually (Figure 9-1).[1]

The classic case of pure PBI is usually seen in a casualty who has been exposed to an underwater detonation. Water transmits blast waves more efficiently than air does; that is, the blast waves' effects do not diminish over distance in water as much as they do over distance in air. An explosion in water has a lethal area that is approximately nine times greater than the lethal area of an airburst using the same amount of explosive.[2] At the same time, water greatly reduces the effective range of any fragments that might be propelled from the detonation site.

In contrast, a casualty who presents with pure PBI from an open-air explosion is likely to have been very close to the explosion but not close enough to have been dismembered by fragments from the exploding device. Pure PBI, particularly to the ear, is more likely when the detonation occurs in a closed space (such as an armored fighting vehicle or a room in a building, in which the blast may reverberate off the walls), or when a special enhanced-blast munition is used.

Pure PBI may be severe when the exposures are repeated, even if the individual blasts are of relatively low intensity. Experimental animals that received repeated blast exposures (commonly called *multiple blast*) had the same types of primary blast lesions that were produced in animals exposed to single blasts.[2] However, repeated exposures to blast *(a)* increased the severity of lesions over those produced by a single blast of the same magnitude, and *(b)* decreased the threshold for injury. These additive effects may be due to the fatigue factor (see Chapter Seven), which describes the lower stress requirement for tissue failure after repeated exposures, and may be important to operators of artillery weapons, for whom the effects of repeated low-level blasts have significant occupational-health implications.

This chapter will focus specifically on PBI. The first section will briefly outline the procedural aspects of the blast casualty's movement through the military health-care system, with particular attention to triage, stabilization, and evacuation. The remaining sections will focus on the most serious manifestations of PBI: *(a)* damage to the respiratory system, *(b)* the production of air emboli, *(c)* gastrointestinal injury, and *(d)* damage to the auditory system. These effects will be discussed in the context of their management at the first level of care at which an evaluative or treatment measure may be performed, although the reader should understand that, under certain conditions, the evaluations may have to be repeated or conducted in greater detail at a higher echelon of care.

ECHELONS OF CARE FOR CASUALTIES WHO HAVE PRIMARY BLAST INJURY

The medical officer is most likely to see PBI when many casualties (some with combined injuries) have survived a civilian blast catastrophe, a terrorist bombing, or a military action. Such a mass-casualty incident will almost certainly cause confusion and chaos. Some of the routine procedures that medical personnel are trained to perform may be impossible to carry out in an ideal sequence under such conditions, and so a certain amount of procedural overlap is built into the evacuation and evaluation system to ensure that important (but perhaps latent) aspects of injury are not overlooked.

The medical evacuation system is designed to move casualties from the site of injury to a definitive-care facility as rapidly as possible. Because the casualties' physical status and the conditions of the battle may both fluctuate, the means of transportation and the health-care destinations may vary as well. Triage (the sorting of casualties according to the severity of their injuries) is done at every level of care.

First Echelon of Care

The first echelon of care occurs on the battlefield, and is usually provided to a casualty by a buddy, a trained combat lifesaver (that is, a member of the unit who has had supplementary first-aid training), a medic, or medics and battalion surgeons at the battalion aid station. First-echelon treatment is limited to essential emergency care, and can range from minimal first-aid interventions that allow a slightly injured soldier to return to duty right away, to crucial stabilizing measures (such as establishing an airway, controlling a hemorrhage, and administering intravenous fluids) that are intended to keep the casualty alive during evacuation to the appropriate care facility. When evaluating blast casualties, medical personnel need to ascertain *(a)* what, if anything, can be done immediately to save the casualty's life and limbs on the battlefield, *(b)* whether the casualty needs to be evacuated, and *(c)* how the casualty should be transported to the next level of care.

Initial Physical Examination and Triage. Blast casualties may have PBI in several anatomical sites and in any degree of severity. They should be evaluated according to normal triage standards. In the military, four triage categories are generally used: *(a) immediate,* which includes casualties who have severe, life-threatening injuries but are likely to survive if they receive the appropriate lifesaving treatment, *(b) delayed,* which includes casualties who can tolerate a delay prior to surgery or other treatment without suffering further damage, *(c) minimal,* which includes casualties who have superficial injuries that can be treated by first-aid procedures, and *(d) expectant,* which includes casualties who are not expected to survive no matter how much medical treatment they receive, or who would not benefit from the limited medical resources available.

Although the care of blast casualties at this echelon will usually center on secondary blast injuries (such as fractures, penetrating wounds, lacerations, and burns), the medical officer needs to be particularly alert for the more subtle signs of PBI. If circumstances permit, medical personnel should carefully examine the casualty for signs of contusion or penetrating wounds.[3] Sometimes, a sentinel (or associated) injury, which may be as dramatic as a traumatic amputation or as relatively minor as a temporary hearing loss, will indicate that the casualty may also have significant PBI. Because some of the most serious manifestations of PBI have few or no overt signs, taking certain preventive measures at this stage may save the life of a blast casualty who is apparently less severely injured.

Triage decisions and the amount of time that can be devoted to them depend upon the nature of the blast incident itself. *Overtriage* may occur when casualties who should be admitted to the MTF for further observation or treatment are instead discharged to duty. *Undertriage* may occur when casualties who have relatively minor injuries are admitted to the MTF for observation, a level of caution that might not have a great effect on a large civilian medical facility, but one that would severely strain available medical resources and result in a significant loss of fighting strength were it to occur in a military mass-casualty situation. During wartime, the military physician or medic may have to return a soldier to combat when *(a)* the underlying severity of the blast injury is not objectively evaluable (that is, radiographic and laboratory screens are unavailable), and *(b)* the risk that a blast lesion would develop later is only problematic (that is, soldiers with only mild symptoms consistent with PBI may be returned to combat despite the theoretical consideration that such activity may worsen the PBI).

Initiation of Life Support. Medical personnel must ensure that the casualty is hemodynamically stable and that the airway is patent. In the PBI casualty, the life-threatening injuries that require immediate stabilization are usually caused by respiratory damage or by blood loss from gastrointestinal hemorrhage.

Respiratory support and mechanical ventilation will be discussed in the section of this chapter that deals with PBI to the respiratory system.

Volume replacement will be discussed in the section that deals with PBI to the gastrointestinal tract, although the reader should understand that a casualty can be hypotensive for many reasons other than blood loss from an abdominal hemorrhage.

The casualty will be stabilized and life-support measures will be continued at the second echelon of care, if necessary.

Establishing a Medical Record. The medic is also responsible for beginning the blast casualty's medical evacuation record, although the realities of the battlefield will determine how complete it will be, or even whether it is done at all. Unlike civilian terrorist bombings, in which the undivided attention of a medical team can be focused on blast casualties, an explosion in combat is unlikely to be an isolated event relatively near an urban medical facility. Even if the medic—who may be working alone—has the opportunity to glean blast-related information, the small size of the medical-record card limits the amount of information that can be conveyed. This limitation is particularly unfortunate in blast incidents, because the casualty's buddies may have noticed important details that the casualty (even if conscious) may have missed. Nevertheless, as soon as possible after the casualty is stabilized and if circumstances permit, medical personnel ideally should try to determine the following:

- What type of ordnance was used and how large was the explosion?

- Where was the casualty located with respect to the blast?
- Did the blast occur inside an enclosed space such as a room or vehicle?
- What was the casualty's activity after exposure?
- Were there fires or fumes that might lead to an inhalation injury?
- What was the orientation of the casualty's head and body to the blast?

Evacuation. PBI may complicate the medical evacuation of these casualties from the battlefield. The casualty's body position, for example, can affect the severity of some primary blast effects, such as potentially lethal air embolism.[4,5,6]

Because physical exertion after blast exposure can exacerbate the severity of PBI, victims of an explosion should minimize physical activity and, if they are experiencing respiratory distress, should be carried from the battlefield by litter rather than be allowed to leave under their own power.[4,7,8] In World War II, for example, some blast casualties initially appeared to be well, but died after vigorous exercise following their blast exposure. Their comrades, who were initially more severely injured and too ill to move, remained sedentary and survived.[8] In experimental studies, rats were either kept quiet or forced to swim to exhaustion after being exposed to blast.[9] The blast alone killed 30% of the sedentary animals, but those rats that were forced to swim to exhaustion 1 hour after exposure had a 70% mortality. When the swimming was delayed for 4 hours, the rats' mortality was 40%. Although the exhausting exercise seemed to increase the rats' lung injury and mortality, a period of rest before exertion appeared to significantly alter their susceptibility to further injury.

Certain manifestations of PBI—particularly those that involve the respiratory, circulatory, and gastrointestinal systems—are known to be more dangerous when the casualty is evacuated by air. Medical personnel should be aware that even a short helicopter flight might jeopardize the stability of a blast casualty, and should take the precautions that are detailed in the system-specific sections of this chapter. The aircraft should fly at the lowest practical altitude. If possible, blast casualties should avoid long-distance, high-altitude flights for several days.

Second Echelon of Care

At the second echelon, which is the medical company of the brigade or division, the casualty will most likely be seen by a military physician or a physician's assistant, who will glean more details of the casualty's blast-exposure history, if possible. If circumstances permit, routine laboratory tests will be done at this stage.

Stabilization and Life Support. Stabilization measures, such as volume replacement, will be continued or initiated if needed. Personnel at this level of care can monitor the casualty's oxygenation and replace blood volume with intravenous solutions, activities that may have been beyond the scope of the medic. Second-echelon facilities may also have the equipment to provide assisted ventilation.

Definitive Physical Examination. The blast casualty will receive a thorough physical examination, and medical personnel should look for certain sentinel signs, such as a ruptured tympanic membrane, hypopharyngeal contusions, hemoptysis in the absence of external chest trauma, or subcutaneous emphysema. Aspects of the examination that focus on particular anatomical areas will be discussed in those sections of the chapter.

Diagnostic Screening. As soon as the blast casualty is hemodynamically stable, medical personnel should take a chest roentgenogram, regardless of the casualty's symptoms. Failure to do so can be disastrous. In one case, a soldier who was injured by a mine explosion had a bilateral tympanic-membrane rupture and abdominal pain.[10] He was rushed to surgery, during which military physicians found diffuse intestinal petechiae and a subcapsular splenic hematoma. The surgeons had failed to obtain a chest roentgenogram before operating, however, and the patient—who also had an unsuspected pulmonary contusion from the blast—rapidly deteriorated into a state of respiratory insufficiency.

If the casualty has complications but is stable enough both to cooperate and to be transported to an MTF that has radiologic facilities, medical personnel may order a computed axial tomography (CAT) scan of the chest, abdomen, or head.

Serial hemoglobin determinations are important guides to blood replacement in all casualties who have severe bleeding, including those with hemorrhage into the lungs or gastrointestinal tract from PBI.

Most routine laboratory studies add little to the evaluation of blast-injured patients. Researchers have used animals to evaluate potential PBI markers, including a multichannel blood-profile chemistry analysis.[11] Both sedentary and exercise-stressed animals were exposed to blast intensities that ranged from trivial to LD_1 (that is, a lethal dose, or fatal injury, for 1% of cases), and their blood was drawn prior to and 90 minutes after exposure. Unfortunately, none of the putative markers proved to be useful as early indicators of either the presence or the degree of blast injury in any organ system.

However, serial monitoring of hematological and biochemical parameters may be useful in following the complicated medical course of any seriously injured patient. In one report from Israel, for example, four out of five patients with PBI to the lung had significant hypokalemia within a few hours of injury.[12] The authors speculated that stress-induced catecholamine release was responsible and were concerned that the electrolyte disturbance might cause or worsen arrhythmias. Three of the patients went on to develop a disseminated intravascular coagulation syndrome with low platelet counts and prolonged coagulation times. The coagulopathies responded to replacement therapy and did not complicate the clinical course.

Treatment. Some manifestations of PBI will resolve on their own, or will require only a continuation of stabilization measures until the casualty is out of danger. Other manifestations will require immediate surgical intervention, or may call for sophisticated equipment that would not be available at the lower echelons of care. In addition, some manifestations of PBI may have long-term sequelae. The following sections will discuss the treatment of PBI as it appears in the most vulnerable systems of the body.

Unless otherwise specified, diagnostic and therapeutic interventions to be discussed require the resources found in a third-echelon MTF or in a level-one civilian trauma service.

PRIMARY BLAST INJURY TO THE RESPIRATORY SYSTEM

The lungs are the vital organs that are most vulnerable to PBI. Damage to the lungs may include *(a)* pulmonary contusions, with or without lacerations, *(b)* pneumothorax, *(c)* traumatic lung cysts, *(d)* interstitial emphysema, *(e)* pneumomediastinum, or *(f)* subcutaneous emphysema. The term *blast lung* is commonly used clinically to refer to PBI to the respiratory tract with pulmonary contusion and respiratory insufficiency, with or without extravasation of air (Table 9-1). Casualties who have pulmonary PBI will experience dyspnea, but those who do not have extrapulmonary air will not usually experience chest pain.

Pulmonary contusions impair gas exchange at the alveolar level. The degree of respiratory insufficiency will depend on the degree of the hemorrhage.[13,14] These contusions develop, stabilize, and resolve relatively rapidly (Figure 9-2). In humans, roentgenographic evidence of lung contusion may appear only hours after exposure; these contusions may resolve in about 1 week.[13,15,16] In animal studies, rats had significant resolution of blast-induced pulmonary hemorrhages after only 24 hours, although there were small residual increases in lung weight after a week (Figure 9-3).[17] The symptoms of significant pulmonary contusion are likely to include *(a)* cough, *(b)* hemoptysis, or *(c)* dyspnea, resulting from widespread alveolar disruption with hemorrhage or pneumothorax or both.

The blood in a pulmonary contusion usually stays within the lung, but if the contusion is complicated by parenchymal laceration, bleeding may occur not only within the parenchyma but also into the pleural space, creating a hemothorax.

Pneumothorax, the most serious form of intrathoracic barotrauma, is the presence of air in the pleural cavity. This extrapleural air interferes with the normal expansion of the lung that occurs when the downward movement of the diaphragm creates negative pressure in the chest cavity. In pneumothorax, the negative pressure acts instead upon the extrapleural air, leaving the lung in its collapsed (expiration) position and thus soon compromising gas exchange. The symptoms of pneumothorax may include *(a)* dyspnea, *(b)* chest pain on one or both sides without signs of external injury, and *(c)* cough. Even more dramatically, the pressure of the air that is trapped in the pleural cavity during expiration can increase so much that it displaces the mediastinal contents, thus decreasing the casualty's venous return to the point of cardiovascular collapse. This condition is called a tension pneumothorax. The casualty will be hypotensive and may exhibit other symptoms of cardiovascular distress, including tachycardia and diaphoresis. A tension pneumothorax can be immediately life threatening.

A blast casualty may have a hemopneumothorax if both blood and air are in the pleural space, and might experience not only the respiratory-distress symptoms of pneumothorax, but also hemoptysis and cardiovascular collapse.

Air may be forced from the alveoli and airways into the interstitium of the lung either as traumatic lung cysts or as interstitial emphysema.[13] These injuries have no overt signs or symptoms, and there is no information available regarding their resolution. The large parenchymal air cysts may also form in casualties who are receiving mechanical ventilation and in whom they have a high risk of rupturing, causing pneumothorax. Interstitial emphysema occurs when air dissects from the airway along bronchial walls.

TABLE 9-1

SYMPTOMS, CLINICAL SIGNS, AND FINDINGS OF PRIMARY BLAST INJURY OF THE RESPIRATORY SYSTEM

Findings	Signs	Symptoms
Nonspecific findings (Common to all primary blast injury)	Cyanosis Tachypnea	Chest pain Dyspnea
Parenchymal Lung Injury (Contusion)	Crackles (rales) Diminished breath sounds Dullness to percussion Tachypnea	Hemoptysis
Pulmonary Barotrauma (Pneumothorax) (Pneumomediastinum)	Diminished breath sounds* Increased resonance* Retrosternal crunch Subcutaneous crepitus Tracheal deviation** or mediastinal shift**	Cardiovascular collapse
Pulmonary Laceration (Hemopneumothorax)	Same as pulmonary barotrauma and dullness to percussion*	Hemoptysis Cardiovascular collapse

* On side of collapse
**Away from the side of collapse

Pneumomediastinum and subcutaneous emphysema can occur when interstitial emphysema decompresses into the mediastinum or the subcutaneous tissue space. These events usually will not cause symptoms and will be detected on radiographs or by the presence of subcutaneous crepitus on physical examination. Neither pneumomediastinum nor subcutaneous emphysema by themselves pose a significant hazard.

Respiratory failure may occur 24–48 hours after blast exposure, but if it does occur that late, it is unlikely to be caused solely by PBI.[18,19] Instead, a combination of blast effects, inhalation injury, massive tissue injury, and transfusion therapy may result in a condition called adult respiratory distress syndrome (ARDS).[18,20,21,22] A discussion of ARDS is beyond the scope of this chapter, and will be found in the TMM textbook *Anesthesia and Critical Care.*

Table 9-2 gives the incidence of respiratory symptoms and findings compiled from two reports of underwater- and air-blast casualties.[13,16]

Initial Physical Examination and Triage

In general, a casualty who has pulmonary PBI will exhibit signs that may include tachypnea, hemoptysis, tachycardia, cyanosis, or an inability to carry on a conversation.[7,13,23,24] Comprehensive emergency care is crucial. The first-echelon medical personnel will not have the opportunity or resources to examine the blast casualty definitively for PBI to the lungs.

Casualties who have *(a)* asphyxia, *(b)* simple or tension pneumothorax, *(c)* cyanosis and extreme dyspnea, *(d)* upper-airway compromise, or *(e)* hypotension from any cause should be placed in the immediate triage category. They should receive emergency stabilization measures and be transported directly to the appropriate echelon of care as soon as possible.

Casualties who *(a)* exhibit lesser degrees of respiratory distress (such as a respiratory rate below 30 breaths per minute), *(b)* are able to carry on a conversation, and *(c)* are hemodynamically stable are in the

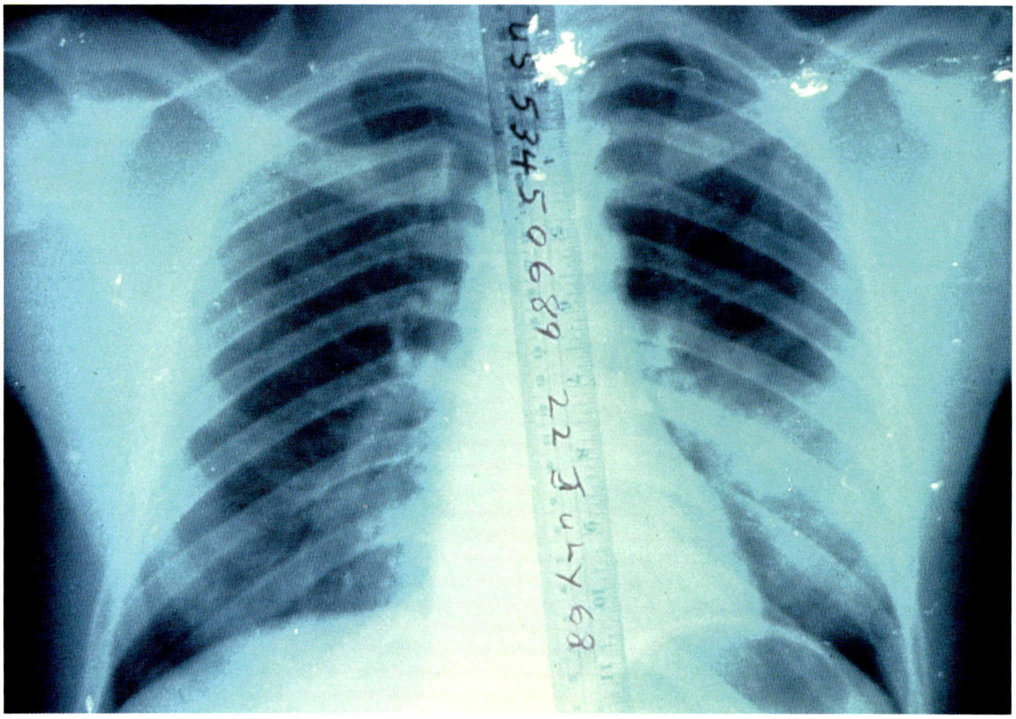

Fig. 9-2. This chest roentgenogram of a soldier who was injured by a bomb blast shows bilateral infiltrates from pulmonary contusions. The patient survived without sequelae.
Source: Wound Data and Munitions Effectiveness Team

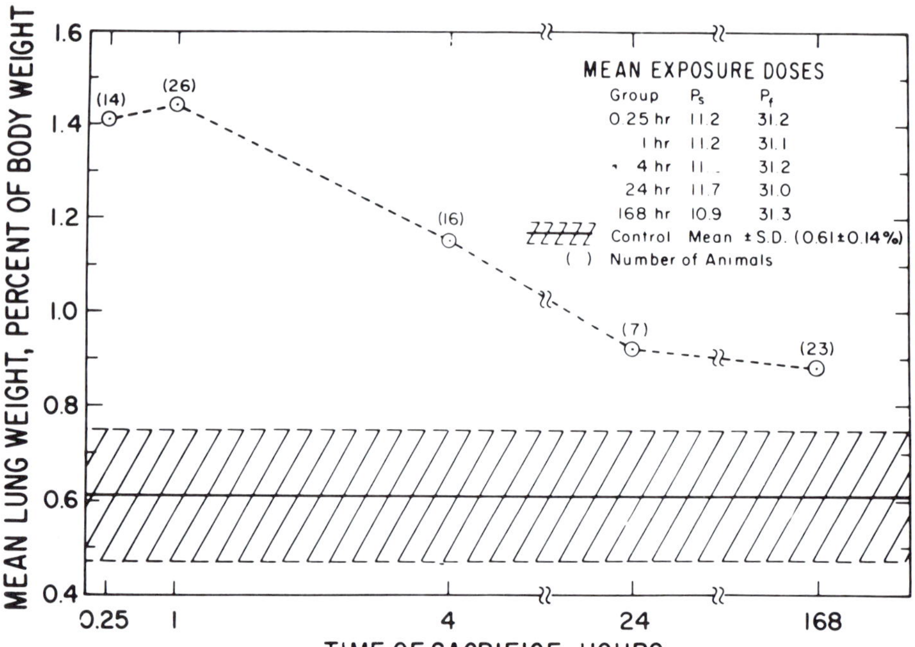

Fig. 9-3. The development and resolution of pulmonary injury in rodents that were exposed to sublethal blast can be measured by their lung weights. Most of the increase in lung weight is secondary to parenchymal hemorrhage.
Source: Reference 18

TABLE 9-2

DISTRIBUTION OF PULMONARY SYMPTOMS AND CLINICAL FINDINGS IN SURVIVORS OF UNDERWATER AND AIR BLASTS*

Clinical Symptoms and Findings	Percentage**
Pulmonary symptoms	
Hemoptysis	55
Dyspnea	38
Chest Pain	22
Pulmonary findings	
Parenchymal infiltrates	84
Crackles (rales)	40
Hemothorax	27
Pneumomediastinum	27
Pneumothorax	4

*Hospitalized survivors of major underwater blast (N=43) and air blast (N=2)

**See Table 9-5 for abdominal injury data from the same incidents. The percent total mortality from pulmonary and abdominal blast injuries was 16%.

delayed triage category, and should be evacuated as soon as the emergency cases have been stabilized and evacuated.

Initiation of Life Support

Establishing an Airway. For blast casualties who are in pulmonary distress, the most crucial emergency measure is the establishment of a patent airway. Inserting a simple oral or nasal airway may suffice, but casualties who have extreme respiratory embarrassment should be intubated endotracheally to handle massive hemoptysis and in anticipation of mechanical ventilatory support.

Inserting Chest Tubes. For either a tension pneumothorax or a simple pneumothorax that has no accompanying contusion or evidence of cardiovascular involvement, an immediate tube thoracostomy is the definitive treatment. The extrapleural air will be evacuated through the tube, allowing the lung to reinflate. This emergency measure may save the casualty's life.

If the casualty has a hemopneumothorax, a foamy mixture of both blood and air will be evacuated through the tube, indicating that a pulmonary laceration exists. The amount of blood that is evacuated should be monitored, but hemothorax from blast is rarely severe enough to lead to hypotension.

Hypotension and Volume Replacement. Hypotension in blast casualties can be ascribed to several different causes, including *(a)* blood loss from secondary blast injuries or other wounds, *(b)* blood loss from a gastrointestinal hemorrhage or solid-organ rupture, *(c)* the sequelae of air embolism, or *(d)* vagal reflexes. A hypotensive casualty must quickly receive sufficient volume replacement to bring the pulse and blood pressure back within normal limits. However, blast casualties who have pulmonary injuries have an increased risk of pulmonary edema when they receive excessive volume replacement.

Because the transudation of hypooncotic fluid is more likely in an injured lung, medical personnel should consider replacing the casualty's lost fluids with blood or a colloid solution rather than with a crystalloid solution.[15,19,22,25,26] Researchers found that the rapid infusion of large volumes of crystalloid solution in dogs that had unilateral lung contusions resulted in a greater impairment of gas exchange and an increase in the weight of the uninjured lung, as compared to infusions of smaller volumes.[27] A German study found less lung damage in pigs that were given furosemide prior to blast exposure, implying that low pulmonary vascular pressures may offer some protection from intrapulmonary hemorrhage or edema after blast.[28] Chinese researchers reported less lung hemorrhage in hypovolemic dogs that had been acutely depleted of 40% of their blood volume before being exposed to a blast, although they did not mention mortality or the nature of the resuscitation protocol after injury.[29]

In casualties with combined burn and relatively mild pulmonary blast injuries, fluids can be replenished according to standard infusion formulae for burn casualties. In Chinese experiments, dogs were given second-degree burns over 40% of their bodies and then were exposed to a large but sublethal blast.[30] To simulate evacuation time from the battlefield, resuscitation began 8 hours after injury. The animals were resuscitated by fluid infusions that were based on a formula of 0.5 ml of colloid and 1.0–1.5 ml of crystalloid per kilogram of body weight per percent of burned body surface area per day. The dogs' lung injuries did not become any worse than what had been expected from the blast effects alone.

Evacuation

Because changes in atmospheric pressure can seriously affect casualties who have suffered respiratory barotrauma, blast casualties have special needs during aeromedical evacuation.

Oxygen Adequacy. Oxygenation problems at air level will be worse at higher altitudes. Both the casualty's level of arterial oxygen (pO_2) and a hematocrit below 30% are other indicators of evacuation risk. If the pO_2 level is below 60 mm Hg, the casualty's amount of dissolved oxygen may be too low to allow safe evacuation. Medical personnel should be aware, however, that casualties may have dangerously low levels of arterial pO_2 even at sea level without showing tachypnea, cyanosis, or other clinical signs of hypoxia. This dangerous situation can become even more so at 35,000 feet, where the aircraft cabin is pressurized to the equivalent of 8,000 feet and the casualty's alveolar air pO_2 may be one-third less than it was at sea level.

If the casualty develops a respiratory emergency during the evacuation, medical personnel should opt for endotracheal intubation, which is safer, quicker, and more easily tolerated by the casualty than a tracheostomy would be. If an endotracheal tube is used promptly, a later tracheostomy may be unnecessary.

Chest-Tube Care. Normally, patients who have chest tubes should not be evacuated by air with the tubes in place, nor should they be evacuated within 72 hours after removal of the tube.

A chest roentgenogram must demonstrate the absence of pneumothorax just before the casualty is transported.[31] However, blast casualties who have pneumothorax must sometimes be evacuated quickly from the battlefield. Because these casualties have a high risk of tension pneumothorax with subsequent cardiovascular collapse, they should receive a tube thoracostomy before being transported—especially if evacuation is by air, regardless of the altitude and distance of the flight. The chest tubes may be left in position during evacuation but should be equipped with functioning valves (such as the Heimlich valve). The aircraft should be pressurized to ground level if such casualties will be aboard.

Casualties who require mechanical-ventilatory assistance should not be evacuated by air.

Definitive Physical Examination

Because pulmonary barotrauma may immediately threaten the casualty's ability to breathe, first-echelon medical personnel will have automatically addressed many of the more serious manifestations of PBI simply by stabilizing the casualty. Second-echelon medical personnel will be able to give the blast casualty a thorough physical examination and should be able to make a directive diagnosis. Examiners should be particularly alert to sentinel injuries that may indicate more serious covert trauma, as well as to those casualties who may be relatively asymptomatic but are at risk for late-developing signs of PBI.

Hypopharynx. The medical officer should examine the casualty's hypopharynx for petechiae or ecchymoses around the larynx, vocal cords, or other hypopharyngeal structures. These small hemorrhages may be associated with significant PBI to the lung.[2,32]

Lungs. Of the organs in the thorax and the abdomen, the lungs are the most vulnerable to PBI, and the examining physician should focus attention on them. The signs of pulmonary PBI are virtually identical to those of pulmonary injuries that occur after blunt chest trauma in motor-vehicle accidents, except that they rarely include rib fractures or aortic and cardiac injuries.[7,13,33,34]

The contused lung will present as a unilateral or bilateral alveolar-filling defect, similar to a pneumonia (Figure 9-2). The medical officer may find dullness to percussion in the presence of crackles or rales. Tachypnea is a common finding; in one study, the average respiratory rate of four patients who had blast lung was 30 breaths per minute.[17] The casualty may also be cyanotic.

If the contused lung is lacerated, then a hemothorax may develop, exhibiting unilateral decrease in breath sounds and dullness to percussion.

A casualty who has developed a pneumothorax that has not yet been treated may exhibit some of the following signs: *(a)* tracheal deviation from the midline, *(b)* increased resonance on the side of collapse when the chest is percussed, *(c)* diminished breath sounds on the side of the collapsed lung, *(d)* a retrosternal crunching from a pneumomediastinum, and *(e)* subcutaneous crepitation, which the examiner will note as a crackling sensation beneath the casualty's skin when palpated. If the pneumothorax has progressed into a tension pneumothorax, a shift of the cervical trachea from the midline will indicate that the mediastinal contents have shifted away from the side of collapse.

Occasionally, the blast casualty's abdominal complaints may distract the examining physician's attention from the presence of pulmonary PBI. For example, only three of twenty-seven survivors who had gastrointestinal injury from an underwater detonation presented with overt respiratory distress, but nineteen were ultimately found to have significant pulmonary compromise.[16] In World War II, naval surgeons suggested that lung damage might be the source of discomfort in an underwater-blast casualty whose pain was limited to the upper-abdominal area.[35]

Diagnostic Screening Procedures

Radiographs are the most useful diagnostic screens for casualties with pulmonary PBI, and some objective measure of respiratory function (such as an arterial blood gas or oximetry) is important. Routine laboratory studies, however, are unlikely to be helpful in either diagnosing or gauging the severity of PBI.

Roentgenography. Because it often reveals a more significant injury than was clinically suspected, a roentgenogram should be taken of any blast casualty regardless of symptoms.[13,36] Routine roentgenographic examinations should include images of both the chest and abdomen, and should be examined carefully for evidence of barotrauma, which will complicate further aeromedical evacuation, mechanical ventilation, and any surgery that requires general anesthesia.

The progression of pulmonary contusion can be tracked by radiographic studies. In uncomplicated PBI, this injury develops quickly. For example, roentgenographic abnormalities were evident in eleven of twelve cases within 9 hours in one series, and within 4 hours of exposure in all five patients of another series.[13,15] In the absence of complications, the roentgenogram should be stable after a day and should improve gradually over the course of about a week.[13,15,16] Radiographic progression after 48 hours suggests another process, such as infection or posttraumatic respiratory distress syndrome.[15]

When pneumothorax is suspected, a chest roentgenogram should be taken immediately. If the casualty exhibits cardiovascular compromise and a tension pneumothorax is suspected, however, an emergency tube thoracostomy has a higher priority than a chest roentgenogram.

The chest film will obviously give the greatest information on lung injury, but it may also show *(a)* free air under the diaphragm (called *pneumoperitoneum*) from the rupture of hollow viscera or *(b)* a long lucent strip to the left of the trachea that may be the result of air extravasated from the esophagus.[13] Interstitial emphysema appears on a roentgenogram as long linear peribronchial lucencies.

The presence of extensive subcutaneous emphysema may make it difficult for the physician to appreciate underlying parenchymal injury, just as pulmonary contusion may make it difficult to identify interstitial air.[26] Conversely, extrapleural air may be difficult to recognize in roentgenograms against the background of parenchymal hemorrhage and subcutaneous and interstitial emphysema (Figure 9-4).[37]

Computed Axial Tomography. A CAT scan may reveal lung injuries that were not apparent on the plain roentgenographic film.[37] It is the most accurate technique for evaluating the lung parenchyma and pleural space (Figures 9-5, 9-6, and 9-7)—even more so than the magnetic resonance imager (MRI)—and is much more likely to be available for combat-casualty care.

A CAT scan can also be used to quantitate the extent of injury based on the amount of parenchyma involved. In one study, for example, all blunt-trauma patients whose CAT scans revealed that more than 28% of their lungs were involved with hemorrhage required ventilatory support.[14] Those who had 45% involvement required mechanical ventilation for an average of 7 days. No patient with less than 18% involvement required a ventilator.

Stabilization and Life Support

Oxygen monitoring and assisted-ventilation measures that were beyond the scope of first-echelon medical personnel can be initiated at a higher echelon.

Restoring Oxygen Adequacy. Even though symptoms of circulatory, respiratory, or neurological dysfunction may not appear immediately, the blast casualty is in a state of relative distress and will need increased oxygen. The adequacy of oxygenation should be evaluated on clinical grounds (Figure 9-8) and with the direct measurement of arterial oxygen saturation by means of either *(a)* pulse oximetry or *(b)* arterial blood gases.

Pulse oximetry (available at the third echelon) is a technique whereby the percentage of oxygenated hemoglobin is noninvasively monitored by infrared reflectometry of the vascular bed in the ear or in a finger. Ideally, pulse oximetry should be continuously monitored in a seriously injured casualty.

An analysis of arterial blood gases reveals the levels of oxygen and carbon dioxide in the blood, and thus gives the medical officer important information on respiratory sufficiency and acid-base status. In general, a blast casualty with uncomplicated PBI can be expected to have a level of arterial pCO_2 that is normal (35–40 mm Hg) or low (hypocarbia). Hypercarbia suggests that something other than PBI may be limiting spontaneous ventilation. For example, the casualty may have muscular or mechanical problems, such as *(a)* flail chest, *(b)* muscle weakness from chemical agents or metabolic derangements, *(c)* airway compromise, or *(d)* diaphragm rupture. An-

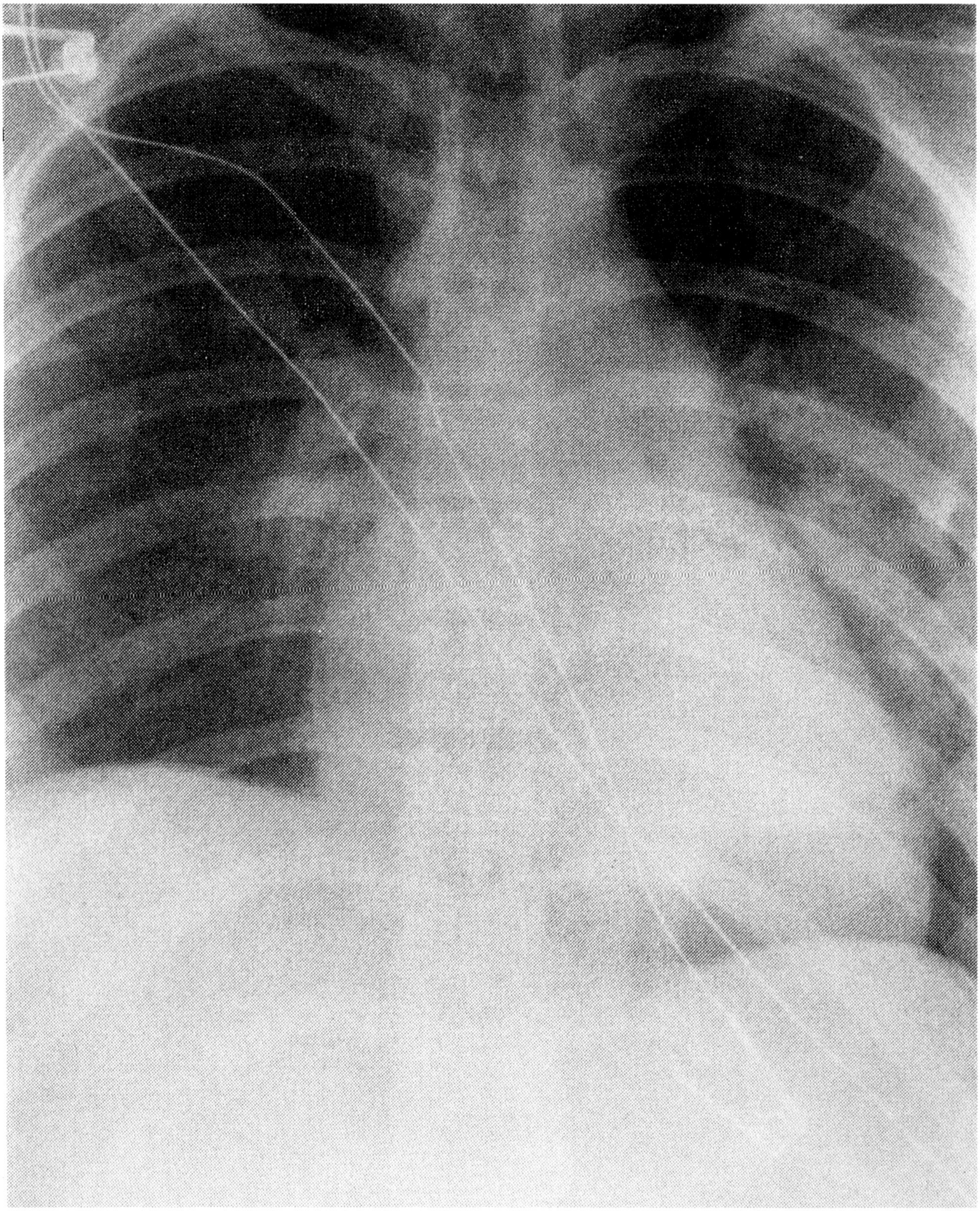

Fig. 9-4. A chest roentgenogram of a patient in the supine position who had blunt thoracoabdominal trauma shows a patchy left midlung infiltrate consistent with pulmonary contusion but shows no evidence of barotrauma.
Source: With permission from reference 36

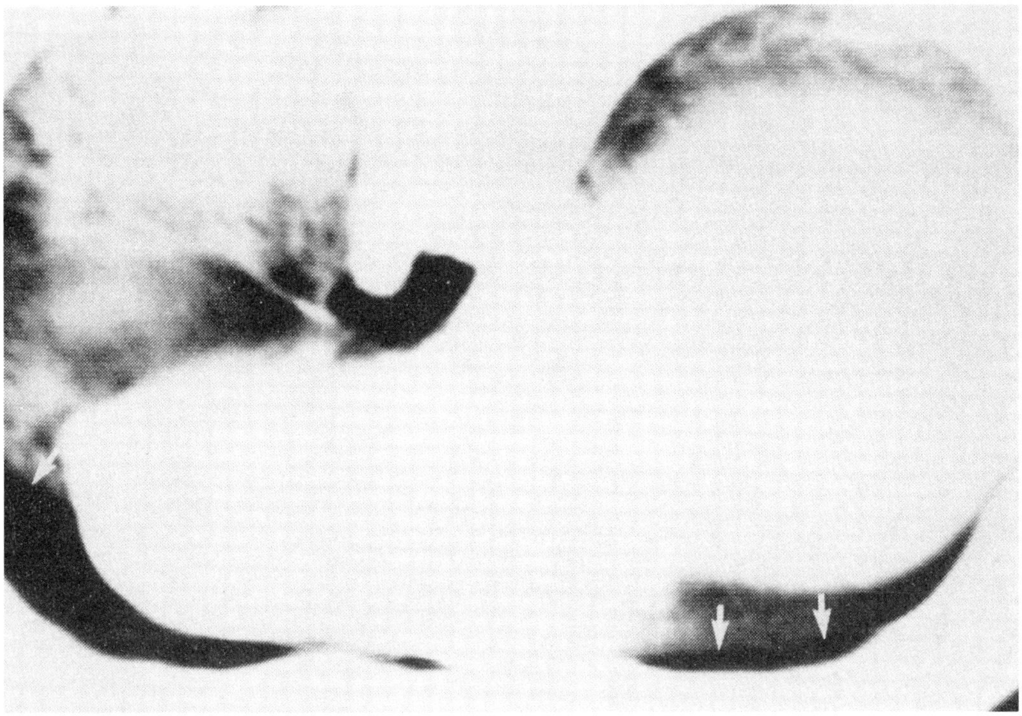

Fig. 9-5. The CAT scan of the same lungs shown in Figure 9-4 not only reveals the air-space consolidation of pulmonary hemorrhage, but also shows unsuspected bilateral pneumothoraces. Arrows indicate the visceral pleural surfaces.
Source: With permission from reference 36

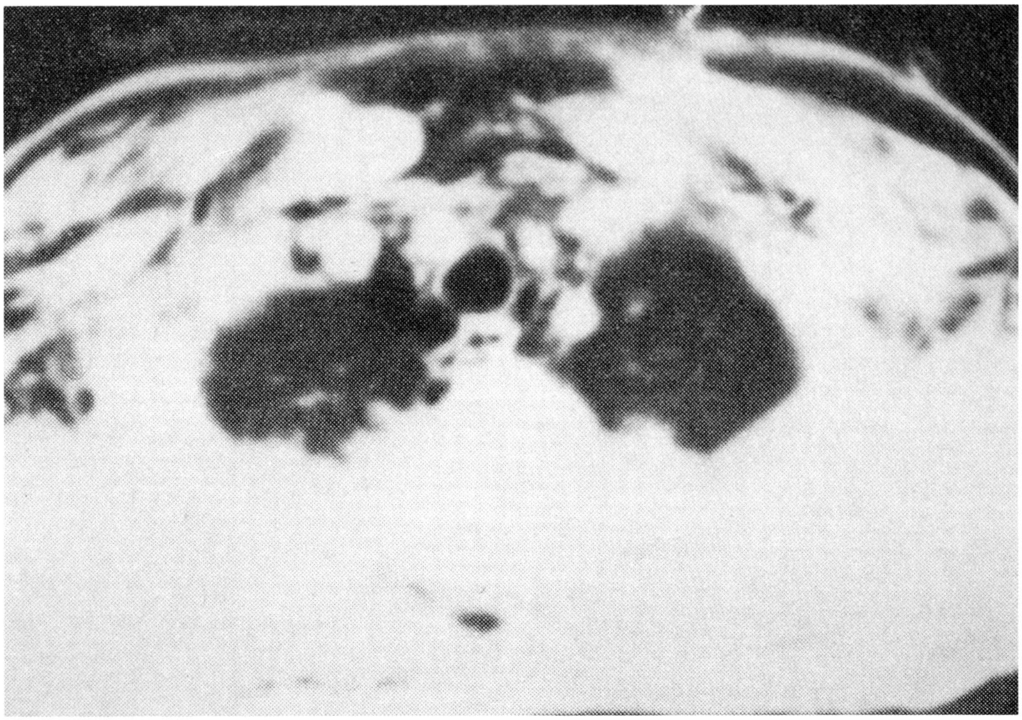

Fig. 9-6. This CAT scan of a blast casualty's thorax shows extensive subcutaneous emphysema that may obscure intrathoracic findings in a more routine roentgenographic evaluation.
Source: With permission from reference 25

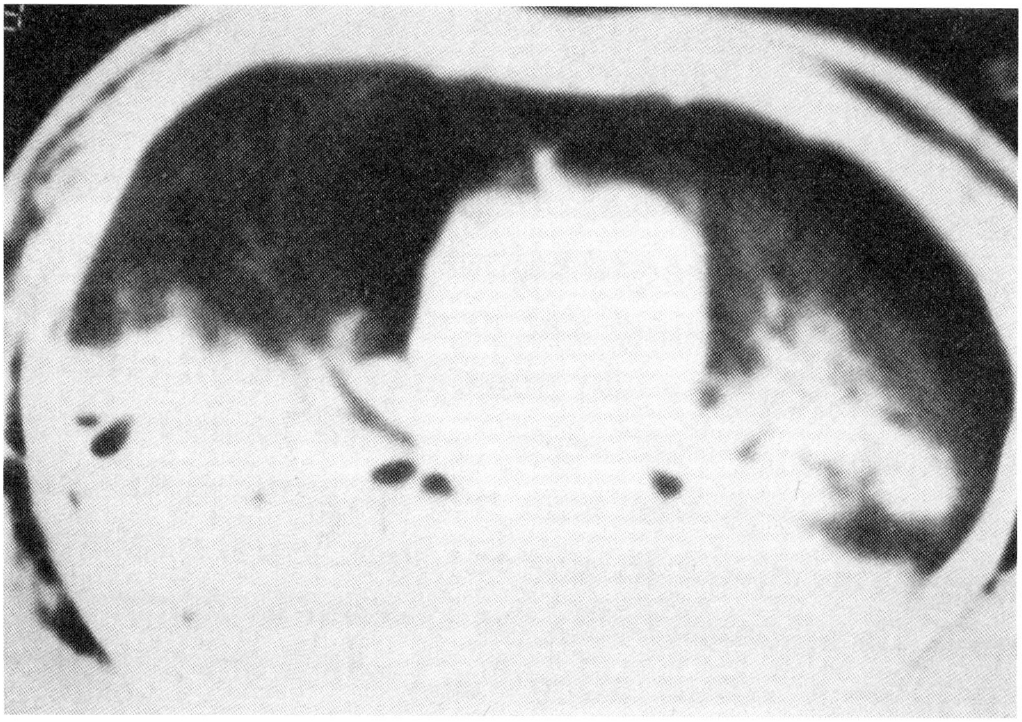

Fig. 9-7. This image reveals bilateral pneumothoraces, pneumomediastinum, and extensive parenchymal consolidation consistent with pulmonary contusion and hemorrhage.
Source: With permission from reference 25

other cause of hypercarbia may be an impairment of the casualty's central ventilatory drive, which may be due to a central nervous system injury from direct trauma, air embolism, or excessive use of analgesic narcotics.

Studies on animals have yielded important information on the sequence of ventilation and oxygenation problems that result from PBI. In studies with sheep,[38,39] dogs,[29,38] and pigs,[33] the animals rapidly became hypoxemic after they were injured by blast. Their immediate response to blast trauma was apnea, which lasted 30–120 seconds.[33,40] The apnea was often accompanied by bradycardia; in animals, both of these responses can be ablated by vagotomy.[40] Within minutes of the injury, the animals' respiratory rate increased greatly over the baseline value, and—although *tidal volume* (the average volume of gas inspired with each breath) was decreased—the *minute volume* (the mean volume of inspired gas per minute) was increased.[41] The increase in the central ventilatory drive may have been caused by either pain or pulmonary mechanoreceptors, and it resulted not only in an increase in oxygen consumption, but also in a decrease in the level of arterial pCO_2.[40] For example, twenty-seven of twenty-nine sheep that had pure PBI but were not in hypovolemic shock had arterial pCO_2 levels that were less than 40 mm Hg.[38]

These animal studies also found that the magnitude of *shunting* (an index of oxygen efficiency that measures the amount of blood passing through the lungs without being oxygenated) was directly related to the degree of lung hemorrhage (Figure 9-9).[39] Although there may be an improvement within 24–48 hours, a measurable decrement in pulmonary gas exchange may last for weeks.

The animals' cardiovascular responses to blast were less dramatic. For example, within a few hours of injury, cardiac output in dogs increased only about 15% because of an increase in both heart rate and stroke volume.[29] These changes returned to a near-baseline level within 24 hours.

The limited data on human trauma victims corroborate the animal experiments. In one report, all five blast casualties were both hypoxemic and hypocarbic, even though they had received supplemental oxygen.[15] In an Israeli report of an explosion on a bus, three patients with simple contusions had pCO_2 values of 26, 27, and 38 mm Hg, whereas two victims with chest-wall injuries were hypercarbic and had pCO_2 values of 46 and 63 mm Hg.[12]

Mechanical Ventilation. Some casualties who have pulmonary contusions will require endotracheal

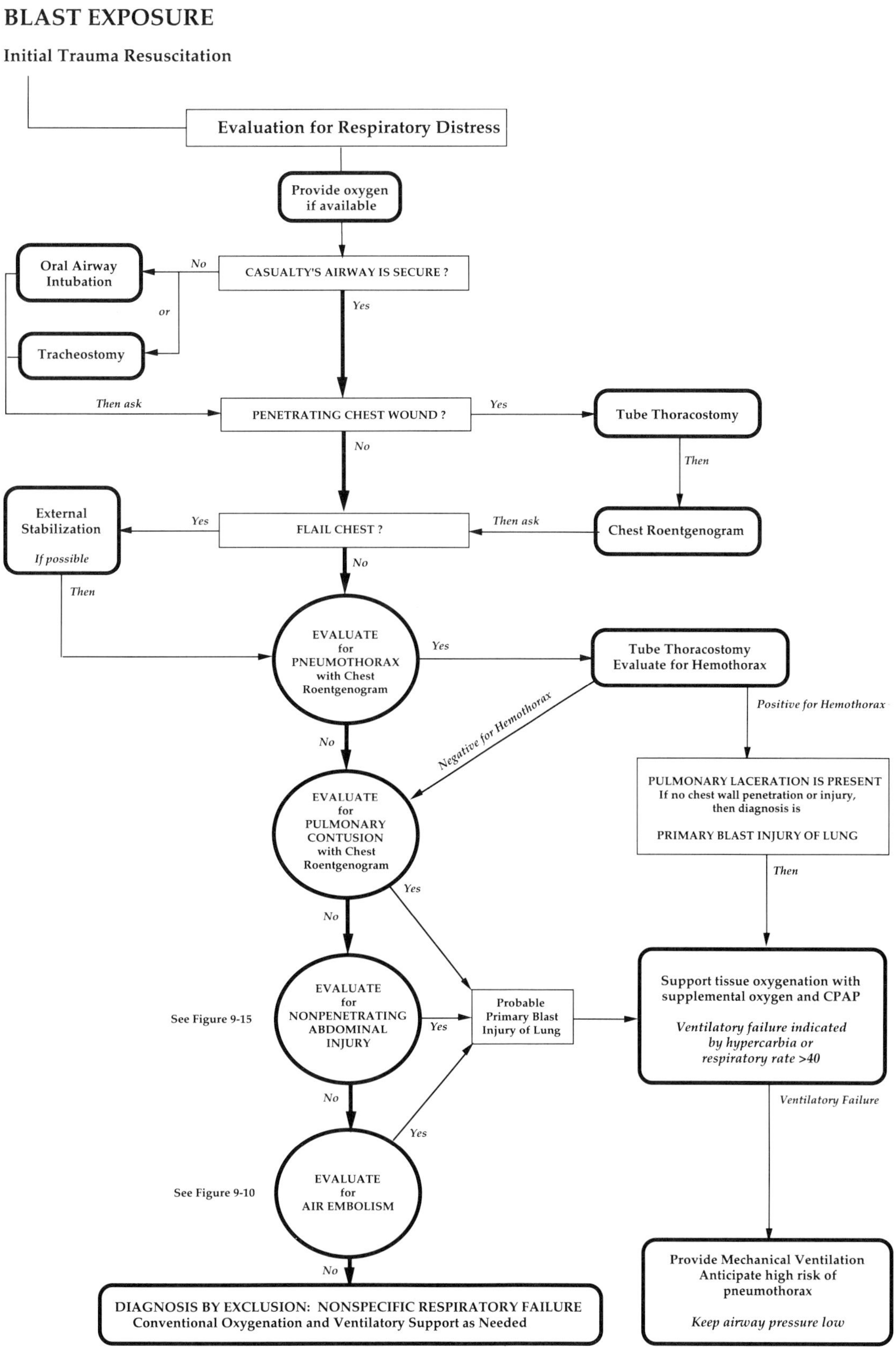

Fig. 9-8. Algorithm for the evaluation of a blast casualty's respiratory distress

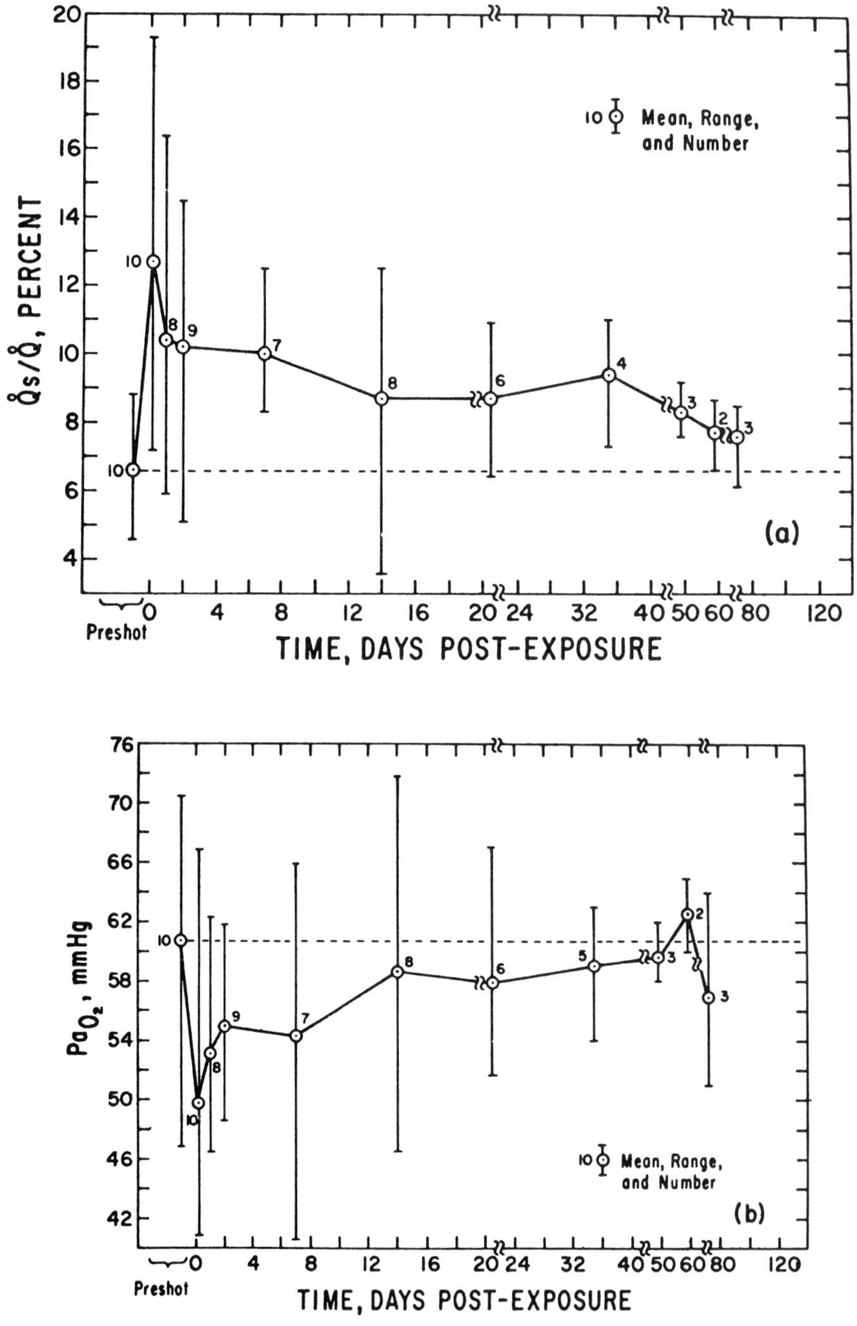

Effects of Blast Pressure on Venous-Arterial Shunt (Q̊s/Q̊) and Arterial Oxygen Tension (Pa_{O_2}) in the Sheep.

Fig. 9-9. These graphs illustrate the magnitude and resolution of arterial oxygenation and shunting in sheep that were exposed to a large but sublethal blast. In the top graph, Qs/Qt is the shunt fraction or venous admixture. In the bottom graph, the preblast PaO_2 is consistent with normal function at the test-site altitude of 1,640 m.
Source: Reference 38

intubation and mechanical ventilation. Ventilatory assistance with a modern positive-pressure ventilator can *(a)* make the work of breathing less strenuous for the casualty, *(b)* correct hypercarbia, and *(c)* improve oxygenation.

Mechanical ventilation is not without risk for the blast casualty. For example, casualties who receive positive-pressure ventilatory support are at a much higher risk for developing tension pneumothorax than spontaneously breathing casualties are. This is a disastrous complication, and some authors have suggested that bilateral prophylactic chest tubes be placed in all blast victims who receive mechanical ventilation.[22,42] In addition, mechanical ventilatory support tends to encourage the production of air emboli from injured lungs.

In spite of these risks, mechanical ventilation should not be withheld in cases of respiratory insufficiency. Instead, the medical officer must take prudent steps to minimize the risks of air embolism and additional barotrauma. For example, the casualty who is hypoxemic but not hypercarbic can be treated with supplemental oxygen or the application of continuous positive airway pressure with an endotracheal tube or a face mask.[25,43,44] When positive-pressure ventilatory support is used, the medical officer should choose parameters for tidal volume, respiratory rate, and inspiratory-flow rate that will minimize the peak airway pressure during machine-delivered breaths. High-frequency jet ventilation may also be useful in lowering airway pressures.[12] Medical personnel should make every effort to keep the airway pressure low and to promote good bronchial hygiene by *(a)* using bronchodilators, *(b)* suctioning, and *(c)* changing the casualty's body position frequently.[45] Ideally, the casualty should be constantly monitored, especially in the intensive-care ward and the operating room.

Extracorporeal membrane oxygenation, a blood-perfusion system that actually takes the place of the injured lung for a time, was used in one heroic but unsuccessful attempt to save an Israeli blast casualty who suffered from both respiratory failure and air emboli.[19] However, this method is unlikely to be useful in a mass-casualty situation because *(a)* it requires massive logistical support, and *(b)* the patient must receive anticoagulants.

Treatment

The treatment of pulmonary blast injury focuses on correcting the effects of barotrauma and supporting gas exchange.

Pulmonary Contusion. Although many simple pulmonary contusions will begin to resolve within 24–48 hours, some patients will need assistance from mechanical ventilation for several days until they have adequate gas exchange and can resume spontaneous respiration.

Most hemorrhages in the airway will subside within a day or two as well. However, if brisk hemoptysis persists or if refractory lobar atelectasis is noted, fiberoptic bronchoscopy should be used to inspect the major airways. For example, in a study of fifty-three patients who had blunt chest injuries, twenty-eight had abnormal bronchoscopies.[46] The findings commonly included unappreciated bronchial fractures and lacerations. Continued hemoptysis without such a proximal lesion may indicate a persistent hemorrhage from a pulmonary contusion or laceration.

Pulmonary lacerations may require both ventilatory support and pleural drainage. A small hemothorax will generally resolve on its own, but surgeons will drain large collections of blood in the pleural space to prevent late complications of empyema and fibrothorax. If the casualty continues to lose blood from a hemothorax, the medical officer should consider surgical exploration.

Pneumothorax. A tube thoracostomy is the definitive treatment for pneumothorax. If the casualty has evidence of an accompanying pulmonary contusion, supplemental oxygen may also be required.

Pneumomediastinum and Subcutaneous Emphysema. By themselves, these injuries are not particularly hazardous to the blast casualty. However, they should prompt the medical officer to be alert to the casualty's increased risk of pneumothorax.

AIR EMBOLISM IN PRIMARY BLAST INJURY

Air emboli may be liberated from the lacerated lung into the arterial circulation, where they may cause occlusions—often with disastrous results. Any organ may be affected by a local vascular obstruction, but the casualty may suffer *(a)* a cerebrovascular accident when cerebral vessels are occluded, or *(b)* a myocardial infarction when coronary vessels are occluded. Air emboli cause most of those deaths that occur within an hour of the blast incident.

Initial Physical Examination and Triage

Air emboli may be produced very soon after blast injury, and their clinical presentation depends upon which vascular bed has been compromised (Table 9-3). Medical personnel should note the following signs and symptoms:

- Does the casualty *(a)* complain of headaches or *(b)* exhibit seizures, changes in mental status, transient blindness, vestibular disturbances, focal neurological deficits, or coma? These symptoms and signs indicate that the central nervous system has been affected (Figure 9-10).[7,15,19,45]
- Is the casualty exhibiting hypotension or other obvious indicators of cardiac distress, such as dysrhythmia, hypotension, or frank ischemic changes?[15,16,19]
- In addition to other symptoms, does the casualty exhibit signs of pulmonary contusion?

The signs of air embolism develop so early that major manifestations are likely to be evident at the initial first-echelon triage, and so medical personnel should evaluate the blast casualty according to present (rather than potential) indications. Only casualties who exhibit clinical evidence of pulmonary contusion will be at risk for air embolism.

Initiation of Life Support

The blast casualty should receive life support measures according to the signs he or she exhibits. Following standard procedures, medical personnel should respond to a blast casualty's respiratory difficulties by making sure that the casualty has a patent airway. Chest tubes should be inserted as warranted to relieve pneumothorax.

As soon as it is available, oxygen should be administered in order to *(a)* support gas exchange in the injured lung, and *(b)* help the tissues to absorb air emboli, a process that occurs faster when the bubbles contain a higher-than-normal proportion of oxygen rather than a predominance of nitrogen. Tissue oxygenation (and hence oxygen reserve) will also be increased.

Air emboli can cause myocardial infarction, and casualties may be hypotensive from this catastrophe as well as from any blood loss they might have suffered. They will require rapid but cautious volume replacement. Medical personnel should be aware that casualties who have extensive pulmonary contusion are at risk for further impairment of lung function if intravenous fluid resuscitation is excessive.[16,26] On the other hand, because lower vascular pressures favor the movement of air from the alveoli into the pulmonary vessels, casualties who do not receive volume replacement will have intravascular volume depletion that may predispose them to air embolism.[5]

TABLE 9-3

CLINICAL SIGNS AND SYMPTOMS OF ARTERIAL AIR EMBOLISM

Signs
Air in retinal vessels
Arrythmias or cardiac ischemia
Focal neurological deficits
Livedo reticularis
Tongue blanching
Symptoms
Blindness
Chest pain
Focal neurological deficits
Loss of consciousness
Vestibular disturbances

Evacuation

As soon as they find the casualty at the blast site, medical personnel can begin to limit air-embolism damage by *(a)* positioning the casualty's body appropriately, and *(b)* ensuring that the casualty is evacuated by litter.

Air emboli in the arterial circulation tend to flow upward in the body and to travel to organs that require a large blood flow.[4,45] Thus, the position of the casualty's body may affect the site of embolism damage. Unless the casualty has a right-lung injury that is obviously more severe than an injury to the left lung, he or she should be kept recumbent in the left-lateral decubitus position with the head down.[4,5,6] An upright posture will direct bubbles to the brain, and the Trendelenburg position may predispose the coronary arteries to air-embolism damage.[45]

If one lung is more severely affected than the other, however, the damaged lung should be in the dependent position.[5] Throughout the dependent lung, alveolar pressures will be lower than vascular pressures. Although this may worsen gas exchange, it will also decrease the risk that air emboli will enter the pulmonary veins.

Stabilization and Life Support

Medical officers who utilize mechanical ventilation must be aware that it can increase the risk of lethal air embolism for blast casualties. Most air emboli

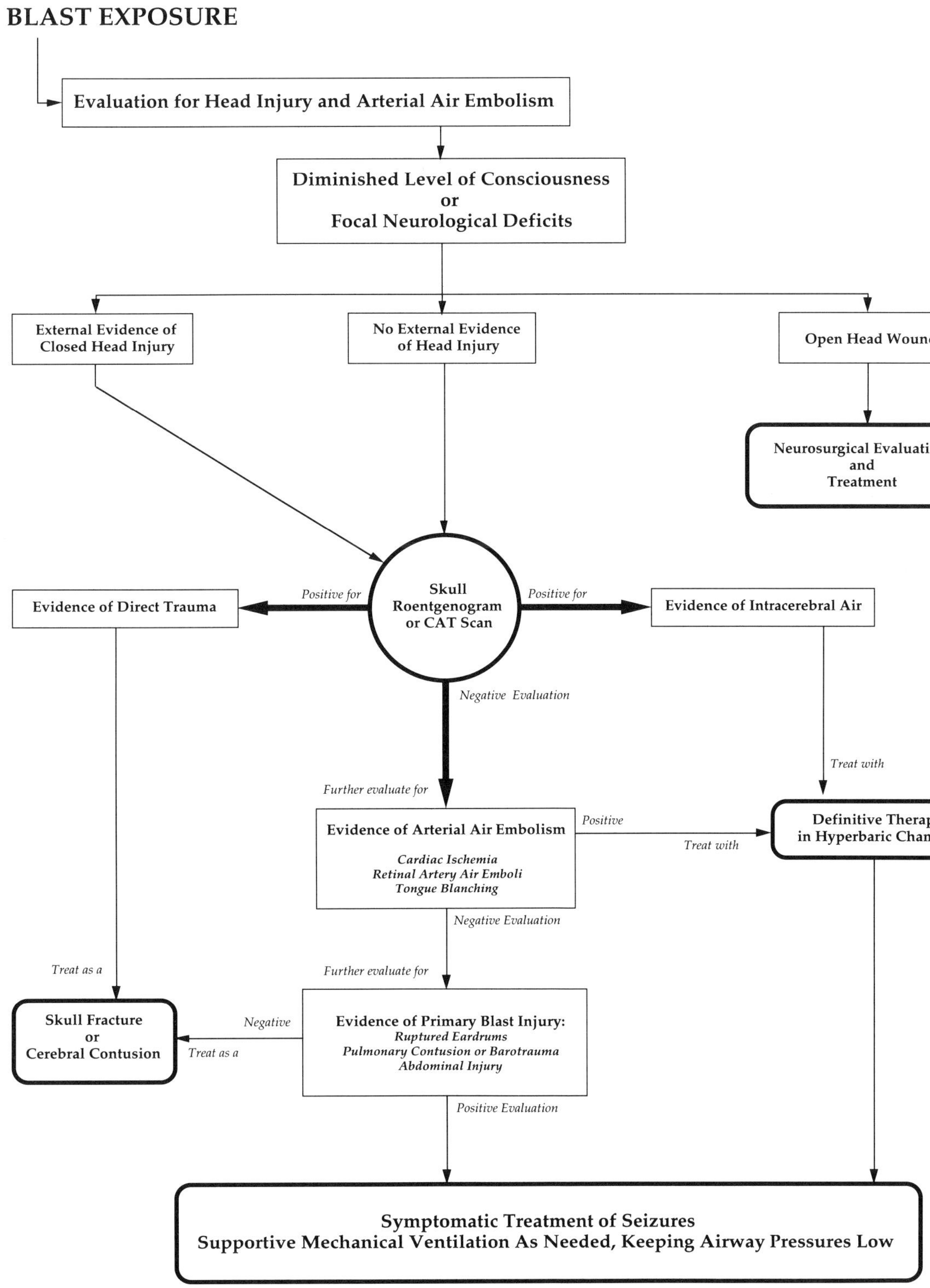

Fig. 9-10. Algorithm for the evaluation of neurological abnormalities in a blast casualty

probably occur within the first 2 hours after the blast exposure, particularly if mechanical ventilation is initiated soon after the injury. In a series of experiments, for example, three groups of dogs received intermittent positive-pressure respiration *(a)* immediately, *(b)* 4 hours after a severe blast injury, or *(c)* not at all (Figure 9-11).[47] Those animals that were ventilated immediately after injury had an 80% mortality, with arterial air emboli found at autopsy in three of ten dogs. The dogs in the second group were treated for 4 hours in a hyperbaric chamber and were then mechanically ventilated for 1 hour. This delayed group had only a 50% mortality and no emboli were detected at autopsy. The control group that received no intervention had a 60% mortality, with one of ten animals exhibiting air emboli at autopsy.

When the lungs are stressed by mechanical ventilation, air emboli can continue to be produced for hours or even days after blast exposure. For example, an autopsy on an Israeli soldier who had received mechanical ventilation revealed cerebral vessel air emboli 60 hours after the blast.[19] Emboli can occur in animals hours after blast exposure once positive-pressure ventilation is initiated (Figure 9-11).[47] In an experiment with dogs that were subjected to a penetrating wound in the chest, for example, the production of air emboli was more extensive if the animals were hypovolemic or if high gas pressures were used to expand their lungs.[5] Even if mechanical ventilation is initiated later, the high airway pressures associated with positive-pressure ventilation may predispose the injured lung to the later reopening of alveolovenous fistulae.[25] For example, two patients with nontraumatic ARDS developed repeated evidence of systemic emboli, which included cerebral infarction, myocardial injury, and cutaneous manifestations.[45]

The age of the casualty may affect the production of air emboli as a result of mechanical ventilation. For example, arterial air embolism is a well-recognized complication of mechanical ventilation in the infant,[48,49] perhaps because of the decreased adherence of peribronchial tissue planes in children.[45] It is less common in older patients on ventilators, despite the common occurrence of other forms of barotrauma in adults.

Definitive Physical Examination

Air embolism is recognized primarily from its effects on specific organs. For example, the physician who examines a blast casualty would recognize the cardiac, cerebral, or other distress that resulted from the air embolism, rather than the embolism itself. One exception might be the presence of retinal-artery air emboli, which have been described as "streaming bubbles or pale silvery sections representing columns of air or, indirectly or later, as pallor of the retina" (Figure 9-12).[19]

Severe or progressive neurological deficits in a casualty who has evidence of PBI should prompt early consideration of hyperbaric therapy (Figure 9-10).

Emboli to the superficial vasculature may cause facial blanching (with later reactive edema), tongue blanching, or *livedo reticularis* (a bluish network-patterned discoloration of the skin).[19,45]

Diagnostic Screening Procedures

Laboratory or roentgenographic studies will not be very helpful in diagnosing arterial air emboli. For example, the chest roentgenogram may show some evidence of PBI. But even though pulmonary damage is a sensitive indicator of air embolism (that is, it is always present when emboli are created), it is not predictive of embolism. Similarly, electrocardiographic monitoring may reveal ischemic changes or rhythm disturbances, but both are nonspecific. A CAT scan of the head may show intracerebral air,[50] but such a study is time consuming and should not be done if the diagnosis is clinically sound and definitive hyperbaric treatment is available.

When medical officers evaluate a blast casualty who has impaired consciousness or a focal neurological deficit, one of the most important differentiations they should make is between cerebral vessel air embolization and closed head injury with cerebral contusion (Figure 9-10). In terrorist bombings, for example, both closed and open blunt traumas to the head are common and are much more likely to be the cause of alterations of consciousness than PBI is. However, if the blast occurred under water or as the result of special military ordnance, then air embolism becomes a more likely diagnosis.[19,51,52,53]

Treatment of Air Emboli

Air emboli that escape from the lacerated lung into the arterial circulation may have the greatest effect on mortality from PBI. They are treated either definitively with hyperbaric therapy or in a less specific supportive manner for clinical manifestations.

Hyperbaric-Chamber Treatment. Treatment in a hyperbaric chamber is the definitive therapy for arterial air embolism.[4,19,54,55] An increase in ambient pressure will decrease the size of the emboli and promote their rapid absorption. The higher partial pressure of oxygen that occurs even without oxygen enrichment of the atmosphere may also play a role in improving

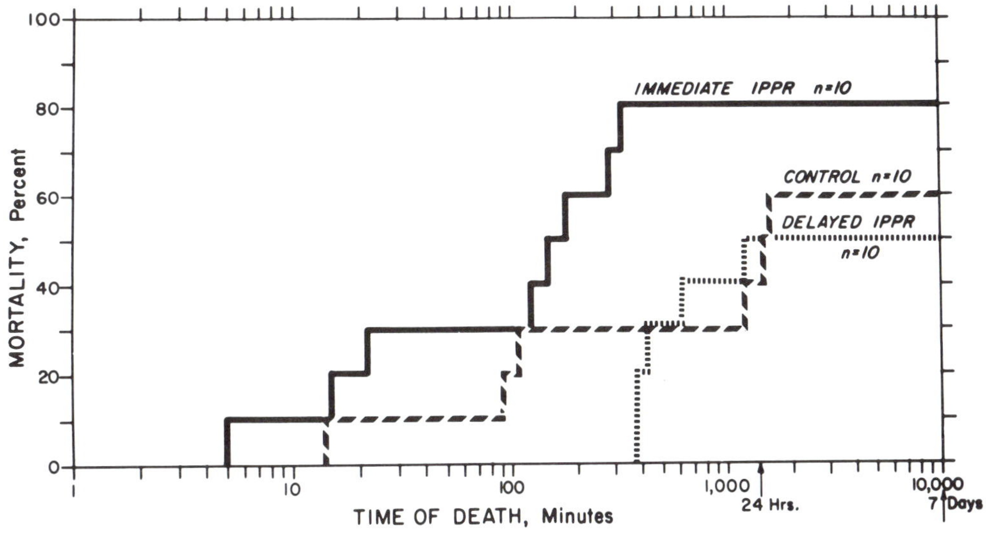

Fig. 9-11. The graph illustrates the mortality following blast injury for beagles that received *(a)* immediate intermittent positive-pressure respiration (IPPR) (——), *(b)* IPPR after a 4-hour delay in a hyperbaric chamber (**IIIII**), or *(c)* no specific treatment at all (– – –). Mortality was greatest with artificial ventilation and was both delayed and lessened by hyperbaric therapy.
Source: Reference 46

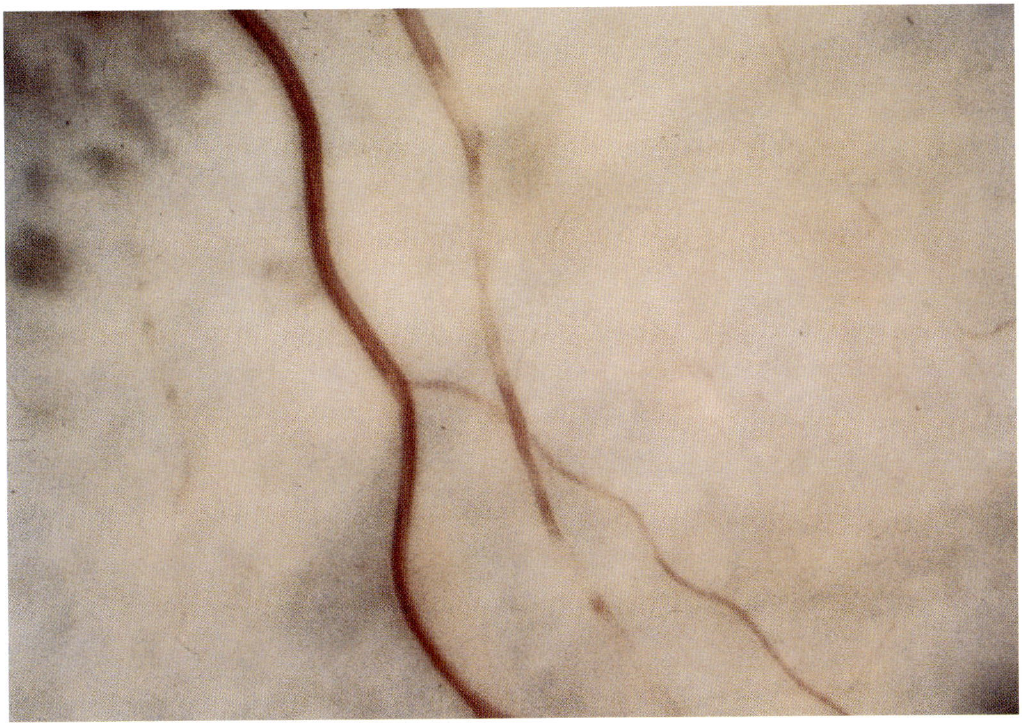

Fig. 9-12. This photograph of the fundus of a sheep that was exposed to intense blast shows air in the retinal artery.
Source: Reference 19

tissue oxygenation by increasing *(a)* the amount of oxygen that is carried dissolved in blood and *(b)* the gradient for diffusion from blood to tissue. The immediate reduction in bubble size, which is dictated by Boyle's law, may be responsible for the rapid response to therapy that has been observed in some cases.[19]

A series of animal experiments demonstrated the effectiveness of hyperbaric therapy in treating PBI (Figure 9-13).[4,56] When hyperbaric therapy was maintained for 29 hours, the blast mortality was reduced from 60% to 0%. The same result was reported for *(a)* hyperoxic therapy at relatively low pressures (15 psi above ambient pressure) and *(b)* a normoxic environment at higher pressures (60 psi above ambient pressure). When pressurization was limited to just 4 hours, deaths were delayed but not prevented. Supplemental oxygen did not improve survival in these studies, but could delay mortality.

The data on the effectiveness of hyperbaric therapy for human arterial embolism are scanty. Most such interventions took place hours after blast exposure and had little effect on outcome.[19,50] As demonstrated by animal studies, hyperbaric treatment must begin as soon as possible after blast exposure. After ten of thirteen swimmers died from a single submersion-blast event, Israeli military physicians advocated the development of helicopter-transportable monoplace compression chambers so that therapy could begin at the site of injury.[19]

Protocols for hyperbaric therapy have been developed by the U.S. Navy for the treatment of decompression sickness (commonly known as the *bends*) and gas embolism.[57,58] They seem to provide a reasonable guideline for the treatment of blast-induced arterial air embolism.[4,6,55] The protocol for the treatment of gas embolism calls for compression to 6 atmospheres (atm) with an air environment. (The initial air environment reduces the risk of oxygen toxicity.) The patient's tolerance of embolic symptoms, which may recur as the chamber's pressure is lowered, guides the rate of decompression. When the pressure has been brought down to 2.8 atm, the air environment should be changed to 100% oxygen and the rate of decompression should again be determined by the medical officer's clinical judgment.

Hyperoxic hyperbaric therapy is not without potential complications.[19,57,58] The elevated pressure may cause pain in ears or sinuses. More importantly, extremely high oxygen concentrations can cause both acute and delayed effects. Symptoms of acute oxygen toxicity include retrosternal burning, muscle fasciculations, paresthesias, and dizziness that may progress to seizures. In the lungs, the very high oxygen concentration may cause serious (but delayed) oxidation damage to the alveolocapillary membrane that may aggravate the patient's pulmonary injury. The high concentration of oxygen can also pose some risk for medical attendants, so the prescribed protocol should be strictly followed.

Most hyperbaric chambers are relatively large and can accommodate the patient and medical attendants. Smaller monoplace chambers, which can be pressurized to about 3 atm, are also available. They offer extremely limited access to the patient and make no provision for sophisticated medical care or mechanical ventilation.[55]

The locations of hyperbaric chambers in the United States can be obtained from the Undersea Hyperbaric Medical Society.[59] In overseas locales, medical societies in host countries or naval medical-liaison groups should be able to provide similar information.

Nonspecific Treatments for Air-Embolism Sequelae. The sequelae of air embolism should be treated as if they had arisen from any impairment in the vascular supply. Such treatments are generally nonspecific and supportive.

Cerebral insults may respond to nonspecific therapies that reduce cerebral edema, such as intravenous dexamethasone (10-mg bolus followed by 4 mg four times daily) or mannitol.[55]

Cardiac-rhythm disturbances should be treated with antidysrhythmics. Significant cardiac ischemia should be treated with nitrates, calcium channel blockers, or beta-adrenergic antagonists to reduce myocardial oxygen demand.

Arterial air emboli that are produced during cardiopulmonary-bypass surgery have been successfully treated with hypothermia, corticosteroids, and barbiturate sedation, although such an elaborate support system is unlikely to be available on a battlefield.[60]

PRIMARY BLAST INJURY TO THE GASTROINTESTINAL TRACT

An injury to the gastrointestinal tract is often overshadowed by the more immediately life-threatening pulmonary contusions and lacerations, as well as by the air emboli that result from them. However, gastrointestinal damage may be the most dramatic injury at the time of presentation. It may also determine the

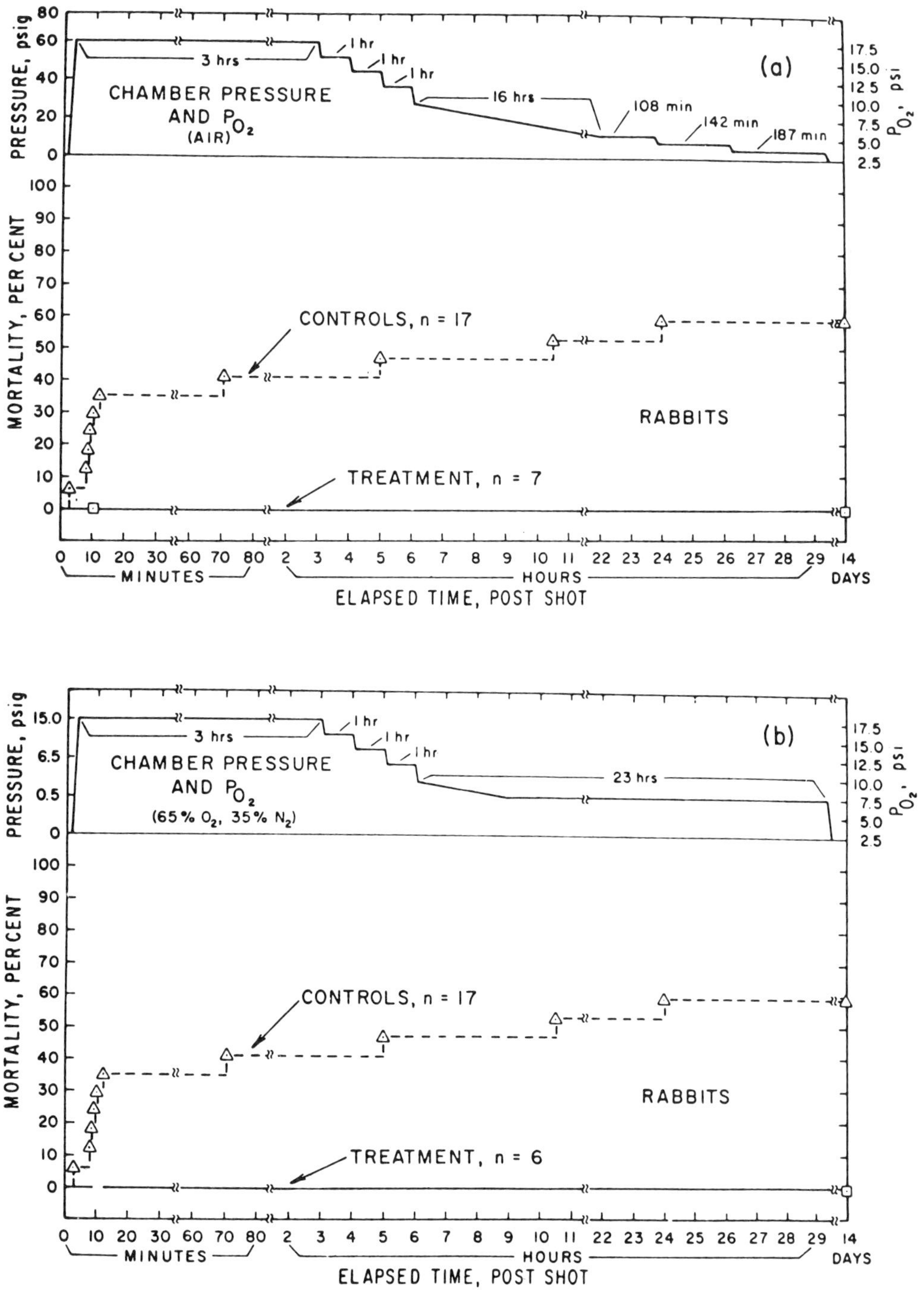

Fig. 9-13. These graphs illustrate the mortality of blast-injured rabbits that were treated with two long-duration hyperbaric protocols. Mortality was 0% for both higher-pressure normoxic therapy (a) and lower-pressure hyperoxic treatment (b).
Source: Reference 56

morbidity of those casualties who survive the first few hours after an exposure to blast. Many of these abdominal injuries will require surgical intervention.

Like injuries to the lungs, the most common primary blast lesions of the gastrointestinal tract are found in the air-containing organs. These lesions commonly include *(a)* hematomas and perforations of the bowel, *(b)* hematomas and tears of the mesentery, and *(c)* ruptures of the hollow abdominal viscera.

Retroperitoneal hemorrhage and damage to the solid abdominal organs are much less common; they are more likely to be secondary blast injuries from fragments, or tertiary blast injuries from bodily displacement.[42] Subcapsular hemorrhage in the liver, spleen, or kidneys is the most common of these injuries; very rarely, the force of the blast will fracture one of these solid organs.[16,23,61]

Blast casualties with gastrointestinal PBI may experience symptoms that include abdominal pain, nausea, testicular pain, an electric-shock sensation, tenesmus, or a temporary loss of motor control in the legs.[16,23,35,62]

Casualties who have pure PBI to the gastrointestinal tract are most likely to have been injured in an underwater blast (Figure 9-14).

Initial Physical Examination and Triage

The physical examination of a casualty with abdominal blast injuries will reveal signs that are similar to those found in blunt abdominal trauma from any cause, except that injury to the solid viscera will be much less common (Table 9-4).

Casualties with abdominal PBI may vomit; a few may even exhibit hematemesis. They may also have signs of peritoneal irritation such as guarding (voluntary or involuntary) or rebound tenderness. Bowel sounds may be absent. Bright-red rectal bleeding may occur later.

Patients who have unimpressive abdominal complaints may temporarily improve, only to develop an abdominal crisis days or even weeks later.[61,63] A soldier who has suffered a significant blast injury and has abdominal complaints should be observed for at least 1 week before being returned to full duty.

Any casualty who is in shock or is hypotensive should receive volume replacement. A blast casualty in shock may also require emergency exploratory laparotomy to control internal bleeding, and should be placed in the immediate triage category if he or she is unresponsive to the initial volume replacement.

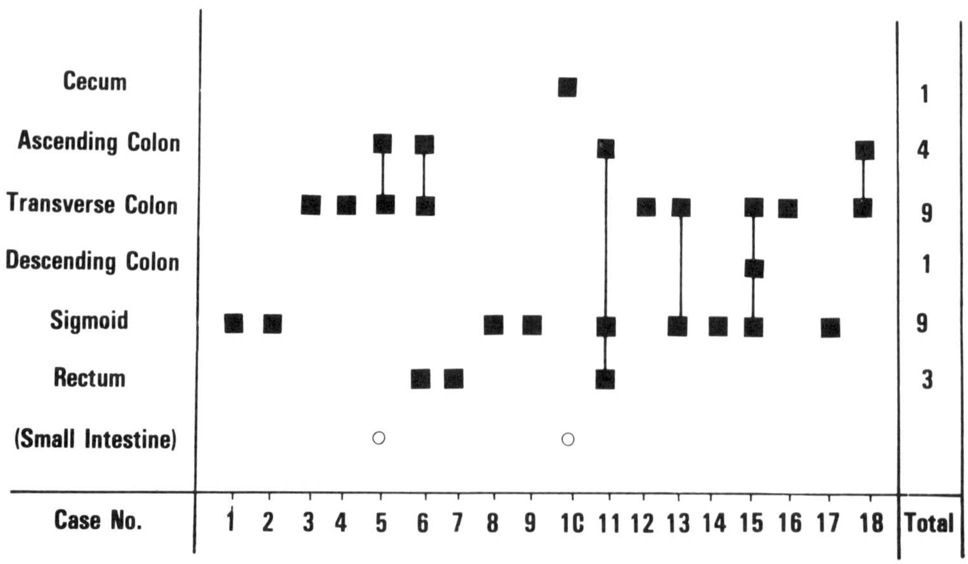

Fig. 9-14. This graph shows the locations of gastrointestinal injuries found at laparotomy in survivors of a large underwater explosion. Three of thirty-two casualties had rectal injuries.
Source: Redrawn with permission from reference 17

TABLE 9-4

CLINICAL SIGNS AND SYMPTOMS OF PRIMARY BLAST INJURY OF THE ABDOMEN

Signs

- Absent bowel sounds
- Bright red blood from rectum
- Hypotension
- Involuntary guarding
- Rebound tenderness

Symptoms

- Abdominal pain
- Nausea and vomiting
- Orthostasis or syncope
- Testicular pain
- Tenesmus

If their blood-pressure levels are within normal ranges, blast casualties should be placed in the delayed triage category.

Initiation of Life Support

Some casualties with PBI may be hypotensive because of blood loss from an abdominal hemorrhage or solid-organ fracture. Secondary blast injuries or other wounds may also cause hypotension.

The hypotension associated with PBI may be multifactorial, with contributions from *(a)* loss of intravascular volume, most commonly because of an abdominal hemorrhage or solid-organ blast fracture, *(b)* bradycardia with or without vasodilation, or *(c)* myocardial ischemia caused by arterial air emboli.[16,26] If the casualty has a vagally associated bradycardia, then medical personnel can administer 0.5–1.0 mg of atropine parenterally.

Initial volume resuscitation should be vigorously pursued according to standard guidelines to maintain an adequate pulse and blood pressure, but the casualty should not be overhydrated. Volume resuscitation should be guided by evidence of adequate tissue perfusion, as assessed clinically by *(a)* blood pressure, *(b)* urinary output, and *(c)* mental status.

In a complicated patient, invasive monitoring of central-venous or pulmonary-artery pressures may be invaluable in guiding volume replacement.

Evacuation

Increased gas in the gastrointestinal tract, which can exacerbate abdominal injuries, can be minimized by nasogastric decompression. This procedure should be performed before the casualty is evacuated.

Definitive Physical Examination

The physical examination plays an important role in evaluating intraabdominal injury. Unequivocal signs of peritoneal irritation, particularly if the casualty is hypotensive, require prompt surgical intervention. Most casualties who will need surgery will exhibit guarding and rebound tenderness, but these signs are not specific and may be found with lesser degrees of injury.[64]

Casualties who have tenesmus or bright-red rectal bleeding should receive a flexible sigmoidoscopy at the first echelon where it is available, which will allow the physician to note rectal tears or perforations.[16]

Table 9-5 summarizes the incidence of abdominal

TABLE 9-5

DISTRIBUTION OF ABDOMINAL SYMPTOMS, SIGNS, AND CLINICAL FINDINGS IN SURVIVORS OF UNDERWATER AND AIR BLAST*

Symptoms, Signs, and Findings	Percentage**
Abdominal symptoms	
Abdominal pain	73
Nausea and vomiting	39
Tenesmus	28
Abdominal signs and findings	
Perforated bowel	67
Isolated bowel hematoma	2
Solid visceral injury	2

*Hospitalized survivors of major underwater blast (N=43) and air blast (N=2)

**See Table 9-2 for pulmonary injury data from the same incidents. The percent total mortality from pulmonary and abdominal blast injuries was 16%.

symptoms and signs in two series of patients who were injured predominantly by underwater blast.[13,16]

The patient who is unconscious or who has a less clear-cut examination will present a diagnostic challenge (Figure 9-15). Military medical officers may find more information on diagnostic evaluations in the extensive civilian literature on blunt abdominal trauma.

Diagnostic Screening Procedures

Serial hemoglobin determinations are essential if the patient might have suffered an intraabdominal blood loss. However, routinely available serum-chemistry and enzyme studies (such as serum transaminases, lactate dehydrogenase, creatine kinase, and alkaline phosphatase) failed to correlate with either the presence or the degree of gut involvement in animals that were injured by blast.[11]

Although routine laboratory screens may not be helpful in evaluating the stable patient who has PBI to the abdomen, *diagnostic peritoneal lavage* (DPL) is a useful procedure.

If abdominal-trauma patients are unstable, medical officers should forego detailed radiologic studies in favor of obtaining only a chest roentgenogram, and should instead perform prompt laparotomy.[65]

Diagnostic Peritoneal Lavage. DPL is an important diagnostic test when abdominal trauma is suspected in blast casualties. For example, in casualties from Northern Ireland's civil conflict, most of whom had penetrating wounds, abdominal lavage was seldom necessary "except in closed injuries due to bomb blast."[20] A recent report of a jejunal transection and duodenal hematoma from a rocket-motor explosion noted that DPL was positive and useful in guiding therapy.[66]

The Nelson-Lazarus DPL technique is relatively simple and can be done in any emergency room or triage ward.[67] First, the casualty's bladder should be drained with a Foley catheter, the gastrointestinal tract should be decompressed with a nasogastric tube, and the abdominal skin should be prepped and draped. An area in the midline that is 2–3 cm below the umbilicus is infiltrated with xylocaine to provide anesthesia and epinephrine to reduce the chance of a false positive tap. Next, an 18-gauge needle is introduced into the peritoneal cavity at a 45° angle towards the pelvis through a small stab wound. A J-wire guide is placed through the needle and a #8 French lavage catheter is passed over the wire into the peritoneal space. If more than 10 cc of nonclotting blood are aspirated, the DPL is positive and urgent laparotomy is indicated. If the aspirate is negative, a liter of normal saline is introduced through the catheter and allowed to drain out by gravity return. More than 100,000 erythrocytes or 500 leukocytes per cc of effluent are considered a positive lavage. If the effluent contains any bacteria, bile, or vegetable fibers, it is also considered positive.[64,67] In equivocal cases, the catheter may be left in place for several hours so that serial lavages can be done.[68]

A positive DPL is not absolutely specific for major abdominal injury. In a review of blunt-trauma injuries, 6%–25% of laparotomies done for a positive DPL were unnecessary because surgically correctable abnormalities were absent.[68] On the other hand, the sensitivity of DPL is said to be as high as 100% for blunt abdominal trauma.[68,69,70] The complication rate in experienced hands is less than 1%; if error occurs, inadvertent bowel aspiration is the most common.[71]

A major drawback of DPL is its insensitivity to retroperitoneal damage and mesenteric hematoma.[64,68,69,71,72] DPL may also fail to detect subcapsular injuries of the liver or spleen.[65,68]

Gastrointestinal Imaging. Radiographic imaging of the blast casualty's abdomen is an important part of the evaluation. The skill with which it is performed and interpreted is crucial.[71]

Noncontrast abdominal roentgenograms may show extraluminal air in about 50% of perforations from blunt trauma.[64] They may also show secondary signs of intraabdominal injury, such as ileus or lumbar scoliosis.[64] Because less than 800 cc of intraperitoneal fluid cannot be reliably detected on noncontrast roentgenograms, these studies are inherently limited in detecting free peritoneal bleeding.[65]

Of the noninvasive imaging procedures, CAT scans and sonograms seem to have the most promise.[65] The CAT scan is likely to be most useful in a patient who is stable enough to permit detailed evaluation.[72] Signs of serious injury that may appear on a CAT scan include *(a)* extraluminal gas or contrast (Figure 9-16), *(b)* hemoperitoneum (Figure 9-17), *(c)* a hypodense accumulation of peritoneal fluid, possibly including bowel contents, and *(d)* bowel-wall hematomas greater than 3 mm in diameter, especially when associated with large fluid collections.[64]

Abdominal CAT scans should be done with both an oral contrast bolus and an intravenous contrast infusion.[65,73] All electrocardiogram leads and other external paraphernalia that might cause artifact should be removed. After the stomach is emptied through a nasogastric tube, 2,300 ml of 1% radiocontrast material should be instilled and the gastric tube should be withdrawn into the distal esophagus. The entire abdomen should be scanned, and 1-cm cuts should be made through the chest as well. If a CAT scan or sonogram is to be done, it must precede any attempt at DPL because the lavage may leave both fluid and air behind

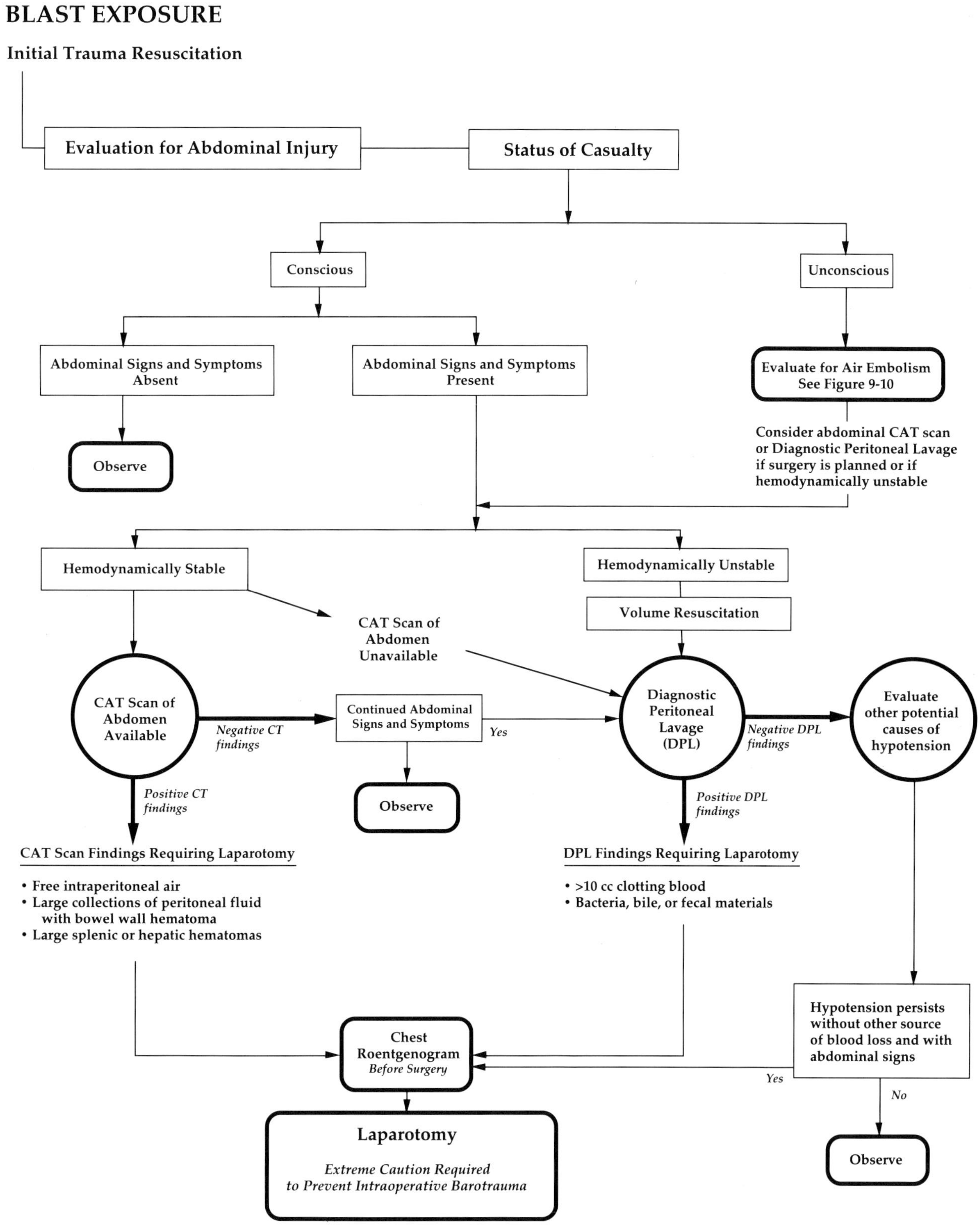

Fig. 9-15. Algorithm for the evaluation of a blast casualty's gastrointestinal injury

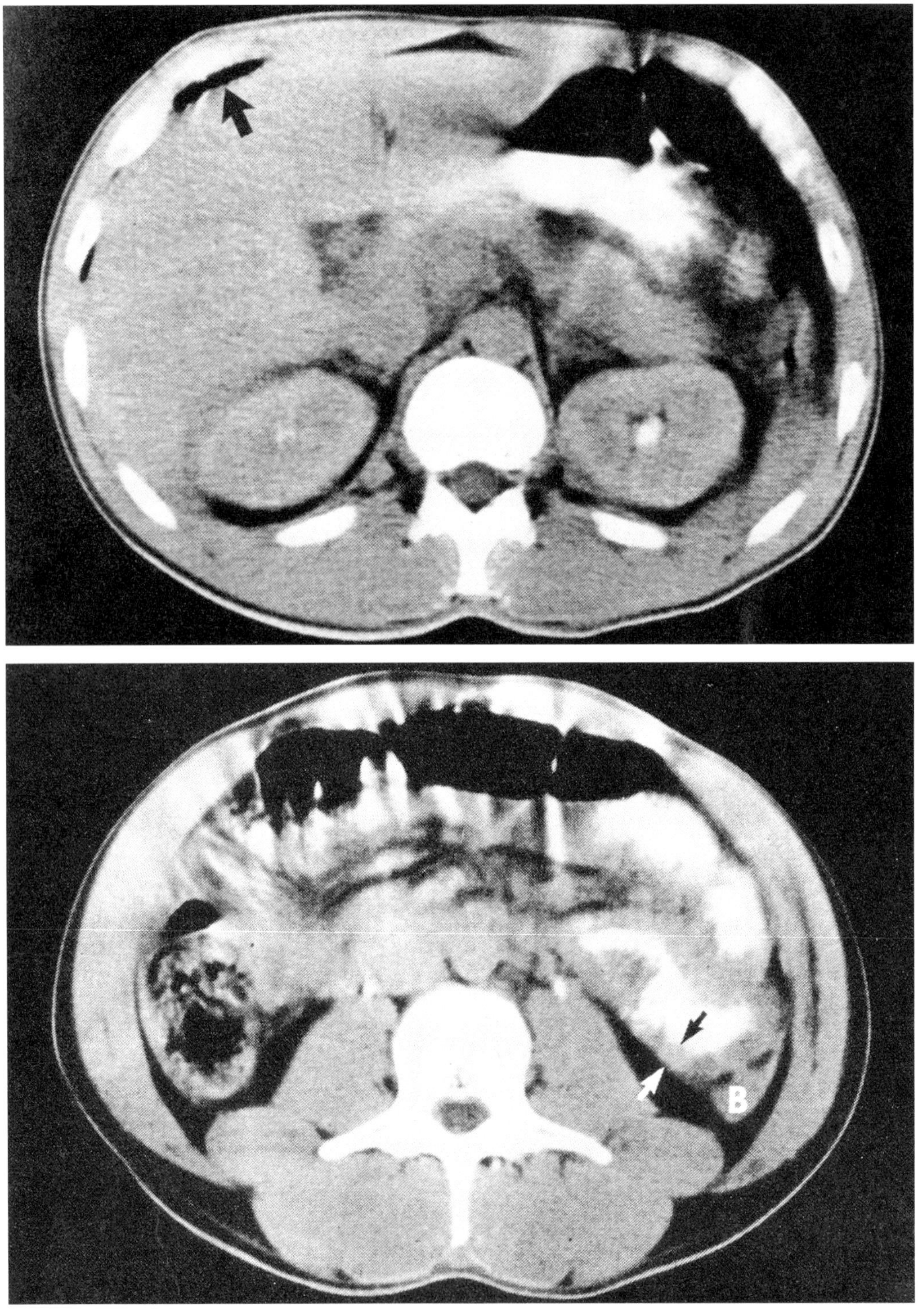

Fig. 9-16. The CAT scan of the abdomen in a blunt-trauma patient shows free intraperitoneal air in the right subphrenic space (arrow in upper image). The lower image shows a thickened jejunal bowel wall (10 mm between arrows); normal walls are 3 mm or less. Free blood is in the adjacent gutter (B).
Source: With permission from reference 64

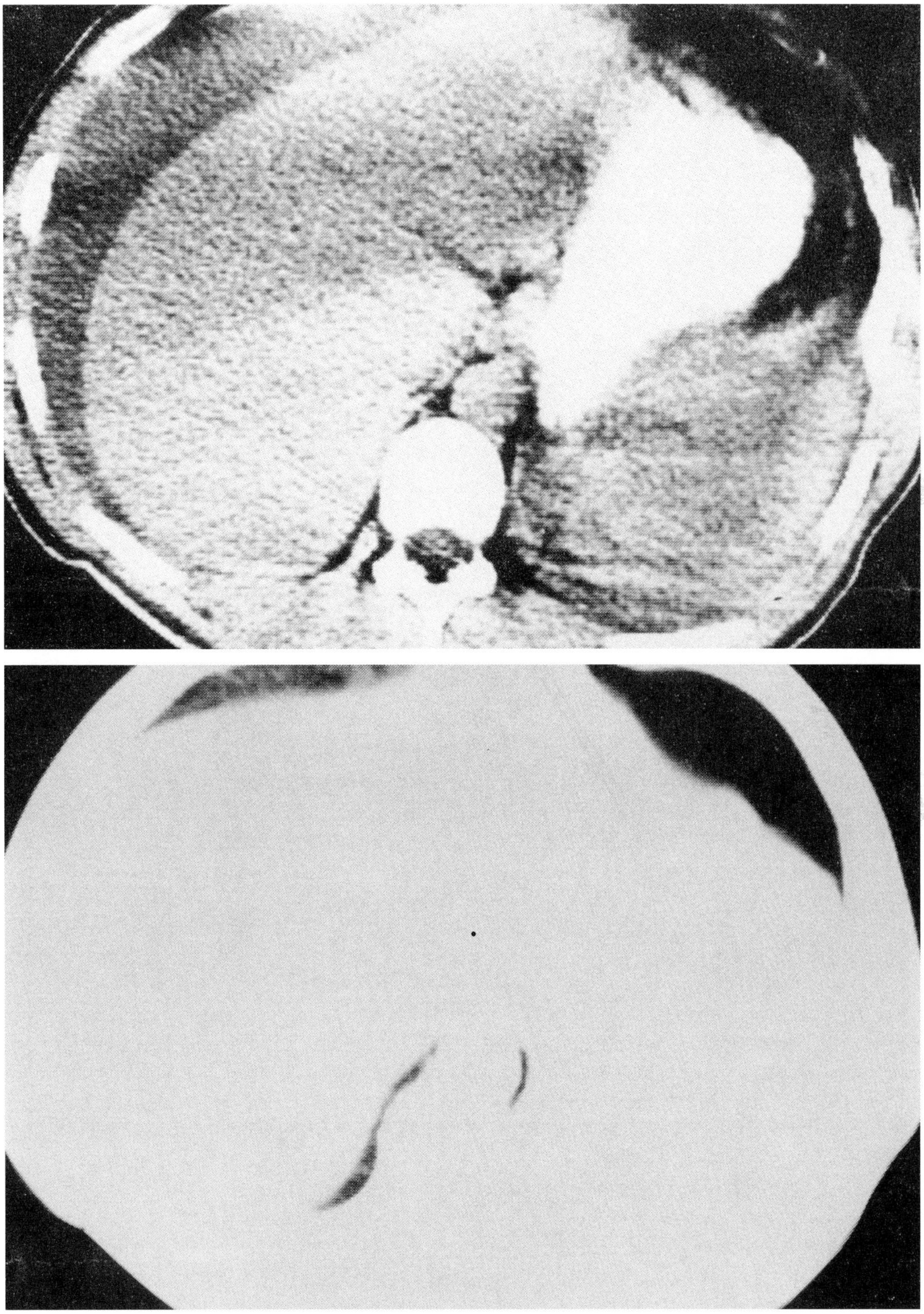

Fig. 9-17. This CAT scan of the upper abdomen of a blunt-trauma casualty was viewed with two windows. The soft-tissue window (upper image) reveals a lacerated spleen and accompanying hemoperitoneum. The lung window (lower image) is the same cut and shows a left pneumothorax. Note the difference between lung parenchyma in the right hemithorax and air in the left chest.
Source: With permission from reference 36

in the peritoneal cavity, thereby causing a false-positive imaging study.[64,73]

Most investigators have concluded that CAT scans are less sensitive than DPL for blunt abdominal injury. According to some studies, the radiologic technique identified only 25%–74% of patients who ultimately required laparotomy.[69,70] It was also insensitive to hollow-viscus injury.[71] Nevertheless, the CAT scan is the probably the imaging procedure of choice for blast casualties in whom gastrointestinal disruption is suspected.[73]

Ultrasound examinations of the abdomen may reveal small quantities of free peritoneal fluid or blood. For example, in civilian accident victims, sonograms detect 84% of injuries that require surgery.[65,68]

Radiologic studies of blunt abdominal injury may reveal unanticipated lung injury. For example, in more than 500 CAT scans of the abdomen, thirty-five pneumothoraces were evident, ten of which had not been apparent on the chest roentgenogram.[37] All CAT scans for abdominal trauma should be extended to include the lower chest, and should use both soft-tissue and lung windows (Figure 9-17).

Treatment of Gastrointestinal Injury

Unlike respiratory barotrauma and air embolism, significant PBI to the abdomen often requires surgical exploration and repair.

Surgical Treatment. The surgical approach to abdominal blast injuries is identical to that for any other blunt abdominal injury. The surgeon must be aware that pulmonary compromise may occur suddenly during general anesthesia and should take the appropriate precautions (discussed below). Copious saline irrigation will be required if the peritoneal cavity has been soiled by intestinal contents.

Bowel that contains a large intramural hematoma should be resected. Failure to do so may result in delayed perforation of the bowel. For example, in one blast casualty undergoing laparotomy, surgeons found only multiple hematomas and took no reparative steps. At a subsequent operation a week later, the bowel in proximity to several of the hematomas contained perforations.[16] A gut segment that includes a mesenteric hematoma that appears likely to compromise bowel-wall circulation should be resected. Small hematomas that do not appreciably thicken the bowel wall should be left alone.[66]

A disruption of the large bowel should lead to exteriorization of the colon. Simple perforations of the small intestine should be closed primarily; more extensively damaged intestine should be resected and reanastomosed. If surgery is greatly delayed, the devitalized small bowel should be resected and exteriorized.[3,20,42,66,74]

Lacerations of solid organs should be oversewn or resected as indicated by the injury's complexity.

The most important adjunct to surgical care is simple gastric decompression with a nasogastric tube, particularly in patients who receive mechanical ventilation.[61]

Complications of General Anesthesia. Blast casualties tend to suffer a high morbidity rate when they receive general anesthesia.[15,16,19,55] For example, three of twenty-four victims of an underwater blast who underwent laparotomy died intraoperatively or shortly after surgery.[16] In another review, one of nine patients undergoing laparotomy died in the operating room.[13] In yet another report, one of three casualties who had blast lung died during a simple tracheostomy as the result of bilateral pneumothoraces.[15]

Both barotrauma and arterial air embolism increase the intraoperative risk, but their incidence and severity may be decreased by keeping airway pressures low during the procedures. Whenever possible, local or regional anesthesia should be used instead of general anesthesia, and the duration of surgery should be kept short. The risk of added injury will be much less if surgery can be delayed for 24–48 hours after the blast event.

If barotrauma is apparent or suspected on the casualty's preoperative roentgenograms, chest tubes should be placed before surgery begins. Medical officers should note the presence on the roentgenogram of intraparenchymal lung cysts, which may predispose the patient to both pneumothorax and air emboli.[45] Periodic intraoperative chest roentgenograms may be useful during an extended surgical procedure. At any time during the procedure, the surgical team should be prepared to decompress the pleural spaces rapidly with chest tubes.

Even though access to the blast casualty may be very restricted during operations that require general anesthesia, monitoring is particularly essential during these procedures to decrease the risk of intraoperative arterial air embolism and respiratory insufficiency.[15] Such monitoring should include a continuous recording of *(a)* arterial saturation, *(b)* cardiac rhythm, *(c)* blood pressure, and *(d)* airway pressure.

The neurological effects of air emboli will be impossible to detect when the patient is under general anesthesia. Therefore, medical personnel should note any cardiac-rhythm or ischemic-electrocardiographic changes that may herald an embolic catastrophe. The anesthesiologist should periodically examine the patient's fundi for evidence of air emboli in the retinal artery (Figure 9-12).[5] If Doppler ultrasound probes are available, medical officers should monitor carotid-artery blood flow for evidence of embolic bubbles.[45]

Drug Therapy. The role of histamine-2 antagonists and prophylactic antibiotics in the treatment of abdominal blast injury is unknown. However, if surgery must be delayed for tactical, logistic, or technical reasons, the patient should receive antibiotic coverage for anaerobes, Gram-negative aerobes, and enterococci.

PRIMARY BLAST INJURY TO THE AUDITORY SYSTEM

The modern military environment depends heavily upon communication. The soldier must acquire and process a great deal of aural information and act upon it quickly and decisively. However, the nature of the combat environment may hinder the soldier from communicating effectively. High levels of background noise, the complex content of the messages, and the increasingly common possibility that neither the speaker nor the listener may be fluent in English make communication difficult enough for soldiers with normal hearing. A hearing-impaired soldier on guard duty or assigned to radio communication may be more of a liability than an asset.

The very nature of the auditory system makes it particularly vulnerable to injury during combat. Pressure waves in the air are collected by the pinna of the ear and are focused in the external auditory canal to act upon the tympanic membrane. The resulting pressures on one side of the eardrum cause it to distort; this movement is amplified by the ossicular chain and is transduced into the fluid-filled inner ear where it is converted into electrical impulses by the hair cells. In the normal acoustic range of pressures, this process is an efficient means of collecting and amplifying a weak air-pressure wave into a physiologically detectable variable (that is, sound).[2,17,75] However, the powerful pressure wave caused by a blast does not normally occur in nature, and it may overwhelm the extremely delicate structures within the ear. The tympanic membrane may rupture, the ossicles may fracture or dislocate, and so much energy may be transmitted to the inner ear that permanent damage will be done.

Aural injuries from blast may range from a trivial insult to a major disruption of middle- and inner-ear structures. Under the stress of combat, a soldier who has been stunned by a nearby explosion may initially be unaware of any aural injury.

The most common injury will be hearing loss, with or without tympanic-membrane rupture. The hearing loss may be *(a) conductive, (b) sensorineural,* or *(c)* a combination of the two.

A conductive hearing loss is defined as decreased hearing sensitivity to sounds transmitted through the air with normal bone conduction of sound. This loss is usually caused by a tympanic-membrane rupture, although ossicular damage and serous otitis can also cause a conductive deficit.[76,77] The amount of conductive hearing loss depends on the size and location of the tympanic-membrane perforation. In the past, medical officers considered the mere presence of perforation to mean that the soldier was unfit for duty. However, many soldiers can function well in spite of it, provided they have no other incapacitating injuries from the blast.[78,79,80]

Sensorineural hearing loss results from damage to the inner ear, and may be the most incapacitating aural symptom in the moments immediately after the blast. It is more prevalent in the high frequencies, but because it can also affect speech frequencies, it may compromise the ability of these casualties to communicate and may seriously disorient them with respect to their environment. Initially unaware of the deficit, they may notice the loss only when they see people talking to them but hear little or no sound.[81]

Sensorineural loss usually resolves within the first few hours, but permanent loss may occur in as many as 30% of blast victims.[18,82,83,84]

Blast-related sensorineural losses range widely in severity. Relatively minor injury may cause a *temporary threshold shift* (TTS) as measured by standard audiometric testing. TTS is a change in hearing acuity that ultimately recovers and that is presumed to be secondary to a transient and reversible biochemical or subtle mechanical cochlear dysfunction. More severe injury may cause longer-lasting or permanent hearing losses from *(a)* loss of hair-cell integrity, *(b)* labyrinthine or perilymphatic fistulae, *(c)* labyrinthine- or basilar-membrane ruptures, or *(d)* other defects.

Either conductive or sensorineural hearing loss may be a permanent complication in a significant number of patients. For example, in one study of seventy-seven military blast casualties, hearing loss was tracked for 1–3 years following injury.[84] Residual sensorineural hearing loss was found in 29% of these casualties' ears, 5% showed a persistent conductive loss, and 7% had a mixed hearing loss.

Tympanic-membrane rupture or perforation can be caused by a blast force as low as 2.5 kg/cm^2, and a blast force of 6.75 kg/cm^2 will rupture half of adult tympanic membranes.[85,86] By comparison, the blast would have to be about ten times stronger to cause severe lung damage.[2] Thus, tympanic-membrane rupture may be the only significant blast consequence for casualties of relatively small-scale terrorist bombings, and in fact does affect as many as one-third of these casualties.

However, the absence of tympanic-membrane damage does not preclude a significant blast exposure, particularly when the ear was not as exposed as other parts of the body, such as *(a)* during an underwater blast, *(b)* when a helmet shielded the ear, or *(c)* when hearing protection was worn.[2] Although almost two-thirds of blast casualties who have nonauditory PBI that is significant enough to warrant hospital admission will also have tympanic-membrane rupture, one-third of such casualties will have intact tympanic membranes.[18,36]

Other less common symptoms of auditory damage include *(a)* persistent otalgia, *(b)* distracting tinnitus, or *(c)* vestibular dysfunction, which manifests itself as vertigo.

Otalgia after blast may have numerous etiologies, including tympanic-membrane rupture, ossicular disruption, or concussive injury from other blast effects. The delayed infectious complications of middle-ear barotrauma might also cause otalgia, although it would probably not be incapacitating. Surprisingly, pain is not a common spontaneous complaint of blast casualties, although most do report ear discomfort when specifically asked.[81]

Tinnitus is a tone or ringing in the ears that may be caused by a persistent signal (in the absence of any sound input) from a damaged acoustic organ. It can be an unpleasant sensation that may distract a soldier from his or her tasks. Tinnitus tends to parallel sensorineural hearing loss, and will generally resolve as the hearing loss does.

Vertigo is the sensation of dizziness or irregular whirling motions that a casualty may feel after blast injury, although it is more commonly a symptom of blunt trauma to the head from secondary or tertiary blast effects rather than a symptom of PBI. Rarely, vertigo may result from PBI when both the cochlea and labyrinthine apparatus are disrupted by blast.[81,82] Such a loss of equilibrium can be expected to completely incapacitate a soldier.

Late sequelae of PBI to the auditory system may include *(a)* permanent hearing loss, *(b)* a predisposition to infection secondary to tympanic-membrane perforation, *(c)* persistent tympanic-membrane defects, and *(d)* cholesteatoma.[76,77,82,83] Cholesteatoma is a granulomatous mass lesion of the middle ear that may ultimately destroy middle-ear structures and cause a conductive hearing loss.

Initial Physical Examination, Triage, and Evacuation

The evaluation of a blast casualty with auditory damage may differ dramatically depending on the situation in which it occurs. Ideally, the casualty would be evacuated to a third-echelon facility and would there be evaluated by an otolaryngologist according to subjective and objective data as well as audiological and microscopic examination. In wartime, these procedures would be luxuries.

In combat, soldiers who suffer isolated blast injury of the ear would be evaluated according to their ability to continue their combat mission. The medical officer should weigh the casualty's current auditory injury, related performance decrement, and risk of suffering further impairment against the unit's need for the casualty's continued participation. For example, a soldier who has a small perforation of the tympanic membrane with no subjective hearing deficit could expect spontaneous healing within 2 weeks, and therefore would not be transferred to an evacuation hospital. On the other hand, a soldier who has severe hearing loss imposed by significant TTS might be nonfunctional in combat.

If the ears of these casualties are not protected from further damage while the initial auditory injury is healing, their hearing impairment may become worse or even permanent. If possible, they should be reassigned to quieter military duties. For example, 433 Israeli soldiers who had hearing loss or tinnitus or both were divided into two groups: *(a)* those who were transferred to a quieter noncombat unit and *(b)* those remaining in the noisy combat units.[80] The hearing of 30.8% of those soldiers who were transferred to less noisy environments improved; the hearing of 4.0% of the soldiers in this group deteriorated. In the group of soldiers who were not transferred, only 8.7% of the injured ears improved, whereas 30.4% deteriorated.

Even if an active combat situation demands that these casualties not be reassigned to quieter environments, they should at least wear hearing protection (either insertional or circumaural) whenever possible after injury. The protectors will decrease the effects not only of subsequent blasts and the sustained impulse noise of weapons, but also the continuous noise of engines, helicopters, and armored-vehicle tracks.

Once the blast casualty is stabilized and any other blast-related injuries (such as PBI to other areas of the body, lacerations, fractures, burns, or penetrating wounds) are assessed, medical officers may have the opportunity to note the following signs and symptoms of possible PBI to the ear:

- The size and location of any tympanic-membrane perforation that may be visible upon otoscopic examination
- The hearing level, using any subjective or objective means available
- The presence of any foreign material in the ear
- Any dislocation of ossicles that may be seen behind a torn tympanic membrane
- The presence of tinnitus, otalgia, or bleeding from the ear
- The pressure sensation of eustachian-tube blockage
- Vertigo

Medical personnel should also note information about any pre-existing hearing loss that the casualty might have had. After the casualty's record has been established, the time course of the hearing loss from this injury and any spontaneous resolution must be noted and, if possible, documented audiometrically.

Casualties who have suffered only auditory PBI should be placed in the delayed or minimal triage categories.

Although significant pain may result from inadequate decompression of the middle ear during a nonpressurized flight, no special precautions need to be taken when evacuating blast casualties who have suffered auditory damage.

Definitive Physical Examination

The signs of blast-related aural injury are usually clearly visible to the examining physician, and include *(a)* tympanic-membrane perforation, *(b)* foreign material in the ear, *(c)* ossicular damage, and *(d)* inner-ear damage.

If the casualty is experiencing vertigo in the absence of other aural signs, then the medical officer should suspect closed head injury and look for other evidence of neurological compromise. Closed head injury is potentially serious and requires more sophisticated evaluation than a cursory examination can provide.

Tympanic-Membrane Perforation. By far, the single most common aural injury is tympanic-membrane perforation. Although these ear problems are usually symptomatic (with otalgia, hearing loss, or tinnitus), they may also be silent.[87,88] The ear nearest the explosion is usually more severely damaged, but the blast wave can reflect off nearby walls to damage the contralateral ear.[81] The most susceptible portion of the tympanic membrane is the pars tensa; the least susceptible seems to be the pars flaccida.

The size of perforation appears to be related to the spontaneous healing rate and thus may be a useful criterion for surgical intervention. Table 9-6 lists the incidence of tympanic-membrane perforation and the spontaneous healing rate reported in the various studies.[89] One study found that as many as 90% of casualties who had a perforation that was smaller than one-third of the tympanic membrane healed by themselves, whereas the spontaneous healing rate of casualties who had a perforation larger than one-third of the membrane was less than 25%.[90] In another study, when perforations involved more than 80% of the tympanic membrane, none of the membranes healed spontaneously. All perforations that were smaller than 80% of the membrane, however, did heal by themselves.[81] One useful index for physicians who need to estimate the likelihood of spontaneous healing might be the loss of half of the tympanic-membrane area.

The presence of a ruptured tympanic membrane indicates that the cochlea may have been damaged as well. The casualty's hearing acuity should be evaluated as soon as audiometric equipment is available.

By itself, the rupture of a tympanic membrane by a blast overpressure is not likely to be the cause of significant acute disability. Fewer than 5% of such cases will involve incapacitating pain or balance disturbance. Barring infection, the vast majority will heal without intervention. Some 10%–20% will ultimately require surgical closure, and a small percentage may be chronically infected or develop cholesteatoma.

Foreign Matter. The medical officer should examine both the external auditory canal and the middle-ear space (if perforation has occurred) for foreign matter, which may include material from the soldier's external environment or material that the soldier placed in the ear as a form of self-protection.

In addition, because the disruption of the tympanic membrane is caused by the positive phase of blast overpressure, squamous epithelium from a ruptured tympanic membrane may have been blown into the middle-ear space. The edges of the tympanic-membrane perforation may have been inverted under the remaining portion of the membrane, and the inwardly folded perforation edges may provide an avenue for the later ingrowth of squamous epithelium.

Either the inverted edges of the perforation or squamous epithelium that has been driven into the middle ear may result in the formation of cholesteatoma over time, and the medical officer should consider this complication when planning the management of blast-injury perforations.

TABLE 9-6

TYMPANIC MEMBRANE PERFORATION

Blast Incidents	Number of Patients	Number of Perforated Tympanic Membranes	Percentage of Ears with Perforations	Percentage of Ears that Healed Spontaneously
Restaurant in Belfast, Ireland (1972)	101	66	33	83
Two pubs in Birmingham, England (1974)	111	29	13	82
Police station in Shaker Heights, Ohio (1970)	7	11	79	*
Indo-Pakistani conflict (1965)	41	52	63	78
Two explosions: sinking of destroyer by missiles (1967); explosion of truck carrying explosives (1970)	77	82	53	88
Combat-related blast incidents: truck bombing, rocket-propelled grenade, and landmine explosions	37	39	53	**

*All repaired surgically
**Not reported
Source: *Ann. Oto. Rhinol. Laryngol.* 98: 9–12, 1989

Ossicular Damage. The medical officer should carefully evaluate the integrity of the ossicular chain. Although ossicular damage is generally associated with large tympanic-membrane perforations, the ossicles may be fractured or dislocated even if the tympanum is intact.

In a study of ossicular damage in casualties who had tympanic-membrane ruptures during the Vietnam War, the most common abnormality (25%) was medial displacement of the malleus handle with disruption of the incudomalleolar joint and adherence of the tip of the malleus to the promontory.[77] Of the incus and stapes abnormalities (8.4% of cases), incudostapedial joint separation (four cases) was most common, followed by incudostapedial joint separation with fracture of the stapes superstructure (one case). In one case of ossicular damage that was sustained when a shell burst 50 yards away from a soldier, his incudomalleolar joint was dislocated, the incus was lying free in the hypotympanum, and both stapedial crura were also fractured.[86]

Inner-Ear Damage. Inner-ear damage (other than hearing loss) as a result of blast is uncommon, but medical officers should be aware that it can occur even without ossicular damage.[76,82,85,91] Inner-ear damage may include *(a)* perilymphatic fistulae in the oval window,[92] *(b)* dislocated stapes,[93] or *(c)* ruptures of the saccule, utricle, and basilar membrane.[76,82,85,91] Such injuries would be associated with a profound hearing loss and the presence of a clear otorrhea.

An otolaryngologist at a rear-echelon facility would have to make a precise delineation of the location and degree of damage.

Cholesteatoma. Most cases of cholesteatoma are believed to be the result of chronic inflammation and the subsequent development of granulomas around ectopic epithelium that has been displaced by trauma or infection. An otologic surgeon should provide long-term follow-up and careful surveillance to blast casualties. Although one study of 5,200 terrorist-blast casualties reported only two cases of cholesteatoma, this complication may be clinically silent for years.[76,82,85,91]

Diagnostic Screening Procedures

Evaluation of hearing sensitivity will often start with the recognition of a hearing deficit at the time of the initial interview, but quantification of aural loss will require formal audiometric testing at a higher echelon.

Audiometric measures of hearing threshold with both air and bone conduction can be used to distinguish sensorineural hearing loss (in which both will be decreased) from conductive loss (in which the bone threshold is normal). In one report, for example, thirty-seven soldiers were victims of a truck bombing, rocket-propelled grenade detonations, or landmine explosions.[79] Twenty-six of the thirty-seven soldiers (70.3%) suffered either unilateral (thirteen soldiers) or bilateral (thirteen soldiers) tympanic-membrane perforations. Thus, 52.7% of the seventy-four ears at risk were ruptured. When the soldiers were given routine audiometric testing, 6.8% of them had pure conductive loss, 44.6% of them had pure sensorineural hearing loss, and 41.9% of them had a mixed hearing loss.

Auditory brainstem response (ABR) audiometry may help the medical officer evaluate blast injuries of the ear. This sophisticated technique uses a machine that measures brain-wave response to sound. ABR audiometry studies have correlated the types of hearing loss after blast injury with the prognosis for recovery.

The field surgeon is unlikely to have audiometric testing equipment available and will have to assess the degree of hearing impairment subjectively. The examiner can make a gross estimate of the casualty's global hearing by standing out of sight and testing the patient's ability to comprehend phrases spoken with varying degrees of loudness, from a conversational tone to a whisper.

Treatment

There is no specific therapy that has been shown to aid recovery from acoustic trauma, although some authorities would administer a course of dextran or corticosteroids in an attempt to limit the damage.[82]

Hearing Loss. If possible, casualties who have severe hearing loss should *(a)* avoid high noise levels, *(b)* be assigned to duties that do not require sensitive hearing, if possible, and *(c)* wear hearing protection.

Casualties who have less severe hearing losses will require individual disposition. They will likely be returned to duty, but should be advised to avoid noise and to use hearing protection to whatever degree they can in their duties.

Tympanic-Membrane Rupture. Basic treatment for a simple tympanic-membrane rupture consists of *(a)* removing debris from the external canal and *(b)* gently irrigating the canal with antiseptic solution.[21,85] In general, this injury does not require immediate attention in a combat setting. Care can be delayed for hours or days without serious adverse consequences.

Although blast-induced ruptures often resolved without surgical intervention, the chances of spontaneous healing and delayed complications were affected by *(a)* size, *(b)* location, and *(c)* time elapsed after the injury.[18,81,84,86,94]

Most perforations involving less than one-third of the tympanum will close spontaneously.[77] Blast casualties with this injury may be returned to duty that does not require sensitive hearing or expose the casualty to further auditory damage. If the perforation is small, isolated, and uncomplicated, the casualty should observe *water precautions* (that is, ensure that water or other nonsterile material is not introduced into the canal) to prevent infection during the course of healing. Neither antibiotics nor ear drops are recommended unless the casualty has an infection or drainage.[85] Auditory blast casualties will need to receive otologic examinations at regular intervals until the rupture is healed. As a rule, 1 month is usually required to heal each 10% of the tympanic membrane.[81] In some studies, perforations larger than 30% had significantly lower spontaneous-healing rates (0%–22%); definitive tympanoplastic surgery would be recommended for ruptures of this size.[81,95]

Posterior-superior perforations may later develop retraction pockets on the healing membrane or cholesteatoma.[97] The medical officer should carefully remove visible debris from the middle ear.

If no healing is evident 10–15 days after the injury, then complete spontaneous healing at any later time is unlikely.[82,96] Some clinicians, however, advocate waiting as long as 6 months to make this determination. An observation period of 2–3 months seems reasonable as long as there are no infectious complications.

If the rupture does not close spontaneously, the physician can treat it definitively by *(a)* patching it with paper or Gelfilm or *(b)* tympanoplasty with fascial grafting, with or without ossicular reconstruction.

A perforated tympanic membrane can be patched under a local anesthetic. The medical officer should clean the ear and remove any fragments of tympanic membrane from the middle ear. Torn edges should be everted and reapproximated under sterile conditions. A Gelfoam bed should be laid in the middle ear for support and a patch of Gelfilm or paper should then be applied over the perforation. This method results in consistent healing rates of more than 90%.[86] The possibility of late cholesteatoma may also be lessened by debridement and eversion of torn membrane edges.

Additional measures may include *(a)* cauterizing the edges of the perforation with trichloroacetic acid (especially if the patching is done long after the blast event), *(b)* relaxing incisions to permit better approximation of edges, and *(c)* using fascial grafts instead of paper or Gelfilm patches.[96]

Tympanoplasty is recommended for perforations that have not healed after 3–6 months or in failed attempts at patching. Tympanoplasty with a medially placed fascial graft alone has a success rate that is greater than 90%.[96] The techniques are beyond the scope of this chapter and would be done by an otologic surgeon in a rear-echelon referral facility.

Ossicular Damage, Inner-Ear Damage, and Cholesteatoma. The casualty will receive definitive therapy at a rear-echelon facility from an experienced otolaryngologic surgeon.

SUMMARY

Although most of our current understanding of PBI comes from animal experiments and terrorist bombing incidents, the medical officer will need to understand PBI in a more complicated military context. Blast casualties in war will enter a medical system that will differ considerably from what civilian casualties would experience. For example, the number of litters that can be allocated on the battlefield—if they can be used at all—may be few, and combat casualties with PBI may have to exert themselves at levels that would be discouraged among civilian casualties, even though to do so might exacerbate their pulmonary injury and the risk of air embolism. Unlike casualties of terrorist bombings, who would most likely be transported to nearby emergency rooms in ambulances, military blast casualties would probably be evacuated by air, and would require special precautions to prevent further barotrauma from air-pressure changes. Military personnel are more likely than civilians to be in an underwater environment that is threatened by blast, and thus are at greater risk of PBI to the gastrointestinal system. Aural injuries from blast might have serious personal implications for civilian casualties, but in a military setting the loss of the ability to communicate could pose a hazard to other personnel as well.

All medical personnel should be aware that excessive volume resuscitation may worsen the casualty's gas exchange, mechanical ventilation support may exacerbate both pulmonary barotrauma and air embolism, and general anesthesia for the blast casualty will be poorly tolerated.

REFERENCES

1. Yelverton, J. T.; Damon, E. G.; Jones, R. K.; Chiffelle, T. L.; and Luft, U. C. 1971. *Effects of irradiation and blast on pulmonary function in sheep* [Technical Report 2630]. Washington, DC: Defense Atomic Support Agency.

2. Phillips, Y. Y III. 1986. Primary blast injuries. *Ann. Emerg. Med.* 15:1446–1450.

3. Pyper, P. C., and Graham, W. J. H. 1982. Analysis of terrorist injuries treated at Craigavon Area Hospital, Northern Ireland. *Injury* 14:332–338.

4. White, C. S. 1968. *Rationale of treatment of primary blast injury to the lung* [Technical Progress Report DA-49-146-XZ-372]. Albuquerque, NM: Lovelace Foundation for Medical Education and Research.

5. Ponn, R. B.; Zatarain, G.; Gerzberg, L.; Hottinger, C. F.; Haase, W.; and Nelsen, T. 1977. Systemic air embolism in experimental penetrating lung injuries. *J. Thorac. Cardiovasc. Surg.* 74:766–773.

6. Phillips, Y. Y III, and Graeber, G. M. 1988. Blast injuries. In *Emergency War Surgery,* 2d U.S. ed. of *The Emergency War Surgery NATO Handbook,* edited by T. E. Bowen and R. F. Bellamy, 74–82. Washington, DC: U.S. Department of Defense.

7. Hutton, J. E., Jr. 1986. Blast lung: History, concepts and treatment. *Curr. Concepts in Trauma Care* 9:8–14.

8. Whelan, T. J. 1981. Surgical lessons learned in the care of the wounded. *Med. Bull. of the U.S. Army, Europe* 38:1–9.

9. Yelverton, J. T.; Viney, J. F.; Jojola, B. III; and Jones, R. K. 1971. *The effects of exhaustive exercise on rats at various times following blast exposure* [Technical Report DASA 2707]. Washington, DC: Headquarters, Defense Nuclear Agency.

10. Van Achterbergh, S. M. 1985. Anaesthesia for a patient injured in a landmine explosion. *S. Afr. Med. J.* 67:858–859.

11. Harmon, J. W.; Sampson, J. A.; Graeber, G. M.; Phillips, Y. Y III; and Richmond, D. 1988. Readily available serum chemical markers fail to aid in diagnosis of blast injury. *J. Trauma* 28:S153–S159.

12. Melzer, E.; Hersche, M.; Fischer, D.; and Hershko, C. 1986. Disseminated intravascular coagulation and hypopotassemia associated with blast lung injury. *Chest* 89:690–693.

13. Hirsch, M., and Bazini, J. 1969. Blast injury of the chest. *Clin. Radiol.* 20:362–370.

14. Wagner, R. B., and Jamieson, P. M. 1989. Pulmonary contusion: Evaluation and classification by computed tomograpy. *Surg. Clin. North Am.* 69:31–40.

15. Caseby, N. G., and Porter, M. F. 1976. Blast injuries to the lungs: Clinical presentation, management and course. *Injury* 8:1–12.

16. Huller, T., and Bazini, Y. 1970. Blast injuries of the chest and abdomen. *Arch. Surg.* 100:24–30.

17. White, C. S.; Jones, R. K.; Damon, E. G.; Fletcher, E. R.; and Richmond, D. R. 1971. *The biodynamics of airblast* [Technical Report DNA 2738T]. Washington, DC: Headquarters, Defense Nuclear Agency.

18. Cooper, G. J., Maynard, R. L.; Cross, N. L.; and Hill, J. F. 1983. Casualties from terrorist bombings. *J. Trauma* 23:955–967.

19. Weiler-Ravell, D.; Adatto, R.; and Borman J. B. 1975. Blast injury of the chest: A review of the problem and its treatment. *Isr. J. Med. Sci.* 11:268–274.

20. Roy, D. 1982. Gunshot and bomb blast injuries: A review of experience in Belfast. *J. R. Soc. Med.* 75:542–545.

21. Hadden, W. A.; Rutherford, W. H.; and Merrett, J. D. 1978. The injuries of terrorist bombing: A study of 1,532 consecutive patients. *Br. J. Surg.* 65:525–531.

22. McCaughey, W.; Coppel, D. L.; and Dundee, J. W. 1973. Blast injuries to the lung. *Anaesthesia* 28:2–9.

23. Cope, Z. 1953. The general effects of blast. Chapt. 18, part 1 of *Surgery*, edited by Z. Cope, 652–664. London: Her Majesty's Stationery Office.

24. The Joint United Kingdom–United States Maritime and Marine Combat Casualty Care Workshop. 1981. *Ballistic injuries.* Alverstoke, England: Institute of Naval Medicine.

25. Uretzky, G., and Cotev, S. 1980. The use of continuous postive airway pressure in blast injury of the chest. *Crit. Care Med.* 8:486–489.

26. Adler, O. B., and Rosenberger, A. 1988. Blast injuries. *Acta Radiol.* 29:1–5.

27. Fulton, R. L., and Peter, E. T. 1973. Physiologic effects of fluid therapy after pulmonary contusion. *Am. J. Surg.* 126:773–777.

28. Wuensche, O., and Scheele, G. 1970. Die anwendung des diureticums Lasix bei druckstossverletzungen (The use of the diuretic Lasix in blast injuries). *Wehrmedizin und Wehrpharmazie* 9:113–117.

29. Wang, Z.-G. 1990. Research on blast injury in China. *Chuang Shang Tsa Chih* 6:222–228.

30. SCITRAN, trans. *Treatment and cure of blast injuries* (in Chinese) [Report HT 061-83]. Fort Detrick, MD: Armed Forces Medical Intelligence Command.

31. Bowen, T. E., and Bellamy, R. F., eds. 1988. *Emergency war surgery.* 2d U.S. ed. of *The emergency war surgery NATO handbook.* Washington, DC: U.S. Department of Defense.

32. Buffe, P.; Cudennec, Y. F.; Baychelier, J. L.; and Grateau, P. 1987. Les lésions laryngées par explosion (Laryngeal lesions caused by explosions). *Ann. Otolaryngol. Chir. Cervicofac.* 104:379–382.

33. Cooper, G. J.; Maynard, R. L.; Aldous, F. A. B.; Evans, V. A.; and Kenward, C. E. 1983. *Nonpenetrating injury to the chest: An experimental study of the biomechanical principles of lung injury, the pathology of pulmonary contusions and their acute physiological effects (U)* [Technical Paper 344]. Porton Down, England: Chemical Defense Establishment.

34. Jönsson, A. 1979. *Experimental investigations on the mechanisms of lung injury in blast and impact exposure.* Ph.D. diss. no. 80, Department of Surgery, Linköping University, Stockholm, Sweden.

35. Gordon-Taylor, G. 1953. Abdominal injuries due to underwater explosion (immersion blast). In *Surgery,* edited by Z. Cope, 664–672. London: Her Majesty's Stationery Office.

36. Rignault, D. P., and Deligny, M. C. 1989. The 1986 terrorist bombing experience in Paris. *Ann. Surg.* 209:368–373.

37. Wall, S. D.; Federle, M. P.; Jeffrey, R. B.; and Brett, C. M. 1983. CT of unsuspected pneumothorax after blunt abdominal trauma. *Am. J. Roentgenol.* 141:919–921.

38. Damon, E. G.; Yelverton, J. T.; Luft, U. C.; Mitchell, K., Jr.; and Jones, R. K. 1971. Acute effects of air blast on pulmonary function in dogs and sheep. *Aerospace Med.* 42:1–9.

39. Damon, E. G.; Yelverton, J. T.; Luft, U. C.; and Jones, R. K. 1970. *Recovery of the respiratory system following blast injury* [Technical Report DASA 2580]. Albuquerque, NM: Lovelace Foundation for Medical Education and Research.

40. Clemedson, C.-J. 1957. Respiratory and circulatory vagal reflexes in rabbits exposed to high explosive shock waves. *Am. J. Physiol.* 190:467–472.

41. Clemedson, C.-J.; Hultman, H.; and Gionberg, B. 1953. Respiration and pulmonary gas exchange in blast injury. *J. Appl. Physiol.* 6:213–220.

42. Mellor, S. G. 1988. The pathogenesis of blast injury and its management. *Br. J. Hosp. Med.* 39:536–539.

43. Hoff, B. H.; Flemming, D. C.; and Sasse, F. 1979. Use of positive airway pressure without endotracheal intubation. *Crit. Care Med.* 7:559–562.

44. Greenbaum, D. M.; Millen, J. E.; Eross, B.; Snyder, J. V.; Grenvik, A.; and Safar, P. 1976. Continuous positive airway pressure without tracheal intubation in spontaneously breathing patients. *Chest* 69:615–620.

45. Marini, J. J., and Culver, B. H. 1989. Systemic gas embolism complicating mechanical ventilation in the adult respiratory distress syndrome. *Ann. Intern. Med.* 110:699–703.

46. Hara, K. S., and Prakash, U. B. S. 1989. Fiberoptic bronchoscopy in the evaluation of acute chest and upper airway trauma. *Chest* 96:627–630.

47. Damon, E. G.; Henderson, E. A.; and Jones, R. K. 1973. *The effects of intermittent positive pressure respiration on occurrence of air embolism and mortality following primary blast injury* [Technical Report DNA 2989F]. Washington, DC: Headquarters, Defense Nuclear Agency.

48. Kogutt, M. S. 1978. Systemic air embolism secondary to respiratory therapy in the neonate: Six cases including one survivor. *AJR Am. J. Roentgenol.* 131:425–429.

49. Brown, Z. A.; Clark, J. M.; and Jung, A. L. 1977. Systemic gas embolus: A discussion of its pathogenesis in the neonate, with a review of the literature. *Am. J. Dis. Child* 131:984–985.

50. Hwang, T.-L.; Fremaux, R.; Sears, E. S.; MacFadyen, B.; Hills, B.; Mader, J. T.; and Peters, B. 1983. Confirmation of cerebral air embolism with computerized tomography. *Ann. Neurol.* 13:214–215.

51. Hill, J. F. 1979. Blast injury with particular reference to recent terrorist bombing incidents. *Ann. R. Coll. Surg. Engl.* 61:4–11.

52. Frykberg, E. R., and Tepas, J. J. III. 1988. Terrorist bombing: Lessons learned from Belfast to Beirut. *Ann. Surg.* 208:569–576.

53. Mellor, S. G., and Cooper, G. J. 1989. Analysis of 828 servicemen killed or injured by explosion in Northern Ireland 1970-84: The Hostile Action Casualty System. *Br. J. Surg.* 76:1006–1010.

54. Stapczynski, J. S. 1982. Blast injuries. *Ann. Emerg. Med.* 11:687–694.

55. Stapcynski, J.S. 1985. Blast injuries. In *Current Emergency Therapy '85,* edited by R. F. Edlich and D. A Spyker, 293–298. Rockville, MD: Aspen Systems Corporation.

56. Damon, E. G., and Jones, R. K. 1971. *Comparative effects of hyperopia and hyperbaric pressure in the treatment of primary blast injury* [Technical Report DASA 2708]. Washington, DC: Headquarters, Defense Nuclear Agency.

57. Bond, G. F. 1977. Arterial gas embolism. In *Hyperbaric Oxygen Therapy,* edited by J. C. Davis and T. K. Hunt, 141–152. Bethesda, MD: Undersea Medical Society, Inc.

58. Leitch, D. R., and Green, R. D. 1986. Pulmonary barotrauma in divers and the treatment of cerebral arterial embolism. *Aviat. Space Environ. Med.* 57:931–938.

59. The Undersea Hyperbaric Medical Society is located at 9650 Rockville Pike, Bethesda, Maryland 20814 (telephone 301-571-1818).

60. Spampinato, N.; Stassano, P.; Gagliardi, C.; Tufano, R.; and Iorio, D. 1981. Massive air embolism during cardiopulmonary bypass: Successful treatment with immediate hypothermia and circulatory support. *Ann. Neurol.* 32:602–603.

61. Harmon, J. W., and Haluszka, M. 1983. Care of blast-injured casualties with gastrointestinal injuries. *Milit. Med.* 148:586–588.

62. Pugh, H. L. 1943. Blast injuries. In *The Surgical Clinics of North America,* edited by W. H. Cole, 1589–1602. Philadelphia: W. B. Saunders Company.

63. Katz, E.; Ofek, B.; Adler, J.; Abramowitz, H. B.; and Krausz, M. M. 1989. Primary blast injury after a bomb explosion in a civilian bus. *Ann. Surg.* 209:484–488.

64. Donohue, J. H.; Federle, M. P.; Griffiths, B. G.; and Trunkey, D. D. 1987. Computed tomography in the diagnosis of blunt intestinal and mesenteric injuries. *J. Trauma* 27:11–17.

65. Jones, T. K.; Walsh, J. W.; and Maull, K. I. 1983. Diagnostic imaging in blunt trauma of the abdomen. *Surg. Gynecol. Obstet.* 157:389–398.

66. Stigall, K. E., and Dorsey, J. S. 1989. Transection of the first portion of jejunum from blast injury in accidental discharge of a (2.75 inch aircraft) rocket from an F15. *Milit. Med.* 154:431–433.

67. Sherman, J. C.; Delaurier, G. A.; Hawkins, M. L.; Brown, L. G.; Treat, R. C.; and Mansberger, A. R., Jr. 1989. Percutaneous peritoneal lavage in blunt trauma patients: A safe and accurate diagnostic method. *J. Trauma* 29:801–805.

68. Grüessner, R.; Mentges, B.; Düber, Ch.; Rückert, K.; and Rothmund, M. 1989. Sonography versus peritoneal lavage in blunt abdominal trauma. *J. Trauma* 29:242–244.

69. Marx, J. A.; Moore, E. E.; Jorden, R. C.; and Eule, J., Jr. 1985. Limitations of computed tomography in the evaluation of acute abdominal trauma: A prospective comparison with diagnostic peritoneal lavage. *J. Trauma* 25:933–937.

70. Meyer, D. M.; Thal, E. R.; Weigelt, J. A.; and Redman, H. C. 1989. Evaluation of computed tomography and diagnostic peritoneal lavage in blunt abdominal trauma. *J. Trauma* 29:1168–1172.

71. Peitzman, A.; Makaroun, M. S.; Slasky, B. S.; and Ritter, P. 1986. Prospective study of computed tomography in initial management of blunt abdominal trauma. *J. Trauma* 26:585–590.

72. Federle, M. P. 1983. Computed tomography of blunt abdominal trauma. *Radiol. Clin. North Am.* 21:461–475.

73. Fischer, R. P.; Miller-Crotchett, P.; and Reed, R. L. II. 1988. Gastrointestinal disruption: The hazard of nonoperative management in adults with blunt abdominal injury. *J. Trauma* 28:1445–1449.

74. Parks, T. G. 1986. Gunshot and bomb blast injuries of the large intestine. *Brit. J. Clin. Pract.* 40:7–10.

75. Phillips, Y. Y III; Mundie, T. G.; Hoyt, R.; and Dodd, K. T. 1989. Middle ear injury in animals exposed to complex blast waves inside an armored vehicle. *Ann. Otol. Rhinol. Laryngol. Suppl.* 140:17–22.

76. Kerr, A. G., and Bryne, J. E. T. 1975. Concussive effects of bomb blast on the ear. *J. Laryngol. Otol.* 89:131–143.

77. Sudderth, M. E. 1974. Tympanoplasty in blast-induced perforation. *Arch. Otolaryngol.* 99:157–159.

78. Anderson, J. 1984. An audiometric survey of royal artillery gun crews following "Operation Corporate." *J. R. Army Med. Corps* 130:100–108.

79. Brown, J. R. 1985. Noise-induced hearing loss sustained during land operations in the Falkland Islands campaign. *J. Soc. Occup. Med.* 35:44–54.

80. Melinek, M.; Naggan, L.; and Altman, M. 1976. Acute acoustic trauma—A clinical investigation and prognosis in 433 symptomatic soldiers. *Isr. J. Med. Sci.* 12:562–569.

81. Pahor, A. L. 1981. The ENT problems following the Birmingham bombings. *J. Laryngol. Otol.* 95:399–406.

82. Kerr, A. G., and Bryne, J. E. T. 1975. Blast injuries of the ear. *Br. Med. J.* 1:559–561.

83. Pratt, H.; Goldsher, M.; Netzer, A.; Shenhav, R. 1985. Auditory brainstem evoked potentials in blast injury. *Audiology* 24:297–304.

84. Ziv, M.; Philipsohn, N. C.; Leventon, G.; and Man, A. 1973. Blast injury of the ear: Treatment and evaluation. *Milit. Med.* 8:811–813.

85. Kerr, A. G. 1980. Trauma and the temporal bone: The effects of blast on the ear. *J. Laryngol. Otol.* 94:107–110.

86. Messervy, M. 1972. Unilateral ossicular disruption following blast exposure. *Laryngoscope* 82:372–375.

87. Walby, A. P., and Kerr, A. G. 1986. Hearing in patients with blast lung. *J. Laryngol. Otol.* 100:411–415.

88. Brismar, B., and Bergenwald, L. 1982. The terrorist bomb explosion in Bologna, Italy, 1980: An analysis of the effects and injuries sustained. *J. Trauma* 22:216–220.

89. Chait, R. H.; Casler, J.; and Zajtchuk, J. T. 1989. Blast injury of the ear: Historical perspective. *Ann. Otol. Rhinol. Laryngol.* 98:9–12.

90. Singh, D., and Ahluwalia, K. J. S. 1968. Blast injuries of the ear. *J. Laryngol. Otol.* 82:1017–1028.

91. Kerr, A. G. 1978. Blast injuries to the ear. *Practitioner* 221:677–682.

92. Strong, S. 1975. *Proceedings of the Irish Otolaryngological Society.*

93. Ruedi, L., and Furrer, W. n.d. *Das akustische Trauma.* Basel: S. Karger.

94. Gapany-Gapanavicius, B.; Brama, I.; and Chisin, R. 1977. Early repair of blast ruptures of the tympanic membrane. *J. Laryngol. Otol.* 91:565–573.

95. Ruggles, R. L., and Votypka, R. 1973. Blast injuries to the ear. *Laryngoscope* 83:974–976.

96. Kanimturk, E. 1979. Clinical evaluation of traumatic perforations of the tympanic membrane. *Int. Rev. Army Navy Air Force Med. Serv.* 6:523–526.

Chapter 10

A BRIEF HISTORY AND THE PATHOPHYSIOLOGY OF BURNS

WILLIAM G. CIOFFI, Jr., M.D.,* LORING W. RUE III, M.D.,** TERESA M. BUESCHER, M.D.,*** AND BASIL A. PRUITT, Jr., M.D., FACS****

*Major, United States Army; Chief, Burn Study Branch, United States Army Institute of Surgical Research
**Captain, United States Army; Burn Study Branch, United States Army Institute of Surgical Research
***Major, United States Army; Burn Study Branch, United States Army Institute of Surgical Research
****Colonel, United States Army; Commander and Director; United States Army Institute of Surgical Research, Fort Sam Houston, San Antonio, Texas 78234-5012

A BRIEF HISTORY OF BURN CARE

Burns have been recognized as threats to our well-being since fire was discovered. The Ebers and Smith Papyri (about 1600–1500 B.C.) contain the earliest known accounts of the treatment of burns. They describe the agents that the ancient Egyptians used, which included various oil preparations, plant extracts, and amalgams of animal tissue, and emphasize their proper sequence of application. The recommendation in the Ebers papyrus that a warmed, oiled frog be rubbed on the burn wound may establish a certain ancestral claim for not only topical therapy but also the brief application of a biological dressing. More importantly, these early accounts stress the need for regular wound examination, because the application of these various treatment agents depended upon the wound's appearance.

The Greeks in the fifth century B.C. stressed the importance of avoiding suppuration in the burn wound, and thought that cleansing and proper care of the wound were of paramount importance. The Roman physician Cornelius Celsus referred to burn care in his book *De Medicina*. This work is also notable for the earliest reference to the surgical care of burns, specifically the excision of burn scars. As the ancient Egyptians had done, Greek and Roman physicians employed poultices of various animal tissues—and even animal excreta—to care for burn wounds.

When gunpowder was introduced to warfare, the incidence of burn wounds sustained during conflict greatly increased. This stimulated a number of surgeons such as Ambroise Paré to propose various treatment regimens for gunpowder burns and projectile wounds. The first systematic evaluation of burns was outlined in Guilhelmus Fabricius Hildanus's book *De Combustionibus* in 1607. Hildanus, the father of German surgery, classified burns on the basis of their appearance; he was probably the first to ascribe the variations in wound appearance to the depth of the burn. He described the most superficial burns as red and blistered, deeper burns as withering but not charring the skin, and the deepest as those with eschar and charred skin.

Treating the Burn Wound

Modern care of burns involves either closed dressings or open exposure. In 1887, the Alabama surgeon W. P. Copeland first proposed an open technique of burn-wound treatment. He stressed a marked improvement in patient comfort, and many other physicians enthusiastically adopted this approach. The exposure method fell into disfavor because of the unavoidable problems of infection, and it was not until the late 1940s that Wallace of Edinburgh reintroduced the notion of open wound care, which is used by many centers today.

Local burn-wound care was greatly advanced when topical antimicrobial agents were introduced. These limited microbial proliferation and invasion through the burned tissue, and significantly reduced mortality due to invasive burn wound sepsis. In 1965, Moyer described using a solution of 0.5% silver nitrate applied as soaks; contemporaneously, at the U.S. Army Institute of Surgical Research, Moncrief described using topical mafenide acetate (Sulfamylon) burn cream. Subsequently, Fox introduced silver sulfadiazine in 1969. The effectiveness of each of these three agents has been documented through extensive clinical use, and together they comprise the therapeutic armamentarium available for topical antimicrobial therapy of burn wounds.

Developments in Fluid Resuscitation Therapy

Baron Dupuytren was the first physician to describe the importance of fluid therapy in burns, and made the first statistical study of burn patients in 1828, when he reported the mortality of fifty patients treated at the Hotel Dieu based upon their age, sex, and extent of burn. In 1854, Buhl made the association between the hemoconcentration that occurred in burn patients and that in cholera patients, due to their fluid loss. Modern concepts of fluid resuscitation did not appear until the beginning of the twentieth century, when the Sicilian physician Tomasoli, in 1897, and the Italian physician Parascandolo, in 1901, described treating severe burns with saline infusions. The first modern scientific evaluation of fluid management was conducted by researchers at Yale University under the direction of Dr. Frank Underhill. This study was based on about twenty patients who were burned in the 1921 Rialto Theater fire in New Haven, Connecticut. These investigators demonstrated that burn shock was the consequence of fluid and electrolyte shifts that occurred after the thermal injury, a concept that served as the basis for resuscitative fluid therapy following a thermal injury.

Subsequent studies by Cope and Moore, performed while treating patients who were burned in the 1942 Coconut Grove nightclub disaster in Boston, provided further information on the fluid, electrolyte, and protein losses that developed after a thermal burn. They demonstrated that the fluid losses that caused hypovolemia not only occurred through the burn wound itself, but also were a consequence of internal fluid shifts throughout the body. They concluded that large volumes of salt-containing solutions were important for adequate fluid resuscitation and proposed a "burn-budget" formula for estimating the fluid needs of patients with extensive burns, relating the patient's colloid-containing fluid needs to body weight.

Another specific formula for determining fluid requirements after a burn injury was reported by Evans in 1952. This formula, based upon the surface area of the burn and the weight of the patient, resulted from a combined research effort between the Medical College of Virginia and the U.S. Army Medical Research and Development Command. The Brooke formula, proposed in 1953, was a modification of the Evans formula. These early formulae recommended administering a volume of colloid-containing fluid that equalled or exceeded the amount of the crystalloid fluid component. It remained for Curtis P. Artz and associates at the U.S. Army Institute of Surgical Research to demonstrate the relative importance of crystalloid fluid and recommend a 3:1 ratio of crystalloid to colloid-containing fluid as the Brooke formula. In recent years, additional resuscitation regimens, such as the Parkland formula, the modified Brooke formula, and the hypertonic salt formula have been recommended to avoid the complications of either over- or underresuscitation that were associated with the early formulae.

Advances in Skin Grafting

Although Celsus, in about the first century A.D., first mentioned a surgical approach to burn injury, it was not until the 1870s that George Pollock performed the first free skin graft to treat a chronic burn wound. Wilms first excised a burn wound in the early twentieth century; he used skin grafting for later closure of the excised areas. The usual approach to the closure of burn wounds was *(a)* local debridement, to permit an adequate bed of granulating tissue to develop and *(b)* subsequent skin grafting. Dr. John Stage Davis, of The Johns Hopkins University, first employed the pinch-graft technique in 1914. This technique employed the application of many small (approximately 1 cm^2) full-thickness grafts, which were applied to a wound bed of granulation tissue, with the expectation that these grafts would eventually expand to cover the wound. Subsequently, surgeons observed that broad, thin sheets of split-thickness graft provided not only more rapid closure of the wound but also were less disfiguring cosmetically than the pinch-graft technique.

Blair first popularized the use of a long, thin knife to obtain these skin grafts. Padgett, Hood, and Reese improved on this and developed drum-type dermatomes. Dr. Harry Brown, while he was a prisoner of war in the Philippines during World War II, conceived the notion of an electric dermatome, and this instrument has greatly facilitated the harvesting of split-thickness skin grafts. In the early 1960s, Tanner developed a meshing device that permits up to a ninefold expansion of split-thickness skin grafts and reduces the need for multiple reharvesting of the few available donor sites on patients with extensive burns.

In 1970, Janzekovic described tangential excision, used to remove only the eschar and to produce a wound bed of bleeding dermis or viable subcutaneous fat, which would be immediately covered by split-thickness skin grafts. Although no prospective randomized studies have documented statistically that excising the burn wound improves the survival of extensively burned patients, tangential excision has been widely employed, and is now considered integral to burn-wound care.

Wound closure becomes a problem when the extent of the full-thickness burns exceeds the area of available donor sites. A variety of biological dressings and skin substitutes have been used to overcome such wound-to-donor-site disproportion and to provide temporary coverage of the burns until the donor sites can be reharvested. Allograft skin, first used by the French surgeon Riverdin in 1869, is the standard of biological dressings, but its storage requirements, limited shelf life, limited availability, and the possible transmission of disease from cadaver to recipient restrict its use. Other biological dressings have been used to avoid or overcome these limitations and to provide temporary coverage when autografting is not possible. In 1682 Canady reported on the use of water-lizard skin for wound closure and, since then, the membranous lining of eggs, and the skins of chickens, guinea pigs, rabbits, and pigs, and amniotic membranes have been used in the treatment of burn wounds. Porcine cutaneous xenograft, the most commonly used biological dressing, achieves biological union when infiltrated by the host's fibroblastic tissue and, if it is left in place long enough, it undergoes necrotic slough but not a true rejection reaction.

Burn Research and Modern Treatment

Studies that clinicians and investigators at the U.S. Army Institute of Surgical Research have performed over the past four decades have yielded many additional improvements in burn care, including:

- documenting the pathophysiology of tissue injury due to electric current, which has led to improved care of patients with high-voltage electrical injury
- demonstrating the complications of using copper sulfate to treat white phosphorus burns, which has led to abandoning that treatment modality
- identifying the stereotypical gastrointestinal-mucosal response to burn injury that defined the central role of intraluminal acid in the pathogenesis of Curling's ulcers; antacid prophylaxis has essentially eliminated that cause of life-threatening upper-gastrointestinal hemorrhage in burn patients
- developing accurate diagnostic techniques that have permitted the early identification of inhalation injury in burn patients and the prompt initiation of therapy
- identifying the neurohormonal changes that orchestrate postburn hypermetabolism, in an extensive program of metabolic studies conducted by Soroff, Wilmore, Mason, and others, which has prompted the development of effective metabolic-support regimens
- revealing the immunosuppressive effects of burn injury on all limbs of the immune system, which serve as the basis for present evaluations of immunomodulation therapy

THE PATHOPHYSIOLOGY OF BURNS

Assessing the Extent of Thermal Burns

Various parts of the body account for roughly 9% (or a multiple) of the total body surface, and burn size can be estimated using the Rule of Nines: 9% of the body surface for the head and each upper extremity, 18% for each lower extremity, the anterior trunk, and the posterior trunk, and 1% for the perineum (Figure 10–1). The patient's palm represents approximately 1% of the body surface area, and that relationship can be used to estimate the size of small, irregular burns. A Lund-Browder diagram, which takes into consideration age-related differences in the proportions of body parts, allows a more accurate burn-size estimate, and is used by most burn centers (Figure 10-2). The patient's weight must be either measured or estimated.

The severity of thermal injury in terms of both the casualty's physiological response and survival depends upon *(a)* the size and depth of the injury, *(b)* the casualty's age, and *(c)* the presence or absence of inhalation injury. The LA_{50} (that is, the lethal area or extent of burn that is associated with a 50% mortality) is 53% for ages 0–14 years, 76% for ages 15–40 years, and 44% for those older than 40.[1] Depending upon the age of the patient and the extent of the burn, mortality may increase by as much as 20% if inhalation injury is present.[2] (These survival figures are based upon peacetime data with all patients receiving full care at a tertiary referral center that is utilizing essentially un

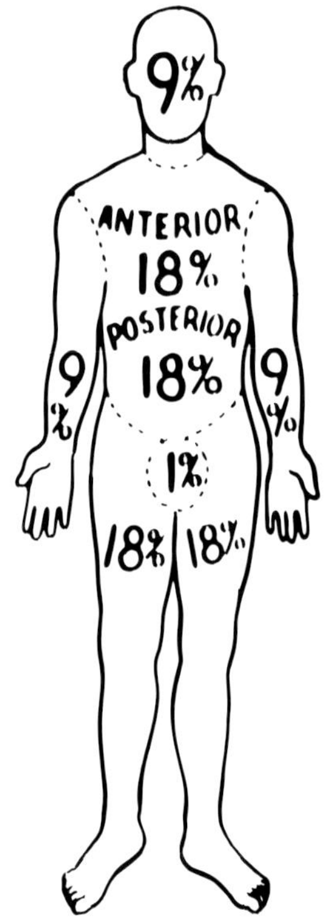

Fig. 10-1. The Rule of Nines can be used to estimate burn size. The surface area of various anatomical regions represent 9% (or multiples) of the body surface.

BURN ESTIMATE AND DIAGRAM

AGE vs AREA

Area	Birth 1 yr	1–4 yr	5–9 yr	10–14 yr	15 yr	Adult	2°	3°	Total	Donor Areas
Head	19	17	13	11	9	7				
Neck	2	2	2	2	2	2				
Ant Trunk	13	13	13	13	13	13				
Post Trunk	13	13	13	13	13	13				
R Buttock	2½	2½	2½	2½	2½	2½				
L Buttock	2½	2½	2½	2½	2½	2½				
Genitalia	1	1	1	1	1	1				
R U Arm	4	4	4	4	4	4				
L U Arm	4	4	4	4	4	4				
R L Arm	3	3	3	3	3	3				
L L Arm	3	3	3	3	3	3				
R Hand	2½	2½	2½	2½	2½	2½				
L Hand	2½	2½	2½	2½	2½	2½				
R Thigh	5½	6½	8	8½	9	9½				
L Thigh	5½	6½	8	8½	9	9½				
R Leg	5	5	5½	6	6½	7				
L Leg	5	5	5½	6	6½	7				
R Foot	3½	3½	3½	3½	3½	3½				
L Foot	3½	3½	3½	3½	3½	3½				
						TOTAL				

BURN DIAGRAM

AGE ____________

SEX ____________

WEIGHT _________

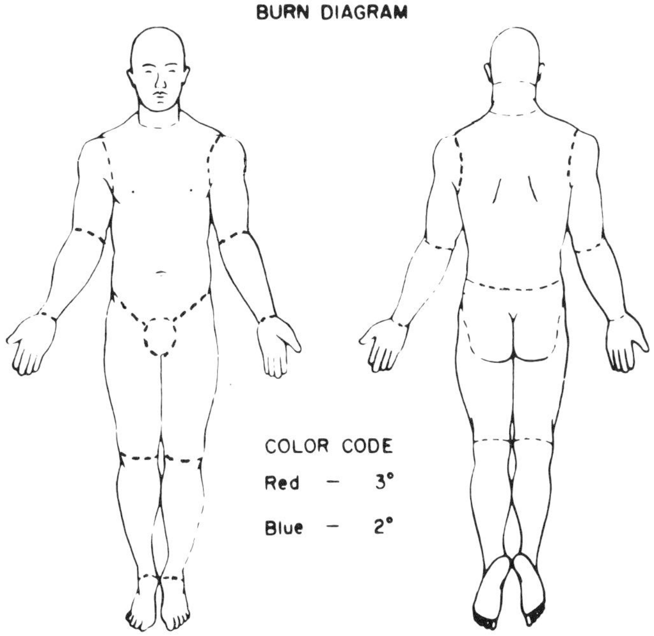

BAMC Form [illegible] NS
1 May 74

Fig. 10-2. A Lund-Browder diagram permits more precise estimates of burn size, based on age-related changes in anatomical surface area.

limited resources. They may not pertain in wartime.)

During combat, available resources must be expended on those individuals with the greatest chance for survival. Casualties at the extremes of age (that is, those under 10 or over 60 years old) or those with 70% of their total body surface area burned (TBSAB) will, in general, do poorly, and should be allocated a lesser share of the resources. The care of those casualties with less than 20% TBSAB can safely be delayed pending either their evacuation to a higher-echelon medical treatment facility (MTF) or the availability of more resources.[3]

Depth of Burns

The depth of thermal injuries may vary from involving only the superficial epidermal elements to the entire epidermis, the entire dermis, and even subcutaneous tissues (Figures 10-3, 10-4, 10-5, and Table 10-1). Superficial partial-thickness burns (that is, first-degree injuries) are erythematous, painful, involve only the superficial layer of the epidermis, and commonly heal within 3–5 days. Medium to deep partial-thickness burns (that is, second-degree injuries) are also erythematous, quite painful, and frequently have bullae. Because some epidermal elements such as hair follicles and sweat glands remain uninjured, these burns, if protected from infections, will heal primarily, although the time required for their healing increases with the depth of the injury. Full-thickness burns (that is, third-degree injuries) are white or charred, leathery textured, insensate, and involve the entire thickness of the epidermis and dermis.

Often, the depth of the injury cannot be ascertained immediately. Thermal injury results in concentric rings of varying degrees of tissue damage. A central zone of necrosis is surrounded by a zone of stasis, which, depending on the adequacy of the resuscitation, can either remain viable or proceed to cell death. This, in turn, is surrounded by a zone of hyperemia (Figure 10-6).[4]

Physiological Response to Thermal Injury

Thermal burns lead to alterations in the function of all organ systems. Their magnitude and duration are proportionate to the size of the burn, but reach a plateau when 50%–60% of the body is burned (Figure 10-7).[5]

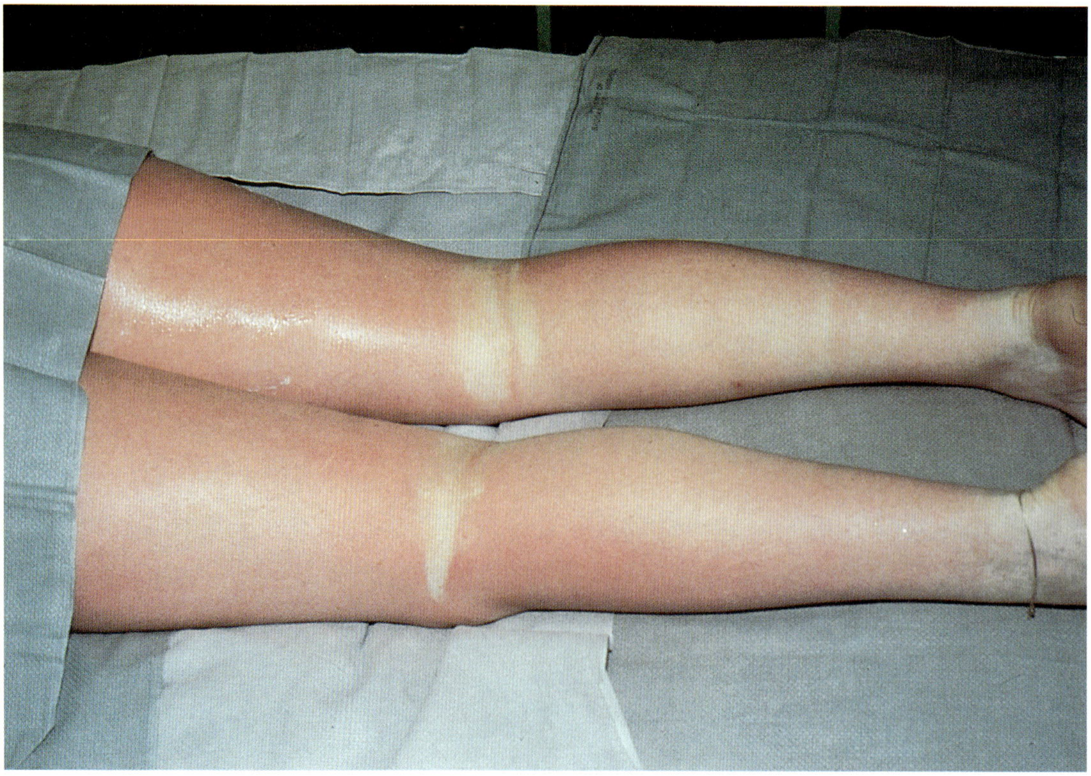

Fig. 10-3. A severe first-degree burn. The characteristic erythematous lesions (usually a sunburn) involve only the epidermis.

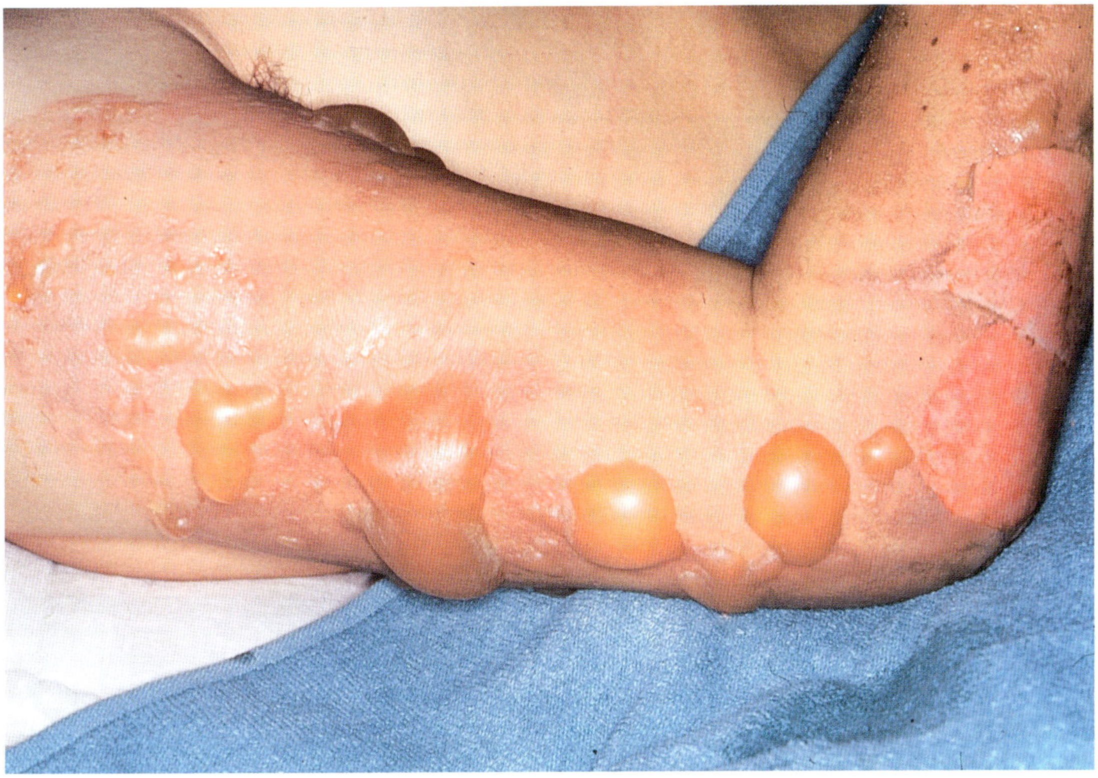

Fig. 10-4. A second-degree burn. Intact and debrided bullae characteristic of a superficial partial-thickness burn involving the entire epidermis and the upper layers of the dermis. These injuries should heal spontaneously in less than 21 days.

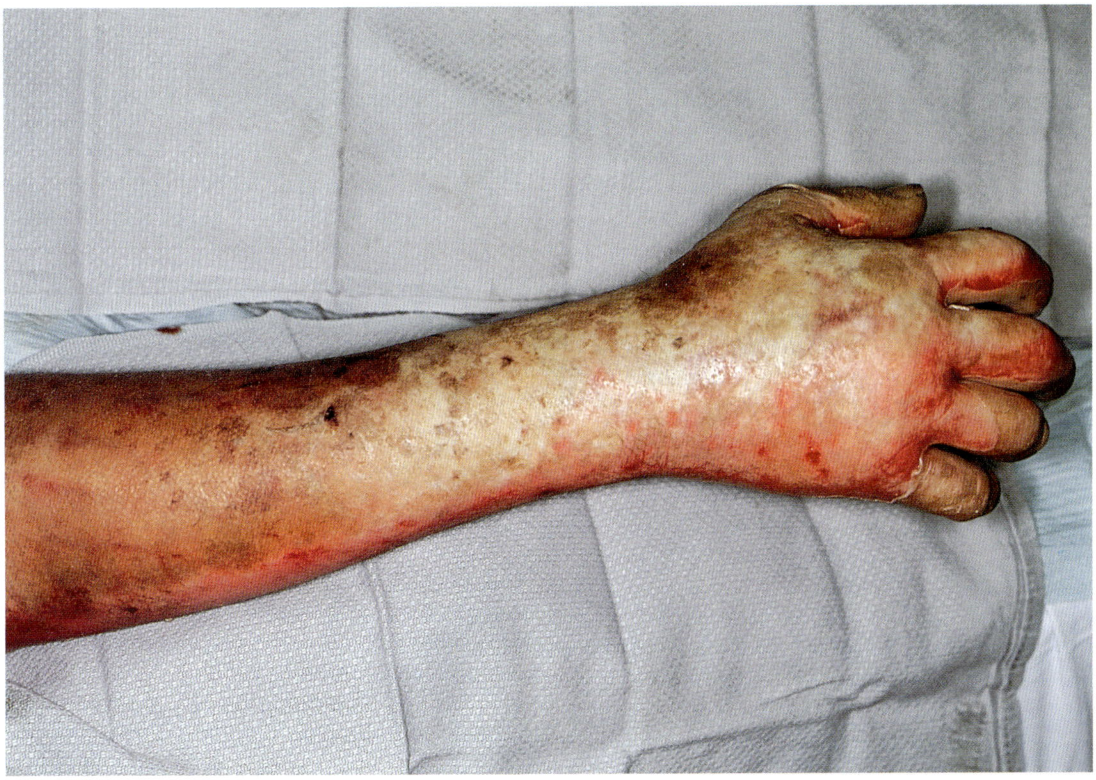

Fig. 10-5. A third-degree burn. The mixed deep-partial and full-thickness injury will require excision and grafting for optimal cosmetic and functional results.

TABLE 10-1

CLINICAL CHARACTERISTICS OF PARTIAL-THICKNESS AND FULL-THICKNESS BURN WOUNDS

		Second-Degree Burns		
	First-Degree Burns	Superficial	Deep Dermal	Full-Thickness or Third-Degree Burns
Cause	Sun, minor flash	Hot liquids, flashes of flame, brief exposure to dilute chemicals	Hot liquids, brief exposure to flame, longer exposure to dilute chemicals	Flame, high-voltage electricity, exposure to concentrated chemicals or hot metal
Color	Pink or light red	Bright red or mottled red	Dark red or yellow-white	Pearly white or charred, translucent and parchmentlike
Surface	Dry or small blisters	Variably sized bullae, moist and weeping	Large bullae, often ruptured, slightly moist	Dry with shreds of nonviable dermis, thrombosed vessels visible
Texture	Soft with minimal edema and later superficial exfoliation	Thickened by edema, but pliable	Moderate edema with decreased pliability	Inelastic and leathery
Sensation	Hypersensitive	Hypersensitive	Decreased pinprick sensation, intact deep pressure sensation	Skin insensate deep, deep pressure sensation present
Healing	3–6 days	10–21 days	>21 days	Grafting required

Typically, the physiological response to thermal injury is biphasic.[6] The initial period of hypofunction manifests as *(a)* hypotension, *(b)* low cardiac output, *(c)* metabolic acidosis, *(d)* ileus, and *(e)* hypoventilation. Serum glucose increases, oxygen consumption decreases, and the patient is unable to thermoregulate. This ebb phase, which typically extends for a variable portion of the first 24 hours, responds to fluid resuscitation. The flow phase, resuscitation, is characterized by gradual increases in *(a)* cardiac output, *(b)* heart rate, *(c)* oxygen consumption, and *(d)* temperature increase to supranormal levels. This hypermetabolic hyperdynamic response peaks 10–14 days after the injury and then slowly recedes toward normal as the burn heals naturally or is surgically closed by applying a skin graft.

Circulatory System. The alteration in capillary permeability that accompanies thermal injury is proportionate to the size of the burn and is greatest in the burned tissue itself.[7] The coagulation and complement cascades, white-cell products, histamine, serotonins, leukotrienes, and prostaglandins alter transvascular-pressure relationships and vascular integrity, and edema and volume depletion result.

Cardiac output falls as a result of both decreased preload induced by these fluid shifts and the increased systemic vascular resistance caused by both hypovolemia and systemic catecholamine release. Blood flow preferentially shifts from the integument to the viscera, although perfusion may be significantly altered in all organ systems.[6]

The goal of resuscitation is to minimize these effects. With successful resuscitation, cardiac output will return to normal within 12–18 hours, and during the second day after the injury, it may increase up to two- and- one-half times normal and remain elevated

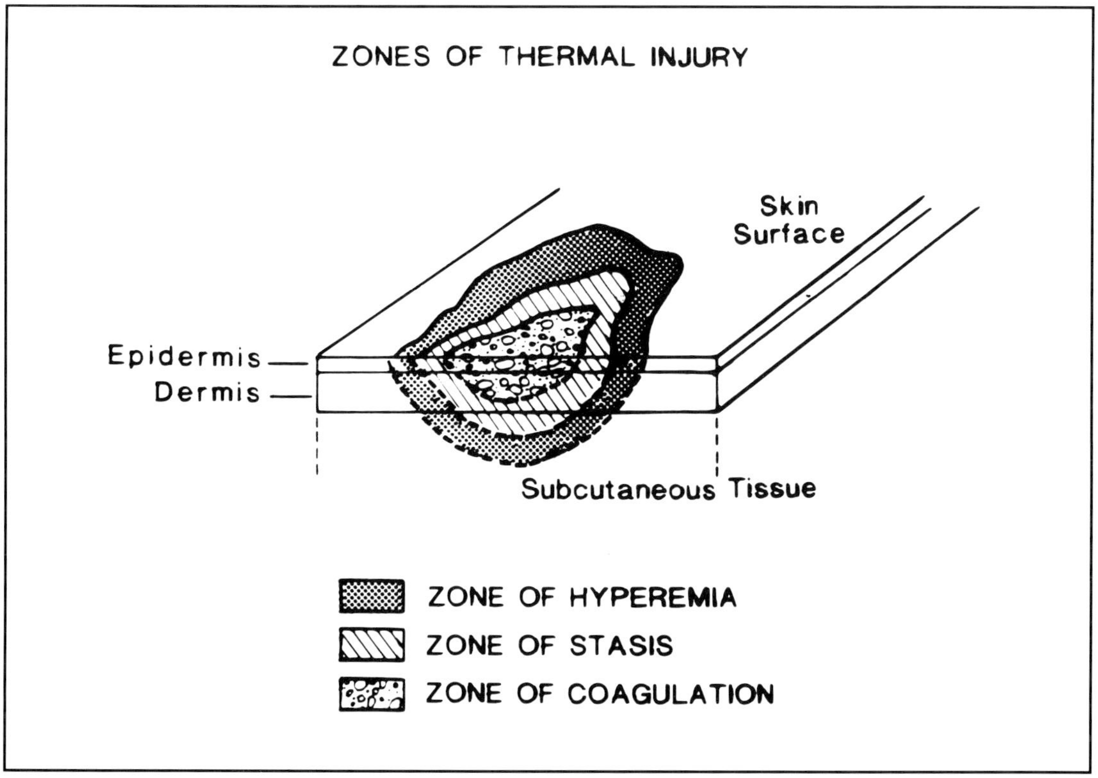

Fig. 10-6. Concentric zones of injury characteristic of the tissue damage caused by thermal energy. In full-thickness burns, the zone of coagulation involves the entire epidermis and dermis; in partial-thickness injury, only part of the dermis is involved.

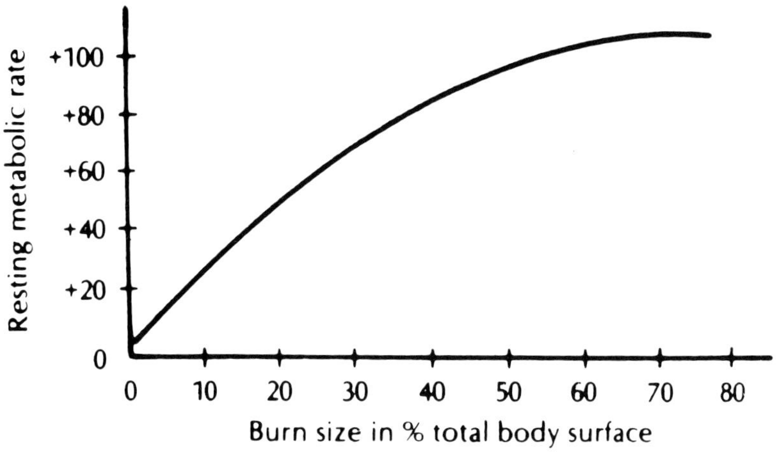

Fig. 10-7. The metabolic effects and all other physiological alterations caused by thermal injury are related to the extent of the burn, but usually plateau when burns cover greater than 60% of the body surface area.

until several months after the burn is closed (Figure 10-8).[5] After the casualty is resuscitated, the burn itself may receive a tenfold elevation in blood flow. This increase is due to the lack of autoregulation in injured vessels, and is also in reaction to both inflammatory mediators and the byproducts of anaerobic metabolism. Because the metabolism of burned tissue is largely anaerobic, local oxygen consumption does not increase similarly.

The red-cell mass decreases after the injury due to direct losses in the burn. Damaged cells are removed from the circulation during the first 4–5 days after the burn, which results in further net loss of red cells. Sampling for laboratory measurements can also cause iatrogenic losses of as much as 1–2 units of packed red cells weekly. Thrombocytosis and elevated fibrinogen, factor V, and factor VIII levels commonly occur, and a "normal" platelet or fibrinogen level may be an early sign of disseminated intravascular coagulation. In this setting, sepsis should be suspected, prompting medical officers to search for the source.

Renal Function. Renal blood flow and glomerular filtration decrease soon after the burn occurs due to *(a)* hypovolemia, *(b)* decreased cardiac output, and *(c)* elevated systemic vascular resistance.[8] Initial oliguria is followed by a usually modest diuresis as the capillary leaks seal, plasma volume normalizes, and cardiac output increases after successful resuscitation. This diuresis becomes most evident as peripheral edema is mobilized. The increased renal blood flow and glo-

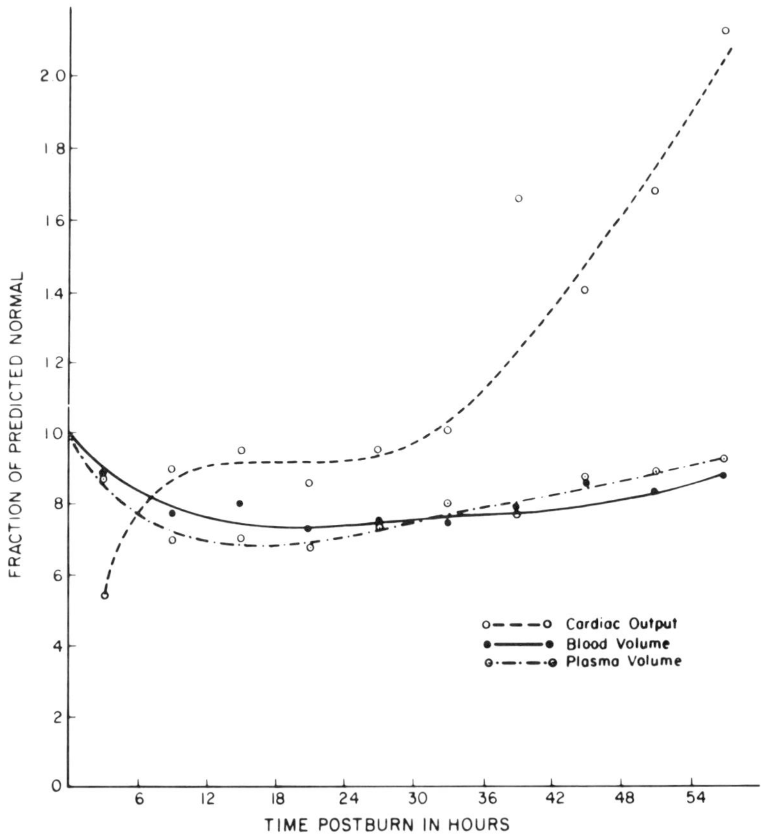

Fig. 10-8. The initially depressed cardiac output returns to normal 12–18 hours after the injury during fluid resuscitation, while blood and plasma volumes are still decreasing. After 24 hours cardiac output rises to supranormal levels, where it remains until wound closure is complete.

merular filtration rate associated with the persistently hyperdynamic circulation increase the rate of renal drug clearance. Consequently, increased dosages of drugs that are principally excreted by the kidneys are required.[8]

Gut Motility. Gut motility decreases in virtually all thermally injured patients whose burns cover more than 20% TBSAB, and manifests as ileus, which typically resolves 3–5 days after the casualty is burned.[9] Focal mucosal erosions may occur in the stomach and proximal small bowel because of splanchnic ischemia and progress to ulceration and perforation if their gastric-acid content is not adequately neutralized. Enteral alimentation, H_2 blockers, and antacids titrated to maintain gastric pH above 5 can virtually eliminate the life-threatening complications (bleeding and perforation) of stress ulcers.[10]

Pulmonary Function. Acute thermal injury alters pulmonary function in many ways. Elevation of pulmonary vascular resistance occurs to a proportionately greater extent than the increase in systemic vascular resistance and may protect against early pulmonary edema during resuscitation.[11] However, this increase in right-ventricular afterload may also alter right-ventricular cardiac performance. The lung parenchyma appears to be spared from diffuse capillary leakage because the ratios of pulmonary lymph-to-plasma protein are unchanged after a thermal injury.[12]

A small increase in minute ventilation occurs in response to the early hypovolemia. As resuscitation proceeds, minute ventilation continues to increase, and it peaks at levels proportionate to the size of the burn. The elevated minute ventilation is sustained by an increase in both tidal volume and respiratory rate. Infection, blood loss, fever, or using carbonic anhydrase inhibitors such as mafenide acetate may cause further increases in minute ventilation.

Endocrine System. Plasma levels of catecholamines, glucagon, and cortisol all increase, reaching maximal levels in patients with a 50–60% TBSAB, while insulin and thyroid hormone levels decrease.[13, 14] Mild hyperglycemia and obligatory nitrogen wasting occur. The metabolic rate may increase by as much as 2.5-fold and remain elevated for months after the burn is closed.[15] Catecholamines are partially responsible for this hypermetabolism; their levels are proportionate to the size of the burn, and the hypermetabolic response is partially abrogated by beta adrenergic blockade. As cortisol levels rise, the normal diurnal variation is deranged, and the response to adrenocorticotropic hormone is altered.

Thermoregulation. Alterations in hypothalamic function result in a readjustment of the thermal regulatory set point, with the zone of thermal neutrality elevated to an ambient temperature between 31–33° C. If an extensively burned casualty is inadvertently cooled and is unable to further increase his or her already maximally stimulated metabolic rate, both hypothermia and cardiovascular collapse may result.

Immune Response. Because the integrity of the skin is lost, this mechanical barrier to infection is impaired. Many immunological defects occur in burned casualties. Immunoglobulin levels are decreased and leukocyte chemotaxis, phagocytosis, and cytotoxic activity are impaired. The reticuloendothelial system's depressed bacterial clearance is thought to be secondary to decreases in opsonic function.[16, 17] These changes, together with a nonperfused, bacterially colonized eschar overlying a wound full of proteinaceous fluid, place the patient at significant risk for infection.

REFERENCES

1. Pruitt, B. A., Jr. 1985. The universal trauma model. *Bulletin of the American College of Surgeons* 70(10):2–13.

2. Shirani, K. Z.; Pruitt, B. A., Jr.; and Mason, A. D., Jr. 1988. The influence of inhalation injury and pneumonia on burn mortality. *Ann. Surg.* 205:82–87.

3. Bowen, T. E., and Bellamy, R. F., eds. 1989. Burn injury. Chapt. 3 in *Emergency War Surgery*, 2d U.S. rev. of *The emergency war surgery NATO handbook*, 35–56. Washington, DC: U.S. Department of Defense.

4. Jackson, D. M. 1969. Second thoughts on the burn wound. *J. Trauma* 9:839–862.

5. Pruitt, B. A., Jr.; Mason, A. D., Jr; and Moncrief, J. A. 1971. Hemodynamic changes in the early postburn patient: The influence of fluid administration and a vasodilator. *J. Trauma* 11:36–46.

6. Asch, M. J.; Meserol, P. M.; and Mason, A. D., Jr. 1971. Regional blood flow in the burned unanesthetized dog. *Surg. Forum* 22:55–56.

7. Arturson, G., and Soeda, S. 1967. Changes in transcapillary leakage during healing of experimental burns. *Acta Chir. Scand.* 133:609–614.

8. O'Neill, J. A., Jr.; Pruitt, B. A., Jr.; and Moncrief, J. A. 1971. Studies of renal function during the early postburn period. In *Research in Burns*, edited by P. Matter and T. L. Barclay, 95–99. Bern: Hans Huber Publishers.

9. Aulick, L. H.; Goodwin, C.; and Becker, R. C. 1981. Visceral blood flow following thermal injury. *Ann. Surg.* 193:112–116.

10. McElwee, H. P.; Sirinek, K. R.; and Levine, B. A. 1979. Cimetidine affords protection equal to antacids in prevention of stress ulceration following thermal injury. *Surgery* 86:620–626.

11. Asch, M. J.; Feldman, R. J.; and Walker, H. L. 1973. Systemic and pulmonary hemodynamic changes accompanying thermal injury. *Ann. Surg.* 178:218–221.

12. Demling, R. H.; Wong, C.; and Jin, L. J. 1985. Early lung dysfunction after major burn: Role of edema and vasoactive mediators. *J. Trauma* 25:959–966.

13. Pruitt, B. A., Jr.; and Goodwin, C. 1983. Nutritional management of the seriously ill burned patient. In *Nutritional Support of the Seriously Ill Patient,* edited by R. W. Winters, 63–84. New York: Academic Press.

14. Wilmore, D. W. 1979. Nutrition and metabolism following thermal injury. *Clin. Plast. Surg.* 1:603–619.

15. Wilmore, D. W.; Long, J. M.; and Mason, A. D., Jr. 1974. Catecholamines: Mediator of the hypermetabolic response to thermal injury. *Ann. Surg.* 180:653–669.

16. Alexander, J. W., and Wixon, D. 1970. Neutrophil dysfunction in sepsis in burn injury. *Surg. Gynecol. Obstet.* 130:431–438.

17. Allen, R. C., and Pruitt, B. A., Jr. 1982. Humoral-phagocyte axis of immune defense in burn patients. *Arch. Surg.* 117:133–140.

Chapter 11

THE MANAGEMENT OF BURN INJURY

WILLIAM G. CIOFFI, Jr., M.D.,* LORING W. RUE III, M.D.,** TERESA M. BUESCHER, M.D.,*** AND BASIL A. PRUITT, Jr., M.D., FACS****

**Major, United States Army; Chief, Burn Study Branch, United States Army Institute of Surgical Research*
***Captain, United States Army; Burn Study Branch, United States Army Institute of Surgical Research*
****Major, United States Army; Burn Study Branch, United States Army Institute of Surgical Research*
*****Colonel, United States Army; Commander and Director, United States Army Institute of Surgical Research, Fort Sam Houston, San Antonio, Texas 78234-5012*

INTRODUCTION

The interest that medical officers currently have in burns is disproportionately greater than the previous incidence of combat-related burns. One reason for this heightened interest is that, although the incidence of combat-related burns has historically been about 3%, in recent wars the incidence is higher because mechanized modern warfare—tanks and other armored vehicles—actually places soldiers at higher risk of being burned than they were previously. During the the Yom Kippur War, burns comprised 10.5% of all injuries; during the Falkland Islands Conflict, 18% of British casualties were burned.[1,2] Furthermore, medical officers should know that in the United States military, burns and inhalation injuries have always been far more important sources of morbidity and mortality in both the navy and the air force than in the army.

Another reason that burns receive greater attention in military medicine than their numbers would predict is that medical officers spend more time per casualty caring for burn patients than they do for other casualties. Many ballistic casualties will die within a few minutes from exsanguination, and blast casualties from air embolism, unless they receive immediate attention on the battlefield. Because the morbidity and mortality of surviving casualties evolve more slowly with burns than they do with other types of combat injuries, burn treatment is prolonged. Therefore, more extensive measurements can be made of the pathophysiology of burn injuries, and a comprehensive body of knowledge on burn trauma exists as a result. In fact, the pathophysiology of the human response to burns can perhaps serve as a model for the human response to all traumas.[3]

This chapter goes beyond considering the treatment of a typical combat casualty. The same fires and chemical or electrical incidents that injure soldiers may also cause collateral damage, and American medical personnel may be called upon to treat civilian casualties at the extremes of age—children and the elderly—in addition to the soldier population. Therefore, this chapter contains information that medical officers may require to treat these additional casualties.

Descriptions of the biophysics of thermal burn injury and the equipment available to protect soldiers from burns can be found in the TMM volume *Battlefield Environment*, and the epidemiological aspects of burns are discussed in great detail in *The Casualty*.

TREATMENT OF BURNS

One of the characteristics of military medicine is its provision of medical care by echelon. As this concept applies to caring for casualties with thermal burns, the first and second echelons have as their responsibilities *(a)* assuring that the airway is open and *(b)* covering the burn to prevent further environmental contamination. While the immediate care for burned casualties consists of not only that treatment necessary for any trauma patient, but also that treatment specific for burns, the care the casualty actually receives before being evacuated from the battlefield to a first- or second-echelon MTF depends upon the battlefield conditions. Ideally, the first responder will administer 100% oxygen, and if ventilatory exchange is impaired, place an endotracheal tube.

On the battlefield, thermal burns may occur in association with mechanical trauma and chemical and electrical burns, which can not only complicate the treatment but also increase both the morbidity and the mortality of patients with these combined injuries. Maintaining both the airway and the hemodynamic stability are priorities in treating burned casualties, as they are with any other trauma patient. Life- or limb-threatening injuries must be treated first, with the burn addressed only after the life-threatening problems have been adequately stabilized. The burning process must be stopped: Extinguish the flames, dilute and wash away the chemicals, or remove the casualty from contact with the electrical current. Initiate cardiopulmonary resuscitation if indicated.

After field emergency care, casualties with significant burns should promptly be transported to an MTF. If the casualty can be evacuated promptly, and if the evacuation will require no more than 35–40 minutes, initiation of intravenous fluid therapy can be delayed until evacuation is completed. If evacuation from the field echelons will be delayed, begin fluid resuscitation with Ringer's lactate. Most casualties are already dehydrated, not only because of their injuries but also because field conditions predispose to dehydration.

Burns should be covered with a clean sheet or dressing to prevent further contamination, and the casualty should be covered with a blanket to conserve body heat. If evacuation from the first or second echelons is likely to be delayed, consider applying a topical antimicrobial like Sulfamylon before dressing the burn. Wet dressings may decrease the casualty's body temperature and should be avoided. Burned extremities should be elevated, if possible, to prevent edema.

Although all U.S. troops should have been actively immunized against tetanus, foreign nationals may not have been; they may require both tetanus toxoid and immune globulin. Administer absorbed tetanus toxoid, 0.5 ml, and human tetanus immunoglobulin, 250 or more units, at separate sites and complete the casualties' active immunization in standard fashion.

Because careful wound observation is difficult during the evacuation period, administer prophylactic penicillin to attempt to prevent beta-hemolytic streptococcal infections.

Burn care at third and higher echelons consists of definitive fluid resuscitation, which is discussed below. Definitive wound care may be started at the third echelon, but will not be completed there. Most casualties with second- and third-degree burns and more than 20% TBSAB will require a longer time to recuperate than the combat-zone evacuation policy allows. They will need to be evacuated to a fourth-echelon MTF or CONUS, where excision and grafting will take place. Because burns frequently occur in accidents that may occur in proximity to third- and fourth-echelon hospitals, these facilities also must be prepared to render emergency, as well as definitive, care.

Fluid Resuscitation

Either in the field or upon the casualty's arrival at the closest aid station or larger facility, medical personnel should quickly establish intravenous access by inserting a large-caliber venous cannula in the largest available vein. The cannula should be placed through unburned skin, if possible, but if such a site is unavailable, then the intravenous line will have to be placed through the burn. Central venous access is not required for the immediate resuscitation of the thermally injured patient. Commence resuscitation by administering lactated Ringer's solution or another balanced salt solution.

Children with burns of less than 10% TBSAB and adults with burns of less than 20% TBSAB can often be successfully resuscitated with oral fluids only. However, even patients with such limited burns may have emesis if they drink large volumes of fluid rapidly. Oral fluids should be given in small amounts over an extended period of time. If emesis occurs, oral fluids should be restricted and resuscitation continued parenterally.

Burns greater than 20% TBSAB produce significant plasma-volume deficits that can lead to shock if untreated. The ileus that accompanies burns usually precludes oral resuscitation and mandates using intravenous therapy. Burn patients' fluid needs are related both to the extent of the burn and the size of the patient (Figures 10-1 and 10-2 in Chapter 10).

Fluid Resuscitation—Colloid or Crystalloid? Many formulae exist for estimating the fluid needs of burn patients in the first 24–48 hours after they are injured, all based upon the weight of the patient and the extent of burns (Table 11-1). Each formula recommends different amounts of electrolyte-free water, salt-containing fluids, and colloid-containing fluids, and each has proven to be effective in treating a large number of patients.

Because capillary leakage occurs in burned tissue, no discernible benefit has been noted when colloid-containing solutions were administered during the first 24 hours after the injury; some investigators have also reported that colloid-containing solutions have a detrimental effect on late pulmonary function.[4] Proponents of colloid resuscitation claim that *(a)* cardiac output is restored to normal sooner, and *(b)* the plasma-volume deficit is reduced earlier. However, by 24–48 hours after the injury, no clinically significant difference in cardiac output or plasma-volume deficit can be seen between those patients resuscitated with colloid-containing fluids and those given crystalloid fluids, and this treatment remains controversial.

The U.S. Army Institute of Surgical Research recommends using a balanced electrolyte solution, such as Ringer's lactate, during the first 24 hours of resuscitation and estimate the amount of fluid required by an adult as 2 ml/kg of body weight/% TBSAB. Because the capillary leakage is greatest during the first 8 hours, one-half of this volume is given during that period, with the second half administered during the next 16 hours. Fluid needs of children (who have a greater surface area per unit of body mass) are estimated as 3 ml/kg of body weight/% TBSAB.[5]

Regardless of which formula is used to resuscitate the patient, the rate that the fluid is administered must be adjusted according to the patient's response (Figure 11-1). The goal of fluid resuscitation is adequate tissue perfusion.

TABLE 11-1

COMMONLY USED BURN RESUSCITATION FORMULAE FOR ADULT PATIENTS

	First 24 Hours			Second 24 Hours		
Formula	Electrolyte-Containing Solution	Colloid-Containing Fluid Equivalent to Plasma*	Glucose in Water	Electrolyte-Containing Solution	Colloid-Containing Fluid Equivalent to Plasma*	Glucose in Water
Burn budget of F.D. Moore	Lactated Ringer's 1,000–4,000 ml 0.5 normal saline 1,200 ml	7.5% of body weight	1,500–5,000 ml	Lactated Ringer's 1,000–4,000 ml 0.5 normal saline 1,200 ml	2.5% of body weight	1,500–5,000 ml
Evans	Normal saline 1.0 ml/kg/%TBSAB	1.0 ml/kg/ %TBSAB	2,000 ml	One-half of first 24-hour requirement	One half of first 24-hour requirement	2,000 ml
Brooke	Lactated Ringer's 1.5 ml/kg/%TBSAB	0.5 ml/kg/ %TBSAB	2,000 ml	One-half to three quarters of first 24-hour requirement	One half to three quarters of first 24-hour requirement	2,000 ml
Parkland	Lactated Ringer's 4.0 ml/kg/%TBSAB	—	—	—	20%–60% of calculated plasma volume	As necessary to maintain urinary output
Hypertonic sodium solution	Volume of fluid containing 250 mEq of sodium per liter to maintain hourly urinary output of 30 ml	—	—	One-third isotonic salt solution orally up to 3,500 ml limit	—	—
Modified Brooke	Lactated Ringer's 2.0 ml/kg/% TBSAB	—	—	—	0.3–0.5 ml/kg/ %TBSAB	As necessary to maintain urinary output

*Administered as 5% albumin solution in lactated Ringer's

Hypertonic Resuscitation. Some investigators use hypertonic saline to decrease resuscitation volume in patients at the extremes of age.[6,7] The goal, in these volume-sensitive patients, is to limit the fluid loading that occurs during resuscitation. Only partial success has been achieved with this method, because either hypernatremia or cellular dehydration may occur. Both sodium levels in excess of 160 mEq/dl and cellular dehydration in excess of 15% appear to be detrimental. A study comparing standard resuscitation using isotonic salt solutions to resuscitation using hypertonic salt solutions showed that by 48 hours after the burn, most patients had received the same amount of free water and salt, regardless of the formula that was used.[8]

Assessing the Adequacy of Resuscitation. Urinary output, as an index of renal and overall tissue perfusion, is used to monitor resuscitation. In adults, a urinary output of 30–50 cc/hour indicates adequate renal perfusion. In children, a goal of 0.5–1.0 ml/kg body weight/hour is optimal. Urinary output greater than these amounts suggests excess fluid administration, and the rate of intravenous flow should be decreased if an osmotic diuresis can be excluded. The rate should be decreased by approximately 10% per hour until the urinary output falls within the guidelines mentioned above. Conversely, oliguria in the first 24–48 hours after the injury is almost always secondary to inadequate volume resuscitation and not to acute renal failure, and thus the rate of fluid administration should be increased. Blind adherence to any resuscitation formula will cause some patients to be either over- or under-resuscitated, with the morbidity that accompanies each.

Invasive monitoring is rarely indicated during routine fluid resuscitation of patients with thermal injuries. Periodic scheduled assessments of the patient's mental status, hourly urinary output, and vital signs usually indicate its adequacy. A tachycardia above 130 beats per minute usually indicates a volume deficit,

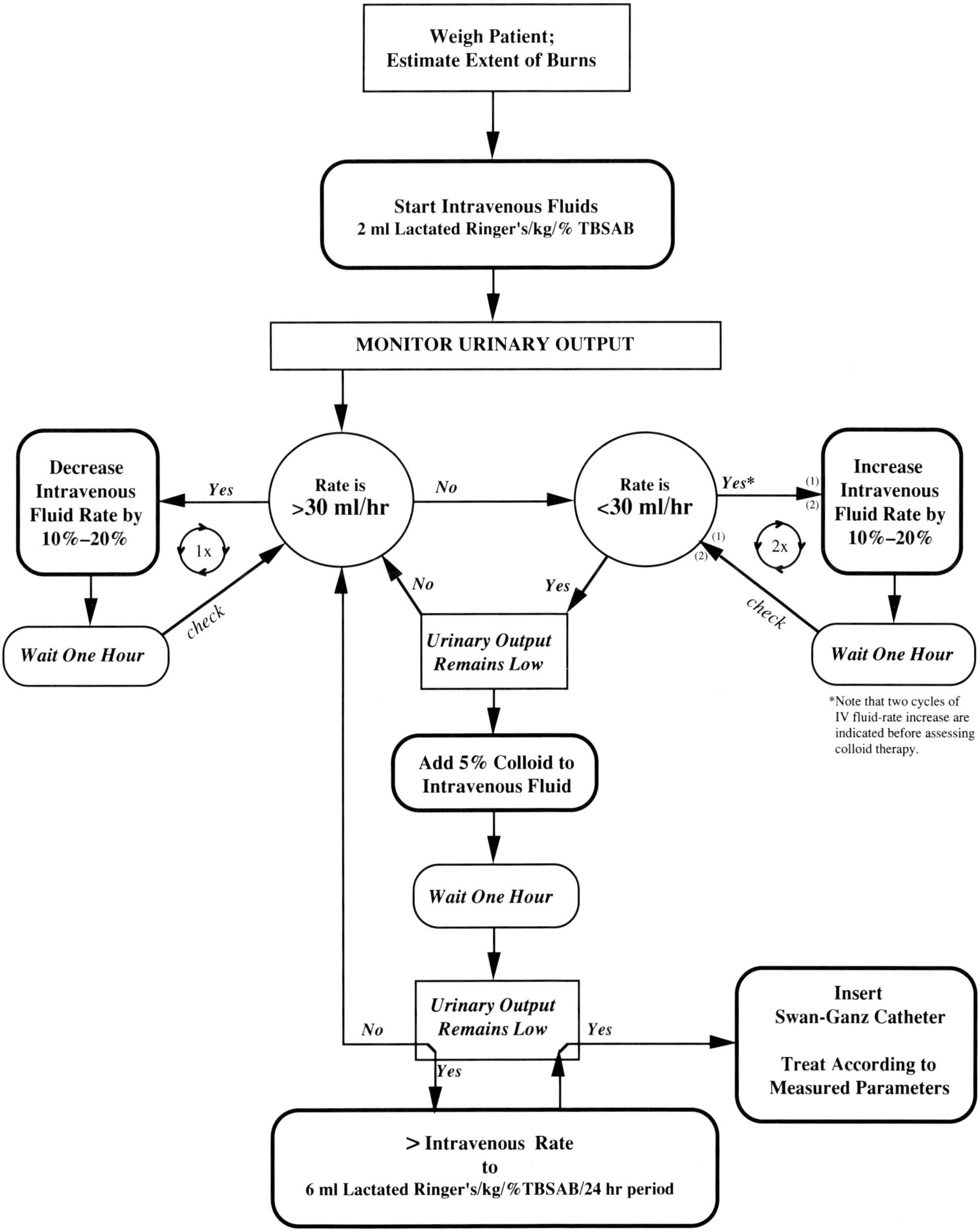

Fig. 11-1. Algorithm for fluid therapy during the first 24 hours after thermal injury

while rates of 110–130 beats per minute are commonly observed in adequately resuscitated adult burn patients. Noninvasive blood pressure measurements are unreliable in a burned extremity, and intraarterial monitoring may be required. However, this invasive monitoring should be reserved for elderly patients with cardiopulmonary disease, polytrauma patients, and those patients who fail to respond within 4–6 hours to hourly intravenous infusion rates that should have resulted in infusion of 6 or more ml/kg body weight/% TBSAB in the first 24 hours after the injury.

Resuscitation during the Second Day. In the second 24 hours after the injury, 5% dextrose in water is administered in an amount necessary to maintain an adequate urinary output. In addition, administering colloid-containing solutions will replace the plasma-volume deficit. The U.S. Army Institute of Surgical Research recommends using physiological concentrations of albumin reconstituted in lactated Ringer's solution. The volume of colloid administered depends upon the size of the burn, with 0.3 cc/kg body weight/% TBSAB administered to patients with up to 50% TBSAB, 0.4 cc/kg body weight/% TBSAB to patients with 50–70% TBSAB, and 0.5 cc/kg body weight/% TBSAB to patients with greater than 70% TBSAB. The patient's serum electrolytes should be frequently monitored, and both the infusion rate and the salt concentration of the administered fluid adjusted if necessary to prevent a precipitous drop in the serum sodium. In pediatric patients, who have a relatively small blood volume, urinary output is maintained during the second 24 hours with 5% dextrose in half-normal saline in place of 5% dextrose in water. Hyponatremia during this time is usually secondary to total body water excess and not to total body sodium deficit, and should be treated by decreasing the rate of intravenous fluid administration.

After the casualty has been resuscitated, fluid therapy should facilitate the excretion of the large sodium and fluid loads that were administered during the resuscitation phase, with the expectation that the patient's weight will return to normal by the tenth day after the burn. Electrolyte-free evaporative water losses should be replaced with 5% dextrose in water. Total daily water losses in resuscitated burn patients may reach 3.0 cc/kg body weight/% TBSAB, with daily losses as great as 6–10 liters possible in patients with large burns.

Insensible water losses can be estimated by the formula: Insensible water loss (ml/hr) = (25 + % body surface area burn) x (m^2 of total body surface area).[9]

Elevated serum sodium usually indicates a free-water deficit, not a total-body sodium excess, and should be treated by administering more free water.

Miscellaneous Early Care

A nasogastric tube should be inserted to decompress the stomach and to decrease the likelihood of emesis and subsequent aspiration.

The analgesic requirements of burn patients are inversely related to the depth of the burn. While full-thickness burns are insensate, partial-thickness burns can be especially painful. Analgesia should be administered by the intravenous route and should be carefully titrated, using small-bolus injections of narcotics. Intramuscular or subcutaneous injections of narcotics should be avoided during the period of systemic hypovolemia and hypoperfusion, since these injectates will not be absorbed in a predictable fashion. Once perfusion has been established, the mobilization of multiple doses of a drug can result in respiratory depression and cardiovascular collapse.

Using anesthesia during resuscitation is hazardous. The vasodilatory effect of general anesthesia may precipitate cardiovascular collapse if the burned casualty is only marginally resuscitated. Anesthesia, if needed, should be delivered at the level of the evacuation hospital or higher and requires close physiological monitoring.

When the casualty reaches a general hospital or burn center, routine admission laboratory tests to be obtained include *(a)* arterial blood gases with a carboxyhemoglobin level, *(b)* electrolytes, including blood glucose and blood urea nitrogen, *(c)* hematocrit, and *(d)* hepatic and renal profiles.

Escharotomy

Circumferential third-degree burns of an extremity may impede blood flow to underlying or distal unburned tissue. As edema develops beneath the inelastic eschar, tissue pressure will increase until it exceeds capillary pressure and may approach arteriolar pressure. This will restrict blood flow not only to this area but also to distal tissue, and ischemia and cell death will occur. Constant elevation of the affected extremity and active exercise of the extremity for 5 minutes every hour are required to minimize edema.

Although the value of escharotomy in relieving compression and restoring blood flow is well established,[10] the precise indications for performing escharotomy are not. The pulses should be monitored hourly in circumferentially burned extremities with the Doppler Ultrasonic flow meter. The most common signs that identify patients who will benefit from escharotomy are diminution or loss of pulses in the palmar arch of the upper extremity and the posterior tibial artery in the lower extremity, but one should be certain that reduced blood flow is not secondary to hypovolemia before proceeding to escharotomy. Some authorities advocate using compartmental-pressure measurements to identify the limbs that will benefit from escharotomy earlier. A compartment pressure above 30 cm H_2O has been identified as the critical level at which escharotomy should be performed.[11]

Escharotomy can be performed as a ward procedure using either a scalpel or an electrocautery. Since the incision is made only through the burned skin in an area of insensate full-thickness burn, anesthesia is unnecessary. The incision should be made in the midlateral or midmedial line of the anatomically positioned burned limb or digit, and should extend from the distal to the proximal margin of the encircling full-thickness burn (Figure 11-2). The depth of the incision should be limited to the eschar, just exposing the underlying subcutaneous tissue (Figure 11-3). Since bacteria will rapidly colonize the exposed unburned subcutaneous tissue, their proliferation should be controlled by applying the topical antimicrobial agent that is being used on the burn.

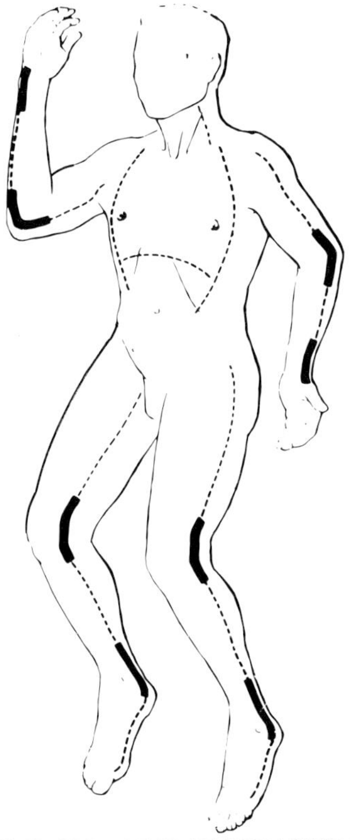

Fig. 11-2. The preferred sites for placing escharotomies. Note that escharotomies should extend across the major joints.

Occasionally, escharotomies of the neck, penis, or chest may be necessary because of encircling full-thickness burns. If full-thickness circumferential burns of the chest impair ventilation, bilateral, anterior, axillary-line escharotomies extending from the clavicle to the costal margin should be performed and, if abdominal-wall eschar necessitates, the axillary-line incisions should be connected by a costal-margin escharotomy. If the burn includes the hand, midlateral and midmedial escharotomy should be extended to the base of the metacarpophalangeal joint of the thumb or the little finger, or both. Longitudinal incisions on the dorsum of the hand and digits may only expose the extensor tendons and should be avoided.

Escharotomy should always be performed when indicated, but prophylactic escharotomies should not be performed, especially during the early phase of resuscitation. Inappropriate escharotomies extending deep into the subcutaneous tissues can risk increased blood loss as resuscitation procedes and intravascular volume is restored. Extensive bleeding may occur but be unrecognized as the casualty progresses through the evacuation chain. If the tactical situation delays evacuation and escharotomies are clinically indicated, they should be performed even if the casualty is at a treatment level at which replacement blood is not available. These patients' incisions should be monitored for bleeding on a scheduled basis (for example, hourly), and a pressure dressing should be applied if bleeding is excessive.

Burn-Wound Management

Initial Wound Care. Initial wound care should be performed at the level of the combat-support hospital or higher. It includes *(a)* cleansing of all wounds with any available surgical disinfectant, *(b)* debriding all nonviable tissue that can easily be removed, and *(c)* shaving the body hair from the areas involved. Bullae greater than 2 cm should be excised to prevent their serving as infection nidi. If the patient is to be transferred to another treatment facility after the burns have been cleansed and debrided, the burns should be covered with lightweight, sterile dressings impregnated with the topical antimicrobial agent of choice, if available. If the patient is at the level of definitive burn care, the wounds can be covered with a topical antimicrobial agent and left exposed if environmental temperatures permit.

Controlling Infection. The goal of burn care is to control infection until the injury either spontaneously heals or is surgically closed. Nonviable tissue within the injury predisposes it to bacterial colonization and

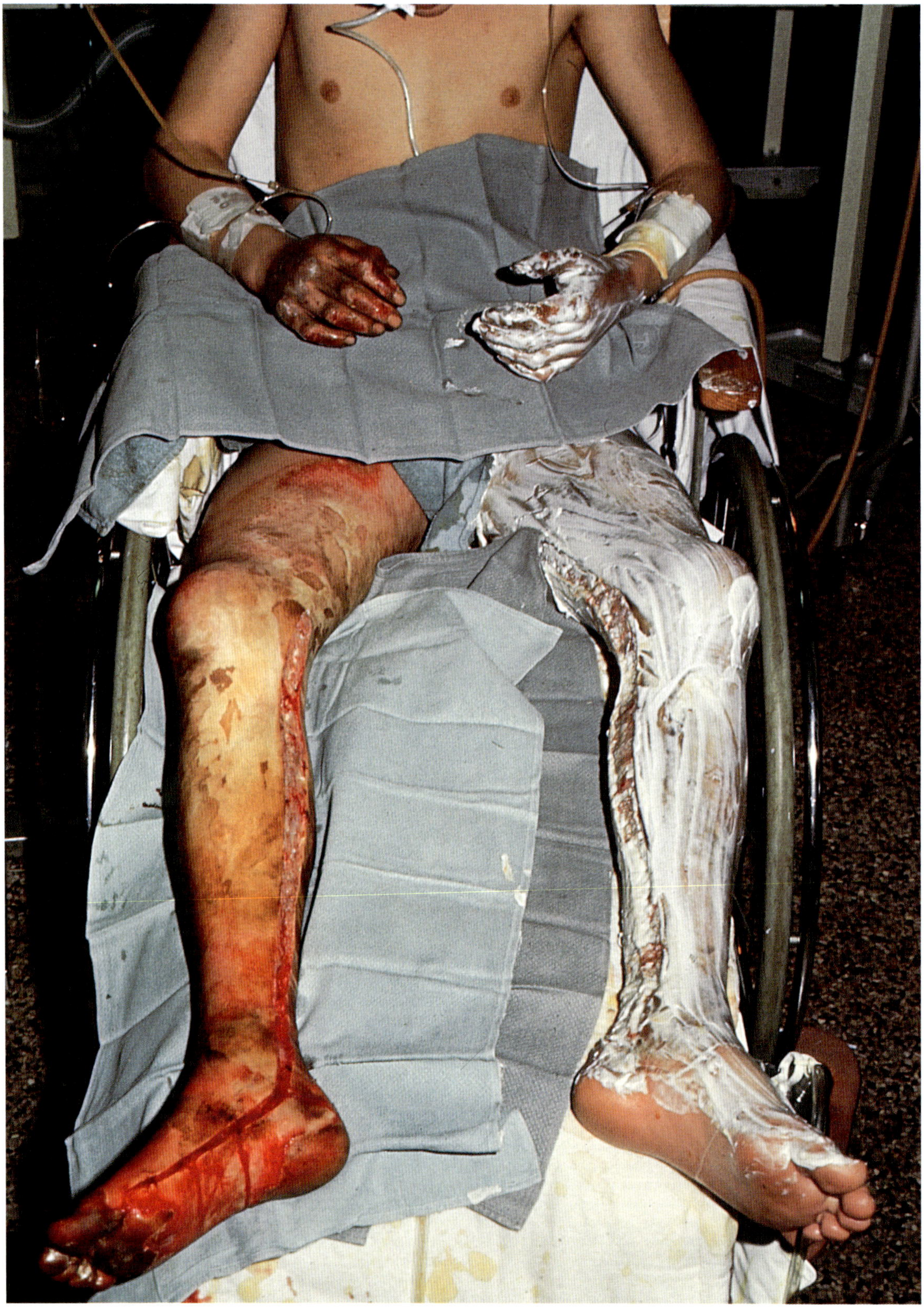

Fig. 11-3. Appropriately placed escharotomies were performed to relieve decreased distal perfusion, indicated by diminished pedal pulses. Edema beneath the encircling full-thickness eschar caused this condition. Note that the incision extends only through the superficial fascia, permitting the wound edges to separate. Liberal application of a topical antimicrobial agent is necessary to control bacterial proliferation in the incision.

subsequent infection. Topical antimicrobial agents decrease the incidence of invasive infections in burns. Three effective chemotherapeutic agents that are frequently used to treat burn infections (Table 11-2) are Sulfamylon, Silvadene, and silver nitrate.

Sulfamylon burn cream is an 11.1% suspension of mafenide acetate in a hydrophilic cream. Mafenide acetate is water soluble, bacteriostatic for both Gram-positive and -negative organisms, and is particularly effective against pseudomonal and clostridial infections. Its solubility allows mafenide acetate to penetrate the eschar. There are significant disadvantages to using Sulfamylon, including pain following its application to partial-thickness burns and carbonic anhydrase inhibition, which may lead to renal bicarbonate wasting and a metabolic acidosis.

Silvadene burn cream is a 1% suspension of silver sulfadiazine in a hydrophilic base. Its solubility is limited and it does not penetrate the eschar well. *Enterobacter* and *Pseudomonas* are frequently resistant to this agent. Furthermore, neutropenia and occasionally pancytopenia may occur during its use. Silvadene's major benefits include the absence of post-application pain and freedom from acid-base disturbances.

Silver nitrate is used as a 0.5% solution. It is painless upon application and is active against a broad spectrum of bacteria. Because of its total lack of penetration, however, silver nitrate must be applied before a dense microbial population develops within the eschar. In addition, silver nitrate has a significant major side effect: It leaches excessive amounts of sodium, chloride, potassium, and calcium from the burn. Silver nitrate also irreversibly stains tissue, clothing, and equipment.

Managing Burn-Wound Infections. Despite their current reduced incidence, invasive burn-wound infection remains the most common cause of morbidity and mortality in patients with extensive burns.[12] Diagnosing these infections is difficult, due to a variety of wound and systemic factors. Hyperthermia, tachycardia, and hyperventilation are characteristic of the hypermetabolic response to burns and are not reliable signs of sepsis. The finding of leukocytosis is likewise unreliable, since postburn leukocytosis typically is followed by leukopenia and subsequent rebound leukocytosis.

Scheduled surveillance is the best way to identify changes indicative of invasive infection in the wound (Figure 11-4). Changes consistent with burn-wound infection (Table 11-3) should prompt immediate wound biopsy to verify the diagnosis. Quantitative cultures taken from the burn wound merely identify the resident flora and are useful only for epidemiological monitoring.[13,14,15] Furthermore, even quantitative cultures of a biopsy specimen do not enable a differentiation to be made between contamination and invasive

TABLE 11-2

TOPICAL CHEMOTHERAPEUTIC AGENTS FOR BURN-WOUND CARE

	Mafenide Acetate	Silver Nitrate	Silver Sulfadiazine
Active component concentration	11.1% in water- miscible base	0.5% in aequeous solution	1.0% in water- miscible base
Spectrum of anti-bacterial activity	Gram-negative: good Gram-positive: good Yeast: minimal	Gram-negative: good Gram-positive: good Yeast: good	Gram-negative: selectively good Yeast: good
Method of wound care	Exposure	Occlusive dressings	Exposure or single-layer dressing
Advantages	Penetrates eschar, wound appearance readily monitored, joint motion unrestricted, no Gram-negative resistance	Painless upon application, no hypersensitivity reactions, no Gram-negative resistance, dressings reduce evaporative heat loss, requires painful dressing changes	Painless, wound appearance readily monitored and joint motion unrestricted when exposure method used
Disadvantages	Painful on partial-thickness burns, acidosis as a result of inhibition of carbonic anhydrase, hypersensitivity in 7% of patients	Deficits of sodium, potassium, calcium, and chloride, no eschar penetration, limitation of joint motion by dressings, methemoglobinemia: rare, argyria: rare, staining of equipment and environment	Neutropenia, hypersensitivity: infrequent, limited eschar penetration, resistance of certain Gram-negative bacteria and clostridia

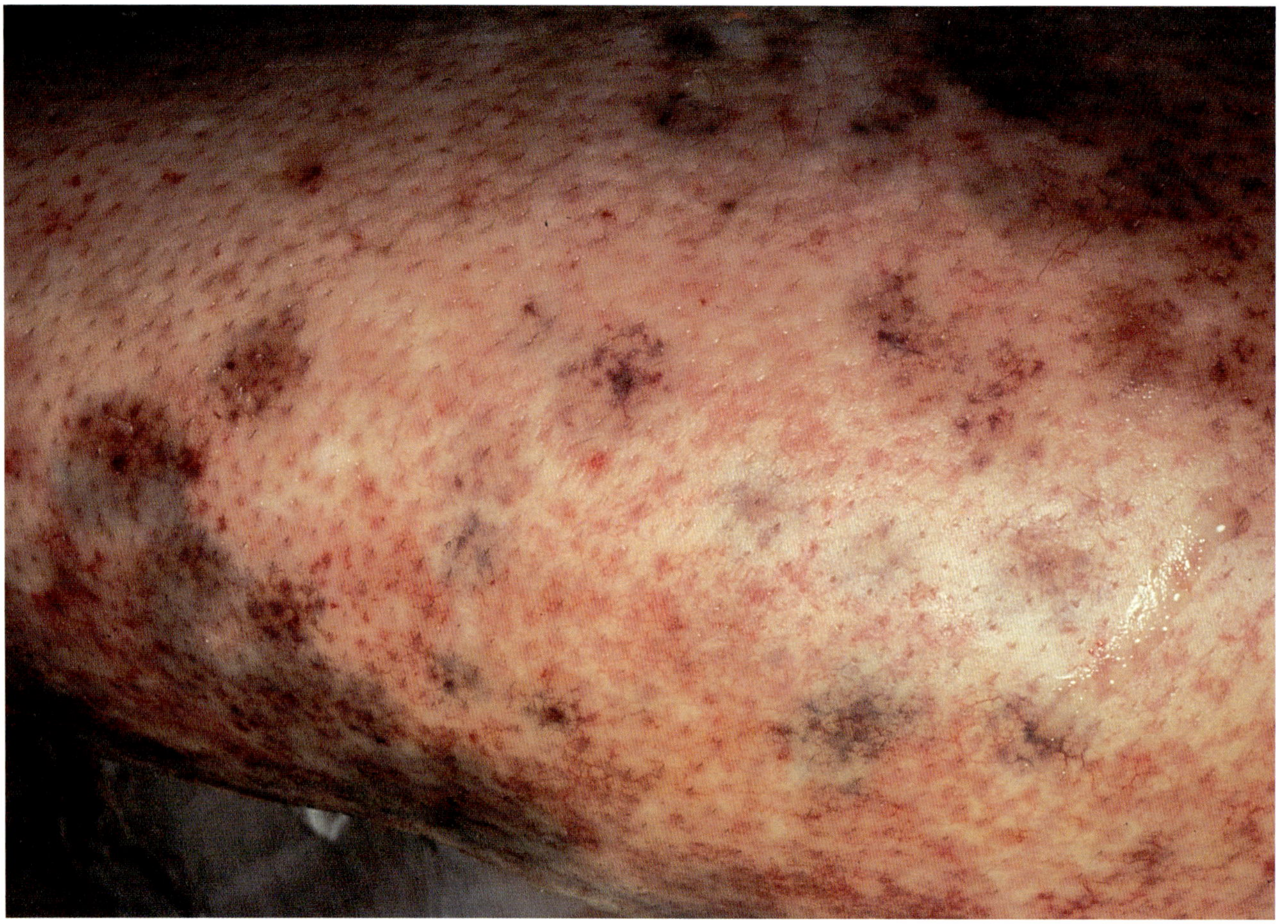

Fig. 11-4. The foci of discoloration in this full-thickness wound characterize invasive wound infection and should prompt immediate burn-wound biopsy.

infection, since high microbial counts are frequently observed in the absence of invasive infection.[16] Histological examination of biopsied tissue is the most rapid and reliable method of diagnosing an invasive burn-wound infection (Table 11-4).

The incidence of invasive infection in burns has steadily decreased over the past decade. However, once generalized sepsis has developed, the patient's chance for survival is markedly reduced. In general, invasive infection is rarely encountered during the first 2 weeks after the burn.

The treatment of burn-wound infection depends upon the invading organism.[17] Streptococcal infections do not deeply invade the tissues and usually are manifested by erythema and lymphangitis. Systemic penicillin administration controls most of these infections promptly. Staphylococcal infections invade more deeply, but are often surrounded by a thick membrane that *(a)* prevents further spread of the infection but *(b)* also prevents parenteral antibiotics from reaching the focus of infection. Local excision is essential for adequate management. Gram-negative infections have the propensity to spread widely via the hematogenous and lymphatic routes. Once the diagnosis of invasive Gram-negative infection has been made, mafenide acetate should be applied (if it is not already being used). Systemic antibiotics to which the invading organism is sensitive should be administered.

Treating the burn wound with subeschar injections of one-half of the recommended total daily dose of a broad-spectrum semisynthetic penicillin 6–12 hours prior to, and again immediately before, surgery limits further microbial proliferation and decreases the risk of hematogenous dissemination during the excision.[18] If all nonviable and infected tissue has been excised, the wound should be covered with a biological dressing to prevent desiccation. If nonviable tissue remains, dressings soaked in either 0.5% silver nitrate or 5% mafenide acetate solution should be used. Autografting of the wound should be delayed until the surgeon is certain that the wound infection has been adequately controlled.

Invasive fungal infections are rare and usually occur late in the course of treatment. Typically, the

TABLE 11-3

CLINICAL SIGNS OF INVASIVE BURN-WOUND INFECTION

- Focal areas of dark red, brown, or black eschar discoloration
- Conversion of partial-thickness injury to full-thickness necrosis
- Hemorrhagic discoloration of sub-eschar tissue
- Green pigment visible in subcutaneous fat*
- Erythematous, necrotic lesions (ecthyma gangrenosum) in unburned skin*
- Edema and/or violaceous discoloration of unburned skin at wound margin
- Accelerated separation of eschar**
- Rapid centrifugal expansion of subcutaneous edema with central necrosis**
- Vesicular lesions in healing or healed partial-thickness burns***
- Crusted, serrated margins of partial-thickness burns of the face***

*Characteristic of *Pseudomonas* infection
**Characteristic of fungal infection
***Characteristic of herpes simplex infection

TABLE 11-4

HISTOLOGIC STAGING OF MICROBIAL STATUS OF BURN WOUNDS

Stage	Characteristics
I. Colonization	
A. Superficial	Microorganisms present on wound surface
B. Penetration	Microorganisms present in variable thickness of eschar
C. Proliferation	Multiplication of microorganisms in subeschar space
II. Invasion	
A. Microinvasion	Microscopic foci of microorganisms in viable tissue adjacent to subeschar space
B. Generalized	Multifocal or widespread penetration of microorganisms deep into viable subcutaneous tissue
C. Microvascular	Involvement of small blood vessels and lymphatics

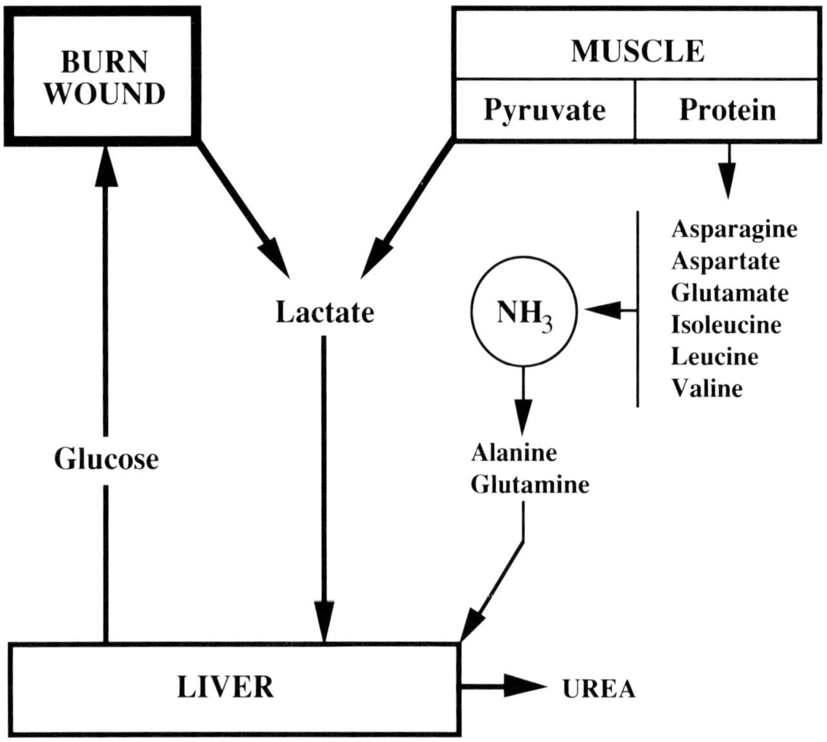

Fig. 11-5. The wound uses glucose (principally by anaerobic, glycolytic pathways) as its primary energy source. This produces large amounts of lactate. In the liver, lactate is extracted and used for glucose synthesis via the Cori cycle. Amino acids from the casualty's peripheral muscle mass are the major source of the three-carbon fragments needed for hepatic gluconeogenesis. After they are deaminated, the amino acids alamine and glutamine are shuttled to the liver for glucose production. This cycle also yields increased ureagenesis.

process is localized and the definitive treatment is excision, with the addition of topical antifungal therapy. Systemic amphotericin is reserved for patients with either fungemia or evidence of vascular invasion in the excised tissue.

Metabolic Support of Burned Patients

Severely burned patients may lose as much as 40 g of protein per day in the form of urea nitrogen, secondary to the extensive peripheral proteolysis that accompanies the hypermetabolic response.[19, 20] This erosion of lean body mass provides alanine and glutamine to the liver, where they are utilized as three-carbon-fragment substrates for gluconeogenesis (Figure 11-5). Wound-produced pyruvate and lactate are utilized in the Cori cycle to provide additional substrate for glucose production. Although catabolism continues until the wound is closed, appropriate nutritional support may increase the synthesis of visceral and muscle protein and protect lean body mass. Nutritional support should be delayed until the casualty reaches an MTF, where he or she can be properly monitored for both the therapy's adequacy and any complications. Nutritional support should be administered enterally, if gastrointestinal function has returned to normal. Parenteral nutrition, which is not usually available until the patient reaches a general hospital, can be used, but it requires more extensive monitoring and is associated with a higher rate of mechanical and infectious complications.

Caloric requirements can be estimated by any of several commonly used formulae (Table 11-5) or measured by indirect calorimetry. Proteins should be administered in sufficient quantity to promote positive nitrogen balance. A calorie-to-nitrogen ratio of 100–150:1 is usually required to achieve this goal. Carbohydrates should supply the major portion of the patient's caloric requirement, but administration rates should not exceed 5–7 mg/kg body weight/min.[21] Rates that exceed this level may cause both hepatic lipogenesis and fat deposition, which not only may impair hepatic function but also are associated with a marked increase in carbon dioxide production. Lipids should supply the remaining calories. Enterally administered medium-chain triglycerides are well tolerated and serve as an effective source of energy. Because mitochondrial oxidation is impaired after a casualty is

TABLE 11-5

FORMULAE FOR ESTIMATING DAILY CALORIC REQUIREMENTS IN ADULT BURN PATIENTS

Curreri

(25 kcal x body weight in kg) + (40 kcal x % TBSAB)

Artz, Moncrief, and Pruitt

(2,100 kcal x body surface area m^2) For patients with burns of > 40 TBSA.

Galveston

(1,800 kcal x body surface area m^2) + (2,000 kcal) (m^2 burn)

U. S. Army Institute of Surgical Research

54.33782 - (1.9961 x age) + (0.025488 x age^2) - (0.00018 x age^3)
[2.33764 - (11.33764 x $e^{-0.02866}$ x burn area)] (body surface area m^2) (24) (1.25)

burned, the long-chain triglycerides contained in parenterally administered lipid emulsions cannot be efficiently utilized as energy sources.[22] Almost all burn patients with greater than 30% TBSAB will require nutritional supplements to meet their increased metabolic demands.

Burn-Wound Closure

Historically, burn wounds were closed by placing cutaneous autografts on the granulation tissue that had formed after the eschar spontaneously separated. Current treatment includes excising the burn wound and then covering the viable tissue below with autograft skin, which decreases the risk of burn-wound infection and shortens the patient's stay in the hospital. However, excision and grafting require that considerable resources such as blood products be expended[23] and should be reserved as a treatment modality employed at fixed hospital facilities such as a general hospital or higher-echelon facility.

Excision. Full-thickness or deep partial-thickness burns (wounds that will not heal within 21 days) are amenable to surgical excision. Once resuscitation is complete and the patient is hemodynamically stable, excision should be considered if the hospital can support the procedure. These limits should not be exceeded unless invasive wound infection has been documented.

Excessive blood loss and hypothermia are the two most significant factors limiting excision. Blood loss associated with scalpel excision is surprisingly large; the surgeon should anticipate a two-blood-volume replacement in children with a 30%–50% excision and a one-half-blood-volume replacement in adults with a 30% excision. The blood loss is even greater with tangential excision, and up to 9% of the blood volume can be lost per 1% of the body-surface area excised.[24] Accordingly, the extent of each surgical excision should be limited to either 20% of the total body-surface area or 2 hours of operative time, whichever occurs first.[24] The operating room should be kept warm and the infused fluids should also be warmed to minimize the loss of body heat and to prevent hypothermia from developing during the operation. If possible, excision should be performed during the first week after the burn, since the blood loss from more mature wounds will be greater. Using tourniquets during limb excisions can limit blood loss, but their use requires that the surgeon have significant experience in determin-

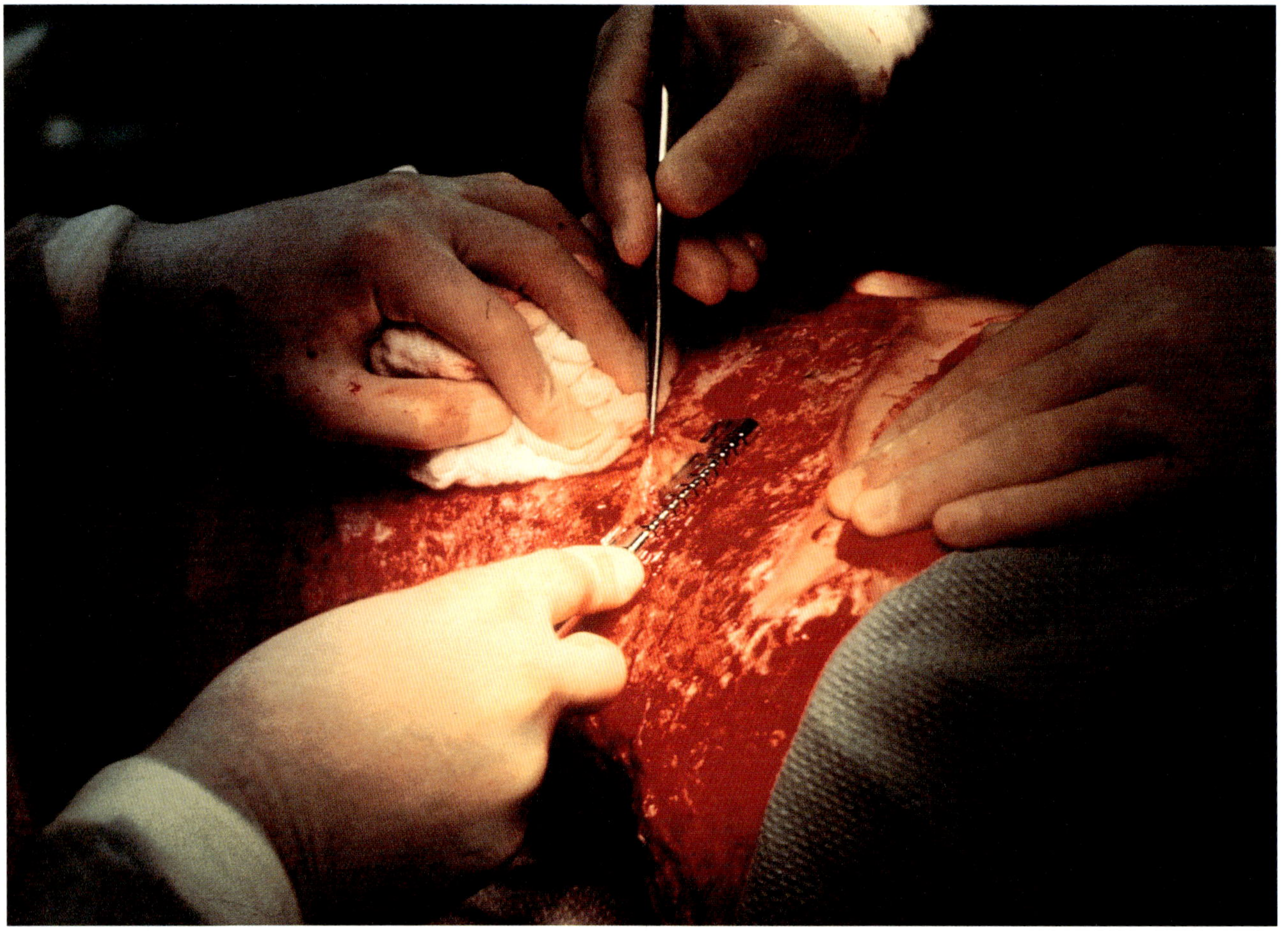

Fig. 11-6. Burns that *(a)* are deep dermal or *(b)* extend just into the superficial fat are best treated by tangential excision with guarded knives or dermatomes. A dense bed of brisk capillary bleeding indicates viable tissue and adequate wound excision.

ing tissue viability, since capillary bleeding is also abolished.

The depth of the injury and the stability of the patient dictate the method of excision that the surgeon should use. Tangential excision is utilized for partial-thickness burns and is accomplished using a guarded skin knife or a dermatome to remove thin layers of eschar until viable tissue is encountered (Figures 11-6 and 11-7). The benefit of this form of excision is maximal salvage of uninjured subcutaneous tissue.

Deep full-thickness burns are best treated by scalpel or electrocautery excision at the level of the investing fascia (Figure 11-8). This technique can be performed more rapidly and with less loss of blood than tangential excision. The major disadvantage of this form of excision, however, is its final cosmetic result, because all subcutaneous fat and lymphatics are removed. However, the percentage of *graft take* (that is, deeper layers of tissue establish continuity with the graft, supply it with nutrients, and assure its survival) on the excised fascial bed is usually excellent, especially when compared to those grafts that are placed on subcutaneous fat.

Early surgical intervention in patients with extensive burns should be directed toward excising and covering large planar areas, in an attempt to reduce complications related to the size of the burn. This should be followed first by excising the extremities, and then specific body parts such as the hands. Early excision and grafting of third-degree burns of the hands should be performed only in patients with small burns that are not life threatening. The goal is to elicit early motion and to minimize functional deficits.

Deep burns of the face should not be excised. Because of the thickness of facial skin, many deep-appearing burns will heal spontaneously and save facial tissue, which will maintain contour and may improve later cosmetic results.

Burns to the perineum are a particularly difficult challenge. The cutaneous injury should be treated conservatively, with definitive closure accomplished after the wound has formed granulation tissue. Di-

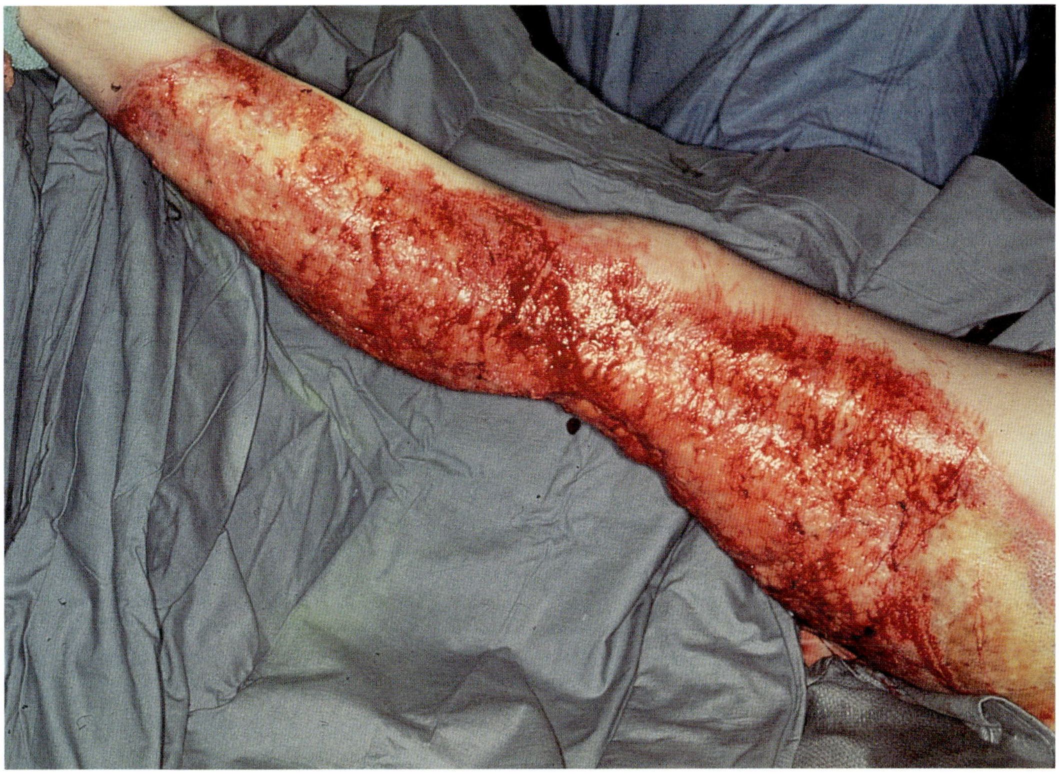

Fig. 11-7. After hemostasis has been achieved, areas of viable dermis intermingled with fat may be covered with autograft or any other readily available biological dressing.

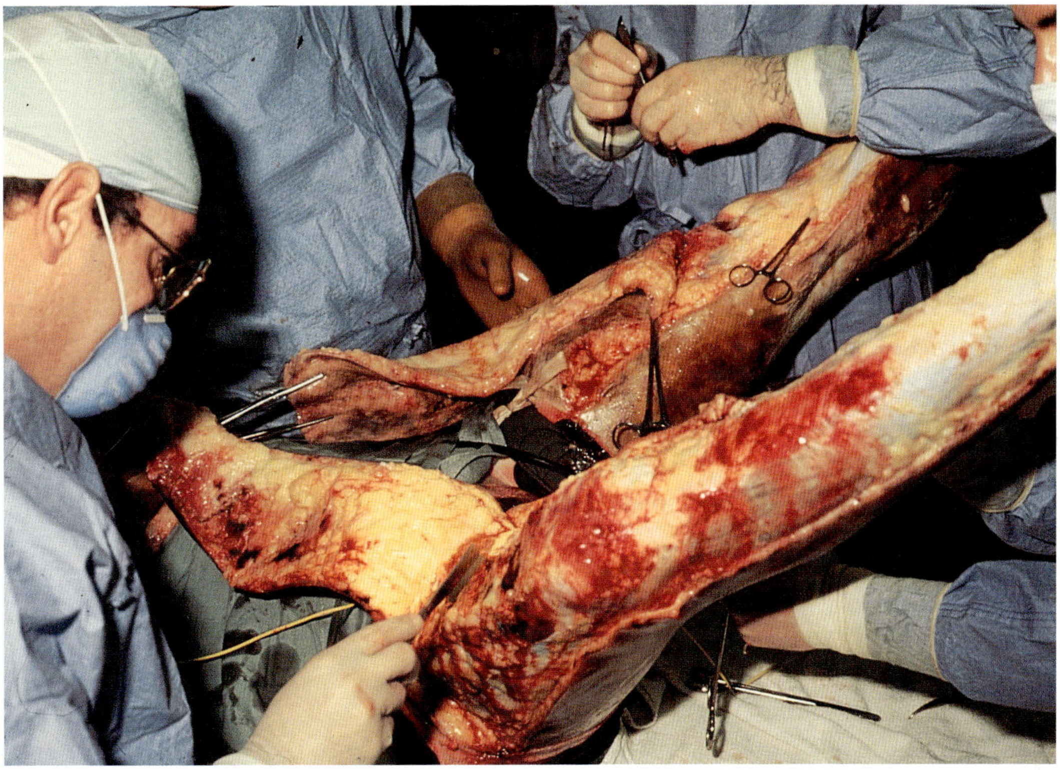

Fig. 11-8. Extensive, deep, full-thickness burns are best treated by excising to the level of the investing muscle fascia. This excision can be performed rapidly with minimal blood loss, but it leaves a significant cosmetic deformity.

verting colostomies are not required either to achieve wound closure or to prevent wound infection. Diversion of the fecal stream usually results in significant anal stenosis, which then requires surgical correction.

Skin Grafts. After a burn wound has been excised, optimal closure is accomplished by the use of cutaneous autografts. However, this is possible only when *(a)* the wound bed is unequivocally viable and *(b)* available donor sites exist. In extensively burned patients, the size of the burn wound often exceeds that of the available donor sites.

Meshed autograft skin is the most commonly used permanent covering after burn-wound excision. The most common expansion ratios are 1.5:1, 2:1, and 3:1, although up to ninefold expansion is possible (Figures 11-9 and 11-10). Because so long a time is required for the interstices of either six- or ninefold expanded skin grafts to re-epithelize, they are seldom employed. To prevent desiccation of the tissues underlying the open interstices of meshed cutaneous autografts, occlusive dressings soaked in either 0.5% silver nitrate solution or 5% mafenide acetate solution are applied until epithelial closure is complete. For widely expanded meshed autograft skin or meshed autograft skin over fat, overlays of cutaneous allograft, xenograft, or Biobrane have proven successful in both increasing graft take and decreasing the time to interstitial closure. In patients with smaller burns involving 30% TBSAB, covering the functional and cosmetically important areas such as the face, feet, neck, and ears may be accomplished with sheet grafts.

The care of donor sites is critical. In extensively burned patients, these areas may need to be reharvested as soon as possible. Donor-site care should maximize re-epithelization and minimize trauma in an environment that promotes epithelial growth. Fine-mesh gauze remains the simplest, most inexpensive donor-site dressing, and when re-epithelization has occurred beneath, the gauze is easily peeled from the wound. Using a synthetic skin substitute such as Duoderm as a donor-site dressing has decreased the healing time of donor sites,[25] but such dressings are expensive, more difficult to use, and will in all likelihood be unavailable in a wartime setting.

When donor sites are limited, the burn wound is frequently closed temporarily, using material other than the patient's own skin. The goals of temporary wound coverage are to decrease the physiological impact of the open wound and to prevent bacterial colonization. Various biological dressings and skin substitutes now exist for achieving this goal. Cutaneous allograft, harvested from cadavers, is the most effective biological dressing and is the standard to which all other biological dressings and skin substitutes

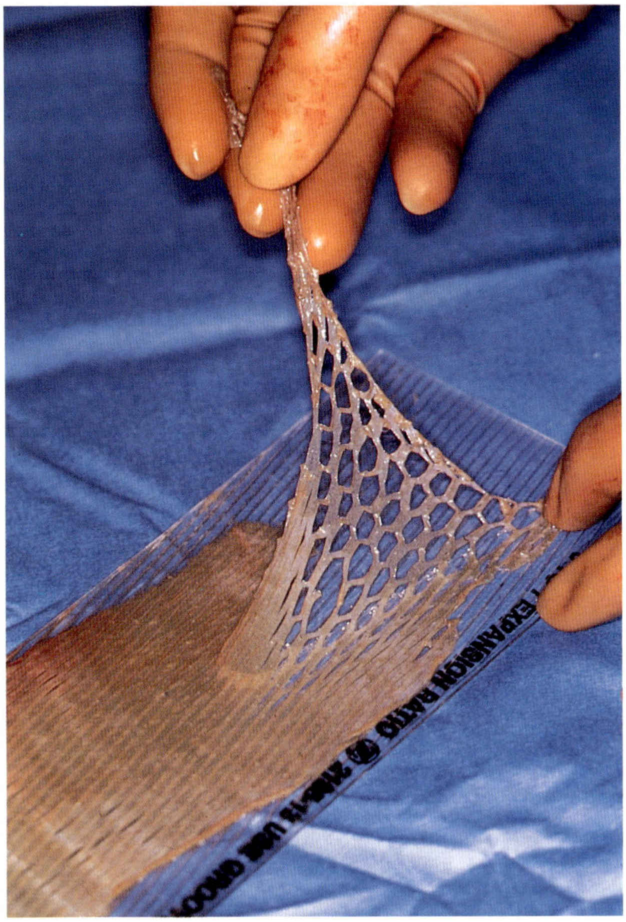

Fig. 11-9. When a casualty's donor sites are limited, a meshed autograft, which can expand, allows a greater portion of the burned body surface to be covered.

must be compared. Frozen cutaneous allograft and porcine cutaneous xenograft are the two most readily available skin substitutes, but they are *(a)* less adherent to the wound bed than fresh allograft, *(b)* less able to control the bacterial population of the underlying wound, and *(c)* usually do not become well-vascularized from the underlying wound bed. Synthetic skin substitutes exist but have met with only limited success. An effective synthetic skin substitute should *(a)* be compatible with the patient's own tissue, *(b)* have no antigenicity or toxicity, *(c)* have water vapor permeability similar to that of skin, *(d)* be impermeable to microorganisms, *(e)* adhere to the wound, *(f)* be readily vascularized, and *(g)* have an indefinite shelf life. The available skin substitutes need to be modified to increase their clinical usefulness by enhancing both their resistance to infection and their ability to accelerate the formation of either neodermis or granulation tissue.

The use of culture-derived epidermal sheets has

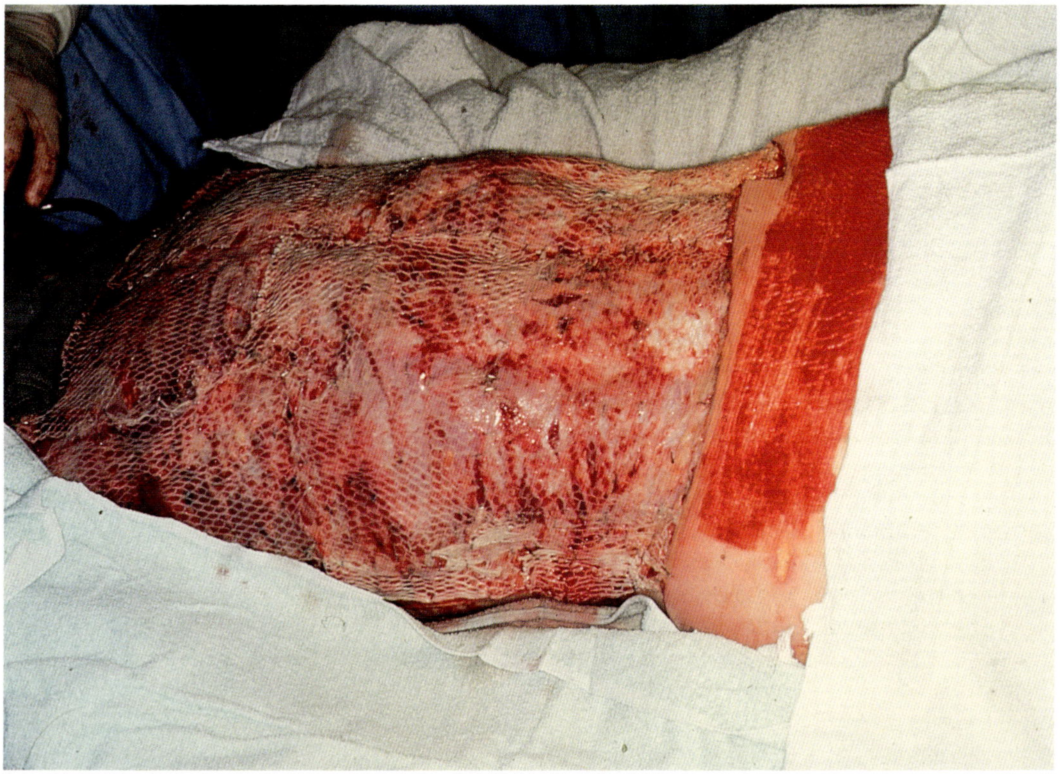

Fig. 11-10. The investing fasciae of this chest and abdomen have been covered with meshed autograft expanded 3:1.

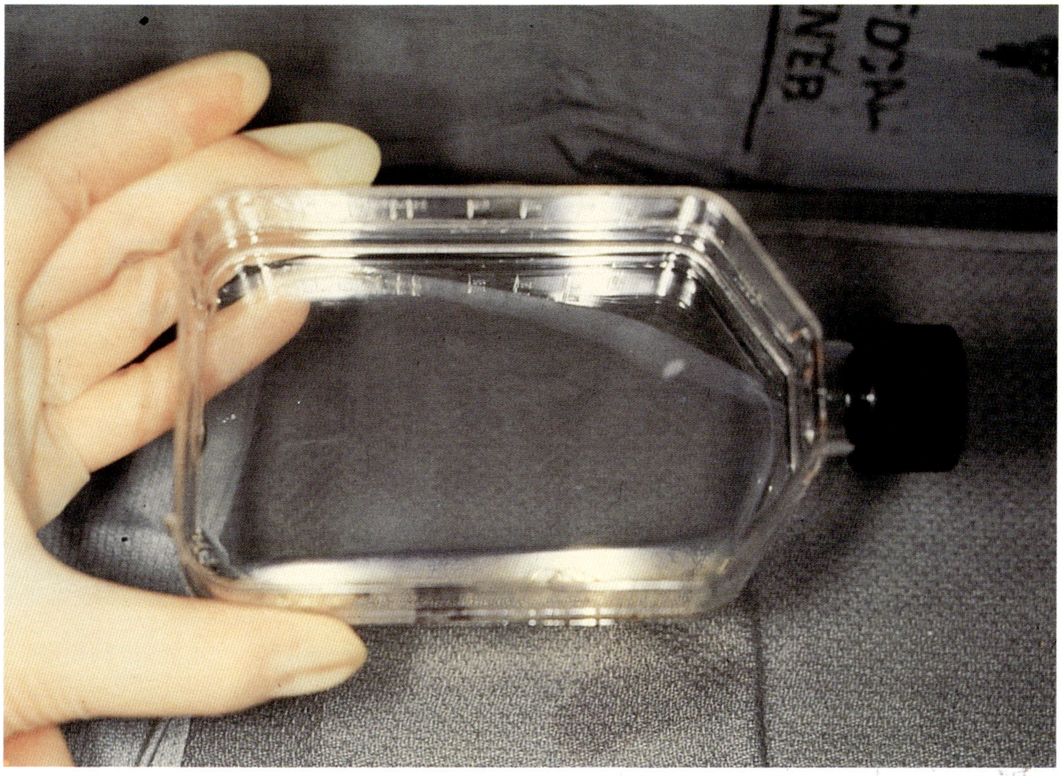

Fig. 11-11. Epidermal sheets derived from culturing autologous keratinocytes are currently being investigated for use as a substitute for split-thickness skin grafts. The extremely thin sheets average only 5–10 cells thick and are exceptionally vulnerable to mechanical trauma. However, a 2 x 2-cm biopsy can be expanded to 1.5–2 m^2 in 25–30 days, allowing for significant wound coverage.

recently gained wide popularity (Figure 11-11).[26] Epidermal sheets are generated from autogenous keratinocytes and are used in place of split-thickness autografts. However, the use of culture-derived keratinocytes now appears to be limited by *(a)* the 3–4 weeks necessary to grow the epidermal sheets, *(b)* the fragility of the tissue, and *(c)* its susceptibility to infection.

Complications

The first complications in burn patients are those associated with resuscitation. Timely institution of resuscitation and infusion of adequate volumes of fluid make acute renal failure infrequent early in the postburn period. However, significant delays in initiating fluid resuscitation may result in a significant plasma-volume deficit, which will lead to hypoperfusion of the kidneys and subsequent renal failure. Later-occurring sepsis, multiple organ failure, and nephrotoxic antibiotics are now the most common causes of renal dysfunction. Dialysis should be initiated to correct volume overload, hyperkalemia, uncontrollable acidosis, a blood urea nitrogen greater than 100, and creatinine greater than 10. Oliguria during the first 24 hours after the burn typically reflects inadequate fluid replacement and should be treated by increasing the rate that the resuscitation fluid is infused.

Complications such as pulmonary edema associated with excess fluid administration may occur if the patient's response to resuscitation is not properly monitored. If resuscitation requirements are grossly overestimated, excessive wound edema may develop and otherwise unnecessary escharotomies may be required.

Early gastrointestinal complications, once common, are now quite rare. Emesis secondary to the ileus that typically occurs after a thermal burn is easily prevented by gastric decompression with a nasogastric tube. Curling's ulcer, the progression of the acute, punctate, shallow, mucosal erosions throughout the proximal stomach and duodenum, may occur in over 80% of patients with greater than 30% TBSAB.[27] Consequently, significant bleeding from acute ulcerations has largely been eliminated by prophylactic measures—including antacids or H_2 blockers or both—to keep the intragastric pH greater than 4.5. Since these preven-

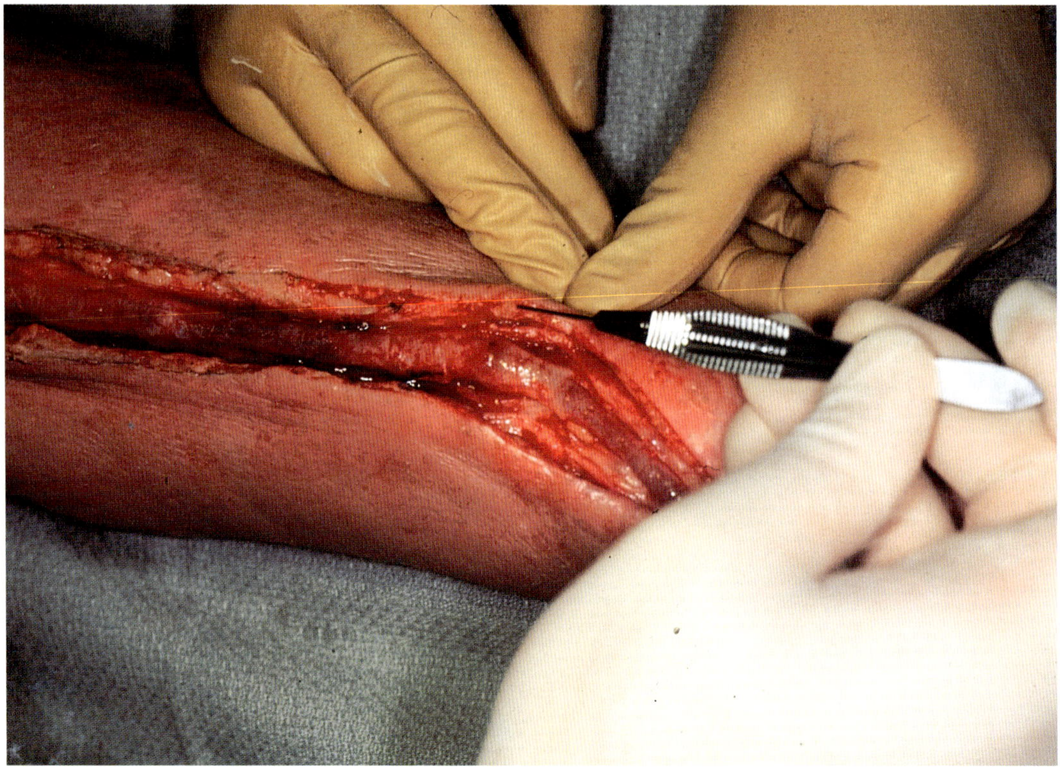

Fig. 11-12. Suppurative thrombophlebitis can occur in any previously cannulated vein. The infected vein should be excised to a point at which it is either grossly normal or has become a tributary of the next-larger order of veins. Note the infected vein's distension, discoloration, and thrombosis.

tive measures have been employed, the need to operate for upper gastrointestinal hemorrhage has markedly decreased.

Sepsis remains the most common complication that occurs after the burn patient's successful resuscitation. Extensive bacterial colonization of the burn wound, as well as the patient's immunosuppressed condition, increases the likelihood that significantly burned patients will develop infectious complications.

Pneumonia has replaced invasive burn-wound infection as the most frequent source of sepsis in thermally injured patients. Hematogenous pneumonia is caused by the systemic dissemination of an infecting organism from a remote source. Its radiographic hallmark—a solitary, nodular, pulmonary infiltrate that may progress to multiple infiltrates—should prompt a search for the source of infection. Common sources include an infected burn wound, endocarditis, and suppurative thrombophlebitis, all of which require immediate treatment. Airborne vectors of infection have surpassed hematogenous spread as the most common sources of pneumonia. The presence of inhalation injury and the requirement for endotracheal intubation increase the likelihood that pneumonia will develop. Fever, sputum leukocytosis, and the presence of infiltrates on chest roentgenograms are sensitive, but nonspecific, indicators of pneumonia.

Suppurative thrombophlebitis can occur in any previously cannulated vein. Microbial seeding at the time of insertion, the composition of the catheter, injury to the vein at the insertion site, and the duration of cannulation all predispose the patient to intraluminal infection. Limiting the time a cannula is in place to a maximum of 72 hours has significantly reduced the incidence of this complication in thermally injured patients from 6.9% to 1.4% in recent years.[28] Any venous cannula inserted under less-than-ideal sterile conditions should be removed as soon as possible. If no other obvious source can be identified, the diagnosis of suppurative thrombophlebitis should be considered in any patient with septicemia. If local signs do not indicate an obvious source, then all previously cannulated veins should be surgically explored (Figure 11-12). The treatment of suppurative thrombophlebitis includes *(a)* administration of systemic antibiotics and *(b)* complete excision of the infected vein to the point at which the vein wall is unequivocally normal and blood can be expressed from the lumen, or to the level at which the vein becomes a tributary of the next-larger order of veins.

EVACUATION OF CASUALTIES WITH THERMAL INJURIES

Criteria for Evacuation

The accepted criteria for transferring patients to a burn center include: *(a)* partial-thickness burns of 20% TBSAB or greater in adults, or 10% in children and those over 50 years old; *(b)* full-thickness burns exceeding 5% TBSAB; *(c)* burns involving the face, feet, hands, perineum, or major joints; *(d)* thermally injured patients with significant preexisting medical problems or polytrauma; *(e)* patients with electrical or lightning injuries; and *(f)* the presence of inhalation injury.[29]

During armed conflict, however, the indications for evacuation are modified.[30] For triage purposes, the presence of inhalation injury or associated major trauma may each be counted as an additional 10% burn. Casualties with small burns involving the hand, foot, or perineum should be considered for early evacuation since their activity will be disproportionately limited, but if the burns are superficial, rapid healing may permit the casualty's relatively early return to duty. If resources are severely limited, the upper burn-size limit for those receiving maximum care can be decreased by 10% increments from 70% until patient-care demands match available resources.[30]

Care During Evacuation

If the casualty will reach a combat-support or higher-echelon hospital within 24–48 hours after the burn, no topical agent need be applied at the lower echelons, but the wounds should be kept clean, dry, and covered. If several days' delay is anticipated, Silvadene, if available, should be applied before the casualty is evacuated. Before and during evacuation, the wound should be managed with closed dressings *(a)* to protect from exogenous contamination and *(b)* to prevent hypothermia. Once the casualty arrives at the combat-support hospital, Silvadene should be applied to the wound after it has been debrided. Extensive burns with a significant full-thickness component should have Sulfamylon applied when the casualty reaches a general hospital. At least once a day, all burn wounds, whether treated by the open-exposure or the closed-dressing method, should be cleansed with a surgical disinfectant to permit inspection and evaluation of the wound for evidence of infection.

The successful evacuation of thermally injured soldiers to fixed treatment centers requires the understanding of simple, but commonly misunderstood, principles.[31] If the local environment and the tactical situation permit, hemodynamic and respiratory stabilization should be achieved before the casualty is evacuated, so that resuscitation can be continued relatively simply. Thermally injured patients are best moved during the first 48 hours after being injured, before they have developed the complications of infection, pulmonary insufficiency, and acid-base abnormalities that can follow resuscitation, all of which can make stabilization and safe transport more difficult. Control of the airway and fluid resuscitation should be initiated as soon as conditions permit, preferably before evacuation.

Casualties with significant inhalation injuries, extensive head and neck burns, or decreased levels of consciousness should be intubated before transfer is begun. Fluid resuscitation should be initiated and the patient should demonstrate an adequate response to fluid infusion before evacuation begins.

Although definitive treatment of the wound is not necessary until the casualty arrives at a burn center or other definitive treatment site, a topical antimicrobial chemotherapeutic agent, if available, can be applied to the wound to prevent its desiccation and to limit microbial proliferation during a prolonged, multistop transfer. Escharotomies should be performed in extremities with circumferential full-thickness burns, but only if the indications discussed previously are present.

Under ideal circumstances, these guidelines for evacuation should be strictly adhered to in order to insure the casualty's morbidity- and mortality-free transfer. However, evacuating the patient from the battlefield or the unit level of care to a third-echelon MFT is usually accomplished by helicopter under less-than-ideal circumstances. Before the decision is made to move an unstable patient by helicopter, medical personnel must realize that it is impossible either to monitor such a patient adequately or to perform lifesaving interventions while in flight.

There are few absolute contraindications to moving patients by air. Active hemorrhage must be controlled before the patient is transported, because bleeding during the flight may be uncontrollable and blood for transfusion is usually unavailable during transport. In patients with marginal respiratory reserve and problems with either ventilation or oxygenation, the underlying causes should be corrected before the casualties are evacuated.

Unique Features of Long-Distance Aeromedical Evacuation

Several medical problems are inherent in air transportation. While most military aircraft are pressurized to an altitude of 5,000–8,000 feet above sea level, the ambient pressure of oxygen will fall as the aircraft's altitude increases. Ambient pressure at 8,000 feet, which is the maximum cabin altitude to which one may be exposed, is 516 mm Hg, and would result in an alveolar oxygen tension of approximately 65 mm. Despite the administration of oxygen, lower atmospheric pressures might produce significant hypoxia in patients with impaired oxygenation.

Decreases in ambient pressure present other problems, as explained by Boyle's Law. At 8,000 feet of altitude, gases expand approximately 30%, compared to sea level. The patient with an untreated pneumothorax that is well tolerated at sea level will require a tube thoracostomy to be placed before being transported by air, because even a small pneumothorax may expand during the flight. Because air in the cuff of an endotracheal tube will also expand, low-pressure, high-volume cuffs should be routinely utilized in order to maintain their pressure no higher than 20 mmHg. Since ileus is the natural consequence of an extensive burn, gastric decompression before the casualty is transported is of utmost importance to avoid emesis and possible aspiration. Air splints that may be used for extremity fractures may become tense enough to obstruct circulation in the limb even at altitudes of 15,000–20,000 feet above sea level unless the excess pressure is relieved.

Patients evacuated in large transport aircraft may require an increase in the rate at which their intravenous fluid is administered to compensate for the low humidity in the cabin. Providing humidified gas through a face mask or an endotracheal tube is necessary to prevent the formation of desiccated and inspissated secretions, which may occlude the airway.

Particular attention to the ambient temperature is necessary in order to maintain normothermia in those casualties who are prone to both hypo- and hyperthermia. Controlling acute problems before evacuation begins, such as maintaining the airway, securing the intravenous lines, and decompressing the gastrointestinal tract, and continually monitoring the adequacy of both hemodynamic and pulmonary functions during the flight ensure the safe transport of the most extensively burned, severely injured patients.

INHALATION INJURY

True inhalation injury is a chemical injury caused by the products of incomplete combustion, and many casualties with thermal burns will also suffer such injury. True thermal damage to the tracheobronchial tree is rare and most often is caused by steam, which can contain 4,000 times more heat than air can. The diagnosis of inhalation injury is based on both history and physical examination, and can be confirmed by bronchoscopic examination and ^{133}Xenon scan.[32] Hypoxemia and hypercapnia develop as the casualty's ability to clear secretions decreases because of *(a)* bronchociliary damage, *(b)* alveolar collapse due to decreased production of surfactant, and *(c)* alveolar filling with fluid because of alterations at the endothelial-epithelial interface. Impaired alveolar expansion and clearance of secretions place the patient at significant risk for pneumonia. The treatment includes *(a)* ventilatory support as indicated, *(b)* frequent endotracheal suctioning, and *(c)* bronchodilator therapy and racemic epinephrine if bronchospasm is present. Antibiotics should be reserved to treat diagnosed infections and should not be administered prophylactically to patients with inhalation injury.[33] Patients without respiratory distress but suspected of having a significant inhalation injury (facial burns and singed hairs, or the mechanism of injury—such as fire in an enclosed space—makes inhalation injury likely) should be prophylactically intubated and placed on mechanical ventilation before being evacuated, if such support is available. These patients may experience tracheobronchial mucosal slough and will require frequent endobronchial toilet, bronchoscopy, or even tracheostomy for adequate pulmonary toilet.

Carbon monoxide is a byproduct of organic material combustion with an affinity for hemoglobin 200-fold greater than oxygen's. Carbon monoxide has little direct effect on the lung, but it reduces the oxygen-carrying capacity of blood by *(a)* binding to hemoglobin, *(b)* shifting the oxygen-hemoglobin dissociation curve to the left, *(c)* binding to myoglobin, and *(d)* binding to the terminal cytochrome oxidase, all of which impair the delivery and utilization of oxygen at the cellular level. Headache, confusion, and irritability are associated with carboxyhemoglobin levels greater than 20%. Levels greater than 40% are usually associated with coma.[22] The diagnosis of carbon monoxide poisoning must be made by direct oximetric measurement of carboxyhemoglobin levels. Routine arterial blood gases, which measure dissolved oxygen, will not exclude this disorder. If measurement is not possible, then all patients suspected of having either carbon monoxide poisoning or of sustaining injury within an enclosed space should be treated with 100% oxygen administered through a tight-fitting face mask or an endotracheal tube. This treatment reduces the half-life of carboxyhemoglobin to approximately 30 minutes, down from 4–6 hours while breathing room air.[34]

COMBINED MECHANICAL AND THERMAL TRAUMA

Although their occurrence is uncommon in civilian trauma, thermal injuries complicated by associated mechanical trauma do occur in a combat environment. In managing patients with combined thermal and orthopedic injuries, the surgeon's principal objective is to achieve bony union in an optimal position while preserving maximal function. The open burn wound must also be treated to *(a)* prevent infection, *(b)* preserve uninjured soft tissue, and *(c)* maximize functional recovery.

Initial management of these complicated injuries involves cleansing the burn wound (as previously described) and, if the associated fracture is open, copiously irrigating and surgically debriding the devitalized tissue. Topical antimicrobial agents and intravenous antibiotics are also recommended for patients with open fractures and overlying burn wounds.

The actual method utilized for stabilizing fractures depends on *(a)* the type of fracture encountered, *(b)* the adequacy of the debridement, and *(c)* the patient's overall condition. Early operative intervention, before the adequacy of resuscitation has been established, should be avoided. After a simple transverse fracture has been reduced, a bivalve cast should be applied, which will permit the surgeon to routinely inspect and treat the overlying burn wound. Open or closed fractures of the humerus or femur can be managed with balanced skeletal traction, which permits local burn-wound care and also reduces the fracture. Unstable fractures involving the shafts of long bones can be managed by placing traction pins through the tissues above and below the fracture, preferably through unburned skin, and applying external fixation devices. This approach permits direct observation and care of the overlying burn. Using internal fixation devices like intermedullary rods or plates should be avoided, because microbial seeding of the prosthesis may occur, secondary to the repetitive bacteremias that occur in patients with extensive thermal injuries. Once the fracture has been stabilized, the burn wound can be closed whenever clinically appropriate.

The combination of significant torso trauma and thermal injury represents a difficult challenge. Although operative intervention cannot be delayed when it is indicated, it should be limited specifically to the one that most quickly and safely addresses the problem. The surgeon must be cognizant of the burn's fluid requirement as well as the associated trauma, and continue burn-related resuscitation during the procedure. Abdominal wounds should be closed with retention sutures in an effort to avoid a potentially catastrophic wound dehiscence.[35] The skin and subcutaneous tissue superficial to the investing fascia of the incision should be left open.

CHEMICAL INJURY

Chemical burns require a sequence of care different from the care that thermal burns receive. Wound care takes initial priority following the American College of Surgeons' Advanced Trauma Life Support ABCs (that is, airway, breathing, and circulatory problems), in an attempt to limit the tissue damage that the chemical causes. Since the severity of the injury is directly related to both *(a)* the amount and concentration of the chemical and *(b)* the duration of the tissue's contact with the chemical, immediate and copious water lavage is essential. All clothing, including gloves and shoes, that have been contaminated with the chemical must be removed during the lavage, and the exposed skin must be well irrigated (Figure 11-13). After the irrigation, however, the topical care for chemical burns is the same as the care for other burns.

Injuries caused by specific agents such as strong alkali powders, hydrofluoric acid, and white phosphorus require that this general treatment plan be modified. Do not attempt to neutralize acid or alkali solutions; the heat that the neutralization reaction generates may cause further tissue damage.

Hydrofluoric Acid

Therapy for hydrofluoric acid burns consists of water lavage followed by specific treatment to detoxify the fluoride ion, which is absorbed through the skin into subcutaneous tissue. Tissue damage can be limited by either *(a)* applying topical 2.5% calcium gluconate gel or *(b)* injecting a 5% solution of calcium gluconate, both of which will combine with the fluoride ions to form an insoluble calcium salt.[36]

White Phosphorus

White phosphorus is an incendiary that oxidizes to phosphorus pentoxide when it is exposed to oxygen. Particles are usually driven into the skin and subcutaneous tissue during explosions and can ignite, causing further tissue damage if allowed to oxidize (Figure 11-14). The casualty's clothing and the visible particles of white phosphorous should be expeditiously removed. The patient's wounds should be kept moist with saline until all particles can be removed. Historically, a 0.5% solution of copper sulfate has been used as a specific agent; it forms a coating of cupric phosphide that both impedes oxidation and facilitates identification of the white phosphorus particles. Since copper sulfate is readily absorbed through the burn, and even through unburned skin, however, significant toxicity—including hemolysis and renal failure—may occur with prolonged exposure. If copper sulfate is used, it should be *(a)* freshly made, *(b)* applied only as a brief wash, and *(c)* promptly lavaged from the wound with a copious volume of water. At present, water lavage and prompt removal of all visible white phosphorus particles is the preferred treatment. Using a Wood's lamp or other sources of ultraviolet light will facilitate the identification of white phosphorus particles in wounds.

While the casualty is being evacuated, the wounds should be kept in moist saline dressings to avoid the further oxidation and possible ignition of the remaining white phosphorus particles. All particles of white phosphorus that are removed should be kept immersed in water to prevent fires in the operating room.

Napalm

The wounds caused by napalm are no different from common flame burns and require no special treatment. The composition of napalm is discussed in Chapter One.

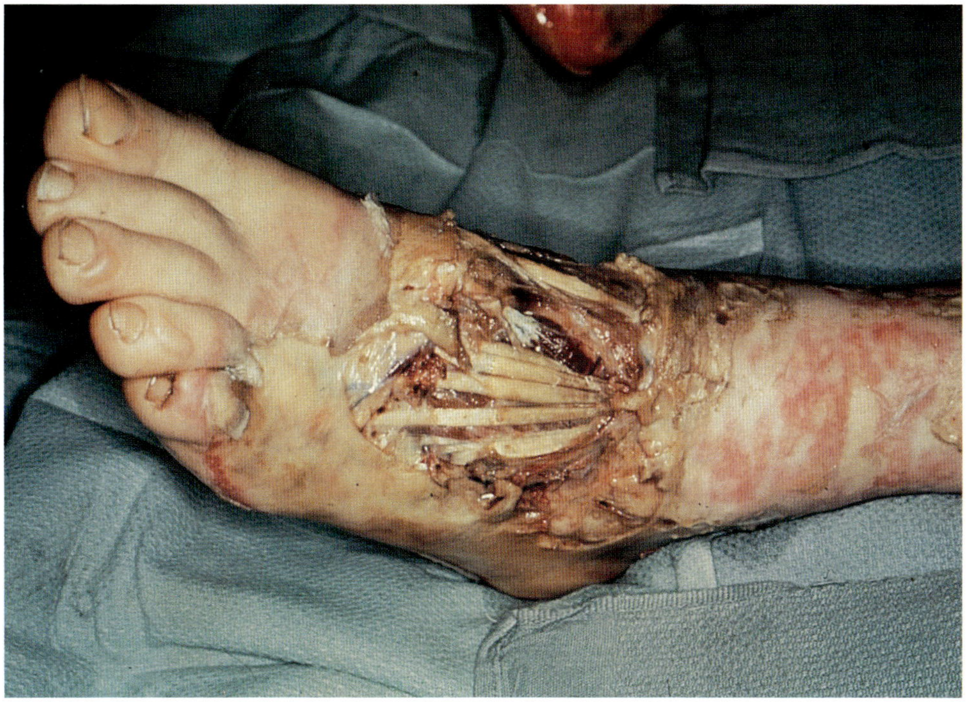

Fig. 11-13. This casualty's footwear was not promptly removed after his foot was exposed to acid. The significant soft-tissue damage should emphasize early wound care to medical officers who may need to treat casualties who have chemical burns.

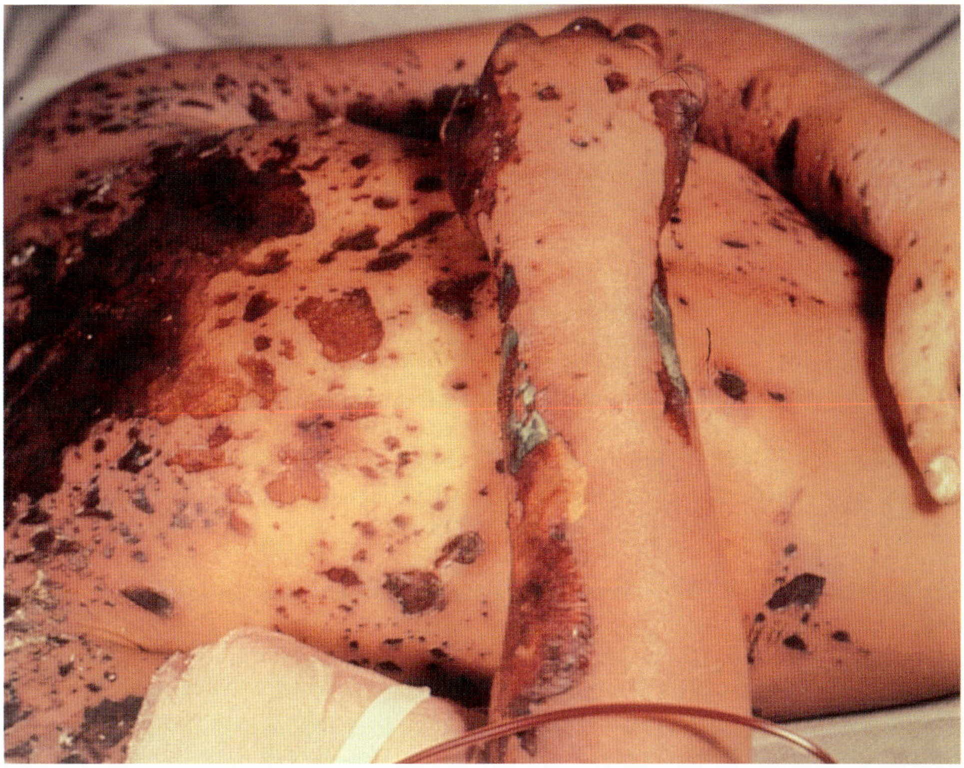

Fig. 11-14. This serpiginous, speckled pattern is typical when particles of white phosphorus are imbedded in the skin and subcutaneous tissues after a white phosphorus-containing munition has exploded. Fragments from the exploding munition can also cause significant soft-tissue injury. During treatment, all wounds must be kept moist to prevent further ignition of the imbedded particles of white phosphorus.

Vesicants

Vesicants, or blistering agents, include mustards, nitrogen mustards, other arsenicals, and mixtures of these compounds. These agents may cause significant damage to the eyes, mucous membranes, pulmonary system, skin, and hematopoietic system. In general, vesicants are odorless and cause little pain upon contact, except for the common arsenical vesicants, such as phenyldichloroarsine and chlorovinyldichloroarsine. As with all chemical injuries, casualties who are contaminated with vesicants place the medical personnel at significant risk of injury; they must take precautions to avoid direct contact with the chemical agent. Unhydrolized vesicants on a casualty's skin may persist for a prolonged period of time, representing a special hazard to medical personnel.

Mustard Gas. Mustard gas is easily aerosolized. Upon contact with a moist surface, the gas hydrolizes to hydrochloric acid, which injures tissue. Mustard gas can be either inhaled or absorbed through the skin or conjunctiva; the eyes are more vulnerable to injury than either the respiratory tract or the skin. Ocular injury may range from mild conjunctivitis and keratitis to significant corneal ulceration and globe perforation, depending upon the duration of exposure. Severe corneal involvement occurs in less than 0.1% of casualties, however. Ophthalmic injuries are treated like any other ocular chemical injury, by rapidly irrigating the eyes with copious amounts of water.

The severity of cutaneous lesions and the rapidity with which they develop depend entirely upon both the concentration of the mustard exposure and its duration. Hot, humid weather increases mustard gas's potential to injure, because high humidity increases the hydrolysis of the parent compound. Cutaneous exposure is followed by a latent period, after which the skin gradually becomes erythematous, resembling a first-degree burn. Except in mild exposures, the erythema is followed by vesication, which is caused by progressive necrosis of the superficial epidermal layers. These lesions are typical superficial, partial-thickness burns. Wound treatment consists of local irrigation and topical antimicrobial burn-wound therapy. Since the wounds are superficial, excision and grafting are rarely needed.

Inhalation injury caused by mustard gas is predominantly a tracheobronchial mucosal injury, with pulmonary parenchymal injury occurring only in the most severe cases. In general, this injury is typical of inhalation injury caused by smoke, and the treatment is the same.

Nitrogen Mustards. Nitrogen mustards are more volatile than mustard gas, but also are significantly less active as vesicants. They are less readily hydrolized than is typical mustard. The eye injuries that nitrogen mustards cause tend to be more severe than those that mustards cause; however, the treatment is the same and requires a rapid decontamination of the eye by irrigation with water. The cutaneous and pulmonary effects of nitrogen mustards are typically less severe than those caused by mustards, and their treatment is also the same.

Arsenical Vesicants. Arsenical vesicants are more volatile than mustards; they react rapidly with water to yield solid arsenoxides, however, which decreases their vesicant activity. Exposure to liquid arsenical vesicants causes severe eye damage. Pain and blepharospasm occur almost instantly. The injury will be severe if the exposure is prolonged.

Liquid arsenical vesicants cause a more severe injury to the skin than liquid mustards. Pain occurs almost immediately upon contact, and there is no latent period following exposure. The burn tends to be a deep, partial-thickness injury, but may progress to a full-thickness injury that will require excision and grafting for definitive wound closure.

While vesicant injuries should generally be treated like all other chemical injuries, medical officers must be cognizant of these compounds' propensity to cause significant ocular and pulmonary injuries.

Chemical injuries to the eyes require prompt irrigation, first with water, then continued with a saline solution until the patient has arrived at the site of definitive care and is examined by a physician experienced in the treatment of such eye injuries.

In addition to the direct toxic effects, vesicant exposure can lead to generalized systemic derangements. With extensive exposure to mustard gas, particularly in amounts approaching a lethal dose, hematopoietic tissues such as bone marrow, lymph nodes, and the spleen sustain significant injury. Marked leukopenia and thrombocytopenia may develop with their associated complications. Nitrogen mustards have greater systemic toxicity. Exposure to these agents can produce degenerative changes in the bone marrow, often within 12 hours of exposure, and can actually progress to severe marrow aplasia. The thymus, spleen, and lymph nodes are also vulnerable target organs, and severe granulocytopenia, lymphopenia, thrombocytopenia, and even anemia may develop after exposure.

The arsenical vesicants can also cause systemic poisoning, which manifests as a change in capillary permeability, giving rise to significant fluid shifts, hemoconcentration, and even hypovolemic shock. Those agents that are oxidized in the liver and then excreted in the bile are also markedly toxic to the hepatobiliary system. Focal necrosis of the liver, biliary mucosal necrosis, and even injury to the gastrointestinal mucosa may occur as a consequence of arsenical vesicant poisoning.

It has also been reported that fishermen exposed to leaking mustard-gas shells that had been discarded after World War II and inadvertently brought aboard their ships have demonstrated chromosomal mutagenicity that presumably increases their risk for developing neoplasia.

ELECTRICAL INJURY

The characteristics of electrical injury require that the treatment plan normally employed for patients with thermal injuries be modified. Tissue damage is caused by a combination of the electrical current's conversion from electrical energy into heat and the ignition of clothing as a result of electrical arcing. The amount of tissue damage depends upon the current's *(a)* voltage, *(b)* type, *(c)* pathway, and *(d)* duration of contact with the casualty.

Resuscitation

Cardiopulmonary arrest is frequently seen in patients who sustain high-voltage injury, and immediate initiation of cardiopulmonary resuscitation is required.

Using the standard resuscitation formulae—based on the extent of cutaneous injury—may result in grossly underestimating the fluid requirements for patients with significant electrical injury, whose extensive deep-tissue injury may be associated with only limited cutaneous injury. Oliguria should be treated with an increased rate of fluid administration until the desired hourly urinary output is achieved. Myoglobinuria secondary to damaged muscle increases the risk of acute renal failure. Unless a brisk urinary output is maintained, myoglobin may precipitate in the renal tubules. The presence of myoglobin in the urine mandates maintaining a urinary output of 75–125 ml/hr. Administering 12.5 g of Mannitol per liter of resuscitation fluid and alkalinizing the urine are indicated only if increased fluid infusion fails to clear the urine of hemochromogens.

Hyperkalemia secondary to extensive tissue damage may also occur. This is treated by administering hypertonic glucose, insulin, and calcium gluconate intravenously. Ion-exchange resins such as Kayexalate may be necessary and, rarely, hemodialysis may be indicated.

Compartment Syndrome

Edema beneath the muscle fascia may impair blood flow to the muscle and to distal tissue, resulting in a compartment syndrome (Figure 11-15). The indications for escharotomy and fasciotomy following electrical injury are the same as those following conventional thermal injury. While fasciotomy is seldom required to restore circulation to a circumferentially burned extremity, it may be necessary in patients with a high-voltage electrical injury, associated skeletal trauma, or a severe crush injury. (Ideally, fasciotomy should always be performed in the operating room under general anesthesia, but conditions may permit only local anesthesia and sterile surgical technique.) Limbs with significant electrical injuries should be surgically debrided as soon as the casualty's clinical condition permits. At operation, all obviously necrotic tissue should be debrided, and amputation, if required, should be carried out at a level proximal to the injury. The deep muscles and vital structures should be explored and their viability assessed, because nonviable tissue may underlie superficial viable tissue. Some authors have proposed ^{133}Xenon washout kinetics and tissue-uptake of technetium pyrophosphate as methods of identifying deep-tissue injuries, but the clinical usefulness, accuracy, and reliability of these techniques remain to be proven.[37,38] Surgical exploration remains the standard for delineating tissue viability.

The patient should be returned to the operating room within 48 hours after the initial debridement or amputation, where the wound is inspected and further debridement carried out as necessary. Upon completion of debridement, the wound can be closed by skin grafting or delayed primary closure, or it can be allowed to form granulation tissue and be autografted later.

Neurological Complications

Neurological sequelae may have early or delayed onset after electrical injury, thus mandating a thorough neurological examination on admission and at scheduled intervals later. Inasmuch as spinal fractures can be produced by tetanic contraction of the paraspinal muscles or by a fall at the time the injury occurred, anterior-posterior and lateral radiographs of the cervical, thoracic, and lumbar spine should be performed on all patients with electrical injuries.

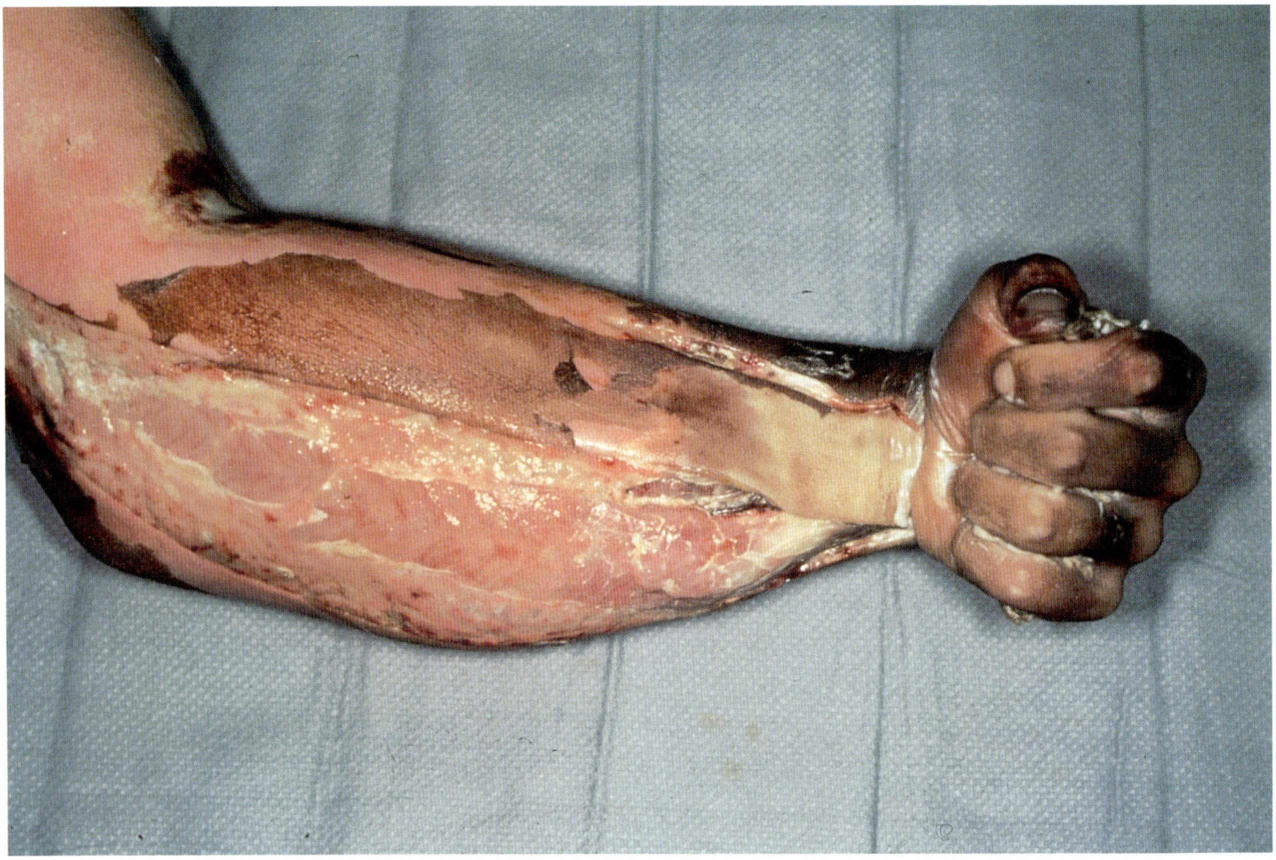

Fig. 11-15. Extensive subfascial edema necessitating fasciotomy may occur after electrical injury. The flexed wrist and hand occurs as a consequence of the nonviable muscle, seen herniating through the fasciotomy incision.

CURRENT RESEARCH AND FUTURE DIRECTIONS OF BURN CARE

The techniques of burn care that have been developed during the past four decades have significantly improved the survival of young-adult burn patients. This progress has both revealed previously unappreciated physiological consequences of burn injury and resulted in the emergence of new complications upon which current research is focused. Research programs sponsored by the U.S. Army Medical Research and Development Command and other agencies address the general systemic effects of severe injury as well as the organ-specific effects of burns.

Diagnostic systems employing spectral reflectance and other physical modalities are being evaluated for use in making early accurate diagnoses of burn depth and in identifying those wounds that require surgical debridement. Hemodynamic and shock studies at the U.S. Army Institute of Surgical Research include using plasmapheresis to produce a model of the acute plasma-volume changes that occur after a burn, and to describe *(a)* the biochemical changes that occur in the burn wound and *(b)* how the composition of the resuscitation fluid affects those changes. The neurohormonal changes that occur soon after a burn and influence salt and water balance are being described in detail to identify pharmacological interventions that might be effective in patients who do not respond to resuscitation as anticipated.

Ongoing correlative laboratory and clinical studies that seek to identify the prevalence and increased mortality of inhalation injury in burn patients have investigated *(a)* the pathogenesis of inhalation injury and *(b)* the interaction of cutaneous and inhalation injuries, and have evaluated synthetic surfactant-replacement therapy and high-frequency ventilation.

Epidemiological studies have documented the ever-changing ecology of infection in burn patients and the emergence of nonbacterial opportunistic agents as the causes of infections in extensively burned patients, whose survival has been prolonged by current treatment techniques. The difficulty of diagnosing infection in hypermetabolic burn patients has focused attention on identifying infection-specific, blood-borne indicators that will permit early, reliable diagnosis of infections.

The effects that burn injury, burn treatment, and infection have on the patient's defenses are also being assessed. Researchers are studying the effects of thermal injury on:

- the number and function of lymphocyte subpopulations
- the immunosuppressive effects of blood transfusions
- the effectiveness of exogenous interleukin-2 therapy
- the relationship between intestinal permeability and bacterial translocation in burn patients
- the effectiveness of hematopoietic growth factors in restoring the immunocompetence of burn patients, and
- the role of prostaglandins, various cytokines, and other products of cell metabolism in the patient's susceptibility to endotoxin and bacterial challenges after a burn

Several investigators are studying the effectiveness of various growth factors as accelerants of burn-wound healing. Studies at the U.S. Army Institute of Surgical Research are documenting that low-amperage direct current, with silver-impregnated nylon used as an anode applied to the burn wound, exerts both prophylactic and therapeutic effects on invasive burn-wound infections and also accelerates healing of deep partial-thickness burns, split-thickness skin grafts, and split-thickness graft-donor sites.

Many investigators continue to define the pathogenesis and characteristics of postburn hypermetabolism. Studies of thyroid function have identified altered iodothyronine feedback as an important factor in the disturbed secretion of thyroid-stimulating hormone that occurs after a burn. Other studies have lead to the proposal that the circadian sympathetic unresponsiveness of the pineal gland serves as a model of the sympathetic unresponsiveness observed in critically ill, burned, and injured patients.

Nutritional research at the U.S. Army Institute of Surgical Research has been directed towards defining injury-specific nutritional needs including: *(a)* trace-metal metabolism, *(b)* nutritional efficacy of medium-chain triglycerides, and *(c)* the interrelationship between vitamin metabolism and plasma amino acid levels.

In other laboratories, investigators are studying the effects of *(a)* various fatty acids on immune function, *(b)* glutamine on intestinal integrity, and *(c)* pharmacological manipulations of nutritional balance.

Another area of active research concerns the development of new and improved biological dressings and skin substitutes. Researchers are *(a)* evaluating collagen-based skin substitutes with varying permeability characteristics and *(b)* seeding the dermal analogues of skin substitutes with autologous epidermal cells and fibroblast, to try to effect permanent wound closure with these membranes. Improved techniques for growing sheets of epithelial cells *in vitro* and producing composite tissue cultures for definitive closure of the burn wound are also being evaluated.

Incorporating the results of these research programs into the clinical care of burn patients will further improve their chances for survival and functional recovery. Such improvements will undoubtedly reveal other previously unapparent pathogenetic effects of burn injury and result in the emergence of yet other complications of both injury and treatment. These emerging problems will then form the basis for future research initiatives.

SUMMARY

Not only are burns common in modern warfare, but combat involving armored fighting vehicles and aircraft is also likely to result in combined thermal and mechanical trauma, which increases the complexity of the care that the burned casualty requires. Successful salvage of the severely burned soldier requires a broad base of knowledge and expertise including critical care, infection control, wound management, respiratory care, metabolism, nutrition, and surgical technique.

Immediate early care consists of maintaining vital organ function and treating the potentially life-threatening associated injuries. Fluid resuscitation, the cornerstone of initial burn therapy, will prevent many of the early complications associated with thermal injury, provided it is promptly initiated and carefully monitored. After they have been resuscitated, patients with significant burn injury are best cared for at fourth-echelon or CONUS MTFs.

Early operative intervention is rarely required to treat thermal injuries, and, if performed within the resuscitative phase, it places the patient at increased risk for cardiovascular collapse. Early care of the burn wound consists of applying a clean, dry dressing (changed as necessary) until the patient can be transported to a third- or fourth-echelon facility. Topical antimicrobials are essential to proper management of the burn wound.

Salvaging a thermally injured soldier is resource-intensive and requires an aggressive team approach. While this is best achieved at specialized treatment centers, it may not be possible during mass-casualty wartime situations. All medical officers need to know the basics of caring for burned casualties.

REFERENCES

1. Nebraska Burn Institute. *Advanced Burn Life Support Manual, 18 Delta.* 1989. Lincoln: Nebraska Burn Institute.

2. Eldad, I., and Torem, M. 1990. Burns in the Lebanon War 1982: "The blow and the cure." *Milit. Med.* 155:130–132.

3. Pruitt, B. A., Jr. 1985. The universal trauma model. *Bulletin of the American College of Surgeons* 70(10):2–13.

4. Goodwin, C. W.; Dorethy, J.; and Lam, V. 1983. Randomized trial of efficacy of crystalloid and colloid resuscitation on hemodynamic response and lung water following thermal injury. *Ann. Surg.* 197:520–531.

5. Graves, T. A.; Cioffi, W. G.; McManus, W. F.; Mason, A. D.; and Pruitt, B. A., Jr. 1988. Fluid resuscitation of infants and children with massive thermal injury. *J. Trauma* 28:1656–1659.

6. Monafo, W. S. 1970. The treatment of burn shock by the intravenous and oral administration of hypertonic lactated saline solution. *J. Trauma* 10:575–586.

7. Caldwell, F. T., and Bowser, B. H. 1979. Critical evaluation of hypertonic and hypotonic solutions to resuscitate severely burned children: A prospective study. *Ann. Surg.* 189:546–552.

8. Shimazaki, S.; Yoshioka, T.; and Tanaka, N. 1977. Body fluid changes during hypertonic lactated saline solution therapy for burn shock. *J. Trauma* 17:38–43.

9. Alexander, J. W., and Wixon, D. 1970. Neutrophil dysfunction in sepsis in burn injury. *Surg. Gynecol. Obstet.* 130: 431–438.

10. Pruitt, B. A., Jr.; Dowling, J. A.; and Moncrief, J. A. 1968. Escharotomy in early burn care. *Arch. Surg.* 96:502–507.

11. Saffle, J. R.; Zeluff, G. R.; and Warden, G. D. 1980. Intramuscular pressure in the burned arm: Measurement and response to escharotomy. *Am. J. Surg.* 140:825–831.

12. Pruitt, B. A., Jr. 1984. The diagnosis and treatment of infection in the burn patient. *Burns* 11:79–91.

13. Pruitt, B. A., Jr., and Foley, F. D. 1973. The use of biopsies in burn patient care. *Surgery* 73:887–897.

14. Kim, S. H.; Hubbard, G. B.; and McManus, W. F. 1985. Frozen technique to evaluate early burn wound biopsy: A comparison with the rapid section technique. *J. Trauma* 25:1134–1137.

15. Kim, S. H.; Hubbard, G. B.; and Worley, B. G. 1985. A rapid section technique for burn wound biopsy. *J. Burn Care Rehab.* 6:433–435.

16. McManus, A. T.; Kim, S. H.; McManus, W. F.; Mason, A. D., Jr.; and Pruitt, B. A., Jr. 1987. Comparison of quantitative microbiology and histopathology in divided burn-wound biopsy specimens. *Arch. Surg.* 122:74–76.

17. McManus, W. F.; Goodwin, C. W.; and Mason, A. D., Jr. 1981. Burn wound infection. *J. Trauma* 21:753–756.

18. McManus, W. F.; Mason, A. D., Jr.; and Pruitt, B. A., Jr. 1980. Subeschar antibiotic infusion in the treatment of burn wound infection. *J. Trauma* 20:1021–1023.

19. Pruitt, B. A., Jr.; and Goodwin, C. 1983. Nutritional management of the seriously ill burned patient. In *Nutritional Support of the Seriously Ill Patient,* edited by R. W. Winters, 63–84. New York: Academic Press.

20. Wilmore, D. W. 1979. Nutrition and metabolism following thermal injury. *Clin. Plast. Surg.* 1:603–619.

21. Wolfe, R. R.; O'Donnell, T. F., Jr.; Stone, M. D.; Richmond, D. A.; and Burke, J. F. 1980. Investigation of factors determining the optimal glucose infusion rate in total parenteral nutrition. *Metabolism* 29:892–900.

22. Crocker, P. J. 1984. Carbon monoxide poisoning, the clinical entity and its treatment: A review. *Milit. Med.* 149: 257–259.

23. Curreri, P. W.; Wilmore, D. W.; and Mason, A. D., Jr. 1971. Intracellular cation alterations following major trauma: Effect of supranormal calorie intake. *J. Trauma* 11:390–396.

24. Canizaro, P. C.; Sawyer, R. B.; and Switzer, W. E. 1964. Blood loss during excision of third degree burn. *Arch. Surg.* 88:800–802.

25. Roberts, L. W.; McManus, W. F.; Mason, A. D.; and Pruitt, B. A., Jr. 1985. Duoderm in the management of skin graft donor sites. In *Surgical Research: Recent Development. Proceedings of the First Annual Session of the Academy of Surgical Research,* edited by C. W. Hall, 55–58. New York: Pergamon Press.

26. Gallico, G. G. III; O'Connor, N. E.; and Compton, C. C. 1984. Permanent coverage of large burn wounds with autologous cultured human epithelium. *N. Engl. J. Med.* 311:448–451.

27. Czaja, A. J.; McAlhany, J. C.; and Pruitt, B. A., Jr. 1974. Acute gastroduodenal disease after thermal injury: An endoscopic evaluation of incidence and natural history. *N. Engl. J. Med.* 291:925–929.

28. Pruitt, B. A., Jr.; Stein, J. M.; and Foley, F. D. 1970. Intravenous therapy in burn patients: Suppurative thrombophlebitis and other life threatening complications. *Arch. Surg.* 100:399–404.

29. Committee on Trauma. 1990. Resources for optimal care of patients with burn injury. In *Resources for Optimal Care of the Injured Patient.* 57–60. Chicago: American College of Surgeons.

30. Bowen, T. E., and Bellamy, R. F., eds. 1989. Burn injury. Chapt. 3 in *Emergency War Surgery,* 2d U.S. revision, 35–56. Washington, DC: U.S. Department of Defense.

31. Cioffi, W. G., Jr., and Pruitt, B. A., Jr. 1989. Aeromedical transport of the thermally injured patient. *Med. Corps Internat.* 4:23–27.

32. Hunt, J. L.; Agee, R. N.; and Pruitt, B. A., Jr. 1975. Fiberoptic bronchoscopy in acute inhalation injury. *J. Trauma* 15:641–649.

33. Levine, B. A.; Petroff, P. A.; and Slade, C. L. 1978. Prospective trials of dexamethasone and aerosolized gentamicin in the treatment of inhalation injury in the burned patient. *J. Trauma* 18:188–193.

34. Halebian, P.; Robinson, N.; and Barie, P. 1986. Whole body oxygen utilization during carbon monoxide poisoning and isocapneic nitrogen hypoxia. *J. Trauma* 26:110–117.

35. Goodwin, C. W.; McManus, W. F.; Mason, A. D., Jr.; and Pruitt, B. A., Jr. 1982. Management of abdominal wounds in thermally injured patients. *J. Trauma* 22:92–97.

36. Caravati, E. M. 1988. Acute hydrofluoric acid exposure. *Am. J. Emerg. Med.* 6:143–150.

37. Clayton, J. M.; Hayes, A. C.; and Hammel, J. 1977. Xenon^{133} determination of muscle blood flow in electrical injury. *J. Trauma* 17:293–298.

38. Hunt, J.; Lewis, S.; and Parkey, R. 1979. The use of Technetium-99m stannous pyrophosphate scintigraphy to identify muscle damage in acute electric burns. *J.Trauma* 19:409–413.

AFFILIATIONS

Ronald F. Bellamy
Associate Professor of Military Medicine,
Associate Professor of Surgery,
The Uniformed Services University of the Health Sciences,
Bethesda, Maryland

Teresa M. Buescher
Clinical Assistant Professor of Surgery,
Department of Surgery, University of Texas Health Science Center,
San Antonio, Texas

William G. Cioffi, Jr.
Clinical Assistant Professor of Surgery,
Department of Surgery, University of Texas Health Science Center,
San Antonio, Texas

Donald P. Jenkins
Associate Professor of Surgery,
Department of Surgery, Georgetown University,
Visiting Associate Professor of Anatomy,
Department of Anatomy, The Uniformed Services University of the Health Sciences,
Bethesda, Maryland

Basil A. Pruitt, Jr.
Professor of Surgery,
Department of Surgery, University of Texas Health Science Center,
San Antonio, Texas

Loring W. Rue III
Clinical Assistant Professor of Surgery,
Department of Surgery, University of Texas Health Science Center,
San Antonio, Texas

Yancy Y Phillips III
Associate Professor of Medicine,
Department of Medicine,
The Uniformed Services University of the Health Sciences,
Bethesda, Maryland

Joan T. Zajtchuk
Professor of Surgery,
Chairman, Division of Otolaryngology,
The Uniformed Services University of the Health Sciences,
Bethesda, Maryland

Russ Zajtchuk
Professor of Surgery,
Associate Dean for Academic Affairs,
The Uniformed Services University of the Health Sciences,
Bethesda, Maryland

INDEX

☆ U. S. GOVERNMENT PRINTING OFFICE : 1991 O - 250-233 : QL 1
PIN : 066946-000